Handbook of Biological Therapeutic Proteins

Since 1972, which marks the invention of recombinant engineering, more than 500 therapeutic proteins have been approved for clinical use. Today, biological drugs constitute almost 70% of all new drugs and have a biological origin. The first edition of this book dealt with biosimilars, and this edition (i.e., the second edition) focuses on new drugs, yet limits to therapeutic proteins. Newer technologies for drug development represent the updated topics in the book and include repurposing, AI-driven identification of newer designs, novel expression systems, manufacturing using these systems, rapidly changing regulatory pathways, and legal hurdles. This edition discusses how to identify, develop, manufacture, and take multibillion dollar products to market within the shortest possible time.

Features:

- Complete and thorough coverage of the regulatory and technological challenges of developing generic therapeutic proteins
- Comprehensive analysis, discovery to market, newer technologies, regulatory planning and intellectual property–related hurdles are included, and this information is not found elsewhere
- Expanded volume that must be in the hands of every company interested in biological drugs, including mRNA-based biopharmaceutical companies that quickly enter into the market
- Discusses how to identify, develop, manufacture, and take multibillion dollar products to market within the shortest possible time
- Renowned author and entrepreneur in the field of drug discovery and production

Handbook of Biological Therapeutic Proteins

Regulatory, Manufacturing, Testing, and Patent Issues

Second Edition

Authored by

Sarfaraz K. Niazi

Adjunct Professor at the University of Illinois

CRC Press
Taylor & Francis Group
Boca Raton London New York

CRC Press is an imprint of the
Taylor & Francis Group, an **informa** business

Second edition published 2024
by CRC Press
2385 Executive Center Drive, Suite 320, Boca Raton, FL 33431

and by CRC Press
4 Park Square, Milton Park, Abingdon, Oxon, OX14 4RN

CRC Press is an imprint of Taylor & Francis Group, LLC

Library of Congress Cataloging-in-Publication Data
Names: Niazi, Sarfaraz, 1949– author.
Title: Handbook of biological therapeutic proteins : regulatory, manufacturing, testing, and patent issues / authored by Sarfaraz K. Niazi.
Other titles: Handbook of biogeneric therapeutic proteins Description: Second edition I Boca Raton : CRC Press, 2024. I Preceded by Handbook of biogeneric therapeutic proteins / Sarfaraz K. Niazi. 2006. I Includes bibliographical references and index. I Summary: "Since 1972 when recombinant engineering was invented, over 500 therapeutic proteins have been approved. Today, biological drugs constitute almost 70% of all new drugs and are of biological origin. The first edition of this book dealt with biosimilars, the second focuses on new drugs yet limits to therapeutic proteins. The newer technologies for development represent the updated topics in the book and include repurposing, AI-driven identification of newer designs, novel expression systems and manufacturing, fast changing regulatory pathways, and legal hurdles. Discusses how to identify, develop, manufacture and take multibillion dollar products to market in the shortest possible time"– Provided by publisher.
Identifiers: LCCN 2023044890 (print) I LCCN 2023044891 (ebook) I ISBN 9781032489605 (hardback) I ISBN 9781032490540 (paperback) I ISBN 9781003392026 (ebook)
Subjects: MESH: Recombinant Proteins–therapeutic use I Biosimilar Pharmaceuticals I Technology, Pharmaceutical I Drug Industry
Classification: LCC RM300 (print) I LCC RM300 (ebook) I NLM QU 55 I DDC 615.1–dc23/eng/20240108
LC record available at https://lccn.loc.gov/2023044890
LC ebook record available at https://lccn.loc.gov/2023044891

ISBN: 9781032489605 (hbk)
ISBN: 9781032490540 (pbk)
ISBN: 9781003392026 (ebk)

DOI: 10.1201/ 9781003392026

Typeset in Times
by Newgen Publishing UK

Contents

Preface

The first chemically synthesized drug was chloral hydrate in 1832; aspirin was first synthesized in 1899. Since then, millions of new drug molecules have been synthesized, many of which have ended up as effective drugs, ranging from modulating immune systems to inactivating viruses, to treat nearly every ailment. However, the discovery of insulin in 1922 revolutionized biological medicine. Insulin was also the first biopharmaceutical drug developed by applying recombinant technology. Penicillin became available in 1928, thanks to Fleming and Waksman. The use of individual enzymatic transformation phases by employing microorganisms in chemical manufacturing pathways, such as the biotransformation of steroids in 1950, expanded the scope of biotechnological pharmaceutical manufacturing.

The term "therapeutic protein" refers to the process of joining DNA obtained from two or more different species to form the recombinant DNA (rDNA) product that is subsequently inserted as the hybrid DNA into a host cell, often a bacterium or mammalian cell, to express the target protein. Therapeutic proteins replace an abnormal or deficient protein in a particular disease or augment the supply of a beneficial protein to the body to help reduce the effect of disease or chemotherapy. Genetically engineered proteins can closely resemble the natural proteins they replace or be enhanced by adding sugars or other molecules in order to extend the protein's duration of activity. UC San Francisco and Stanford researchers created this molecular chimera in 1972. Stanley Cohen of Stanford and Herbert Boyer of UCSF received a US patent in 1980. On July 26, 1974, ten researchers, including six future Nobel Laureates (James Watson, Paul Berg, Stanley Cohen, David Baltimore, Ronald Davis, and Daniel Nathans), wrote a letter to the magazine *Science* urging that the National Institutes of Health should regulate rDNA technology.

The first rDNA product came into light in 1982, which was when rDNA insulin was approved; now, hundreds of recombinant proteins are approved by regulatory agencies. Examples of this diverse class of compounds include interferons, cytokines, interleukins, thrombocytes, growth factors, coagulation factors, blood factors, anticoagulants, Fc fusion proteins, monoclonal antibodies, etc. The global biologics market is expected to reach an income of approximately USD 719.94 billion by 2030, valued at USD 366.50 billion in 2021 and growing at a compound annual growth rate of 7.15% from 2022 to 2030. The current market of therapeutic proteins exceeds USD 380 billion.

The first edition of the book, which is the first book dedicated to biosimilars, was entitled, *Handbook of Biogeneric Therapeutic Proteins: Regulatory, Manufacturing, Testing, and Patent Issues*, published in early 2002, long before the term "biosimilar" came into vogue. Calling these biologicals "biogeneric" was intentional to invoke a similar approval process as that currently available to generic chemical drugs. The United States (US) Food and Drug Administration (FDA) recommended me that legal issues are involved when using the term "biogeneric" because "generic" is associated with a specific Act of Congress. We selected the term "biosimilar" to indicate that these products will be "biologically similar," not necessarily chemically or otherwise. Because pharmacology, toxicology, and clinical responses to biological drugs are related to receptor binding, the term "biosimilar" fulfils the critical need for a clear definition. However, many regulatory agencies use different labels, but currently, all of them seem to converge into one label, "biosimilars."

Biosimilars evolved 18 years ago, and currently, they account for 76 products granted approvals in the European Union (EU) and 41 in the US, and hundreds more worldwide. The European Medicines Agency introduced the first biosimilar guideline and approved the first product in 2006; the US guidelines came into use in 2019. Tables 1.2 and 1.3 list the approved (also rejected and withdrawn) products in the US and EU.

Now that more than two decades have passed since I wrote the first book on this subject, there appears a need to revise the perspective presented earlier, as there may be changes in the views over time, let alone for technology that is most rapidly advancing. Apart from technology, the regulatory process has also changed significantly. The second edition, entitled, *Handbook of Biosimilar Therapeutic Proteins: Regulatory, Manufacturing, Testing, and Patent Issues*, describes the major changes, which would be of great importance to the developers, as did the first edition of this book. My initial goal was to introduce this technology to new developers, mostly in developing countries, and this edition will be handy and continue to provide advice and suggestions on how to reduce development cost, starting from the technology stage to the regulatory filing planning stage.

The first edition was introduced by a dear friend, Francisco Baralle, who was the head of ICGEB, Trieste, Italy, and was pivotal in developing and transferring recombinant technologies to many countries. Francisco Baralle has left ICGEB, and I am pleased and honored to have him write an introduction to this second edition.

I wish to express my gratitude to my scientific and professional colleagues, particularly to those whom I know from the field's seminal literature and those whom I have never met. Given that I may have unknowingly cited their research, assuming that it was available in the public domain, I hope that I would be excused for taking this liberty, as it would be highly challenging for me to recognize such citations. Finally, I also hope that I would be excused for any errors, as mentioned in the first edition of *Encyclopedia Britannica* (1786): "With regard to errors, in general, whether falling under the denomination of mental, typographical, or accidental, I am conscious of being able to point out a greater number than any critic. Men acquainted with the innumerable difficulties attending the execution of a work of such an extensive nature will make proper allowances. To these, we appeal and shall rest satisfied with the judgment they pronounce."

I would appreciate your suggestions and comments, especially with regard to any errors in the book, as they will help me to improve this treatise in the future.

Disclaimer: The author does not accept responsibility for any technical or legal suggestions or advice provided in this book; all views expressed in this book are those of the author in his capacity and not as the Patent Agent of the US Patent and Trademark Office, as an officer of any company or in any academic positions held, or in any capacity as advisors to regulatory agencies.

Author Biography

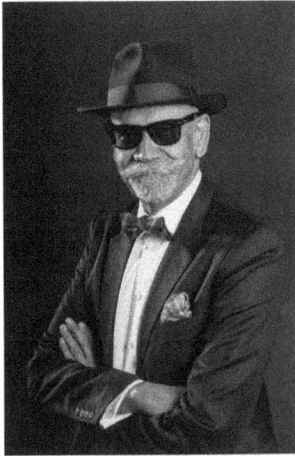

Sarfaraz K. Niazi, PhD, is an adjunct professor at the University of Illinois. He has authored 60+ major books, 100+ research papers, and 100+ patents, mainly in the field of bioprocessing. He has hands-on experience in biopharmaceutical projects, starting from concept preparation to drug entry into the market, including setting up the first biosimilar company in the US and acquiring several FDA approvals. He serves as an advisor to several regulatory agencies, including the FDA.

Introduction by Professor Francisco Baralle

I am pleased to see the second edition of the epic book on biosimilars authored by Professor Sarfaraz K. Niazi, wherein I have introduced him and his work. At the time of writing this book, I was heading the International Centre for Genetic Engineering and Biotechnology (ICGEB), a unique intergovernmental organization initially established as a particular project of UNIDO. The ICGEB has been an autonomous organization since 1994, and it has run over 45 state-of-the-art laboratories in Trieste (Italy), New Delhi (India), and Cape Town (South Africa). It is an interactive network with almost 70 Member States, with operations aligned to those of the United Nations System. It plays a crucial role in biotechnology, especially in promoting research excellence, training, and technology transfer to industry to achieve a concrete contribution to sustainable global development. I became acquainted with Professor Niazi when he began his career in biotechnology in the early 1990s. I am pleased that the ICGEB was able to fulfill many needs of a recombinant startup manufacturing globally, in several instances, in collaboration with Professor Niazi.

In my 2006 introduction to his excellent book, *Handbook of Biogeneric Therapeutic Proteins: Regulatory, Manufacturing, Testing, and Patent Issues*, I called it a significant milestone in furthering biotechnology applications, and in this case, the milestone is manufacturing of recombinant therapeutic proteins, worldwide. Now that Professor Niazi has fulfilled his ambition of securing the registration of biosimilars globally, he has revised his book to add decades of experience that has made this book a practical handbook for startups and established companies. In addition, this handbook will be helpful for anyone involved in the development, regulatory filing, and manufacturing of biosimilars, especially with regard to the term he has proposed in his book. He soon discovered that the term "generic" has legal constraints; hence, the best term would be "biosimilars." This term is almost a universal representation of the copies of biological drugs that have "no clinically meaningful difference" with their reference products.

One of the most significant breakthroughs in the field of biotechnology was achieved in the third quarter of the past century when scientists could clone the gene and combine it with the host DNA to produce the desired target molecules; thus, recombinant technology evolved. Insulin was the first endogenous hormone that was produced through recombinant technology and that benefited millions of patients worldwide. Indeed, today, the only major source of insulin is synthesis through recombinant technology in *Escherichia coli* cells. However, the recombinant techniques became useful only after the US Supreme Court ruling that a recombinant bacterium or a life form can be patented; since then, hundreds of endogenous molecules have been produced by recombinant techniques to bring a solution to humanity for diseases that were once thought of as incurable. Indeed, mortality from diseases related to the deficiency of endogenous proteins in patients has significantly decreased; yet, these drugs are very expensive, mainly because of the high investment required to develop and manufacture drugs. Delays also occur in the introduction of biosimilars owing to intellectual property constraints. Professor Niazi is also a patent law practitioner in the US, and he has described many strategies for managing IP risks effectively in this book.

The teachings in this book should go a long way in helping generic companies worldwide establish more efficient manufacturing systems while delivering a comparable quality product at a fraction of the price of the current innovator products. This can lead to a better quality of life and, therefore, an overall reduction in healthcare costs worldwide, which is one of the most serious concerning issues of global healthcare organizations such as the United Nations and the World Health Organization.

The *Handbook of Biogeneric Therapeutic Proteins* was the first comprehensive treatise on every aspect of manufacturing recombinant drugs; it was remarkable how such a large volume of information has been condensed into only a few hundred pages. After almost two decades, information, knowledge, and perspectives in the development and manufacturing of recombinant drugs have changed drastically; the second edition involves a change in the title from "generic" to "similar" but maintains the proven convenient and informative structure. This is a handbook, not a textbook; therefore, the emphasis remains on practical applications rather than the theories underlying the processes and methods. However, it is inevitable not to discuss some theory when describing these details. The book provides just the right balance between science and practical applications.

It was a pleasure to review this book authored by Professor Niazi, who has an eloquent style of expression and the ability to condense a large volume of data into a lucid format. I hope that more people will benefit from the emerging field of biotechnology through this book and from the experience of Dr. Niazi in this field. I particularly hope that developers in the developing world, which is the primary focus at ICGEB and, in particular, its Biotechnology Unit, will benefit from the timely, up-to-date information provided in this book to develop products that are now off-patent and make these products available to the public at a price they can afford while maintaining quality standards. Furthermore, I hope that prospective manufacturers will gain extensively from the discussion of quality systems in the book and, accordingly, build facilities of the highest standards; this is the only way to ensure the safety of biological products.

Professor Francisco Baralle
Trieste, Italy
baralle@fegato.it

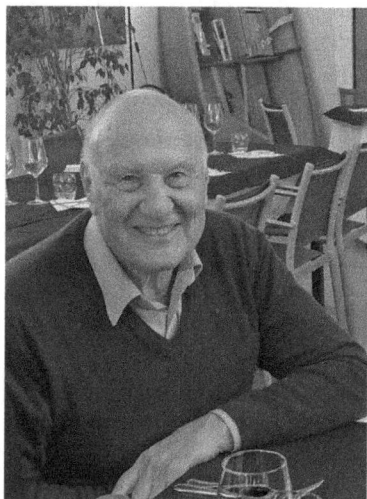

Professor Francisco Baralle is the president of the Scientific Committee, IRNA Metabolism Group, Italian Liver Foundation, Trieste, Italy. He was the second director general of the International Centre for Genetic Engineering and Biotechnology (ICGEB) in Trieste, Italy, since the institute's inception under a charter of the United Nations in 1984. Professor Baralle has motivated hundreds of scientists worldwide to develop applications of biotechnology to resolve the endogenous problems of developing countries. He has made substantial contributions to the science of molecular biology, proteomics, and recombinant techniques. A former professor of pathology at the University of Oxford, member of Magdalen College, and elected member of the Molecular European Biology Organization, Professor Baralle has pioneered cloning techniques and developed several new biological drugs. Under his supervision, the ICGEB developed programs for extensive training in constructing genetically modified cells and has offered global assistance in recombinant therapeutic protein manufacturing.

1 Overview of the Development of Biosimilar Biopharmaceuticals

1.1 INTRODUCTION

The cost involved in the development of a new drug has currently reached billions of United States dollars (USD), and the price has remained high for at least 5 years for a new chemical and 12 years for a new biological drug. Additionally, the stringent regulatory guidelines have increased the cost involved in the approval of a new biological drug to hundreds of million USD, resulting in the high price of these products (Table 1.1) to amortize the investment over 12 years of exclusivity for biological drugs.

As patents expire at the time of approval of a new drug, its biosimilars enter the market, a history that is not only remarkable in its lifetime but also shaky in terms of the extent to which the biosimilars have entered the market. A severe deficiency in the biosimilar landscape is the dearth of molecules entering the market; thus far, only 14 molecules are available in the US and 14 in the European Union, while many remarkable choices await entry (Tables 1.2–1.4).

The first tranche of biosimilar approval guidelines raised an abundance of caution for biosimilars (e.g., new biological drugs), especially through extensive analytical comparisons, animal pharmacology and toxicology, clinical pharmacology, and clinical safety and efficacy studies. The only exception from those studies was the extrapolation of the indications. A comparative clinical efficacy testing in one indication would be sufficient to qualify all other indications allowed for the reference product. To further assure safety and efficacy, biosimilars must be used with the same dose, strength, route of administration, and mechanism of action (MOA); however, the formulations may differ. Additionally, the prescribing information must be the same; guidelines for writing the prescribing information for biosimilars are available.

Over time, the agencies became more convinced of the safety of biosimilars in response to challenges against the guidelines. It became well accepted that animal testing of biosimilars is redundant; since recently, even new biological products may not require such testing because the MOA of biological drugs involves receptor binding that is often unavailable in animal species. The significance of clinical efficacy testing has also been criticized for scientific reasons because such studies cannot demonstrate negative results; if the studies aim to overcome the lack of similarity in the analytical or clinical pharmacology profiles, then it leads to a higher possibility for safety risk when such studies are considered for biosimilar approval. An excellent example of progressive changes to guidelines is the Medicines and Healthcare products Regulatory Agency of UK (MHRA). Last year, as the Brexit transition period ended, the MHRA published its first comprehensive guideline on May 14, 2022, and it deviated from all other guidelines by providing a clear rationale for not requiring animal and clinical efficacy testing.

Clinical pharmacology studies, including those comparing pharmacokinetics (PK) and pharmacodynamics (PD), are part of the analytical methodology, wherein similarities can be established

DOI: 10.1201/9781003392026-1

TABLE 1.1
Most Expensive Treatment Costs

Drug	Active	Indication	Cost, USD
Actemra	**Tocilizumab**	**Rheumatoid arthritis and cytokine release syndrome**	**6,000–9,000/month**
Acthar Gel	Repository corticotropin	Multiple sclerosis, infantile spasms, and nephrotic syndrome	40,000–60,000 per vial
Actimmune	**Interferon gamma-1b**	**Chronic granulomatous disease and severe, malignant osteopetrosis**	**157,000/yr**
Alecensa	Alectinib	Non–small cell lung cancer	159,000–178,000/yr
Almita	Olorinab	Breast cancer	150,000/yr
Amondys 45	Casimersen	Duchenne muscular dystrophy	300,000/yr
Blenrep	**Belantamab mafodotin**	**Multiple myeloma**	**400,000/yr**
Blincyto	**Blinatumomab**	**Acute lymphoblastic leukemia**	**178,000/trt**
Braftovi	Encorafenib	Melanoma	174,000/yr
Brineura	**Cerliponase alfa**	**Late infantile neuronal ceroid lipofuscinosis type 2 (CLN2)**	**350,000/yr**
Bylvay	Lumasiran	Bile acid synthesis disorders	300,000/yr
Calquence	Acalabrutinib	Chronic lymphocytic leukemia	175,000/yr
Ceredase	**Alglucerase**	**Gaucher disease**	**200,000–300,000/yr**
Cerezyme	**Imiglucerase**	**Gaucher disease**	**350,000/yr**
Darzalex	**Daratumumab**	**Multiple myeloma**	**150,000–170,000/yr**
Elaprase	**Idursulfase**	**Hunter syndrome (MPS II)**	**375,000/yr**
Erwinaze	**Asparaginase *Erwinia chrysanthemi***	**Acute lymphoblastic leukemia**	**14,000–28,000 per vial**
Evrysdi	Risdiplam	Spinal muscular atrophy	340,000/yr
Firdapse	Amifampridine	Lambert–Eaton myasthenic syndrome	140,000/yr
Gattex	Teduglutide	Short bowel syndrome	350,000–400,000/yr
Gilenya	Fingolimod	Multiple sclerosis	90,000–100,000/yr
Glybera	Alipogene tiparvovec	Lipoprotein lipase deficiency	1,000,000/trt
Harvoni	Ledipasvir + sofosbuvir	Chronic hepatitis C	94,500/trt
Hemlibra	**Emicizumab**	**Prevention of bleeding episodes in hemophilia A with factor VIII inhibitors**	**482,000/yr**
Ilaris	**Canakinumab**	**Cryopyrin-associated periodic syndromes (CAPS) and systemic juvenile idiopathic arthritis**	**200,000–300,000/yr**
Imfinzi	**Durvalumab**	**Certain types of cancer including lung cancer**	**150,000–170,000/yr**
Isturisa	Osilodrostat	Cushing's disease	295,000/yr
Jakafi	Ruxolitinib	Myelofibrosis and polycythemia vera	12,000–14,000/month
Kalydeco	Ivacaftor	Cystic fibrosis	330,000–360,000/yr
Keytruda	**Pembrolizumab**	**Various types of cancer, including melanoma and lung cancer**	**150,000–170,000/yr**
Kymriah	Tisagenlecleucel	Certain types of non-Hodgkin lymphoma and acute lymphoblastic leukemia	475,000/trt
Kyprolis	**Carfilzomib**	**Multiple myeloma**	**180,000–200,000/yr**
Lumakras	Sotorasib	Non–small cell lung cancer	17,000/month
Luxturna	Voretigene neparvovec	Inherited retinal diseases causing blindness	850,000/trt
Mavenclad	Cladribine	Multiple sclerosis	99,000/yr

TABLE 1.1 (Continued)
Most Expensive Treatment Costs

Drug	Active	Indication	Cost, USD
Monjuvi	**Tafasitamab**	**Diffuse large B-cell lymphoma**	**160,000/yr**
Myalept	Metreleptin	Leptin deficiency in generalized lipodystrophy	700,000/yr
Naglazyme	**Galsulfase**	**Mucopolysaccharidosis VI (MPS VI)**	**375,000/yr**
Nerlynx	Neratinib	Breast cancer	150,000/yr
Ocrevus	**Ocrelizumab**	**Multiple sclerosis**	**65,000/yr**
Olysio	Simeprevir	Chronic hepatitis C	66,000–84,000/trt
Opdivo	**Nivolumab**	**Various types of cancer, including melanoma and lung cancer**	**150,000–170,000/yr**
Opdivo plus	**Nivolumab + Ipilimumab**	**Certain types of cancer, including melanoma and lung cancer**	**250,000–270,000/yr**
Opsumit	Macitentan	Pulmonary arterial hypertension	200,000–220,000/yr
Orfadin	Nitisinone	Hereditary tyrosinemia type 1	275,000/yr
Orkambi	Lumacaftor + Ivacaftor	Cystic fibrosis	260,000–300,000/yr
Orladeyo	Berotralstat	Hereditary angioedema	470,000/yr
Orlissa	Elagolix	Endometriosis and uterine fibroids	30,000/yr
Padcev	**Enfortumab vedotin**	**Urothelial cancer**	**16,000/month**
Pomalyst	Pomalidomide	Multiple myeloma	160,000–180,000/yr
Pulmozyme	**Dornase alfa**	**Cystic fibrosis**	**311,000/yr**
Ravicti	Glycerol phenylbutyrate	Chronic management of urea cycle disorders	350,000–400,000/yr
Remicade	**Infliximab**	**Rheumatoid arthritis, Crohn's disease, and other autoimmune conditions**	**30,000–40,000/yr**
Rozlytrek	Entrectinib	Solid tumors with NTRK gene fusion	450,000/yr
Sandostatin LAR	Octreotide	Acromegaly and neuroendocrine tumors	15,000–20,000/month
Signifor	Pasireotide	Cushing's disease and acromegaly	200,000–300,000/yr
Soliris	**Eculizumab**	**Paroxysmal nocturnal hemoglobinuria and atypical hemolytic uremic syndrome**	**500,000–700,000/yr**
Sovaldi	Sofosbuvir	Chronic hepatitis C	84,000/trt
Spinraza	Nusinersen	Spinal muscular atrophy	375,000 for the first year and 375,000/yr after that
Sprycel	Dasatinib	Chronic myeloid leukemia and acute lymphoblastic leukemia	120,000–130,000/yr
Stelara	**Ustekinumab**	**Psoriasis, psoriatic arthritis, and Crohn's disease**	**30,000–40,000/yr**
Strensiq	**Asfotase alfa**	**Hypophosphatasia**	**300,000/yr**
Synagis	**Palivizumab**	**Prevention of respiratory syncytial virus (RSV) in infants**	**9,000–15,000/month during the RSV season**
Takhzyro	**Lanadelumab**	**Hereditary angioedema**	**488,000/yr**
Tecentriq	**Atezolizumab**	**Certain types of cancer, including bladder cancer**	**150,000–170,000/yr**
Translarna	Ataluren	Duchenne muscular dystrophy	262,000/yr
Trikafta	Elexacaftor + tezacaftor + ivacaftor	Cystic fibrosis	311,000/yr
Ultomiris	**Ravulizumab**	**Paroxysmal nocturnal hemoglobinuria and atypical hemolytic uremic syndrome**	**498,000/yr**

(continued)

TABLE 1.1 (Continued)
Most Expensive Treatment Costs

Drug	Active	Indication	Cost, USD
Vimizim	**Elosulfase alfa**	**Morquio A syndrome**	**375,000/yr**
Vitrakvi	Larotrectinib	Solid tumors with NTRK gene fusion	400,000/yr
Xalkori	Crizotinib	Small-cell lung cancer	149,000–167,000/yr
Xolair	**Omalizumab**	**Severe asthma and chronic idiopathic urticarial**	**32,500/yr**
Xpovio	Selinexor	Multiple myeloma	160,000/yr
Xtandi	Enzalutamide	Prostate cancer	129,000–144,000/yr
Xyrem	Sodium oxybate	Narcolepsy with cataplexy	50,000–75,000/yr
Yervoy	**Ipilimumab**	**Certain types of cancer, including melanoma**	**150,000–170,000/yr**
Yescarta	Axicabtagene ciloleucel	Certain types of non-Hodgkin lymphoma	373,000/trt
Zolgensma	Onasemnogene abeparvovec	Spinal muscular atrophy	2,100,000/trt
Hemgenix	Viral gene therapy	Hemophilia B gene	43,000,000 per dose

Note: Therapeutic proteins are shown in bold.

TABLE 1.2
Forty-One FDA Approvals of Biosimilars

No.	Biosimilar Name	Approval Date	Reference Product
1.	Tyruko (natalizumab-stn)	August 2023	Tysabri (natalizumab)
2.	Yuflyma (adalimumab-aaty)	May 2023	Humira (adalimumab)
3.	Idacio (adalimumab-aacf)	December 2022	Humira (adalimumab)
4.	Vegzelma (bevacizumab-adcd)	September 2022	Avastin (bevacizumab)
5.	Stimufend (pegfilgrastim-fpgk)	September 2022	Neulasta (pegfilgrastim)
6.	Cimerli (ranibizumab-eqrn)	August 2022	Lucentis (ranibizumab)
7.	Fylnetra (pegfilgrastim-pbbk)	May 2022	Neulasta (pegfilgrastim)
8.	Alymsys (bevacizumab-maly)	April 2022	Avastin (bevacizumab)
9.	Releuko (filgrastim-ayow)	February 2022	Neupogen (filgrastim)
10.	Yusimry (adalimumab-aqvh)	December 2021	Humira (adalimumab)
11.	Rezvoglar (insulin glargine-aglr)	December 2021	Lantus (insulin glargine)
12.	Byooviz (ranibizumab-nuna)	September 2021	Lucentis (ranibizumab)
13.	Semglee (Insulin glargine-yfgn)	July 2021	Lantus (Insulin glargine)
14.	Riabni (rituximab-arrx)	December 2020	Rituxan (rituximab)
15.	Hulio (adalimumab-fkjp)	July 2020	Humira (adalimumab)
16.	Nyvepria (pegfilgrastim-apgf)	June 2020	Neulasta (pegfilgrastim)
17.	Avsola (infliximab-axxq)	December 2019	Remicade (infliximab)
18.	Abrilada (adalimumab-afzb)	November 2019	Humira (adalimumab)
19.	Ziextenzo (pegfilgrastim-bmez)	November 2019	Neulasta (pegfilgrastim)
20.	Hadlima (adalimumab-bwwd)	July 2019	Humira (adalimumab)
21.	Ruxience (rituximab-pvvr)	July 2019	Rituxan (rituximab)
22.	Zirabev (bevacizumab-bvzr)	June 2019	Avastin (bevacizumab)
23.	Kanjinti (trastuzumab-anns)	June 2019	Herceptin (trastuzumab)
24.	Eticovo (etanercept-ykro)	April 2019	Enbrel (etanercept)
25.	Trazimera (trastuzumab-qyyp)	March 2019	Herceptin (trastuzumab)

TABLE 1.2 (Continued)
Forty-One FDA Approvals of Biosimilars

No.	Biosimilar Name	Approval Date	Reference Product
26.	Ontruzant (trastuzumab-dttb)	January 2019	Herceptin (trastuzumab)
27.	Herzuma (trastuzumab-pkrb)	December 2018	Herceptin (trastuzumab)
28.	Truxima (rituximab-abbs)	November 2018	Rituxan (rituximab)
29.	Udenyca (pegfilgrastim-cbqv)	November 2018	Neulasta (pegfilgrastim)
30.	Hyrimoz (adalimumab-adaz)	October 2018	Humira (adalimumab)
31.	Nivestym (filgrastim-aafi)	July 2018	Neupogen (filgrastim)
32.	Fulphila (pegfilgrastim-jmdb)	June 2018	Neluasta (pegfilgrastim)
33.	Retacrit (epoetin alfa-epbx)	May 2018	Epogen (epoetin-alfa)
34.	Ixifi (infliximab-qbtx)	December 2017	Remicade (infliximab)
35.	Ogivri (trastuzumab-dkst)	December 2017	Herceptin (trastuzumab)
36.	Mvasi (Bevacizumab-awwb)	September 2017	Avastin (bevacizumab)
37.	Cyltezo (Adalimumab-adbm)	August 2017	Humira (adalimumab)
38.	Renflexis (Infliximab-abda)	May 2017	Remicade (infliximab)
39.	Amjevita (Adalimumab–atto)	September 2016	Humira (adalimumab)
40.	Erelzi (Etanercept-szzs)	August 2016	Enbrel (etanercept)
41.	Inflectra (Infliximab-dyyb)	April 2016	Remicade (infliximab)
42.	Zarxio (Filgrastim-sndz)	March 2015	Neupogen (filgrastim)

Note: There were no reported rejections or withdrawals (www.fda.gov/drugs/biosimilars/biosimilar-product-information).

TABLE 1.3
Biosimilars Approved, Rejected, and Withdrawn in the European Union

No.	Product Name	Active Substance	Authorization Date
1.	Vegzelma	Bevacizumab	March 22, 2023
2.	Sondelbay	Teriparatide	June 16, 2022
3.	Stimufend	Pegfilgrastim	March 12, 2022
4.	Hukyndra	Adalimumab	November 15, 2021
5.	Libmyris	Adalimumab	November 12, 2021
6.	Byooviz	Ranibizumab	August 18, 2021
7.	Abevmy	Bevacizumab	April 21, 2021
8.	Alymsys	Bevacizumab	March 26, 2021
9.	Oyavas	Bevacizumab	March 26, 2021
10.	Yuflyma	Adalimumab	February 11, 2021
11.	Kirsty (previously Kixelle)	Insulin aspart	February 5, 2021
12.	Onbevzi	Bevacizumab	January 11, 2021
13.	Nyvepria	Pegfilgrastim	November 18, 2020
14.	Livogiva	Teriparatide	August 27, 2020
15.	Aybintio	Bevacizumab	August 19, 2020
16.	Zercepac	Trastuzumab	July 27, 2020
17.	Insulin aspart Sanofi	Insulin aspart	June 25, 2020
18.	Nepexto	Etanercept	May 25, 2020
19.	Ruxience	Rituximab	April 1, 2020
20.	Amsparity	Adalimumab	February 13, 2020

(continued)

TABLE 1.3 (Continued)
Biosimilars Approved, Rejected, and Withdrawn in the European Union

No.	Product Name	Active Substance	Authorization Date
21.	Cegfila	Pegfilgrastim	December 19, 2019
22.	Grasustek	Pegfilgrastim	June 20, 2019
23.	Idacio	Adalimumab	April 2, 2019
24.	Zirabev	Bevacizumab	February 14, 2019
25.	Ogivri	Trastuzumab	December 12, 2018
26.	Ziextenzo	Pegfilgrastim	November 22, 2018
27.	Fulphila	Pegfilgrastim	November 20, 2018
28.	Pelmeg	Pegfilgrastim	November 20, 2018
29.	Pelgraz	Pegfilgrastim	September 21, 2018
30.	Hulio	Adalimumab	September 17, 2018
31.	Hefiya	Adalimumab	July 26, 2018
32.	Hyrimoz	Adalimumab	July 26, 2018
33.	Trazimera	Trastuzumab	Jul 26, 2018
34.	Zessly	Infliximab	May 18, 2018
35.	Kanjinti	Trastuzumab	May 16, 2018
36.	Semglee	Insulin glargine	March 28, 2018
37.	Herzuma	Trastuzumab	February 8, 2018
38.	Mvasi	Bevacizumab	January 15, 2018
39.	Ontruzant	Trastuzumab	November 15, 2017
40.	Imraldi	Adalimumab	August 24, 2017
41.	Insulin lispro Sanofi	Insulin lispro	July 18, 2017
42.	Blitzima	Rituximab	July 13, 2017
43.	Erelzi	Etanercept	June 23, 2017
44.	Rixathon	Rituximab	June 15, 2017
45.	Riximyo	Rituximab	June 15, 2017
46.	Enoxaparin BECAT	Enoxaparin sodium	March 24, 2017
47.	Amgevita	Adalimumab	March 21, 2017
48.	Truxima	Rituximab	February 17, 2017
49.	Movymia	Teriparatide	January 11, 2017
50.	Terrosa	Teriparatide	January 4, 2017
51.	Inhixa	Enoxaparin sodium	September 15, 2016
52.	Flixabi	Infliximab	May 26, 2016
53.	Benepali	Etanercept	January 13, 2016
54.	Accofil	Filgrastim	September 17, 2014
55.	Abasaglar	Insulin glargine	September 9, 2014
56.	Bemfola	Follitropin alfa	March 26, 2014
57.	Grastofil	Filgrastim	October 17, 2013
58.	Ovaleap	Follitropin alfa	September 27, 2013
59.	Inflectra	Infliximab	September 10, 2013
60.	Remsima	Infliximab	September 10, 2013
61.	Nivestim	Filgrastim	June 7, 2010
62.	Filgrastim Hexal	Filgrastim	February 6, 2009
63.	Zarzio	Filgrastim	February 6, 2009
64.	Ratiograstim	Filgrastim	September 15, 2008
65.	Tevagrastim	Filgrastim	September 15, 2008
66.	Retacrit	Epoetin zeta	December 18, 2007
67.	Silapo	Epoetin zeta	December 18, 2007
68.	Binocrit	Epoetin alfa	August 28, 2007
69.	Abseamed	Epoetin alfa	August 27, 2007
70.	Epoetin alfa Hexal	Epoetin alfa	August 27, 2007
71.	Omnitrope	Somatropin	April 12, 2006

TABLE 1.3 (Continued)
Biosimilars Approved, Rejected, and Withdrawn in the European Union

No.	Product Name	Active Substance	Authorization Date
Refused or withdrawn biosimilars in Europe			
1.	Alpheon	Interferon alfa-2a	Refused on September 5, 2006
2.	Biograstim	Filgrastim	September 15, 2008; withdrawn on December 22, 2016
3.	Cyltezo	Adalimumab	November 10, 2017; withdrawn on January 15, 2019
4.	Epostim	Epoetin alfa	Withdrawn March 15, 2011
5.	Equidacent	Bevacizumab	September 24, 2020; withdrawn on November 23, 2021
6.	Filgrastim ratiopharm	Filgrastim	September 15, 2008; withdrawn on April 20, 2011
7.	Halimatoz	Adalimumab	July 26, 2018; withdrawn on January 29, 2021
8.	Kromeya	Adalimumab	April 2, 2019; withdrawn on December 17, 2019
9.	Lextemy	Bevacizumab	CHMP positive opinion February 25, 2021; withdrawn on December 14, 2021
10.	Lusduna	Insulin glargine	January 3, 2017; withdrawn on October 29, 2018
11.	Qutavina	Teriparatide	August 27, 2020; withdrawn on January 18, 2021
12.	Ritemvia	Rituximab	July 13, 2017; withdrawn on August 16, 2021
13.	Rituximab Mabion	Rituximab	Withdrawn on March 16, 2020
14.	Rituzena	Rituximab	July 13, 2017; withdrawn on April 10, 2019
15.	Solumarv	Insulin human	Refused on February 11, 2016
16.	Sondelbay	Teriparatide	Withdrawn on June 19, 2020
17.	Solymbic	Adalimumab	March 22, 2017; withdrawn on March 5, 2019
18.	Somatropin Biopartners	Somatropin	September 9, 2013; withdrawn on November 9, 2017
19.	Thorinane	Enoxaparin sodium	September 14, 2016; withdrawn on October 24, 2019
20.	Udenyca	Pegfilgrastim	September 21, 2018; withdrawn on February 15, 2021
21.	Valtropin	Somatropin	April 24, 2006; withdrawn on May 10, 2012

Note: www.gabionline.net/biosimilars/general/biosimilars-approved-in-europe.

TABLE 1.4
Potential Biosimilar Candidates

Abatacept	Abciximab	Aflibercept	Alemtuzumab
Alirocumab	Atezolizumab	Avelumab	Basiliximab
Bedinvetman (V)	Belimumab	Benralizumab	Bevacizumab
Bezlotoxumab	Blinatumomab	Blood factors	Brentuximab vedotin
Brodalumab	Brolucizumab	Burosumab	Canakinumab
Caplacizumab	Cemiplimab	Certolizumab pegol	Cetuximab
Crizanlizumab	Daclizumab	Daratumumab	Darbepoetin alfa
Denosumab	Dinutuximab	Dupilumab	Durvalumab
Eculizumab	Elotuzumab	Emapalumab	Emicizumab
Erenumab	Etanercept	Evolocumab	Follitropin alfa
Fremanezumab	Frunevetmab (V)	Galcanezumab	Gemtuzumab ozogamicin
Golimumab	Guselkumab	Ibalizumab	Idarucizumab
Inotuzumab ozogamicin	Insulin detemir	Insulin lispro	Interferons
Ipilimumab	Isatuximab	Ixekizumab	Lanadelumab
Lokivetmab (V)	Mepolizumab	Mogamulizumab	Moxetumomab pasudotox
Muromonab-CD3	Natalizumab	Necitumumab	Nivolumab

(continued)

TABLE 1.4 (Continued)
Potential Biosimilar Candidates

Abatacept	Abciximab	Aflibercept	Alemtuzumab
Obiltoxaximab	Obinutuzumab	Ocrelizumab	Ofatumumab
Olaratumab	Omalizumab	Palivizumab	Panitumumab
Pembrolizumab	Pertuzumab	Polatuzumab vedotin	Ramucirumab
Ranibizumab	Ravulizumab	Raxibacumab	Reslizumab
Rilonacept	Risankizumab	Romosozumab	Sacituzumab govitecan-hziy
Sarilumab	Secukinumab	Selumetinib	Siltuximab
Teprotumumab-trbw	Tildrakizumab	Tocilizumab	Urofollitropin

Note: www.drugpatentwatch.com.

by simulating the drug assimilation and kinetics observed physiologically. These studies should be promoted and recommended for newer technologies and approaches to develop structural equivalence.

Other misconceptions occur in animal testing and clinical efficacy testing. At the end of 2022, the US government passed a new law, The Food and Drug Administration (FDA) Modernization Act 2.0 removed the term "animal toxicology" and replaced it with the word "nonclinical" to exclude all terms related to animal testing, as animals do not have the receptors to which biological drugs bind. In addition, the MHRA recently announced that animal and clinical efficacy testing might be unnecessary. This will be the first requirement for any universal guideline to remove all procedures related to animal testing; as commonly practiced, animal testing, when used to justify the variability in analytical assessment, creates the risk of approval of unsafe biosimilars.

It is essential to comprehend that immunogenic proteins are used to create biologics and vaccines. Increased immunogenicity of these proteins can result in decreased effectiveness of the vaccine or unfavorable immunological responses such as allergic reactions or the production of neutralizing antibodies. It is well known that all proteins are immunogenic. Acquired or antigen-specific immune response involves T and B lymphocytes (T and B cells). If the immunogenicity profile of the proteins differs but does not influence the disposition profile, then the differences will be meaningless and unnecessary to compare, as in the case of insulins. Data on immunogenicity and safety should be gathered from PK trials. Particularly, the assessments should focus on antidrug antibody (ADA) production rate, kinetics, and their effect on PK (and PD) using a predetermined subgroup study of participants with ADA-negativity and ADA-positivity. Under in vitro conditions, immunogenicity assays might enable functional and analytical assessments, although they cannot replace the immunogenicity assessment in the PK study. The findings of short-term immunogenicity analyses might not reflect the actual usage of biologics, especially biosimilars. Because of the small population exposed and the greater scrutiny of patient care in the clinical trial setting, rare ADA-related side effects may not be identified in the premarketing phase. Therefore, it is recommended that risk management and pharmacovigilance strategies involving monitoring of other medication-related adverse events should also monitor immunogenicity.

The limitations of efficacy testing in patients are well recognized by regulatory agencies. To overcome these limitations, the FDA's Division of Applied Regulatory Science (DARS) has recently published its recommendations to remove efficacy testing for biosimilars based on comparing PD properties between a biosimilar candidate and its reference product. Instead, it is now labeled as clinical efficacy testing in healthy subjects. A PD biomarker does not necessarily be a surrogate endpoint or have an established relationship with clinical efficacy outcomes. For example, the area under the effect time curve for the absolute neutrophil count is a more reliable endpoint than the duration of severe neutropenia as a clinical efficacy endpoint. DARS drew these conclusions based on its investigations and clinical studies; it has defined best practices for characterizing PD biomarkers for various drug classes. Studies on PD biomarkers have evaluated the utility of human plasma proteomics and transcriptomics analyses to identify novel biomarkers for the approval of biosimilars. More efforts are underway to remove efficacy testing of all biological drugs in humans, including monoclonal antibodies (mAbs) that do not show PD markers.

Clinical efficacy trials have not revealed any clinically significant differences between a biosimilar and its reference product. Therefore, these trials have not led to any product withdrawals or recalls from the market. These data are available in the 96 European public assessment reports from the European Medicines Agency and 37 approval documents from the FDA. All these regulatory submissions passed their clinical efficacy assessment. In addition, research published on the ClinicalTrials.gov website substantiates that all 141 studies for which the findings complied with the required standards. The PubMed database contains 435 randomized controlled clinical trials conducted during 2002–2022, and all failed to detect a clinically significant difference.

The main reason to remove clinical efficacy testing is not cost avoidance, but ethical concerns arising from the universal belief that no healthy subject should have unnecessary exposure to the drug as codified in the US 21 CFR 320.25(a)(13), "the universal belief that 'No unnecessary human testing should be performed.'" The hazardous concerns arise from the possibility of approving biosimilars based on clinical efficacy testing overruling the mismatches in analytical and clinical pharmacology profiles.

The FDA now allows waiving clinical efficacy testing in patients based on comparing PD properties between a biosimilar candidate and its reference product. This process is now labeled as clinical efficacy testing in healthy subjects. A PD biomarker is not required to be a surrogate endpoint or have an established relationship with clinical efficacy outcomes. For example, include the area under the effect time curve for the absolute neutrophil count is a more reliable endpoint than the duration of severe neutropenia as a clinical efficacy endpoint. PD biomarkers can be identified using large-scale proteomics approaches and other technologies in situations where PD biomarkers are not readily available. The FDA has also confirmed that PD biomarkers need not necessarily correlate with a clinical response to allow their use to support the claim of biosimilarity. A biosimilar development plan aims to demonstrate similarity between the proposed biosimilar and its reference product, instead of focusing on replicating the reference product, and the safety and effectiveness are established independently. Therefore, a correlation between the PD biomarker and clinical outcomes, although beneficial, is not required.

If discrepancies exist between the proposed biosimilar and its reference product, then PK and PD similarity analyses may be preferred owing to higher sensitivity than an analysis of clinical effectiveness endpoint(s) to establish biosimilarity. The standards for surrogate biomarkers used for supporting the approval of novel drugs are fundamentally different from those for PD biomarkers used for assisting the confirmation of biosimilarity. This provides opportunities for biomarkers used as secondary and exploratory endpoints in new drug development programs to support biosimilar testing. Many opportunities are available to identify new PD biomarkers or fill information gaps on existing PD biomarkers to facilitate the utilization of PD biomarker data in clinical pharmacology studies instead of their utilization in comparative clinical efficacy studies.

Some of the drugs that serve as PD markers and are thus exempt from patient testing are presented in Table 1.5.

For biological products that do not serve as PD biomarkers, such as mAbs, other "omics" technologies such as transcriptomics and metabolomics may offer possibilities to discover novel, sensitive, and robust candidate biomarkers for further exploration as PD biomarkers. However, a more rational approach will be to take a step back in the testing cycle of biosimilars and examine whether ex vivo testing can provide more sensitive and reliable evidence of biosimilarity in terms of identifying a "clinically meaningful difference" in accordance with the FDA guidelines.

TABLE 1.5
Biosimilars With Pharmacodynamics Markers Are Exempted From Clinical Efficacy Testing in Patients

Drug	Patent Expiry
Interferon beta-1b	2004
Parathyroid hormone	2004
Interferon alpha-2b	2004
Chorionic gonadotropin	2007
Interferon alpha-n3	2011
Etanercept	2012
Menotropins	2015
Urofollitropin	2015
Peginterferon alpha-2b	2015
Interferon beta-1a	2020
Insulin regular	2025
Insulin lispro	2014

As the PD response is triggered by receptor binding, cell-based bioassays, or potency assays, such as enzyme-linked immunosorbent assay (ELISA), binding assays, competitive assays, cell signaling, ligand binding, proliferation, and proliferation suppression, should provide a good functional comparison between a biosimilar candidate and its reference product. Furthermore, functional tests for the MOA, such as testing for apoptosis, complement-dependent cytotoxicity, antibody-dependent cellular phagocytosis, and antibody-dependent cellular cytotoxicity, are generally not required and can be added only to provide a higher degree of confidence in terms of safety and efficacy.

mAbs bind to specific protein epitope targets on the target cells, thereby stimulating a therapeutic response. Characterization of the binding affinity of the mAbs includes target antigen and affinity for binding to specific Fc receptors (Fc [RI, Ia, IIa, IIb, IIIa, and IIIb]; Fc [RN]); effector functions such as Antibody dependent cell mediated cytotoxicity (ADCC) and complement dependent cytotoxicity (CDC); molecular properties such as charge, pI, hydrophobicity, and glycosylation; and off-target binding, and these assessments are performed using robust in silico or in vitro techniques such as baculovirus ELISA tools to establish functional similarity of the biosimilar. Additional tests can be performed based on specific applications; for example, for tumor necrosis factor alpha (TNF-α) blockers: C1q; CDC; induction of regulatory macrophages; inhibition of T-cell proliferation (mixed lymphocyte reaction [MLR]); LTα; MLR; mouse TNF-α; off-target cytokines; reverse signaling; soluble TNF-α; suppression of cytokine secretion; transmembrane TNF-α. Functional assays are more robust tools to elicit biomarkers to establish efficacy comparisons rather than testing in human subjects, without the necessity to demonstrate any PD response for mAbs [112,113]. However, the functional tests ADCC, ADCP, and CDC) are of little value when the drug targets a soluble antigen.

A collection of functional assays pertinent to a range of biological activities can be used for a product possessing multiple biological activities. For instance, some proteins have a variety of functional domains that express enzymatic and receptor-binding functions. The metric for biological activity is potency. Analytical studies evaluating these features can be easily performed when the immunochemical properties of the biosimilar contribute to the activity assigned to the product (for instance, antibodies or antibody-based products).

1.2 BIOSIMILARITY

Proteins including antibodies have a large structure that forms the variable region because of its unique nature acquired during synthesis in a living species. It is challenging to demonstrate that the biosimilar and its reference product, both with a variable structure, have equivalent variability because of the inevitable lack of understanding of the relationship between a product's structural attributes and its clinical performance.

1.3 TERMINOLOGY

The regulatory guidelines and standard scientific literature relating to biosimilars use specific terms, which are listed in Table 1.6.

TABLE 1.6
Terminology Related to Biosimilars

Biobetter	A biological product cannot be claimed as a proposed biosimilar product if it demonstrates higher efficacy, has lower dose requirement, causes fewer side effects, enables more convenient drug administration, or has any other difference that is considered an improvement over the reference product. Such products are considered new biological products and not accepted for evaluation by agencies adhering to this guideline.
Comparability testing	Comparability guidance such as ICH Q5E and ICH Q6B applies to a change in the manufacturing process of an approved product. The testing is conducted using the final approved biological product as the reference product. The testing is limited to critical quality attributes that are well known to the manufacturer. These guidelines may serve as overall guidance but do not apply to the development of biosimilars, regardless of the development stage, including the final scale-up. However, the guidance for the agencies may apply once the product has been approved. To avoid any confusion in referring to these guidelines, the current guideline uses the term "comparative testing" rather than "comparability testing."
Product	When used without modifiers, it is intended to refer to the intermediates, drug substance, and drug product, as appropriate. The use of the term "product" is consistent with the usage of this term in ICH Q5E. This should not be confused with the regulatory consideration of a drug's or a biological product's approval pathway. A drug product can be approved as a drug or a biological product. During the development process, a proposed biological drug is labeled with the term "proposed" to differentiate it from a proposed biosimilar that will be an authorized product.
High similarity or highly similar	Similarity is a binomial attribute; a protocol used for testing may either fail or pass. If it fails, a close examination is conducted to determine the cause of failure if any of the failed attributes have clinical significance. Often the terms "high similarity" or "highly similar" are used to indicate that there is residual uncertainty that is clinically meaningful.
No clinically meaningful differences	A proposed biosimilar product is not identical to the reference product. It has differences from the reference product; if the differences do not affect the safety or efficacy of the biosimilar, then we can claim that the proposed biosimilar has no clinically meaningful difference with the reference product.
No residual uncertainty	Every test must meet a pre-determined qualification; however, where the testing fails, it leaves uncertainty about the safety and efficacy of the biosimilar as supported by the given test. When such delays are removed, we can consider that the test has left no residual uncertainty.
No one size fits all	Every test for biosimilars should be specific to the product type and requires highly individualized development protocols.

(continued)

TABLE 1.6 (Continued)
Terminology Related to Biosimilars

Fingerprint-like similarity	At the highest possible level, a similarity level is the only variance remaining among the analytical methodology variations. In most cases, reaching this level of similarity will significantly reduce the burden of additional testing.
Totality-of-the-evidence	Evidence of the safety and clinical efficacy of the biosimilar is accumulated through multiple studies, and when we combine all results, we can establish biosimilarity.
Stepwise	Testing is conducted at pre-defined steps, and only when the testing meets the criterion at one step that the testing can move to the next step, there is significance of a higher value of any test, and a higher step does not resolve residual uncertainties of the lower steps.
Phase 1, 2, and 3 studies	Phase 1–3 studies are either standalone, i.e., Phase 1 and 2, or placebo controlled, as in Phase 3. None of these conditions apply to testing of the proposed biosimilar products; these terms are widely used by regulatory agencies and mostly by the developers. The correct terms are nonclinical pharmacology, clinical pharmacology, or comparative efficacy studies.

2 Regulatory Requirements for a Proposed Biosimilar Product

2.1 QUALIFICATION OF A PRODUCT AS A PROPOSED BIOSIMILAR

To qualify a product as a proposed biosimilar, the product must involve the same administration route, the same dosing, the same strength, and the same mechanism of action (MOA) as those of the reference product. The application for authorization of that product must contain information confirming that the biological product is similar to the reference product notwithstanding minor differences in clinically inactive components (e.g., a proposed biosimilar product formulated without human serum albumin can possibly demonstrate biosimilarity to the reference product formulated with human serum albumin). A product under development may be labeled as "a proposed biosimilar product," and any data claiming that the product has a "high similarity" or is a "biosimilar" may not be available. Such designations are given only by the regulatory agency.

2.1.1 QUALIFIED REFERENCE PRODUCT

To obtain marketing authorization, the developers must first demonstrate that the biosimilar product is proposed as a biosimilar to a single reference product that is first authorized based on a complete dossier in one of the International Council on Harmonisation (ICH+) regions: the European Economic Area following the provisions of Article 8 of Directive 2001/83/EC, as amended; authorized in the United Kingdom, Switzerland, Canada, or Australia, or licensed by the United States (US) Food and Drug Administration (FDA) under a 351(a) Biological License. The dossier should be adequate for the proposed biosimilar to be approved by the country authority where it was developed; generally, a broader qualification will include a product that is approved in one of the stringent regulatory authority countries based on a complete and adequate dossier.

- Only a single reference product can be used as the comparator throughout the comparative testing program for quality, safety, and efficacy assessments during the development of the proposed biosimilar product to allow evaluation of the totality of the evidence.
- Reference standards included in pharmacopoeia may not be used as the reference product.
- If the reference product has different strengths, then the reference product with the same strength as that of the proposed biosimilar product to be compared should be selected.
- To develop a global dossier, the developers may use multiple reference products, but these products may not be obtained from various manufacturing sites, regardless of their current good manufacturing practice (cGMP) compliance status.

DOI: 10.1201/9781003392026-2

2.1.2 Mechanism of Action

In several instances, the MOA of the reference product is known; the MOA may involve multiple mechanisms that may have led to multiple approved indications. A proposed biosimilar product may not claim or demonstrate an MOA that is not established for the reference product. This restriction comes from the correlation between the MOA and the scope of the side effects of the product.

2.1.3 Route of Administration

The application for authorization must include information demonstrating that the route of administration of a proposed biosimilar product is the same as that of the reference product. The developers of a proposed biosimilar product or a supplement to an approved proposed biosimilar may not obtain marketing authorization for a product that has route of administration, dosage form, or strength different from those of the reference product. However, the developers may obtain marketing authorization for all routes of administration of a proposed biosimilar product for which a designated reference product is approved. However, the developers may not be required to conduct studies of all products that have different routes of administration; generally, they will be required to conduct studies of those products for which the route of administration is more likely to show variability, for example, subcutaneous administration vs. intravenous administration.

2.1.4 Dosage Form

The developer must demonstrate that the dosage form of a proposed biosimilar product is the same as that of the reference product. For implementing this provision, the regulatory agency considers dosage form as a physical manifestation containing both active and inactive ingredients that constitute the drug product. In the context of drug administration, the agency considers, for example, "injection" (e.g., a solution) to be a different dosage form from "for injection" (e.g., a lyophilized powder). Thus, if the dosage form of the reference product is "injection," then the developers will be unable to obtain marketing authorization for a proposed biosimilar product with a "for injection" dosage form even though the developers demonstrate that the biosimilar, when constituted or reconstituted, could meet the other requirements for the application for a proposed biosimilar product. The agencies also consider emulsions and suspensions of products intended to be injected as distinct dosage forms. Liposomes, lipid complexes, and products with extended-release characteristics are grouped under a special category owing to their unique composition and perspective. The developer seeking further information should contact the agencies. However, it should be noted that this interpretation regarding the same dosage form is applicable only to biosimilars and is not applicable to generic chemical drugs.

2.1.5 Strength

The developers must demonstrate that the "strength" of a proposed biosimilar product is the same as that of the reference product. Data and information collected as part of the analytical assessment may reveal whether the proposed biosimilar product has the same strength as that of its reference product. Generally, the developers of a proposed biosimilar product with an "injection" dosage form (e.g., a solution) can demonstrate that the product has the same strength as that of the reference product by showcasing that both products have the same total content of drug substance (in mass or units of activity) and the same concentration of drug substance (in mass or units of activity per unit volume). For a proposed biosimilar product that is a dry solid (e.g., a lyophilized powder) from which a constituted or reconstituted solution is prepared, the developers can demonstrate that the product has the same strength as that of the reference product by showcasing that both products have the same total content of drug substance (in mass or units of activity). Although not part of demonstrating the same "strength," if a proposed biosimilar product is a dry solid (e.g., a lyophilized powder) from which a constituted or reconstituted solution is prepared, the application generally should contain affirming information that the concentration of the biosimilar, when constituted or reconstituted, is the same as that of the reference product, when constituted or reconstituted. The developers should determine the total content of the drug substance for both the reference product and the proposed biosimilar product using the same method.

2.1.6 FORMULATION

A proposed biosimilar product may contain different inactive ingredients that are proven safe and do not affect the efficacy of a proposed biosimilar product. Generally, a biosimilar candidate should contain the same inactive ingredients as those of the reference product; the exact composition of the reference product will be available in literature or in portal of the US FDA, European Union (EU), or the Australian Therapeutic Goods Administration (TGA).

2.1.7 DRUG DELIVERY DEVICE

A proposed biosimilar product in a delivery device is considered a combination product. The proposed biosimilar product may have a delivery device or container closure system different from that used for its reference product. Some design-related differences in the delivery device or container closure system used for a proposed biosimilar product may be acceptable. The developers can obtain marketing authorization for a proposed biosimilar product contained in a prefilled syringe or an auto-injector device (both of which are considered the same dosage form), even if the reference product is contained in a vial for the same dosage form, provided that the proposed biosimilar product meets the standard for biosimilarity and that adequate data for the performance of the delivery device or container closure system are provided and available. For a proposed biosimilar product contained in a different delivery device or container closure system, the device or container must demonstrate compatibility for use with the final formulation of the biological product through appropriate studies such as extractable/leachable studies and stability studies. For design-related differences in the delivery device or container closure system, performance testing and a human factors study may be needed. However, the developers will be unable to obtain marketing authorization for the proposed biosimilar product when a design-related difference in the delivery device or container closure system is apparent.

2.1.8 CURRENT GOOD MANUFACTURING PRACTICE COMPLIANCE

A proposed biosimilar product must be manufactured in adherence to the cGMP compliance associated with the manufacturing process to assure its safety and efficacy. Clinical lots of a proposed biosimilar product must be manufactured at-scale in adherence to cGMP compliance, as no changes can be made to the manufacturing process until the authorization of the proposed biosimilar product, without the need for any repeat testing. Once a product has been authorized, the developers can make changes to the manufacturing process, without any limit, using the ICH Q5E guidelines where the reference product is the product manufactured before the changes are made. This allowance is made because the developer now knows the in-process controls and how it may affect the safety and efficacy of the biosimilar.

2.1.9 EXTRAPOLATION AND SUBSTITUTION

All indications approved for the reference product as of date are generally extrapolated to the proposed biosimilar product, and the biosimilar is allowed barring any intellectual property during marketing authorization. The developer should provide a justification document to claim extrapolation in light of the observed similarity; in some situations, extrapolations may not be allowed because of the peculiarities found in a proposed biosimilar product. For instance, the reference product may receive marketing authorization for additional indications without making any changes to the reference product. In that case, the developers may request a modification to their label claim, regardless of the intellectual property involved because this is an issue that has to be resolved by the developer and the innovator company.

The European Medicines Agency (EMA) does not allow automatic substitution of a proposed biosimilar product for the reference product. However, various jurisdictions within the EU make their judgment; in the US, substitution of a proposed biosimilar product for the reference product requires additional testing of the biosimilar to demonstrate no more safety risk and no less efficacy upon switching and alternating; the FDA is yet to approve any product with this designation.

2.1.10 STUDY WAIVERS

Application for the marketing authorization of a proposed biosimilar product may rely upon the previous determination of safety, purity, and potency of the reference product, including any clinical QT/QTc interval prolongation, proarrhythmic potential, and drug-drug interactions. If such studies were not required for the reference product, then these data generally would not be needed for the marketing authorization of the proposed biosimilar product.

The proposed biosimilar product is considered not to have a "new active ingredient," and a pediatric assessment is generally not required if such a waiver has been awarded to the reference product. However, where the proposed biosimilar product has a different formulation, the developer should submit a statement asserting why the formulation does not create any additional pediatric use risk.

Specific studies such as carcinogenicity and reproductive toxicity are not required for biosimilars.

2.1.11 PUBLIC DOMAIN KNOWLEDGE

It is important to collect and analyze all reports that are freely accessible, including the EPARs, the FDA Biologicals Licensing Application (BLA) review documents, and similar documents made available by other agencies. When relying upon published scientific literature, the developers must ensure that the publications do not have any conflict of interest, for instance, a manufacturer publishing data submitted for marketing authorization with conclusions drawn that may differ from the regulatory authorities' decision. While the US FDA makes BLA details available for many new products, the developers may request this information using the Freedom of Information Act provisions on a small fee basis. While these documents are redacted for confidential information, the developer will have sufficient scientific knowledge to make the best use of the available information.

It is also important to collect and analyze all information available on the approved biosimilars to the reference product selected by the developer. The regulatory information, as enumerated above, is also available for biosimilars. In particular, the developers can benefit from prescribing information approved for these products. The developers may also want to create an internal library of all available scientific reports on the reference product, its active ingredient, and the technology employed in the manufacturing and testing of biological products. Regulatory information should be considered only from the following countries: Western Europe, the US, Japan, Canada, or Australia. Some emerging market regulatory authorities have adopted a chemical-generic approach, allow study waivers, and do not assure safety and efficacy of the biosimilar.

In May 2023, the US FDA issued draft guidance, "Generally Accepted Scientific Knowledge in Applications for Drug and Biological Products: Nonclinical Information," suggesting that nonclinical testing can be reduced based on FDA's Generally Accepted Scientific Knowledge (GASK): first, where a product contains a substance (either naturally derived or synthesized) that occurs naturally in the body and has a known effect on biological processes; second, where a sponsor has demonstrated a drug's effect on a particular biological pathway to conclude that certain nonclinical studies are not necessary to support approval and labeling of the drug. For example, some drugs have distinct effects on well-known biological pathways; hence, specific outcomes can be predicted once the drug's effect on the biological pathway is demonstrated. In addition, in some cases, a drug has either on-target or off-target effects on a biological pathway or molecular MOA that is known to result in adverse effects at clinically relevant exposures based on the operation of the biological pathway. Thus, according to the US FDA, it may be appropriate to rely on GASK regarding the effect of the pathway rather than to conduct specific pharmacology and/or toxicology studies intended to measure the effect of the pathway.

2.1.12 REFERENCE PRODUCT

The reference product's MOA, dose, frequency, route of administration, concentration (strength), and safety and efficacy are similar to those of a biosimilar, the conjugates, products, and derivatives that contain polypeptides. These proteins and polypeptides can be defined using proper analytical techniques and finely purified. Peptides, as compared to proteins, are polymers of 40 or fewer alpha-amino acids. Peptides include glucagon, liraglutide, nesiritide, teriparatide, and teduglutide. The peptide of a reference products is matched as a generic medication and is governed as a chemical substance.

To qualify as a reference product, a comprehensive dossier must have been used to approve a biological product, which is still being marketed in the originating country. Only one reference product should be utilized. When a reference product with different strengths or presentations is available, the lowest-strength product should be used. Several batches of the reference product should be obtained directly from the relevant market throughout time (months to years) to account for the reference product's production variability. The reference product batches should undergo testing for the permitted shelf-life and be stored according to the recommendations on the label. It may occasionally be possible to test batches that have been stored for a long period (e.g., frozen at −80°C) or past their intended shelf-life if reliable data demonstrate that the storage conditions have no effect on the critical quality attributes (CQAs). During the analysis, it is important to document how old the reference product batches were (based on their expiry dates) during the testing period.

Some agencies make a mistake and require that the reference product must be registered in the domestic markets and that the samples for testing should come from these batches. This is not only improper but also impractical, as the developer will need multiple batches that may not be available locally. Moreover, some new drugs may not be registered in several countries.

2.1.12.1 Reference Standard

The in-house primary reference material is an adequately documented sample made by the manufacturer from a representative lot or lots and calibrated against the in-house working reference material that is used for the biological assay and physicochemical testing of the following lots. It is the sole source acceptable for use as a working reference material. Reference standards that are freely accessible (such as the European Pharmacopoeia) cannot be used as the reference product to prove biosimilarity, but method certification and standardization can be accomplished by applying these criteria. No information may be used to develop a reference product specification or a biosimilar candidate in any drug substance or product monograph. The testing procedures are followed by verification.

2.2 ANALYTICAL CONSIDERATIONS

The methods defined in ICH Q6B are used to appropriately characterize the reference product. Some of these characterizations involve determining the physicochemical qualities, biological activity, immunochemical properties (if any), purity, impurities, contaminants, and quantity. Developers are encouraged to adopt newer technologies as available. As the quality attributes of the reference product vary from batch to batch, it is essential to establish the range of these variations to allow similar variability in the biosimilar candidate. The variations are either process-related (the expression system) or product-related (the manufacturing system). Generally, any variation in the product-related attributes cannot be resolved, requiring the developer to create a different expression system; the same can be the case for process-related attributes, but these are readily fixed. In both cases, safety studies cannot be submitted to justify a significant difference.

While most attributes are common to many products, in most cases, the criticality also depends on the manufacturing process and its robustness. Developers should know that some quality attributes are compared at the analytical assessment level, while others are evaluated at the release level. The latter includes all manufacturing process attributes such as PTMs, impurities, aggregates, subvisible particles, and physical properties. Impurities form a crucial basis for establishing biosimilarity, as an unidentified impurity, regardless of whether it is product-related (likely to be active) or process-related (unlikely to be active), must be studied for its safety potential. Safety issues are not necessarily related to the quantity of the unidentified impurities; therefore, even a small detectable amount of impurity should be thoroughly studied. Otherwise, the impurities may create only a small difference in the bioactivity of the product. The developers are strongly urged to modify the manufacturing process to remove any unidentified impurity to remove residual uncertainty, which may lead to extensive nonclinical and clinical studies. Other attributes such as aggregates and subvisible particles can affect negatively, and these must be minimized through process changes. Noteworthy, shaking protein products may produce more aggregates, as evident from the warnings on the label of some products such as erythropoietin, which mentions to avoid shaking the product.

It is the applicant's responsibility to demonstrate that the selected methods used in a proposed biosimilar comparability exercise would detect slight differences in all aspects pertinent to the evaluation of quality (e.g., ability to detect relevant variants with high sensitivity). Methods used in the characterization studies form an integral part of the quality data package and should be appropriately qualified for comparability. If applicable, standards and reference materials (e.g., from the European Pharmacopoeia, World Health Organization, etc.) should be used for the qualification and standardization of a method.

For some analytical techniques, direct or side-by-side analysis of a proposed biosimilar and reference product may not be feasible or may provide limited information (e.g., because of the low concentration of the active substance and the presence of interfering excipients such as albumin). Thus, samples could be prepared from the finished product (e.g., extraction, concentration, and other suitable techniques). In such cases, the methods used to prepare the samples should be outlined. Their effect on the samples should be appropriately documented and discussed (e.g., comparing active substances before and after formulation/reformulation preparation).

As analytical similarity evaluation forms the backbone for establishing biosimilarity, the largest investment is likely made in terms of establishing appropriate testing within the laboratories or outsourcing it. Even in case of outsourcing, in-house testing is inevitable to ensure that the process changes are reasonable to ensure compliance. Test methods for the analytical assessment of similarity need not be validated. These must be suitable and sensitive, such as the test methods used for comparing the primary, secondary, and tertiary structure elements. Test methods for the release of the product must be validated. This difference in the need for validation comes from the side-by-side testing of the reference product with a proposed biosimilar product where method variance will be the same for both products. Additionally, some methods such as mass spectrometry, nuclear magnetic resonance spectroscopy, dynamic light scattering/static light scattering, circular dichroism, and isothermal titration are difficult to validate.

Regulatory agencies are particularly sensitive to compliance with 21 CFR Part 11, a consideration where many companies frequently fail. Noteworthy, the agencies do not necessarily require that any IT basis is created; often, a manual record will also qualify, but the developer should always be able to prove that the original data remain intact and that it could not be manipulated.

2.2.1 PHYSICOCHEMICAL PROPERTIES

A physicochemical characterization program should include determining the composition, physical properties, and primary and higher-order structures (HOS) of a proposed biosimilar, using appropriate methodologies. The target amino acid sequence of the proposed biosimilar should be confirmed and is expected to be the same as that for the reference product. The N- and C-terminal amino acid sequences, free SH groups, and disulfide bridges of the proposed biosimilar should be compared with those of the reference product, as appropriate. Any modifications/truncations should be quantified, and any intrinsic or expression system–related variability should be described. Any detected differences between the proposed biosimilar and the reference product should be justified concerning the micro-heterogeneous pattern of the reference product (e.g., C-terminal lysine variability).

The presence and extent of PTMs (e.g., glycosylation, oxidation, deamidation, and truncation) should be appropriately characterized. Carbohydrate structures, if present, should be thoroughly compared, including the overall glycan profile, site-specific glycosylation patterns, and site occupancy. The presence of glycosylation structures or variants not observed in the reference product may raise concerns and require appropriate justification, with particular attention to nonhuman structures (nonhuman linkages, sequences, or sugars).

2.2.2 NONCLINICAL TESTING

Once a product has been scaled up to the development level, developers may consider conducting nonclinical pharmacology studies where needed. Agencies encourage developers to justify waivers for conducting nonclinical studies based on the analytical assessment conducted, prior public knowledge about the product's toxicity, and relevance of animal data to the safety and efficacy of the product. Recently, agencies have begun to accept waivers even for complex molecules.

The Biological Price Competition and Innovation Act (BPCIA) has been amended effective January 2023, wherein the term "animal toxicology" has been removed and the term "nonclinical" testing has been added instead. As biological drugs act by receptor binding and animals may not have these receptors, there is no further need to perform any animal toxicology study. This also means that developers cannot use animal safety data to support any difference in the analytical profile.

The developers should understand that the purpose of animal pharmacokinetic (PK) studies is to remove any structural similarity, as the disposition characteristics of the product may indicate differences in the structure and any immunogenic response that might affect drug clearance from the body.

A proposed biosimilar comparability exercise should include assessing the biological properties of both the proposed biosimilar and the reference product as an essential step in establishing a complete characterization profile. Biological activity is the specific ability of the product to achieve a defined biological effect. Biological assays that use different and complementary approaches to measure the biological activity of the product should be considered, as appropriate. Depending on the product's biological properties, different types of assays can be used (e.g., ligand or receptor binding assays, enzymatic assays, cell-based assays, and functional assays), considering their limitations.

Next, complementary or orthogonal approaches should be performed to address any limitations in the validation characteristics of single bioassays. If relevant, separate assays should be performed to evaluate the binding and activation of receptors. Where appropriate, cross-reference to nonclinical and clinical section(s) of the dossier may be made. Biological assays are sensitive, specific, and sufficiently discriminatory. The results of relevant biological assay(s) should be provided and expressed in units of activity calibrated against an international or national reference standard, when available and appropriate. These assays should comply with appropriate requirements of the European Pharmacopoeia for biological assays, if applicable.

2.2.2.1 Immunochemical Properties

The immunological functions of monoclonal antibodies and related substances (e.g., fusion proteins based on IgG Fc) should be thoroughly compared. This would typically include a comparison of the affinity of the products to the intended target. Moreover, the affinity of Fc-binding ligands to relevant receptors (e.g., FcγR, C1q, FcRn) should be compared unless justified. Appropriate methodologies should also be used to compare the ability of the monoclonal antibodies to induce Fab- and Fc-associated effector functions.

2.2.3 Purity and Impurity Profiles

When developing a biosimilar, impurity profiling is required, and guidelines for product-related variations with the innovator are established. For instance, a biosimilar may contain fewer impurities in terms of type and quantity, but there must be no mismatched contaminant; this cannot be supported by a safety study unless the reference product is shown to contain an impurity that is harmless.

The purity and impurity profiles of a proposed biosimilar and the reference product should be compared qualitatively and quantitatively by combining different analytical procedures. Appropriate orthogonal and state-of-the-art methods should be used to identify and compare product-related substances and impurities. This comparison should consider specific degradation pathways (e.g., oxidation, deamidation, and aggregation) of the proposed biosimilar product and the potential PTMs of the proteins. The age/shelf-life of the reference product at the time of testing should be mentioned, and its potential effect on the quality profile should be discussed, where appropriate. A comparison of the relevant quantitative attributes tested at selected time points and storage conditions (e.g., accelerated or stress conditions) could be used to further support the similarity of the degradation pathways between the reference product and the biosimilar.

Process-related impurities (e.g., host cell proteins, host cell DNA, reagents, and downstream impurities) are expected to differ qualitatively from process to process. Therefore, a qualitative comparison of these parameters may not be relevant in a proposed biosimilar comparability exercise. Nevertheless, state-of-the-art analytical technologies following existing guidelines and compendial requirements should be applied. The potential risks related to these identified impurities (e.g., immunogenicity) will have to be appropriately documented and justified.

2.2.4 Quantity

Quantity should be determined using an appropriate assay and expressed in the same units as those for the reference product. A comparable strength should be confirmed for the proposed biosimilar and the reference product. There is a dispute whether dose strength is an analytical assessment attribute or a release attribute; if it is the latter, then it need not be part of the analytical assessment, although the samples tested must be released based on the specification.

2.2.5 SPECIFICATIONS

As for any biotechnology product, the selection of tests to be included in the specifications (or control strategy) for both drug and drug products is product-specific and should be defined as described in ICH Q6B. The rationale used to establish a proposed range of acceptance criteria for routine testing should also be described.

The product's claimed shelf-life should be justified with full stability data obtained with the proposed biosimilar product. Comparative real-time, real-condition stability studies between the proposed biosimilar and the reference product are not required.

2.2.6 TEST PROCEDURES

Critical variations in the product and process of the biosimilar are compared with those of the reference product to enable appropriately, not necessarily, validated procedures, as some test methods cannot be fully validated. Analytical methods must be qualified, sensitive, and adequately selective to identify potential differences. Where appropriate, the procedures described in the ICH recommendations (ICH Q2A, Q2B, Q5C, and Q6B) for analytical assessment can also be utilized to evaluate quality attributes for batch release. Additionally, the use of appropriate orthogonal methodologies is necessary for obtaining robust data.

2.2.7 FUNCTION-BASED TESTS

CQAs should be identified using analytical and in vitro functional tests. Functional experiments should be pertinent to the potential MOA in all therapeutic indications, including those that determine apoptosis, complement-dependent cytotoxicity, antibody-dependent cellular phagocytosis, and antibody-dependent cellular cytotoxicity. Unless there is compelling evidence to the contrary, a biological occurrence should be considered when determining whether it applies to the MOA. Functional tests (ADCC, ADCP, and CDC) are not necessary for a reference product that primarily targets a soluble antigen.

2.2.8 NUMBER OF BATCHES

Generally, eight batches will be tested, one of which should be the clinical batch. Therefore, the final third-party analytical assessment will include at least three Pharmaceutical Process Qualification (PPQ) lots. More details are found later in the discussion of analytical assessment statistics.

2.2.9 DATA EVALUATION

A visual comparison suffices for test results sent as printed output, such as spectra. Quantitative statistics should be applied to the data of nearly ten batches, and the 3Sigma range, which is derived for the reference product as (ref − 3ref, ref + 3ref), provides the most accurate inference. If the test sample's MinMax range falls within the 3Sigma range, then the 3Sigma test is accepted. With a larger sample size, the 3Sigma technique offers a more workable compromise of error rates.

2.2.10 EXPRESSION SYSTEM

The expression system determines product-related CQAs such as primary structure, HOS, glycosylation (only in eukaryotic hosts), product-related variations, and process-related variations. The primary structure is further broken down into the secondary structure, tertiary structure, and conformational stability. Testing include higher order structure (HOS) in the oligosaccharide pattern, glycopeptide mapping, and monosaccharide/sialic acid content; also tested are the size variations, charge variations, and related proteins created in post-translational modifications (PTMs), as well as product-associated variations.. The expression system for the biosimilar should belong to the same class as that used for the reference product. The developers are also advised to select more steady expression systems; generally, high-yielding cell lines produce more variants. Therefore, cell lines should be qualified according to the ICH Q5D.

2.2.11 POST-TRANSLATIONAL MODIFICATIONS

As the primary sequence of a protein remains constant, it is expected to be precisely the same, except for justified PTMs such as truncation of terminal amino acids in the body. Size-based heterogeneities (aggregates, fragments, and visible/subvisible particles), charge-based heterogeneities (acidic and basic variants), and other product modifications (reduced, oxidized, glycated, misfolded proteins, etc.) are a few examples of heterogeneities produced during the development, management, and storage of biological products. When the environment changes during different stages of the production process, hydrophobic patches of the protein unfurl, causing accumulation or fragmentation, and sometimes, immunogenic responses may occur. The aggregates range from soluble aggregates to visible residues depending on the duration of exposure to various stresses such as shear, thermal, chemical, and freeze-thaw. Protein loss due to interactions in the stationary phase and salt-induced aggregation or dissociation is common during size-exclusion chromatography analysis. To quantitatively evaluate the size distribution, sedimentation velocity-analytical ultracentrifugation, a matrix-free substitute for size-exclusion chromatography, is used.

Charge variations are proteoforms that occur at different stages of the manufacturing process in various colloidal matrices (such as culture medium, in-process buffers, or formulations) and that have varying charges. It is, therefore, preferable to use several types of cation exchange chromatography.

Oxidation, phosphorylation, sulfation, acetylation, methylation, and hydroxylation are some of the nonenzymatic PTMs occurring at various manufacturing stages. Liquid chromatography is preferable for identifying PTMs and detecting associated molecular variations and contaminants.

Cell substrates are process-related variations or residuals, including HCPs, HCDs, cell culture, and downstream processing residuals. Enzyme-linked immunosorbent assay and real-time or quantitative polymerase chain reaction assay are the main HCP and HCD detection and quantitation techniques. These variants are not tested during the drug substance qualifying phase because they are part of the release specification.

2.2.12 QUALITY ASPECTS

Publicly available reference standards (e.g., the European Pharmacopoeia) cannot be used as the reference product to demonstrate biosimilarity. However, the use of these standards plays an important role in the qualification and standardization of a method.

An extensive comparability exercise will be required to demonstrate that a proposed biosimilar has a highly similar quality profile as that of the reference product. This should include comprehensive analyses of a proposed biosimilar and its reference product using sensitive and orthogonal methods to determine similarities and potential differences in quality attributes. These analyses should include side-by-side comparative studies unless otherwise justified. Any differences in the quality attributes will have to be appropriately justified about their potential effect on safety and efficacy.

In case relevant quality differences are confirmed (for which the absence of a clinically relevant effect will be difficult to justify), it may be challenging to claim similarity to the reference product, and thus, a complete application for marketing authorization may be more appropriate. Alternatively, the applicant could consider adequate revision of the manufacturing process to minimize or avoid these differences.

It is not expected that all quality attributes of a proposed biosimilar product should be identical to those of the reference product. However, where qualitative and quantitative differences are detected, such differences should be justified and, where relevant, demonstrated to have no effect on the product's clinical performance. This may include additional non-clinical and clinical data, as outlined in the guidelines on similar biopharmaceutical products containing biotechnology-derived proteins as active substances: nonclinical and clinical issues. Particular attention should be given to quality attributes that might affect immunogenicity or potency or have not been identified in the reference product.

The application should provide information that the desired product (including product-related substances) present in the finished product of a proposed biosimilar is similar to that of the reference product. By contrast, process-related impurities may differ between the reference product and proposed biosimilar products, although these impurities should be minimized. It is preferable to rely on purification processes to remove impurities rather than to establish a nonclinical testing program for their qualification. Differences that may confer a safety advantage (e.g., lower levels of impurities) should be explained but are unlikely to preclude biosimilarity.

Quantitative ranges for a proposed biosimilar comparability exercise should be established, where possible. These ranges should be based primarily on the measured quality attribute ranges of the reference product and should not be wider than the range of variability of the representative reference product batches unless otherwise justified. The relevance of the ranges should be discussed, considering the number of reference product lots tested, the quality attribute investigated, the batches' age at the time of testing, and the test method used. A descriptive statistical approach to establish ranges for quality attributes could be used if appropriately justified.

Acceptable ranges used for a proposed biosimilar comparability exercise versus the reference product should be handled separately from release specifications. It is acknowledged that the reference product's manufacturing process evolves through its lifecycle, which may lead to detectable differences in some of the quality attributes. Such events could occur during the development of a proposed biosimilar product. They may result in development according to a quality target product profile (QTPP), which is no longer fully representative of the reference product available on the market. The ranges determined before and after the observed shift in quality profile could normally support a proposed biosimilar comparability exercise at the quality level. Either range is representative of the reference product. Quality attribute values of a biosimilar located outside or between the quality attribute range(s) determined for the reference product should be appropriately justified about their potential effect on safety and efficacy. There is no regulatory requirement for the re-demonstration of biosimilarity once the marketing authorization is granted.

2.2.13 RELEASE SPECIFICATION

Characterization of the reference product can help establish release specifications that were determined before the analytical assessment. The reference product will be characterized by identifying its physicochemical characteristics, biological activity, immunochemical characteristics, purity, and contaminants using appropriate testing techniques. The lots used during the development phase may be used as the test lots. However, at least one tested lot used for the initial clinical trial in the PK/PD study must included. If a test method is selected from a pharmacopoeia, then it must also be confirmed or verified. Based on inevitabilities, specific variances are allowed for injectable products, such as 3% for protein content, 3% for impurities, 1% for any single contaminant, or 15% for potency testing.

Additionally, comparison tests do not consider pharmacopoeial requirements for the qualification of the dosage form, such as sterility, fill volume, delivered volume, and physical qualities. Other historical characteristics such as sterility, invisible particles (debatable with biosimilars to consider as aggregates), protein content, potency, and physical characteristics unique to the biosimilar candidate are independently established. These standards may be used to specify the biosimilar candidate's release specification.

When a new biological product is developed, the specification is established based on the quality attributes determined from multiple lots. There is rarely any question of why a particular specification is used to release a product, notwithstanding known limitations common to the dosage form. When a proposed biosimilar product is developed, the boundaries of the specifications are already drawn to match despite the realization that the expression systems, upstream process, and downstream process are inevitably different. This decision is mainly chosen with the intent of minimizing the need for studies required to prove that deviations, if any, are not clinically meaningful from the reference product. Biosimilar companies must have a deep understanding of the product, the technology, and the testing methodologies as well as creative thinking to assure the regulatory agencies that there is no clinically meaningful difference between a proposed biosimilar and the reference product.

Multiple reference products should be used to establish specifications required for the qualification of a drug and its products. The number of reference product lots depends on the variability of the quality attributes in the reference product. Generally, considerable variations in protein concentration, bioassay, PTMs, impurities, and other physical properties of the reference product are unlikely to occur because the manufacturer of the reference product had validated the manufacturing process and the corresponding attributes over time. For a proposed biosimilar product, the developer does not have access to the in-process controls; therefore, earlier lots of the proposed biosimilar product may show a higher variation, making it essential to collect extensive data on the variability of quality attributes in the reference product lots. Release specifications should include assay, bioassay, physical attributes, subvisible particles, total impurities, individual impurities, aggregates, and PTMs.

2.2.14 FORMULATION

A proposed biosimilar can have a different formulation from that of the reference product. A formulation with the same number of inactive substances or fewer is recommended, regardless of changes in the constituent composition, unless doing so is banned by the intellectual property guidelines. Addition of excipients that are used to prepare biological products using another formulation is not advisable. The formulation's stability, compatibility (i.e., how it interacts with excipients, diluents, and packaging materials), should be confirmed, along with the active ingredients' integrity, activity, and potency. If the primary packaging that is in contact with the product is different, then further safety tests are required to verify that there is no unexpected leaching of package components into the product. Developers are encouraged to select a primary packaging material that is compatible with the proposed biosimilar, as it is often difficult to defend and justify these findings. The formulation may not contain any unique excipients previously used in a similar product, and all excipients must be free of animal products.

2.2.15 STABILITY

The stability of the biosimilar candidate must be evaluated according to ICH Q5C. Stress stability testing is an analytical evaluation and determines whether the degradation products are comparable to the reference product. Sterility, presence of endotoxins, microbiological restrictions, container volume, homogeneity in dosage units, and permissible particle matter are among the general monographs of pharmacopoeia. These are assessed through release specification tests so that the pharmacopoeial standards can be applied. Accelerated and stress stability experiments are also necessary to further enable a direct assessment of structural similarities and obtain degradation profiles. ICH Q5C and Q1A(R) guidelines should be reviewed when deciding the specifications for stability studies that provide relevant data for possible comparison.

2.2.16 PROCESS QUALIFICATION

Before performing any analytical assessment for similarity, the upstream and downstream processes must be verified. However, on completion of clinical pharmacology studies, no batch size adjustment is permitted; the developer may adjust the batch size only during post-approval, in adherence to ICHQ5E. Bridging studies are needed to validate alterations in the production size.

2.3 ANIMAL TOXICOLOGY

For a proposed biosimilar, no animal toxicological testing has been necessary since January 2023; however, many agencies still require these data.

2.4 CLINICAL PHARMACOLOGY

PK/PD studies are pivotal to establishing analytical similarity; immunogenicity similarity, in some instances; and bioavailability, where applicable. Generally, studies conducted in healthy subjects will be more meaningful for two reasons: first, to recruit subjects with a narrow demographic variation to reduce the inter- and intra-subject variability, and second, to reduce the impact of disease and related treatments on the disposition profile. However, in some instances where the likelihood of the production of antidrug antibodies is very high, more particularly for an endogenous product, it may be unethical to recruit healthy subjects owing to unnecessary drug exposure, requiring the use of a patient population. Regardless of the choice of the population, the goal should be to reduce the number of subjects in the study; in this regard, the developers can conduct a two-arm (two-dose), parallel, two-phase (dose 1 and dose 2) study with a follow-up duration suitable for immunogenicity evaluation; there may be situations where PD determination may restrict the use of this model. The developers may also conduct a post hoc analysis, especially when a study fails to meet the predetermined acceptance criteria, to facilitate the discussion of whether the pre-determined criteria could have been made broader. A post hoc analysis does not aim to change the acceptance criteria retrospectively but rather to determine whether the failed study constitutes a significant residual uncertainty. The post hoc analysis may not include additional characterization of the results that are closer to the midpoint of the acceptance range as erroneously suggested in some guidelines established by other agencies.

2.5 CLINICAL IMMUNOGENICITY

Immunogenicity testing can be preferably combined with PK/PD profiling; however, in some situations, it is necessary to conduct an independent study wherein a specific population or protocol that may not allow combining immunogenicity testing with PK/PD studies should be followed. The developers must first confirm that there is no residual uncertainty regarding the factors responsible for an immunogenicity response before conducting clinical testing. A more important element of these studies is the evaluation of antidrug antibodies, which should be estimated from public domain data; for example, filgrastim induces an extremely low immunogenic response, and PEGylation of the molecules induces an even less immunogenic response; therefore, any studies on filgrastim must provide acceptance criteria that will have clinical meaningfulness. For simpler, low-molecular-weight products where the immunogenic response is not likely to affect the clinical efficacy of the biosimilar, immunogenicity studies will not be needed (e.g., insulin products). The developers may present challenges to conducting immunogenicity testing based on similar or other novel arguments.

The US FDA has recently issued guidelines to remove the requirement to test clinical immunogenicity of insulin if it meets analytical similarity testing; the factors responsible for this waiver are a smaller molecule with less complexity. More waivers of this type can be expected in the future.

PK and pharmacodynamic (PD) studies, which are an extension of analytical evaluation, reflect how the body perceives the chemical and vice versa. For a product used as intravenous administration, PK studies are necessary to evaluate the degree and strength of receptor binding that may alter PK characteristics such as the drug distribution volume and clearance, even if a biosimilar is not administered parenterally, such as a biosimilar injected into the eye. PK/PD studies aim to compare the profiles of the reference product and the biosimilar candidate, not to characterize them; therefore, such studies can be performed on a homogeneous population to decrease inter- and intra-subject variability and reduce study sample size. A robust design should accommodate a crossover or parallel design. A crossover approach can easily reveal changes but might not be appropriate for reference products that are robust inducers of immune responses or long half-lives. Modeling and simulation should be performed to optimize the study design, including selecting the most sensitive dose(s), study population, and sample size PK differences, if relevant population PK or PK-PD models for the reference product are available in the literature. Both linear (nonspecific) clearance and nonlinear (target-mediated) clearance should be considered through dosage choice and assessment of partial areas under the curve (AUCs). The statistical approach should specify any modifications for body weight or additional variables (such as sex/gender) to be used in the statistical analysis of a parallel-group experiment. The equivalence margins must be pre-specified, and the appropriate range is often 80.00%–125.00%. The key PK parameters, typically $AUC_{0-\infty}$ and C_{max}, should be equivalent in the PK experiment. A finding of biosimilarity should be supported by descriptive results from the PK study, which can be utilized to evaluate PD parameters. Comparative PK studies designed to demonstrate similar PK profiles of a proposed biosimilar and the reference product are essential parts of a proposed biosimilar development program.

Although the comparison of target-mediated clearance is of significance in the biosimilarity exercise, it may not be feasible in patients because of major variability in target expression, including variability over time. However, because in vitro studies are expected to show comparable interaction between a proposed biosimilar and its target(s) (including FcRn for a monoclonal antibody), the absence of a pivotal PK study in the target population is acceptable if additional PK data are collected during efficacy, safety, and PD studies to allow evaluation of the clinical impact of variable PK and possible changes in PK over time. These correlations can be made by determining the PK profile in a subset of patients or in a population.

A single-dose cross-over study with full characterization of the PK profile, including the late elimination phase, is preferable. A parallel-group design may be necessary for studies on substances with a long half-life and a high risk of immunogenicity (avoiding second dosing of the same drug substance). The doses in the single-dose comparability PK study of the proposed biosimilar in healthy volunteers may be lower than the recommended therapeutic doses. PK studies are not always feasible in healthy volunteers. In this case, the PK needs to be studied in patients as part of a multiple-dose study if a single-dose study is not feasible. A sensitive model/population, i.e., fewer factors that cause significant inter-individual or time-dependent variation, should be explored.

If the reference product can be administered both intravenously and subcutaneously, then the evaluation of subcutaneous administration will usually be sufficient to cover both absorption and elimination. It is possible to waive the intravenous administration assessment if the proposed biosimilar comparability in both absorption and elimination has been demonstrated for the subcutaneous route. The PK study of intravenous administration needs to be conducted when the molecule has an absorption constant much slower than the elimination constant (flip-flop kinetics).

In a single-dose PK study, the primary parameters are $AUC_{(0-inf)}$ for intravenous administration and $AUC_{(0-inf)}$ and usually C_{max} for subcutaneous administration. Secondary parameters such as t_{max}, volume of distribution, and half-life should also be estimated. In a multiple-dose study, the primary parameters should be truncated AUC after the first administration until the second administration (AUC_{0-t}) and AUC over a dosage interval at steady state. Secondary parameters are C_{max} and C_{trough} at a constant state.

In any PK study, antidrug antibodies should be measured parallel to the PK parameters using appropriate sampling time points.

2.5.1 Pharmacodynamic Studies

It is recommended that PD markers are added to the PK studies whenever feasible. The PD markers should be selected based on their relevance to the clinical outcome. In some instances, comparative PK/PD studies may be sufficient to demonstrate the clinical comparability of a proposed biosimilar and the reference product, provided that the following conditions are met:

- The selected PD marker/biomarker is an accepted surrogate marker. It can be related to the patient outcome to the extent that the demonstration of a similar effect on the PD marker will ensure a similar effect on the clinical outcome. Relevant examples include an absolute neutrophil count to assess the effect of granulocyte colony-stimulating factor (G-CSF), early viral load reduction in chronic hepatitis C to assess the effect of alpha interferons, and euglycemic insulin clamp test to compare two types of insulin in terms of tissue sensitivity to insulin. Magnetic resonance imaging of disease lesions can be used to compare two β-interferons in multiple sclerosis.
- Some PD markers may not be established surrogates for efficacy but are relevant for the pharmacological action of the active substance, and a clear dose-response or a concentration-response relationship has been demonstrated. In this case, a single or multiple dose exposure–response study at two or more dose levels may be sufficient to waive a clinical efficacy study. This study design ensures that a proposed biosimilar and the reference product can be compared within the steep part of the dose-response curve.
- In exceptional cases, the confirmatory clinical trial may be waived if physicochemical, structural, and in vitro biological analyses and human PK studies, together with a combination of PD markers that reflect the pharmacological action and concentration of the active substance, can provide robust evidence for the comparability of the proposed biosimilar.

When evidence to establish the comparability of the clinical proposed biosimilar is derived from PK studies supported by studies with nonsurrogate PD/biomarkers, it is recommended to discuss such ("fingerprinting") approach with regulatory authorities. The plan should include a proposal of the size of the equivalence margin(s) with its clinical justification and the measures for the demonstration of a comparable safety profile.

2.5.1.1 Clinical Immunogenicity

Immunogenicity is an inherent property of proteins, and it is best tested in healthy subjects in clinical pharmacology profiling. However, it is important to note that the immunogenicity of a specific protein can be assessed through preclinical and clinical studies during drug development. These studies evaluate the protein's potential to elicit an immune response, including antibodies production against the protein.

Immunogenicity testing of a proposed biosimilar and the reference product should be conducted within a proposed biosimilar comparability exercise using the same assay format and sampling schedule, which must meet all current standards. Analytical assays should be performed with both the reference product and the proposed biosimilar molecule in parallel (in a blinded manner) to measure the immune response against the product that was received by each patient. The analytical assays should preferably detect antibodies against both the proposed biosimilar and the reference product. Yet, they should at least detect all antibodies developed against a proposed biosimilar molecule. Usually, the incidence and nature (e.g., cross-reactivity, target epitopes, and neutralizing activity) of antibodies and antibody titers should be measured and presented. They should be assessed and interpreted about their potential effect on clinical efficacy and safety parameters.

The duration of the immunogenicity study should be justified on a case-by-case basis depending on the duration of the treatment course, the disappearance of the product from the circulation (to avoid antigen interference in the assays), and the time for the emergence of the humoral immune response (at least 4 weeks when an immunosuppressive agent is used). The duration of follow-up should be justified based on the time course and characteristics of unwanted immune responses described for the reference product, for instance, a low risk of clinically significant immunogenicity or no significant trend for increased immunogenicity over time. In the case of chronic administration, 1-year follow-up data will generally be required pre-authorization. Shorter follow-up data pre-authorization (e.g., 6 months) might be justified based on the reference product's immunogenicity profile. If needed, immunogenicity data for an additional period, that is, for up to 1 year, could then be submitted post-authorization. For specific products, refer to product-specific proposed biosimilar guidelines.

Increased immunogenicity, when compared with that of the reference product, may become an issue for the benefit/risk analysis and question biosimilarity. However, decreased immunogenicity for a proposed biosimilar is also a possible scenario, which would not preclude approval as a biosimilar. In case of reduced development of neutralizing antibodies with the biosimilar, the efficacy analysis of the entire study population could erroneously suggest that a proposed biosimilar is more efficacious than the reference product. Therefore, it is recommended to pre-specify an additional exploratory subgroup analysis of efficacy and safety in people who did not have an antidrug antibody response elicited during the clinical trial. This subgroup analysis could help establish that the efficacy of a proposed biosimilar and the reference product is, in principle, similar if not affected by an immune response.

Immunogenicity depends on several factors, including the route of administration, dosing regimen, patient-related factors, and disease-related factors (e.g., co-medication, type of disease, and immune status). Thus, immunogenicity could differ among indications. Extrapolation of immunogenicity from the studied indication/route of administration to other uses of the reference product should be justified.

2.5.2   CLINICAL EFFICACY IN PATIENTS

No clinical efficacy and safety testing is required for products that have known PD markers; for other products, the developer can submit a rationale for waiving these studies.

In the absence of surrogate markers for efficacy, it is usually necessary to demonstrate comparable clinical efficacy of a proposed biosimilar to that of the reference product in adequately powered, randomized, parallel-group comparative clinical trial(s), preferably double-blind, by using efficacy endpoints. The study population should generally represent approved therapeutic indication(s) of the reference product and be sensitive in detecting potential differences between a proposed biosimilar and the reference product. Occasionally, changes in clinical practice may require deviation from the approved therapeutic indication, such as a concomitant medication used in combination treatment, line of therapy, or severity of the disease. Deviations need to be justified and discussed with regulatory authorities.

In general, an equivalence design should be used. The use of a noninferiority design may be acceptable if justified based on a strong scientific rationale and considering the characteristics of the reference product, for example, safety profile/tolerability, dose range, and dose-response relationship. A noninferiority trial may be accepted only in instances where the possibility of a significant and clinically relevant increase in efficacy can be excluded on scientific and mechanistic basis. However, as in equivalence trials, assay sensitivity must be considered.

Efficacy trials of the proposed biosimilar product do not demonstrate efficacy per se, as this has already been established with the reference product. The purpose of the efficacy trials is to confirm comparable clinical performance between the proposed biosimilar and the reference product.

In developing a proposed biosimilar product, the choice of clinical endpoints and time points of the analysis of endpoints may deviate from the guidelines for new active substances. The Committee for Medicinal Products for Human Use (CHMP) has issued disease-specific guidelines for the development of innovative products. In the absence of such a guideline, comparability should be demonstrated in appropriate, sensitive clinical models and certain study conditions. The applicant should justify that the chosen model is relevant and adequately sensitive to detect potential efficacy and safety differences. Nevertheless, deviations from endpoints recommended in disease-specific guidelines need to be scientifically justified. Clinical data cannot be used to justify substantial differences in quality attributes.

The correlation between the "hard" clinical endpoints recommended by the guidelines for new active substances and other clinical/PD endpoints that are more sensitive in detecting clinically meaningful differences may have been demonstrated in previous clinical trials with the reference product. In this case, it is unnecessary to use the same primary efficacy endpoints as those used in the reference product's marketing authorization application. However, it is recommended to include some standard endpoints (e.g., secondary endpoints) to facilitate comparisons with the clinical trials conducted with the reference product.

Comparability margins should be pre-specified and justified on both statistical and clinical basis using the reference product's data on the choice of the noninferiority margin.

2.5.3 CLINICAL SAFETY

Clinical safety is important throughout the clinical development program and is captured during the initial PK and PD evaluations and as part of the pivotal clinical efficacy study. Comparative safety data should generally be collected pre-authorization, and the amount of data depending on the type and severity of safety issues known for the reference product. The duration of safety follow-up pre-authorization should be justified.

2.6 EXTRAPOLATION

The reference product may have more than one therapeutic indication. When the comparability of the proposed biosimilar has been demonstrated in one indication, extrapolation of clinical data to other indications of the reference product could be acceptable but needs to be scientifically justified. In case it is unclear whether the safety and efficacy confirmed in one indication would be relevant for another indication, additional data will be required. It is expected that the safety and efficacy can be extrapolated when the comparability of the proposed biosimilar has been demonstrated by thorough physicochemical and structural analyses as well as by in vitro functional tests complemented with clinical data (efficacy and safety and PK/PD data) in one therapeutic indication. Additional data are required in certain situations, some of which are listed below:

- The active substance of the reference product interacts with several receptors, which may lead to a difference in the effects on the tested and nontested therapeutic indications.
- The active substance itself has more than one active site, and each site may produce a different effect in different therapeutic indications.
- The studied therapeutic indication is not relevant for the other indications in terms of efficacy or safety, that is, it is not sensitive for differences in all relevant aspects of efficacy and safety.

2.6.1 PHARMACOVIGILANCE

While a pharmacovigilance program does not satisfy any residual uncertainty in biosimilarity, in some cases, pharmacovigilance may provide additional confidence to regulatory agencies; for example, if the formation of antidrug antibodies is dependent on the demographic aspects, then only a large-sample study can provide reliable data, and such information can be collected through a pharmacovigilance plan, among other routine and common attributes.

2.7 INTERCHANGEABILITY AND SUBSTITUTION

A generic drug is generally considered interchangeable with its reference (brand-name) product and other generic products that use the same reference product. However, because a proposed biosimilar is not structurally identical to its brand-name biologic, assessing interchangeability is a separate process. In the US, the FDA regulates the drug product, but the states regulate pharmacies and pharmacy practices. According to the National Conference of State Legislatures (NCSL), as of October 22, 2018, "at least 49 states have considered legislation establishing state standards for substitution of a proposed biosimilar prescription product to replace an original biologic product." The NCSL indicates that 45 states and Puerto Rico have enacted legislation; the provisions of state legislation vary.

The US FDA has issued its final guidelines on demonstrating the interchangeability of a proposed biosimilar with its reference product to assist sponsors in showing that a proposed therapeutic protein product is interchangeable with the reference product. There were two citizen petitions by the author (Niazi), wherein suggestions were mostly considered in the final guidelines.

It is important to reiterate that the FDA guidelines are not binding, and for the same reason, they do not preclude a sponsor from making an alternate proposal to the FDA, even though most sponsors would hesitate to do so.

The FDA is yet to approve the first interchangeable product. As the FDA gains more confidence in the evaluation of interchangeability, after approving a few products, the guidelines will change substantially.

Data from pre-authorization clinical studies are usually insufficient to identify rare adverse effects. Therefore, the clinical safety of the biosimilars must be monitored closely on an ongoing basis during the post-approval phase, including continued benefit-risk assessment.

Within the authorization procedure, the applicant should present a description of the pharmacovigilance system and a risk management plan following the current EU legislation and pharmacovigilance guidelines. The risk management plan should consider identified and potential risks associated with the use of the reference product and should detail how these issues will be addressed in the post-marketing follow-up. Immunogenicity should specifically be addressed in this context. Any specific safety monitoring imposed on the reference product or product class should be adequately addressed in the biosimilar pharmacovigilance plan. Applicants are encouraged to participate in already existing pharmaco-epidemiological studies in place for the reference product. However, new studies might be needed. Risk minimization activities in place for the reference product should, in principle, also be included in the risk management program of the biosimilar.

For suspected adverse reactions relating to biopharmaceutical products, the definite identification of the concerned product about its manufacturing is of particular importance. Therefore, all appropriate measures should be taken to identify any biopharmaceutical product, which is the subject of a suspected adverse reaction report, based on its brand name and batch number.

2.7.1 MISCELLANEOUS

2.7.1.1 Naming

Biosimilars should have a brand name and share the same International Nonproprietary Name as that of the reference product and any additional designations required in the local jurisdiction. Biosimilars should also have a different brand name.

2.7.1.2 Label

The label must, without exception, include all risks related to the reference product and the same indications as well as be formatted and specified following this guideline. All indications issued to the reference product are permissible once a biosimilar candidate is highly comparable to it, so long as they are not covered by market exclusivity or patents. The developer is not permitted to ask for fewer or more indicators.

2.7.1.3 Substitution

The reference product and other biosimilars authorized using the same reference product can be replaced or interchanged with biosimilars as most recently confirmed by the EMA.

2.7.1.4 Pediatrics

For biosimilars, no pediatric compliance studies are necessary.

2.7.1.5 Human Factors Studies

These investigations are necessary to ensure that the appropriate dose is administered when a patient receives a product. However, these studies are not required if the device utilized for the biosimilar is very similar to that of the reference product. Furthermore, no such studies are necessary when a healthcare expert uses the product.

2.7.2 Risk Management

A biosimilar product uses the same risk management strategy as that used for the reference product. Additionally, accurate biosimilar traceability must be ensured using the brand name and batch number. Post-market surveillance data submission is not required. Safety pharmacology, reproduction toxicology, and carcinogenicity are not required for biosimilars. Local tolerance studies are usually not required unless new excipients are introduced, for which no or little experience exists with the intended clinical route of administration.

2.8 DOCUMENTATION

The development and documentation for the proposed biosimilar should cover two distinct aspects:

- Molecular characteristics and quality attributes of the target product profile should be comparable to those of the reference product.
- Performance and consistency of the manufacturing process of a proposed biosimilar on its own.

The QTPP of a proposed biosimilar should be based on data collected on the reference product, including publicly available information and data obtained from the reference product's extensive characterization. The QTPP should form the basis for the development of a proposed biosimilar product and its manufacturing process. This QTPP should be considered a development tool for which some target ranges may evolve during development as further information on the reference product becomes available.

A proposed biosimilar is manufactured and controlled according to its development, considering state-of-the-art-art information on manufacturing processes and consequences on product characteristics. As for any biopharmaceutical product, a proposed biosimilar product is defined by the molecular composition of the active substance obtained from its manufacturing process, which may introduce its molecular variants, isoforms, or other product-related substances as well as process-related impurities. Consequently, the manufacturing process should be appropriately designed to achieve QTPP. The expression system should be carefully selected, considering differences in the expression system that may result in undesired consequences, such as atypical glycosylation pattern, higher variability, or a different impurity profile, than those with the reference product.

The formulation of a proposed biosimilar does not need to be identical to that of the reference product. Regardless of the formulation selected, the suitability of a proposed formulation regarding stability, compatibility (i.e., interaction with excipients, diluents, and packaging materials), integrity, activity, and strength of the active substance should be demonstrated. In case a formulation and container/closure system different from those of the reference product is selected (including any material in contact with the product), then its potential effect on the efficacy and safety of the proposed biosimilar should be appropriately justified.

The stability of a proposed biosimilar product should be determined according to ICH Q5C. Any claims about stability and compatibility must be supported by data and cannot be extrapolated from the reference product.

It is acknowledged that a proposed biosimilar will have its lifecycle. When changes to the manufacturing process (active substance and finished product) are introduced during product development, a comparability assessment (as described in ICH Q5E) should be performed. For clarity, any comparability exercise(s) for process changes introduced during development should be identified in the dossier and addressed separately from the comparability exercise performed to demonstrate biosimilarity versus the reference product. Process-related changes may occur during the development of a proposed biosimilar product. However, it is strongly recommended to generate the required quality, safety, and efficacy data to demonstrate biosimilarity with the reference product using the product manufactured through the commercial manufacturing process and therefore represent the quality profile of the batches to be commercialized.

3 Development of a Master Plan for the Biosimilar

3.1 CHOICE OF THE PRODUCT

Most of the proposed biosimilar developers face a dilemma when choosing to develop the product because of cost and time constraints for taking the product through regulatory approval. Traditional business development teams follow hard rules of the market; competitors, including both pre-approval and post-approval phase competitors; and cost of goods in order to decide which product to manufacture. While these considerations have survived the test of time, there are many reasons why these rules do not always apply to select a proposed biosimilar product for development.

3.1.1 COMPETITION

First, unlike chemical generics, competitors' field will always be much smaller, not so much for a financial reason but for the need for deep science that is not available to many. Hence, regardless of the nature of the product, the competition will always be limited. Given that almost every proposed biosimilar product can become a blockbuster biologic, a different type of projection is required to qualify a product regardless of the competitors.

3.1.2 COST OF GOODS

Cost of goods can be controlled: most products will cost the same within a small range of variation if the development cycle is followed to reduce your future cost of goods. The cost of goods is often considered a selection criterion, but this is a poor indicator because the production cost of biological drugs is relatively uniform, such as 150–300 USD per gram of the proposed biosimilar developed from monoclonal antibodies (mAbs); cytokines have not shown much variation in their category. Most of the production cost is attributed to the cost of cell culture media, as production involves producing a carbon-based entity, since, the carbon-in and carbon-out exchange occurs in carbon cycle. More details about the cost of goods are provided in the section on the manufacturing process.

3.1.3 MANUFACTURING PLAN AND FACILITY

It is important to create a manufacturing plan involving the utilization of a similar cell line as that used for the reference product, although this requirement is unnecessary. The developers should know that using novel cell lines will inevitably increase the burden of proof required to establish the safety and efficacy of a proposed biosimilar product. The developers should also realize that the cell lines used for the reference product are often decades old when the productivity was not high;

DOI: 10.1201/9781003392026-3

however, manufacturers do not change cell lines to avoid safety and efficacy concerns. The use of a similar cell line, despite the availability of cell lines that provide much higher productivity, can be challenging. Two key elements should be considered when choosing a cell line: First, cell lines with lower productivity generally yield more consistent products because of reduced pressure; second, the actual cost savings achieved when using a high productivity cell line may not reduce the overall cost significantly. Most of the production cost is attributed to the cost of the cell culture media used proportionally to the protein output; a higher productivity cell line reduces the capacity of the bioreactor. The developers are advised to carry out a detailed analysis before using newer cell lines with a very high yield.

Developers must assure the regulators that there are no cross-contamination possibilities between the facilities used for bacterial processing and mammalian cell processing to avoid the risk of viral contamination. The upstream and downstream manufacturing areas should be class 100,000 (Class 8) and 10,000 (Class 7) facilities, respectively. Maintaining a single-pass system of personnel and material is recommended. Additionally, innovating clean area engineering designs based on the single-pass system with only minimal air replaced to meet the OSHA requirements can help reduce the CAPEX of heating, ventilation, and air conditioning systems by 50%–70% and the OPEX by a similar margin.

Most of the large pharmaceutical companies will have fixed-pipe stainless steel systems in place and are less likely to adopt the single-pass systems; for newly emerging pharmaceutical companies, the single-pass system should be the only choice, as it eliminates the need for cleaning validation, a process that adds more than just cost—the risk of contamination causing alterations in the molecular structure of the biosimilar is a serious consideration.

3.1.4 EXPRESSION SYSTEM

Generally, some quality attributes are strictly related to the expression of proteins and the selection of cell lines. When a new biological product is developed, the product of the selected cell line is characterized and evaluated through all three phases of product development. For a biosimilar, the cell line must produce a similar product as that of the reference product, and this process can be challenging if the product has many post-translational modifications, a higher molecular weight, and a highly complex structure. When designing mAbs, a single cell (monoclonal) is used to create a uniform cell line, which may not necessarily be the best choice. The developers should first conduct analytical testing of the reference product to establish the quality attributes required before selecting a cell line to avoid extensive testing at a later stage to justify any analytical differences in the expression of proteins from the selected cell line. It is also important to understand that a high-titer cell line reduces only the capacity of the bioreactor; for low-yield products such as cytokines, the titer differences do not affect the size or cost as much as it is touted by the suppliers of new cell lines.

3.1.5 BATCH SIZE

As a proposed biosimilar product may likely be approved without extensive comparative clinical safety and efficacy studies, the first clinical study, that is, pharmacokinetics (PK)/pharmacodynamics (PD) studies, must use a commercial-scale lot. If single-use upstream processing is chosen, then the size of the bioreactors available have limitations. The developers may choose a smaller-sized bioreactor for manufacturing clinical lots, and then, after approval of the product, they may use ICH Q5E to scale up the process. The developers may also combine several smaller-scale upstream lots to remove the scale-up issues and decrease the burden of ICH Q5E compliance. Generally, the downstream process is less likely to cause significant changes to the product than the upstream process, where post-translational modifications to the protein commonly occur.

When conducting similarity testing of the analytical profile, it is recommended to include at least one commercial-scale lot even at this stage, as the lot may not have undergone PPQ qualification.

3.1.6 RESIDUAL UNCERTAINTY

After completing all the testing, the developer should prepare a detailed report to justify to the agency that the proposed biosimilar product possesses the required biosimilarity to allow licensing (in the US) or authorization (in other countries). This is the most critical stage where a developer can save 24–36 months and scores of millions of dollars from securing approval. Most of the proposed biosimilar developers are too eager to carry out safety and efficacy studies to support their marketing efforts based on their archaic understanding of selling biopharmaceuticals through prescribers. If the developer can demonstrate that there is no residual uncertainty through a strong argument, then it is highly likely that any additional clinical testing will not be required, and even if it requires, this may be limited to additional clinical pharmacology studies.

The developers should present an argument affirming that the totality-of-the-evidence provided is sufficient to determine that the proposed biosimilar product is highly similar to the reference product. The arguments should include a description of any differences in the analytical assessment, nonclinical assessment, and clinical pharmacology assessments in this specific order, realizing that any residual uncertainty must be removed (either proving it nonconsequential or demonstrating that it does not affect the clinical safety and efficacy of the biosimilar). One argument favoring the developer is that additional testing may not necessarily remove any marginal residual uncertainty.

3.1.7 CLINICAL SAFETY AND EFFICACY

The developers should realize that if a PK/PD study has failed and any residual uncertainty related to the failure is not resolved, then the agencies will not approve conducting a clinical safety and efficacy assessment to provide additional proof of biosimilarity, regardless of the size of the clinical efficacy study proposed by the developers.

However, where an efficacy study is conducted, the study design must provide justification of the indicators chosen to test the product where multiple indications are allowed through extrapolation. The study size should first present the effect size analysis (M1) based on public domain data. An equivalence interval (M2) was decided based on clinical judgment, and a rational argument was used to justify the M2 value. The choice of the study model, that is, equivalence margin vs. noninferiority, should also be explained. A critical element of these studies is the population demographic, and making it a practical choice is often difficult, particularly for anticancer drugs. While treatment-naïve patients' option is always desirable, it is often not possible to achieve these criteria. Some complications emerging from safety and efficacy studies make the study results less reliable than the outcomes of PK/PD/immunogenicity testing. When safety and efficacy studies are conducted, the developers are encouraged to use clinical markers rather than hard efficacy results where possible, realizing that the study's purpose is not to demonstrate that the proposed biosimilar product is effective, rather that the biosimilar is equally effective to the reference product. Clinical markers that are relatively easier to evaluate provide greater robustness to the study than the hard efficacy results. Finally, the purpose of a safety and efficacy study is to remove any residual uncertainty and not provide proof of biosimilarity based on the study results alone.

3.2 HISTORICAL DATA ON REGULATORY COMPLIANCE

The developers' common practice is to examine the public domain data, particularly the BLA documents available (www.accessdata.fda.gov/scripts/cder/daf/). However, a critical analysis of the developers' studies showed that the data vary widely in number and detail.

A detailed analysis of the regulatory submissions that led to the approval of these products showed high diversity, frequent redundancy, and reliance on studies that may not assure the safety and efficacy of the biosimilars. The paradigm of stepwise development and evaluation suggested by the Food and Drug Administration (FDA) has not worked well. We have sufficient data available to indicate that a significant change in the biosimilar approval guidance is required to remove redundant testing and reduce the risk of approval of unsafe biosimilars.

Until the end of 2020, more than 1100 studies on analytical similarity, 96 studies on animal pharmacology, 42 in vitro/ex vitro studies on pharmacology, 52 studies on clinical pharmacology, and 32 studies on clinical efficacy studies were submitted. The highlights of these submissions are as follows (Table 3.1):

TABLE 3.1
Testing Approaches Submitted for Licensing of Biosimilars Approved by the Food and Drug Administration

Licensed Product	Analytical	Animal Pharmacology	In Vitro/Ex Vitro Pharmacology	Clinical Pharmacology	Clinical Efficacy	Total
Humira						
Adalimumab-atto	41	2	0	1	2	46
Adalimumab-adaz	52	5	1	4	1	63
Adalimumab-adbm	70	6 (2)	26 (10)	2	1	105
Adalimumab-afzb	25	1	0	3	2	31
Adalimumab-bwwd	38	2	0	2	2	44
Avastin						
Bevacizumab-awwb	56	7 (2)	0	1	1	65
Bevacizumab-bvzr	42	2	4	1	1	50
Epogen						
Epoetin alfa-epbx	32	15 (13)	0	4	0	79
Enbrel						
Etanercept-szzs	53	5	0	4	1	88
Etanercept-ykro	52	3	0	1	1	57
Neupogen						
Filgrastim-aafi	38	1	0	3	0	42
Filgrastim-sndz	41	5	0	5	1	52
Infliximab-abda	52	3	0	1	1	57
Remicade						
Infliximab-axxq	61	1	2	1	1	66
Infliximab-dyyb	33	4 (2)	2	4	5	48
Infliximab-qbtx	51	2	0	2	1	80
Neulasta						
Pegfilgrastim-bmez	NA	13 (8)	0	2	2	17
Pegfilgrastim-cbqv	31	1	2	2	0	36
Pegfilgrastim-jmdb	31	2	0	2	1	36
Rituxan						
Rituximab-abbs	50	1	1	1	1	171
Rituximab-pvvr	40	2	0	1	2	98
Herceptin						
Trastuzumab-anns	27	5	2	1	1	111
Trastuzumab-dkst	37	2	2	1	1	84
Trastuzumab-dttb	48	2	0	1	1	99
Trastuzumab-pkrb	44	2	0	1	1	48
Trastuzumab-qyyp	44	2	0	1	1	48

- Twenty-seven animal pharmacology studies were not reviewed by the FDA, labeling them as redundant or unnecessary.
- No animal pharmacology or in vitro/ex vitro study demonstrated failed results.
- A few clinical pharmacology studies had to be repeated to meet the acceptance criteria because of the wrong choice of the study population. However, none demonstrated failed results.
- No clinical efficacy studies have failed, even if the primary endpoints did not meet by conducting post hoc analysis to add scientific justification for their approval. In two cases, higher immunogenicity was overcome by making minor changes to the manufacturing process. No product was rejected based on a failed efficacy study.
- No correlation existed between submissions for the same molecule; a total of 48–111 studies on trastuzumab were conducted by different developers.

In summary, all analytical similarity testing met the acceptance criteria, and animal pharmacology studies contributed only little to available evidence; all clinical pharmacology studies reached the acceptance criteria, and even though differences prevailed among clinical efficacy studies, these were overcome through discussion and consensus decision-making, allowing marketing authorization. Given these observations, the developers of a proposed biosimilar have an opportunity to present testing protocols to the FDA that may not be as extensive as used in the approval of all current products.

Table 3.1 lists the testing approaches used by the developers for licensing of biosimilars approved by the FDA. First, the developers should meet with the FDA at a Biosimilars Advisory Meeting that requires having expressed the biological entity at a small scale with initial analytical similarity testing. This meeting should be followed by type 2 meetings to secure an agreement with the FDA on the minimal testing studies required.

3.3 PLANNING FOR MANUFACTURING

Establishing a manufacturing plan for biosimilars is essential to enable accessibility to biological drugs; unlike chemical generic drugs, there is no option of operating a fill and finish operation, as the drug substance constitutes the main product. This practice, carried out in several developing countries, should be discouraged to ensure safety of the product.

The definitions of terms are provided below:

3.3.1 QUALIFIED PRODUCT

A qualified product is a product that has a reference SRA product currently distributed in the country of origin; the proposed biosimilars should have the same mechanism of action, dose, frequency, route of administration, and concentration (strength).

3.3.2 RAPPORTEUR

Using rapporteurs is a standard practice in the European Union (EU); the FDA also accepts third-party audits. Rapporteurs are members of the Committee for Medicinal Products for Human Use or the Committee for Medicinal Products for Veterinary Use, assigned to assess applications for marketing authorization. They play a critical role in evaluating and monitoring medicines in the EU. The competent national authorities of the EU Member States appoint the rapporteurs. The European Medicines Agency (EMA) generally identifies the rapporteurs and co-rapporteurs for specific medicines in its assessment reports as well as maintaining the identities of the rapporteurs and co-rapporteurs confidential in certain situations. For example, a list of 61 rapporteurs for biosimilars is available at the EMA.

3.3.3 THIRD-PARTY CURRENT GOOD MANUFACTURING PRACTICE AUDIT: DATA AND SAMPLE INTEGRITY

As clinical pharmacology testing for biosimilars is conducted in an at-scale current good manufacturing practice (cGMP) lot (i.e., a final commercial lot), it is imperative that the developer qualifies its cGMP production. The audit is specific to the product and not waived based on previous audits. The audit is conducted by third-party auditors. The auditors also confirm and assure that the samples that will be selected for clinical pharmacology testing are valid and their integrity confirmed.

3.3.4 VALIDATED SAMPLES

The samples used for analytical assessment and clinical pharmacology must be validated for their source, history, and compliance. Generally, during an audit, samples will be collected and provided to a third-party testing facility.

3.3.5 THIRD-PARTY ANALYTICAL ASSESSMENT

The final analytical assessment must be conducted by a third party approved by a newly formed Global Medicines Agency (GMA) as a qualified testing facility.

3.3.6 CERTIFIED SAMPLES RETAINED BY CLINICAL RESEARCH ORGANIZATIONS FOR CLINICAL PHARMACOLOGY TESTING

Clinical research organizations should retain the samples if there is an issue regarding an outlier or later inquiry; the time limit is through the product's shelf-life.

3.3.7 REFERENCE PRODUCT

To qualify a product as a reference product, a comprehensive dossier must be used to approve a biological product, which is still being marketed in the nation of origin. Only one reference product can be utilized. When the reference product has different strengths or presentations, the lowest-strength product should be used. Several batches of the reference product should be used, as it will reach the market at different time points and can be obtained directly from the market. The reference product batches should undergo testing for the required attributes to establish the shelf-life and should be stored as recommended. Occasionally, it may be possible to test reference product batches that have been stored for a long period (e.g., product samples frozen at −80°C) or beyond their intended shelf-life if reliable data demonstrate that the storage conditions have no effect on the critical quality attributes (CQAs).

3.3.8 CHARACTERIZATION

As defined in ICH Q6B, proper methods should be used to perform characterization of the reference product. Some of the characterization studies determine physicochemical qualities, biological activity, immunochemical properties (if any), purity, impurities, contaminants, and amount. Developers are encouraged to adopt newer technologies as available. As the quality attribute values of the reference product can vary from batch to batch, it is essential to establish the ranges of these variations. The variations are either process-related (the manufacturing system) or product-related (the expression system), the latter cannot often be resolved, requiring the developer to create a different expression system; the same can be the case for process-related attributes, but these are readily fixed. However, any difference in both groups of attributes cannot be justified based on any in vivo or ex vivo studies.

3.3.9 IMPURITIES

When developing a biosimilar, impurity profiling is required, and guidelines for product-related variations are established with the developer. For instance, a biosimilar may show fewer impurities in terms of type and quantity, but there must be no mismatched impurity, as it cannot be justified through a safety study.

3.3.10 FUNCTION-BASED TESTS

CQAs should be identified using analytical profiling and in vitro functional levels. Functional experiments should be pertinent to the potential mechanism of action in all therapeutic indications, including those that examine apoptosis, complement-dependent cytotoxicity, antibody-dependent cellular phagocytosis, and antibody-dependent cellular cytotoxicity. Functional tests (ADCC, ADCP, and CDC) are not suitable for a reference product primarily targeting a soluble antigen.

3.3.11 TEST PROCEDURES

Testing of CQAs does not require validated procedures, as some test methods cannot be fully validated. Analytical methods must be qualified, sensitive, and adequately selective to identify potential differences. Where appropriate, the procedures described in the ICH recommendations (ICH Q2A, Q2B, Q5C, and Q6B) for analytical assessment can also be utilized to evaluate quality attributes for batch release. Additionally, the use of appropriate orthogonal methodologies is necessary for robust data.

3.3.12 NUMBER OF BATCHES

Generally, eight batches will be tested, one of which should be the clinical batch. Therefore, the final third-party analytical assessment will include at least three PPQ lots.

3.3.13 DATA EVALUATION

Depending on the type of data output, a visual comparison suffices for test results sent as printed output, such as spectra. Quantifiable data from multiple batches should use the 3-Sigma range, which is derived for the reference sample as (ref − 3ref, ref + 3ref), providing the most accurate inference. If the test sample's MinMax range falls within the 3-Sigma range, then the 3-Sigma test is accepted.

3.3.14 EXPRESSION SYSTEM

The expression system determines product-related CQAs, including primary structure, higher-order structures, glycosylation (only in eukaryotic hosts), product-related variations, and process-related variations. The expression system should be the same class as the one used to express the reference product, even though SRA agencies allow the use of a different expression system; this recommendation comes from the realization that switching an expression inevitably leads to variable post-translational modifications that may be difficult to evaluate in safety and efficacy studies. The developers are also advised to select more steady expression systems; generally, high-yielding cell lines produce more variants. Cell lines should be qualified according to the ICH Q5D.

3.3.15 ANALYTICAL PROFILES

Proteins undergo addition of functional groups after translation (post-translational modifications [PTMs]), which should be comparable, not necessarily identical. In addition to PTMs, these profiles include aggregates, fragments, visible or subvisible particles, acidic and basic variants, and other product modifications such as reduced, oxidized, glycated, and misfolded protein forms. These attributes can change over the product's shelf-life, requiring testing over the shelf-life duration. When the environment changes during different stages of the production process, hydrophobic regions of the protein can unfurl, causing either accumulation or fragmentation, adding to immunogenic responses. The aggregate size ranges from soluble aggregates to visible residues, depending on the duration of exposure to various stresses such as shear, thermal, chemical, and freeze-thaw, among others. The matrix-free size exclusion chromatography substitute analysis helps define size distribution, sedimentation velocity-analytical ultracentrifugation.

Charge variations are proteoforms that occur at different stages of the manufacturing process in various colloidal matrices (such as culture medium, in-process buffers, or formulations) and have varying charges. It is, therefore, preferable to use several types of cation exchange chromatography.

Oxidation, phosphorylation, sulfation, acetylation, methylation, and hydroxylation are examples of nonenzymatic PTMs occurring across various manufacturing stages. Liquid chromatography is preferable for defining PTMs and measuring associated molecular variations and contaminants.

Cell substrates are process-related variations or residuals, including host cell proteins (HCPs), host cell DNAs (HCDs), cell culture, and downstream processing residuals. Enzyme-linked immunosorbent assay and real-time or quantitative polymerase chain reaction assay are the main HCP and HCD detection and quantitation techniques, respectively. These variants are not tested during the drug substance qualifying phase because they are part of the release specification.

3.3.16 RELEASE SPECIFICATION

Release specifications are based on the characterization of the reference product, except for the legacy compendial attributes such as sterility, fill volume, and delivered volume; other characteristics are independently established, such as sterility, invisible particles, protein content, potency, and physical characteristics unique to the biosimilar candidate. These standards may be used to specify the biosimilar candidate's release specification.

3.3.17 FORMULATION

A formulation different from that of the reference product is permissible for biosimilars. A formulation with the same number of inactive substances or fewer is advised, unless constrained by patent protection. The formulation's stability and compatibility (i.e., how it interacts with excipients, diluents, and packaging materials) should be proved, along with the integrity, activity, and potency of the active ingredients. If the primary packaging that is in contact with the product is different, then further safety tests are required to verify that there is no unexpected leaching of package components into the product. Developers are encouraged to select a primary packaging materials as similar as possible, since it is often difficult to justify these findings. The formulation may not contain any unique excipients previously not used in a similar product, and all excipients must be free of animal products.

3.3.18 REFERENCE STANDARD

The in-house primary reference material is an adequately documented sample prepared by the manufacturer from a representative lot or lots and calibrated against which the in-house working reference material is used for biological assays and physicochemical testing of the following lots. It is the sole source acceptable for use as a working reference. Reference standards that are openly accessible (such as European Pharmacopoeia) cannot be used as the reference product for comparison testing.

3.3.19 STABILITY

The stability of the biosimilar candidate must be evaluated according to the ICH Q5C including accelerated and stress stability testing to further enable direct assessment of structural similarities and produce degradation profiles.

3.3.20 PROCESS QUALIFICATION

Before any analytical assessment for similarity, the upstream and downstream processes must be evaluated. However, on completion of the clinical pharmacology studies, no batch size adjustment is permitted; the developer may do this only under ICHQ5E, which applies only post-approval. Bridging studies are needed to validate whether or not the production size changes.

3.3.21 ANIMAL TOXICOLOGY

For biosimilars, no animal toxicological testing is necessary. This conclusion is based on the recent amendment to the BPCIA, wherein "animal toxicology" was removed and replaced with "nonclinical testing." As animals have no binding receptors for biological drugs, this binding results in pharmacological and toxicological reactions. This testing is currently also recommended for new biological drugs.

3.3.22 CLINICAL PHARMACOLOGY

An extension of analytical evaluation, PK, and PD studies reflect how the body perceives the drug molecule and vice versa. Such studies are also conducted for drugs such as aflibercept or ranibizumab that are administered locally into the eyes; these drugs do not enter the general circulation, and hence, they are tested through parenteral administration for the same reason. For most of the chemical generic drugs, PK profiling is not required when the drugs are administered intravenously, intramuscularly, or subcutaneously. However, biosimilars administered through parenteral routes require PK profiling, as PK parameters such as half-life and distribution volume can also correlate with the kinetics of receptor binding, an essential assessment because all biological drugs act by receptor binding.

One misunderstanding in the design of PK/PD lies in the traditional goal of characterizing the profiles in a wide range of subject qualifications such as age, sex, body mass index, body weight, and race. All these variables add much inter-and intra-subject variability that requires a larger population. None of it is necessary for comparative PK/PD profiling, as these studies aim not to characterize but to compare the profile attributes. A robust design should accommodate crossover or parallel designs. A crossover approach is better at identifying differences but might not be appropriate for reference products with robust immune responses or a long half-life. The equivalence margins must be prespecified, and the appropriate range is often 80.00%–125.00%. The key PK parameters, typically AUC_0-_{Cmax}, should be equivalent in the PK experiment.

3.3.23 IMMUNOGENICITY

Immunogenicity is an inherent property of proteins, and it is best tested in healthy subjects during clinical pharmacology profiling. However, the immunogenicity of a specific protein can be assessed through preclinical and clinical studies during drug development. These studies evaluate the protein's potential to elicit an immune response, including production of antibodies against the protein.

3.3.24 CLINICAL EFFICACY

No clinical efficacy and safety testing is required for molecules with a PD response; this will exclude mAbs until similar waivers allow them. Comparative clinical efficacy testing requires hundreds of thousands of patients to obtain statistically meaningful results; thus, such studies have never failed. This requirement will vary in different parts of the world, but over time, a concurrence will be reached that such testing is not necessary.

3.3.25 NAMING

Biosimilars should have a brand name and share the same international nonproprietary name as that of the reference product and any additional designations required in the local jurisdiction. Biosimilars should also have a different brand name.

3.3.26 LABEL

The label must, without exception, include all risks related to the reference product and have the same indications. The developer is not permitted to ask for fewer or more indicators.

3.3.27 SUBSTITUTION

The European Medicines Agency (EMA) very recently approved that the reference product and other biosimilars authorized using the same reference product can be replaced or interchanged with biosimilars.

3.3.28 PEDIATRICS

For biosimilars, no pediatric compliance studies are necessary.

3.3.29 HUMAN FACTOR STUDIES

These investigations are necessary to ensure that the appropriate dose is administered when a patient receives a product. However, these studies are not required if the device utilized is very similar to that of the reference product. Furthermore, no such studies are necessary when a healthcare expert uses the product.

3.3.30 RISK MANAGEMENT

A biosimilar product uses the same risk management plan as that of the reference product.

It is anticipated that a developer is planning to distribute the product globally; while most developers avoid securing the assistance of a rapporteur, the use of a rapporteur is highly recommended to save time and cost. Holding meetings with regulatory agencies with an available rapporteur report will always be helpful and earn greater confidence of the regulatory agencies.

4 Trends in the Manufacturing of Recombinant Proteins

4.1 BACKGROUND

Manufacturing of therapeutic proteins utilizes either unmodified or genetically modified living entities, bacteria, mammalian cells, viruses, and yeast to produce large protein molecules. Some of the manufacturing systems are straightforward, for instance, the manufacturing of naturally produced products such as penicillin, and are therefore not included in this chapter.

To gain a clear understanding of the manufacturing processes for therapeutic proteins, it is important to understand the roles of DNA and RNA in our body. The manufacturing processes are tightly connected at each unit of operation during upstream and downstream processing. Variation in yield, diverse impurities, and protein product potency achieved are the factors that significantly affect the steps involved in the manufacturing process. Therefore, the manufacturing process should be carefully laid out in a lengthy definition and development process in the form of a flow chart that identifies sizing issues.

The manufacturing process starts with establishing a genetically modified cell line through culturing to express the desired therapeutic protein in a bioreactor. The term "bioreactor" refers to a device or vessel that supports the growth of a living entity, and the term "fermenter" also refers to a bioreaction vessel that involves the production of gases and heat; in many cases, these terms are used interchangeably. The correct term that should be used for the production of therapeutic proteins is bioreactors.

In the first step, the living entities are allowed to express the desired therapeutic protein (product), and in the next step, the expressed protein products are removed from the culture media either by filtration (if the therapeutic protein is in solution) or by first disrupting the cells (in case of bacteria) and then removing the protein through a multistep process.

The subsequent steps involve purification of the therapeutic proteins and, in some cases, induction of proper protein folding. If mammalian cells susceptible to virus infection are used as the expression entities, then any viral contamination should be removed.

Finally, the purified therapeutic protein should be labeled as a drug substance when it is diluted with a buffer and stored at $-20°C$.

After production, the drug substance should be formulated into a drug product in the form of a solution in a vial or a prefilled syringe or as a lyophilized powder. Thus far, therapeutic proteins are being administered parenterally, but efforts are being taken such that, in the future, these proteins may be administered orally, transdermally, through inhalation, or other routes.

The therapeutic protein manufacturing process is expensive and subject to strict regulatory control because even subtle changes in the molecular structure can alter their immunogenicity and efficacy. More recent technologies of single-use, continuous manufacturing (CM), and online monitoring

DOI: 10.1201/9781003392026-4

are rapidly changing the manufacturing risk profile. They offer many long-term advantages in the planning of manufacturing facilities, which are described in detail in this chapter.

4.2 PROCESS OPTIMIZATION

4.2.1 CELL LINE DEVELOPMENT

The development of a traditional cell line is time-consuming. A critical step in early-stage manufacturing can take nearly 40+ weeks starting from concept to creation in establishing a high-yielding and high-quality clone. This includes choosing a suitable cell line, construction of an expression vector, transfection of cells, cell sorting, clone selection, and evaluation based on cell growth and productivity. Single-cell isolation and screening are critical in the workflow of cell line development from a regulatory perspective. The conventional screening approach involves seeding a single cell per well in a 96-well plate and then screening multiple plates to choose a high producer.

Several tools available today can accelerate some of the steps involved in cell line development, and they can help reduce the overall timeline. Cell line developers can use an effective targeted transfection process that allows gene insertion into "hot spots" when compared with random transfection events used previously. This specific manipulation allows the creation of a high-yielding cell line and significantly reduces the follow-on screening process. Additionally, instead of screening multiple plates (50–100 plates in traditional processes), wherein each well contains one clone, seeding cells into mini-pools and then selecting a high-performing pool of cells yields a smaller cell population that enables choosing the final single clone. Fluorescence-activated cell sorting together with glutamine synthetase is a rapid clone-screening approach. Today, microfluidics-based technology is being widely used by cell line developers. These systems can sort and deposit single cells and can also provide evidence of clonality, proliferation rates, and specific productivities within a short span (as little as 5 days). When used as a combined technique, they can significantly reduce the overall timeline for cell line development to nearly 8–10 weeks, thus helping the process development progress faster toward early-stage deliverables.

Several manufacturers continue to focus on traditional techniques such as plating into semi-solid media and determining an individual clone's protein titer at the static phase that does not correlate well with fed-batch. The most common enrichment method for potentially higher producers but equally for pre-selection includes, fluorescence-activated cell sorting or vector optimization for sorting.

One of the myths related to bioprocess technology is that the cell line must be forced to produce higher yields. However, the extent to which the cell line is being pushed is limited before it becomes unstable; the cells will produce a higher titer that may not be desirable for monoclonal antibody, but for a monoclonal antibody, variations in glycosylation other DNA-based changes will become inevitable. Developers must therefore calculate the overall cost based on the cost of media serving as the carbon source needed for pilot production before switching over to higher-yielding cell lines. In many cases, a higher-yielding cell line helps reduce the bioreactor size but not necessarily the cost of goods.

4.2.2 CELL CULTURE MEDIA

Cell culture medium is the primary raw material for cell culture and exists in more than 100 different formulations comprising critical components, including amino acids, vitamins, fatty acids, and lipids. The chemical constituents of a medium, formulation, and concentration are crucial factors that determine the suitability of a medium to support cell growth, cellular metabolism, yield, and protein quality. Developments in cell culture media significantly affect cell density, increase specific productivity, and improve product quality (less variability). The following section presents some of the culture media optimization strategies and challenges that can enhance process intensification.

Media optimization approaches cannot be universally applied for all cell lines or clones; a medium that may enhance productivity in one clone may not necessarily enhance the same for another clone. Likewise, product quality can be affected. A platform approach, particularly one that uses a single basal medium, is always unlikely to yield satisfactory results. While it is advantageous to use an available medium (ease of sourcing media components and having a fixed and validated approach) for the production of all monoclonal antibody products using the same host cell line, variations in product quality (glycosylation, charge variants, etc.) may be necessary for the functionality of the final product. As such, having unique solutions, even with a finite number of compounds, is highly recommended.

A traditional approach to the development of a culture medium and evaluation of its suitability for a particular cell line involves changing one component in the media at a time. A design of experiments approach enables the study of the relationship between the components to optimize the composition. Depending on the number of components being used in a medium, multiple iterations are possible, which makes the assessment relatively time-consuming. Media blending, an alternative to the traditional design of experiments approach, allows simultaneous optimization of the several components within a medium, and it has become a commonly used method. Additionally, successful medium formulation requires reliable analytical methods such as capillary electrophoresis, high-performance liquid chromatography (HPLC) coupled with mass spectrometry, and gas chromatography to quantify metabolites present in the culture medium during the entire duration.

However, today's newer technology, for example, high-throughput microarray analysis, involves an integrated approach toward whole-media analysis rather than measuring these metabolites and ions individually. Microarray analysis (EMD MilliporeSigma) can be used to identify medium components to which cells respond, and this approach reduces the need for random testing. Several manufacturers of cell culture media are backed by biotechnological companies and therefore offer high-throughput technologies to drug manufacturers for medium optimization (e.g., MilliporeSigma, Sartorius). Given that modeling has the ability to reduce the need for additional research or experimental analysis, it presents many opportunities to the field of culture medium development that can significantly reduce time and cost. With such stoichiometric models and kinetic models, online or inline analysis during cell culture can provide valuable inputs to these models to optimize media or even feed solutions to establish a more robust process. In view of this approach, companies can create their platform cell culture media specific to their cell lines.

Cell culture medium optimization is further catered to fed-batch processes that utilize intermittent feeding (mostly concentrates of specific media components). However, given the high volumes of media requirements, having a cost-effective solution for medium preparation is of paramount importance for a perfusion culture. A concentrate in a cell culture medium is one option to reduce operational footprint; for instance, a medium whose components are concentrated three to four times their original amount will be equivalent to approximately 60,000–70,000 L, which can easily support a perfusion process, provide significant space, and reduce resource utilization. Alternatively, a medium explicitly designed for the perfusion process is also another option to meet the perfusion process media demands. Such medium will be more suitable to support high-cell densities, improve volumetric productivity, and reduce costs (lower perfusion rates) rather than adapt media used for a fed-batch process (Table 4.1).

4.2.3 High–Cell Density Cryopreservation

Cell bank manufacturing is an optimal opportunity for process intensification. Briefly, in a typical mammalian cell banking process, a vial of cryopreserved cells sourced from a high–cell density cell bank is thawed, and the cells are inoculated into at least a 25-mL culture medium. The seed culture is subsequently expanded to generate adequate cells that can be banked. In industrial practice,

TABLE 4.1
Decision Matrix to Address Bottlenecks and Develop Next-Generation Process

Technology Solution	Pros	Cons	Comment
Bottleneck: Limited facility footprint			
Perfusion	High volumetric productivity	Operational complexity	Needs more process development than fed-batch
Bottleneck: Limited CAPEX			
Perfusion	Smaller bioreactor	Operational complexity	Needs more process development than fed-batch
Bottleneck: Limited capacity in a production bioreactor			
N-1 perfusion	Cell expansion time shifts to N-1; shorter N time with the same titer	Operational complexity, possible effect on process performance	Ensures capacity for shorter turnaround times
Perfusion	High volumetric productivity	Operational complexity	Identify a separation technique that will suit your process
Bottleneck: QC/QA release			
Online sensors and PAT implementations	Reduce number of release methods through tighter process control	Resource demanding to develop	Spectral methods combined with multivariant analysis can offer several process parameters
Multi-attribute release methods	Drastic reduction in release methods	Resource demanding to develop	Still in development
Bottleneck: Low-yield process			
Perfusion	High volumetric productivity	Operational complexity	Identify a separation technique that will suit your process
Concentrated fed-batch	High volumetric productivity	Operational complexity	
Bottleneck: Several products and processes			
Perfusion	Higher level of flexibility	Operational complexity	Scale-out depending on batch volume needed

Source: www.genengnews.com/magazine/324/supplement-next-generation-bioprocess-techniques/

approximately 1 million cells per vial are generally used. Compared with the scale-up of a production bioreactor for commercial purposes, the scale-up factor or the number of seed trains required to generate a sufficient quantity of inoculum from the vial to the production bioreactor is high. This process is time-consuming and may require additional resources and measures to ensure no failure during the seed generation stage. The seed expansion stage can take approximately 20–30 days from a low-density cell bank to a production bioreactor. To negate the additional time and processing, a high-density cell bank is being recently used to accelerate the process by providing a larger working volume at thaw. The use of a high-density cell bank to inoculate the first seed train bioreactor (N-3 bioreactor) can significantly reduce the time. For example, use of a 100- to 150-mL high-density cell bag (cryopreserved) at $50–100 \times 10^6$ cells/mL can reduce the seed expansion process by 10 days to 2 weeks. This innovative process eliminates the need for handling multiple vials, minimizes the variability in the cell density, reduces contamination risks, and, most importantly, significantly decreases the time to start a production bioreactor. In high–cell density cryopreservation, it is preferable to use a specific medium capable of supporting high cell density while ensuring no cell damage due to freeze-thaw. Additionally, modern technologies required to design single-use bag assemblies that can handle large volumes for cell freezing and banking (fluoropolymer 2D bags) are currently under development.

4.2.4 CELL CULTURE OPERATIONS

The last few decades have predominantly focused on fed-batch cultures. While perfusion systems are available, the industry has not widely adopted them, mostly because of the need for a high volume of medium and vessel capacity to support high cell densities and increased productivity. Although cell densities achievable with fed-batch are relatively lower than those in perfusion culture, the advancements made toward increasing productivities have kept the fed-batch process in continuous use for a long time. With the need to reduce manufacturing costs and facilities to gain more flexibility, steady-state perfusion and perfusion-based processes, including concentrated fed-batch, are now being fostered by the increasing adoption of single-use technologies. Perfusion processes in seed train and production phases can result in a threefold increase in volumetric productivity. Upstream process intensification can be achieved through perfusion-based operations such as by compressing the seed train duration by reducing the size and number of bioreactors required, maximizing bioreactor utilization, increasing volumetric productivity, and reducing overall footprint, thereby maximizing facility utilization and efficiency.

N-1 perfusion, a form of seed train intensification, refers to the intensification of cell growth during the step before the production bioreactor (N). In N-1 perfusion, process intensification is carried out by attaching a cell retention device to the N-1 bioreactor to achieve high cell density and viability, thus seeding the production bioreactor at a higher starting cell density and shortening the production bioreactor run time. This modification can dramatically increase the facility output without direct change to the core production process. A robust cell retention device is required to attain a high-density cell inoculum for the production bioreactor.

Benefits of N-1 perfusion include

- Increased fed-batch process efficiency.
- Time-saving and cost-effective.
- Reduced operational risk.
- Smaller bioreactor footprint.

N-1 perfusion can help optimize fed-batch production in two ways:

- High–cell density seeding of the production bioreactor (N), achieved by attaching the cell retention device to the N-1 bioreactor.
- Removal of the N-1 bioreactor, achieved by maintaining continuous attachment of the cell retention device to the N-2 bioreactor, provided the N-2 bioreactor can provide sufficient cells for the production bioreactor (N).

The N-1 bioreactor is the most widely used application for perfusion. Increasing the cell density of the N-1 bioreactor allows for starting the production bioreactor with a high seeding density and possibly reducing the bioreactor's overall cycle time to achieve the desired titers. Higher productivity and the possibility of inoculating multiple production bioreactors from a single N-1 bioreactor can increase overall upstream capacity and production volumes. Such increase in production can also be achieved with a reduced footprint; for example, a traditional process requiring a 20,000-L bioreactor can now be fitted with a 2,000-L perfusion bioreactor. Furthermore, the use of single-use components eliminates the need for cleaning validation, i.e., clean-in place (CIP)/steam sterilization-in-place (SIP). Additionally, the perfusion-based process can be extended further down to the N-3 seed train and high–cell density cryopreservation, as discussed previously. A single-use bag with approximately 150- to 500-mL high–cell density culture can be frozen during storage and can then be thawed to inoculate a seed bioreactor, thereby eliminating shake flasks and a lengthy seed expansion step.

Perfusion can dramatically increase the cell density of the N-1 bioreactor and accelerate the production process to achieve a gain in efficiency. When perfusion culture is introduced into the seed train to increase cell density, it can reduce the number of bioreactors needed or the time required to reach the desired titer at harvest.

Another application that allows process intensification is the intensified fed-batch mode or a concentrated fed-batch mode. A concentrated fed-batch process is much similar to a perfusion culture, except for the recirculation of the cells and the product. The production bioreactor used in the concentrated fed-batch process has a hollow-fiber filter and an alternating tangential flow pump, much similar to the bioreactor used in perfusion. However, the filter pore size should be chosen such that the bioreactor can retain both the cells and the product. For antibody production, a 30-kDa filter is used. The process typically starts in the fed-batch mode, and recirculation of the cells and product begins only toward the end of the production cycle. Similar to perfusion culture, a concentrated fed-batch process is advantageous in terms of the high cell density and the single-operation harvest, which avoids titer dilution. The most widely reported example of the concentrated fed-batch application is PERCIVIA, a collaboration between Crucell and DSM. Experiments with PERCIVIA showed significantly high yields of 27 g/L when PER.C6 cells from the concentrated fed-batch process were used.

The increased productivity allows for the development of smaller facilities and increases the efficiency of the process when coupled with single-use technology (SUT). A drug manufacturer can leverage these advantages into the existing infrastructure while increasing the capacity to remain competitive.

4.2.5 BIOREACTOR CYCLE

The production bioreactor poses a notable limitation during production in a facility. Process duration (commonly approximately 2 weeks for a fed-batch process) is mostly a rate-limiting step in an industrial facility, given that all other upstream and downstream process steps require only up to a few days. Therefore, the utilization of perfusion culture in the bioreactor immediately preceding production should be investigated. The typical net result is higher densities during inoculation at the production stage, shorter process duration, and similar titer and product quality. Thus, the production process is even more productive with higher overall facility volumetric productivity. The challenge lies in optimizing the perfusion medium to generate the necessary cells for the production bioreactor without creating any new burden of infrequent, large-volume medium preparation in a facility. The key parameters are the cell densities achieved over time and the cell-specific productivity, which determine the overall cell and product mass generated during the cell culture process, respectively.

Another application of upstream process intensification is the seed train. Here, an emerging strategy is to use perfusion culture instead of the batch mode in the scale-up process. Briefly, a perfusion culture can be grown to a very high cell density, enabling inoculation of a production-scale reactor with very few intermediate scale-up steps. For example, a 10-L perfusion culture, with 60 million cells/mL, can be used for direct inoculation of a 2000-L reactor at an initial cell density of 0.3 million cells/mL. A more conventional scale-up process with batch cultures would have included intermediate vessels of, for example, 50-L, 200-L, and 500-L scale. Another aspect is that a high-density seed culture enables inoculation of the production culture at a high initial seed cell concentration. This can reduce the production lag phase and shorten the production process considerably. A shorter process can enable more production batches annually and better facility utilization. Specially designed cryo bags eliminate open cell culture operation steps, lead to better reproducibility in seed train expansion, and decouple cell expansion and batch production, allowing for global distribution of cells to production facilities from a central expansion facility.

4.3 SINGLE-USE TECHNOLOGY

The initial reluctance to SUT has rapidly shifted to a broad recognition of the multiple advantages of disposables, including increased flexibility and decreased upfront investment. Manufacturing suites and production plants entirely based on production with single-use technology are becoming more common, and agile and flexible facilities with disposable technology are being constructed in less time.

These upstream technologies should balance media and SUT costs while considering processing times in the overall production process timelines and the annual number of batches produced. The application of smaller bioreactors using SUT could provide flexibility. With fewer limitations on changeover time and cleaning verification, it becomes possible to run more lots and products in a facility.

SUT has evolved significantly over the last few years and has continually undergone innovation. A facility incorporating SUT or a process using single-use components enables rapid configuration for different processes and changeover between batches—this smart implementation presents drug manufacturers with increased capacity and enhanced flexibility.

While SUT revolves around equipment, the facility and its design of SUT are also extremely essential. Facility footprint and ease of operation are key features, and currently, integrating a modular facility has become popular, particularly when manufacturers want to retain some features of a classic facility. Preconfigured setups allow for a faster establishment of a manufacturing site.

SUT facilitates the development of a process in one manufacturing location and easily transfer/relocate it to a second location upon establishing the facility. This is accomplished by coupling platform processes with single-use components, resulting in reduced process development time, and effort for equipment specifications, suitability, and parallel activities.

SUT suppliers are constantly improvising on existing systems, e.g., multi-use of one equipment (Smart Flexware systems from EMD Millipore) for several operations. These systems are compatible with both chromatography and tangential flow filtration (TFF) operations, all of which reduce footprint and investment. Comparative analyses have shown at least a 15% overall cost reduction with SUT versus stainless steel. New technologies in single-use components have shown increased process robustness, better process control due to automation, flexibility, overall cost reduction, and lower cost of goods sold.

A key concern of regulatory agencies in biopharmaceuticals manufacturing is to ensure no cross-contamination of the batches. This cGMP concern is difficult to resolve in the manufacturing of biological products because it is not possible to rely on cleaning validation to ensure that there are only traces of substances from previous batches. Because even a small amount of contaminants can affect protein structure, the issue of cleaning validation is much severe for biological products than for chemical drugs. Additionally, the increase in demand has also necessitated simple, yet faster, and low-cost production systems.

SUT has addressed some of these challenges when compared with conventional stainless-steel systems. Technologies have been developed over the past three decades, with major suppliers such as Pall, Sartorius, and Millipore taking the lead and developing disposable products that are pre-sterilized, gamma-irradiated, eliminating the need to conduct cleaning validation exercises.

The earliest SUT products in this category were as simple as filters. Soon, these products became the standard components: today, more than 95% of filters used in bioprocessing are of the disposable type. The focus then shifted to other process components associated with bioreactors and chromatography technologies for purification. Additional improvements made to the process, including high titers and process intensification, have facilitated runs at a relatively smaller scale (10,000-L stainless-steel bioreactors vs. 2000-L single-use bioreactors). SUT is advantageous in terms of cost-effectiveness, a smaller and efficient facility, a faster turnaround time between batches, and the elimination of CIP and SIP and has therefore gained acceptance during the significant revolution in biopharmaceutical manufacturing.

SUT components support various production stages of biopharmaceutical manufacturing, including clone selection, cell banking, upstream and downstream process development, GMP production, formulation, and fill-finish. The combination of SUT with platform processes makes it possible to quickly progress from clone selection to the production of GMP products. The adoption of SUT is gradually gaining pace, particularly in small-scale or clinical-scale production. Until recently, single-use systems did not have the capacity to handle a large batch size, but newer systems, including TFF and chromatography systems, have this capacity.

While regulatory agencies do not recommend the utilization of single-use or disposable items in manufacturing, it is the manufacturer's responsibility to ensure compliance with cross-contamination limits. When the cost and time needed to meet those requirements become onerous, the cost of single-use or disposable items becomes a serious aspect to be considered. The US Food and Drug Administration (FDA) and European Medicines Evaluation Agency (EMEA) strongly urge manufacturers to create a sterile environment that prevents the entry of contaminants rather than cleaning the area and proving effective cleaning through validation protocols. This stance by the regulatory authorities became sterner in the 1970s as viral contamination in drug preparations from human and animal tissues came to light. Several manufacturers who could not comply with the new requirements had shut down. The breakout of transmissible spongiform encephalopathies further compounded the complexity, and consequently, manufacturing of biological drugs in cGMP-compliant facilities became too expensive. However, one of the foremost challenges with SUT has been the lack of regulatory guidance on the qualification requirements of these systems.

SUT is advantageous in being safer, greener, cheaper (particularly capital costs), and more flexible. However, there are challenges in the mainstream of manufacturing, especially with regard to questions about the quality of materials used, scalability, running costs, extent of automation possible with these components, reliance on supplier chain, testing for extractable and leachable components, and training of staff for assimilating these components in an established bioprocessing system.

While the European Medicines Agency has approved a vaccine manufactured using SUT, the US FDA is yet to approve a product manufactured using SUT, and several applications are pending approval.

4.3.1 Containers and Mixing Systems

Disposable or single-use bag systems are well adopted as alternatives to hard-walled containers. This is because, historically, pharmaceutical products, such as sterile intravenous solutions, blood, plasma, plasma expanders, and hyperalimentation solutions, have been stored and dispensed in disposable bags. A disposable bag would typically have a one-layer film made of polyvinyl chloride or ethylene-vinyl acetate for storing blood. In biomanufacturing, single-use containers include bottles, 2D and 3D bags, two-ply and three-ply bioprocess bags (for storing culture media); cryopreservation bags; tank liners for buffers and solutions; mixing bags; and microcarrier filter bags. Typical process steps in mixing include dissolving components of a buffer or culture medium, refolding of a solution, dispersion of cell culture in bioreactors, and heating or cooling of liquids.

4.3.2 Drums, Containers, and Tank Liners

Tank liners are simple, single-use (disposable) bags used for lining containers and transport carrier systems. In most cases, they are not gamma-sterilized because they are used in open systems, such as in the preparation of buffer solutions and culture media at the initial stage. However, these tank liners are also available as pre-sterilized versions. Tank liners are a cost-effective alternative to dedicated stainless-steel or poly tanks and totes. The container outside the tank liner provides only mechanical support. Contour liners reduce the need for cleaning validation and sterilization of traditional containers. The most important advantage with tank liners is that the potential of cross-contamination between different products is low because they have only single use.

For smaller volumes, single-use containers (capacity range: 50 mL to 20 L) with an integrated handle, integrated hanging capability, and needle-free sampling port are available. These containers may be used with a sterile welder and are known as the manifold system.

Liners for cylindrical tanks (capacity range: 50 to 750 L) are available in 2D and 3D designs and with a top or bottom drain, and they fit most of the industry standard cylindrical tanks. Tank liners are generally manufactured in accordance with cGMP requirements in an ISO-certified sterile room to minimize bioburden and contamination with other particulate matter. The use of tank liners eliminates the need for pre-cleaning and post-cleaning, which consequently reduces cycle times. They are widely used for the hydration of powdered media and preparation of buffers and other nonsterile solutions.

Commercially available overhead mixers can readily be integrated with most of the currently available tank liners because these liners are open systems. However, tank liners are designed to operate only in specific mixing systems for which the impeller is powered from the bottom. Generally, mixing systems that do not involve any mechanical parts inside the bag (2D or 3D bags) are preferred to reduce the cost or to minimize the risk of damage to the bag due to the rotating devices, grinding of the bag, or stirrer inside the bag. Stirring systems that use a magnetic field for stirring provide more sterile conditions than those that are magnetically coupled.

Mixing systems may also be integrated with a load cell such as a temperature sensor. Additionally, tank liners may have provisions for pH measurements (reusable and single-use) and sampling ports. Weight measurement (load cell) is the most important feature of a tank liner. While most manufacturers would use a floor scale, large-scale production requires installing load cells in the outer containers to avoid moving the containers for weighing. Noteworthy, more expensive systems have programming elements that might make the process analytical technology (PAT) work easier. Yet, during buffer and media preparation, there are only a few challenges that can be readily overcome by implementing the most straightforward and cheapest systems.

Several major equipment suppliers provide a complete line of mixing systems. While these systems offer an advantage in handling large volumes consistently, these lines can be designed by the clients and need not secure help of equipment suppliers. Currently, a broad choice of low-density polyethylene (PE) liners for industrial application is available, such as HyPerforma™ (Thermo Fisher Scientific), Mobius® Single-Use Mixing Systems (EMD Millipore), and Flexel 3D (Sartorius).

4.3.2.1 Two-Dimensional Bags

2D bags are sterile, ready-to-use small-volume bags (capacity range: 5 mL to 50 L, beyond which they become difficult to handle). These bags are designed for storage, sampling, filtration, and transportation of culture media, buffer solutions, clarified harvests, intermediate products, drugs, and drug products. These bags are also equipped with ports connected to other sterile single-use systems in a sterile manner. In some instances, 2D bags are used to store powders (such as buffer salts, active pharmaceutical ingredients, and excipients): these bags have a funnel shape and are equipped with large sanitary fittings or aseptic transfer systems and are antistatic and free from additives.

The design of 2D bags creates a limitation at a larger scale; it becomes difficult to maintain their integrity, leading to handling and transportation issues. When filled to the maximum capacity, the seals of 2D bags may not be tight because the fluid weight is transferred to the seams of these bags. This becomes particularly problematic when the 2D bags are shaken during mixing, which adds further stress to the seams.

4.3.2.2 Three-Dimensional Bags

3D bags as liners in hard-walled containers obviate the integrity problems encountered with 2D bags; 3D bags are available in different sizes. The design of 3D bags also provides an additional surface to install ports with complex functions. The 3D bags are made of welding films and are mostly offered in cylindrical, conical, or cube shapes. More often, the shape is determined by how these containers are stored or stacked in outer containers with the same shape, which allows a snug fitting of the 3D bags. These 3D bags are designed for storage and shipping of a large volume of solutions. They are supplied in a sterile state and are ready to use for quick process implementation.

Single-use bags can be readily used to transport or store frozen products, ranging from cell culture as working cell bank for direct introduction into a bioreactor to shipping biologically active pharmaceutical ingredient. By contrast, flexible bags can survive temperature variations; often, it is difficult to detect damage to them during transportation and, thus, require a protective surface around them to prevent this risk.

Plastic disposable containers offer the best alternative solution in the utilization of disposable components, as they remove cleaning and validation requirements. Low-density PE liners in a hard-walled plastic container and a standard mixer make the cheapest combination of pieces to prepare buffers and media. More complex mixing systems are unnecessary and are not expensive proprietary containers to hold these PE liners.

4.3.3 Advantages of Single-Use Technology

The adoption of single-use or hybrid systems represents a faster, more flexible, and less capital-intensive route. The cost and benefits of each option should be weighed against existing infrastructure, technical constraints, and production volume requirements. Single-use manufacturing systems offer multiple advantages versus traditional stainless-steel equipment, which are as follows:

- Increased speed-to-market.
- Reduced capital: Higher utilization of equipment and facility and increased number of batches.
- Reduction/elimination of cleaning and validation costs: A biologic manufacturing facility can consume approximately 800,000 gals of water per day, most of which is to perform SIP/CIP and operate autoclaves—none of these would be needed in the next-generation single-use systems.
- Elimination of carryover.
- Increased flexibility for facilities with multi-products and batch sizes and faster turnaround—lower cost and flexible capacity to easily adapt to changing scales and accommodate new modalities. SUT allows for a plug-and-play approach when coupled with modular facilities.
- Reduce cross-contamination risks: This allows unit operations to be connected, thereby eliminating open processing. This allows concurrent step processing or even consider multiple product processing.

Evaluation of the cost-benefit of considering a single-use option for a particular process step should include the effect it could have on the other process steps (e.g., previous and subsequent steps). Cost analysis should be inclusive of end-to-end process manufacturing costs and compared against the fixed costs of a stainless-steel process. Perhaps, the greatest impediment in the wider acceptance of single-use items comes from manufacturers' inability to discard their large investments made, relatively recently (the 1970s and 1980s), in fixed equipment and systems. Therefore, the changes occur at smaller companies, research organizations, and contract companies. However, this scenario is about to undergo rapid changes. The high cost of production that was acceptable to large pharmaceutical companies must now be challenged as the patents of blockbuster recombinant drugs have begun to expire, which allow smaller companies to compete on cost—the biosimilar business should convince the industry to embrace the future of bioprocessing. Additionally, environmental considerations are involved.

The integration of an innovative single-use approach in upstream and downstream processing provides an opportunity to develop a flexible and small footprint facility, which is, ultimately, advantageous for manufacturing cost-effective and affordable drugs. A start-to-finish facility is built entirely on disposable and single-use systems. Several analyses have reported that a single-use facility has a lesser operating cost (approximately 22%, Levine 2013) than a stainless-steel facility. Figure 4.1 presents a schematic showing all manufacturing operations built from start to finish with single-use systems.

4.3.4 SINGLE-USE BIOREACTORS

The science and the art of bioprocessing dates back thousands of years, incorporating newer modalities for biologics, a diverse range of products, more particularly biopharmaceuticals. The shift in cell culture from a benching technique at a milligram scale to industrial production at a kilogram scale took nearly two decades through trials. The current era of biopharmaceuticals is manifested in producing large quantities of biologics in stainless-steel bioreactors. Today, these large-scale stirred-tank bioreactors (10,000–100,000 L in scale) represent modern mammalian cell culture technology, a significant workhorse of the biopharmaceutical industry.

Stainless-steel bioreactors have been used for bioproduct manufacturing for centuries. The essential elements of these bioreactors, i.e., a vessel to contain culture and media under sufficient mixing and aeration, are readily provided through their traditional designs. Today, a multitude of options in the design of bioreactors are available. These options became available when bioreactors expanded in manufacturing biological drugs requiring many control features that were not needed or required in other industries. With animal, human, and plant cells and viruses being sources to produce therapeutic proteins, vaccines, and antibodies, there arose a need to modify traditional bioreactors to accommodate the growing needs of these new production engines: the application of recombinant engineering technologies has placed these new engines in the forefront of biological drug production. One major recent change in bioreactors' design is the use of single-use bioreactors (SUBs) to avoid challenges in cleaning validation, which reduce the regulatory barriers in drug production. Hundreds of new molecules are under development using disposable bioreactors, and in many instances, disposable bioreactors are used to manufacture clinical supplies.

Almost all of the recombinant drugs currently available in the market were developed by large pharmaceutical companies starting approximately 40 years ago when the traditional bioreactor was the only choice available; even though their process may be less efficient, it was not worth the effort to switch over to another manufacturing method because of the prohibitive cost of changeover protocols that need to be completed.

The dramatic decrease in changeover time with increased flexibility has been a remarkable benefit with single-use bioreactors. For example, a changeover time for a 200-L bioreactor has been reduced to 2–3 hours instead of more than 24–48 hours as with a stainless-steel bioreactor.

SUBs have varied designs and purposes, but all of them are made of class VI plastic films, which are sterilized by gamma radiation and are disposed after use. These bioreactors may have several attachments that allow filtration of media and monitoring of pH, dissolved oxygen (DO), oxygen demand, pCO_2, temperature, and other PAT-related parameters. In SUBs, mixing and aeration inside the bag is achieved through the use of stirrers, paddles, and shaking and rocking of the bags by mechanical or hydraulic means, which is as effective as that in a traditional stainless-steel tank and, in some instances, causes less stress to the culture.

SUBs are available in many sizes, with capacity ranging from milliliters to thousands of liters. Their structure can range from very simple to very complex, i.e., they may also be equipped with control systems, either manual operated or highly automated. They can be as inexpensive as a

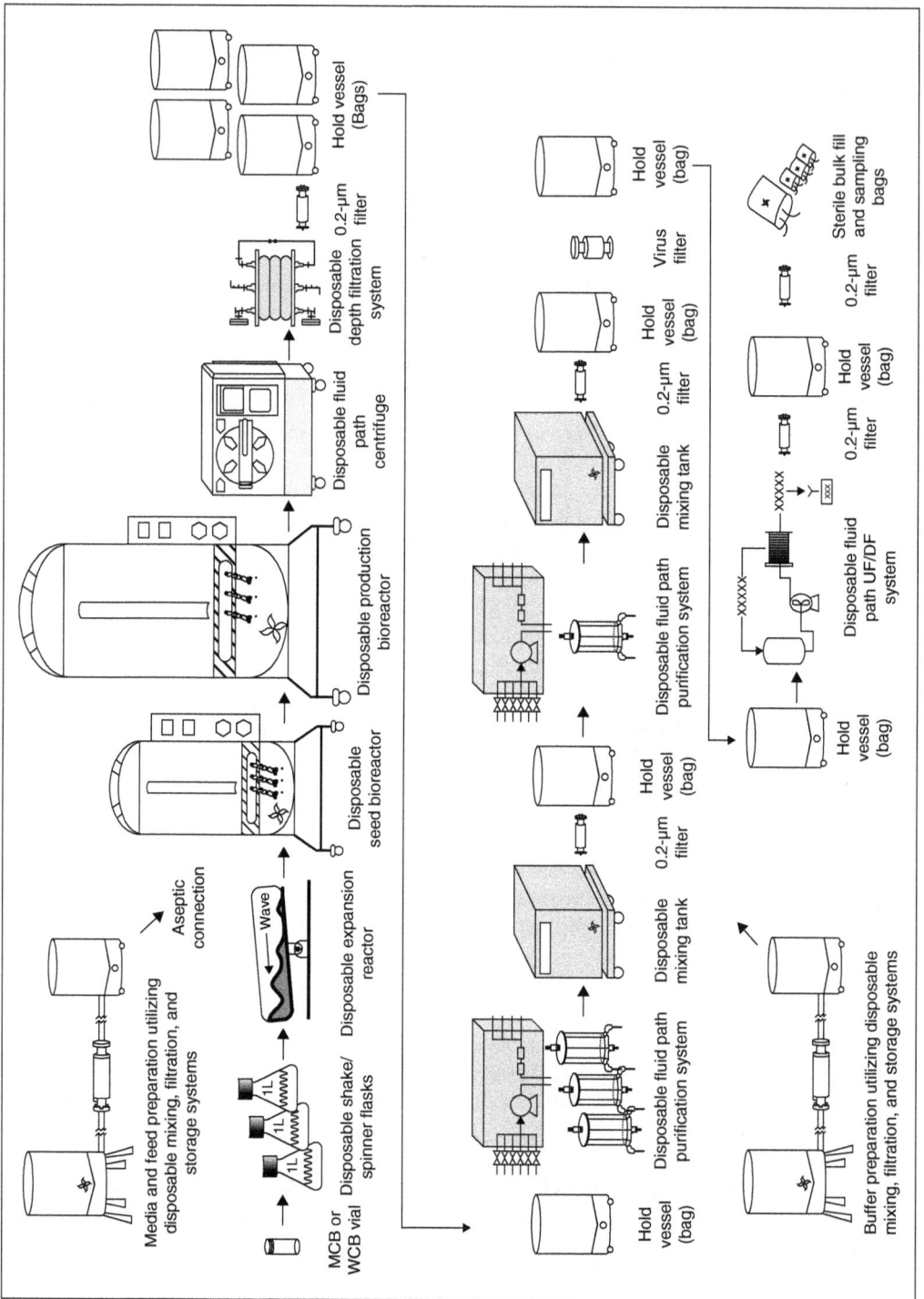

FIGURE 4.1 Single-use systems built for biopharmaceutical manufacturing processes

plastic bag or as expensive as a high-end traditional hard-walled bioreactor. The field of disposable bioreactors is still evolving, with new inventions surfacing almost routinely. One example is the replacement of glass Petri dishes, T flasks, and roller bottles or glass flasks with plastic plates, polypropylene flasks, and Teflon bags, respectively, for small-scale bacterial, yeast culturing, disposable hollow fiber systems, wave bioreactors, and stirred 3D reactors.

Types of stirring mechanisms include mechanical stirrer attached to a motor, magnetically levitating stirrer, stirrer without contact with motor, magnetic stirrer at the bottom, stirrer that rubs off the surface, and mechanical stirrer inserted from the top. Rocking wave motion is the most commonly used stirring mechanism; pioneered by WAVE Bioreactor, several equipment suppliers have adopted this system. The stationary bioreactor concept differs drastically from the usual wave motion that requires moving the plate; here, the bag remains stationary. Instead, a flapper pushes down one edge of the disposable bag.

The 3D single-use stirred tank reactor systems have been successfully able to mimic conventional stainless-steel bioreactors. The dimensions, proportions, sparging systems, and mixing systems of the 3D single-use systems are similar to those of the classical stainless-steel systems (reusable). SUBs are equipped with a sparger ring or a microsparger and two axial-flow three-blade-segment impellers or one axial-flow three-blade-segment and one radial-flow six-blade-segment impeller. The stirring system at the center achieves homogeneous mixing in the bag. All SUBs facilitate mixing, sparging, venting, and temperature monitoring. The bioreactor bags have provisions for pH and DO monitoring (single-use and reusable), sampling, liquid transfer, inoculation ports, and harvest ports. SUBs have a plug-and-play setup and operation through standard sterile connections, coupled with easy integration with most control platforms predominantly used at the industry-wide level. SUBs decrease the need for cleaning and sterilization and reduce the risk of cross-contamination. The wide volume range makes SUBs suitable for process development, clinical manufacturing, and large-scale cGMP manufacturing (Figure 4.2).

2D single-use bioreactors such as Cellbag specific to the WAVE systems have been successfully used. These bioreactor bags use a rocking motion for agitation. These bags are produced from two-layer films, which are welded together at their ends. The resulting structure is a flat chamber

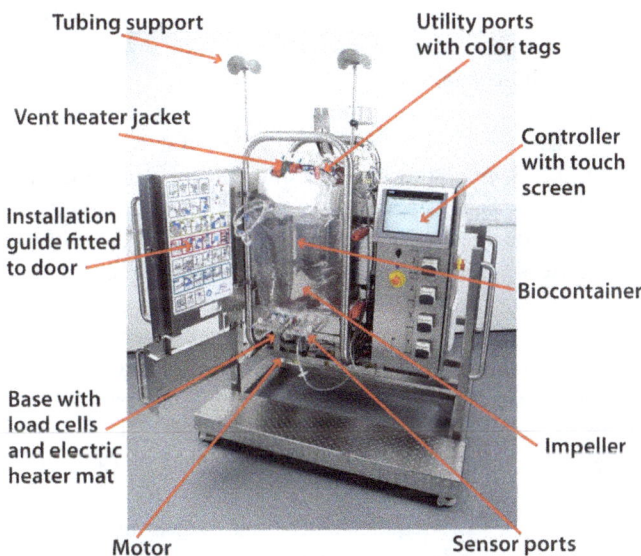

FIGURE 4.2 A single-use bioreactor

Source: https://bioprocessintl.com/2016/design-performance-single-use-stirred-tank-bioreactors/

with ports, whose either face or end is welded. With limitations in volume and challenges related to agitation and aeration at a large scale, these WAVE bioreactors are predominantly used for seed train steps. Furthermore, WAVE bioreactors displace the first disposable bioreactors such as roller bottles, cell factories, and hollow fiber bioreactors. This is because most animal and human cells are cultured in a serum-free medium and in suspension because cell culture bioreactor volumes are currently shrinking owing to increased product titers.

The application of noninvasive optical sensor technology to transparent cultivation containers for animal cells has resulted in highly automated or precisely monitored and controlled disposable micro-bioreactor systems. This has paved the way for a change in early-stage process development from being unmonitored to being well characterized and controlled and has made an important contribution to the accurate replication of larger-scale conditions.

In the pharmaceutical industry, it is assumed that the current drive toward safe, individualized medicines (e.g., personalized antibodies, functional cells for cancer, immune, and tissue replacement therapies) will contribute to the continuing growth of disposable bioreactors. When optimized cell densities and product titers must be achieved in the shortest possible time, cell culture technologists should be willing to deviate from their gold standard approach, that is, use of stirring systems. In addition to highly instrumented, scalable, wave-mixed, and stirred SUBs, orbitally shaken disposable bioreactors and novel approaches such as PBS Biotech or BaySHAKE are increasingly used.

Bioreactor manufacturers (Thermo Fisher Scientific, Cytiva [formerly GE Life Sciences], Eppendorf, and Sartorius) have demonstrated the successful application of SUBs for cultivating bacteria and supporting high-density mammalian culture.

4.3.5 OTHER COMPONENTS

According to the FDA Guidance for Industry (www.fda.gov/media/71012/download), PAT is intended to support innovation and pharmaceutical development efficiency. PAT is a system for designing, analyzing, and controlling manufacturing through timely measurements (i.e., during processing) of critical quality and performance attributes of raw and in-process materials and processes to ensure final product quality. The term "analytical" in PAT is viewed broadly to include an integrated approach of chemical, physical, microbiological, mathematical, and risk analyses.

Single-use sensors, either integrated into the SUB or included in the cover and are disposed with the bioreactor, must fulfill process requirements. They provide a continuous signal and provide information about the cell culture status at any stage.

As disposable bioreactors are new applications in this industry, the first attempt to monitor the bioreactor's product is by using the traditional biosensors used in hard-walled systems to measure bioreactor temperature DO, pH, conductivity, and osmolality. These probes must first be sterilized (autoclaving) and then be attached to penetration adapter fittings welded into bioreactor bags. Not surprisingly, this is a labor-intensive and time-consuming process with the potential to compromise the integrity and sterility of SUB bags. However, owing to technological innovations and advancements in SUBs, the use of reusable biosensors has been largely discarded in favor of genuinely disposable sensors. Critical process parameters that are often monitored include pressure, pH, DO, cell density, and ultraviolet (UV) absorbance. The packages that contain the traditional technologies for monitoring these parameters are not usually compatible with or effective when integrated into single-use assemblies for many reasons: cost, cross-contamination, inability to maintain a closed system, and incompatibility with gamma irradiation. Because of these challenges, some of the measurements are performed offline.

The adoption of disposable sensors requires a keen understanding of their need and utilization. Their suitability and purpose would be determined by their material properties, sensor manufacturing, process compatibility, performance requirements, control system integration, compatibility with treatments before use, and regulatory requirements.

Although these obstacles do not always preclude the use of traditional measurement technologies, single-use solutions for monitoring process parameters eliminate the need for equipment cleaning and autoclaving small parts, reduce the risk and cost associated with establishing process connections, and may be more cost-effective than traditional technologies. For example, a sanitary, autoclavable pressure transducer qualified for a certain number of autoclave cycles and required recalibration may be more expensive to use than a single-use pressure sensor.

Disposable sensors are used in two modes: one where the sensors are placed in situ in contact with the liquid, and the other where the external sensors are in contact with the medium either optically (ex situ) or through a sterile (and disposable) sample removal system (online). Single-use sensors must be sterilizable or be available pre-sterilized if they are in contact with the media, cost-effective, and reliable. Newer designs use inexpensive sensing elements placed inside a disposable bioreactor and combined with reusable (and more expensive) analytical equipment outside the reactor. Inexpensive, single-use sensors can be placed on transistors or inside the headspace, inlet, outlet, or cultivation broth for liquid-phase analysis (for monitoring temperature, pH, and pO_2). These single-use sensors can also be optical sensors, which allow noninvasive monitoring through a transparent window.

4.3.5.1 Optical Sensors

Optical sensors work on the principle of the effect of electromagnetic waves on molecules. The use of optical sensors is an entirely noninvasive method and can provide continuous results of many parameters simultaneously. It is relatively easy to use them, as they can be seen through a transparent window in the bioreactors. The detector part of the system can be physically separated, which facilitates the utilization of expensive analytical devices, allowing optical sensors to be used in situ or online.

Fluorescence sensors can be optimized for nicotinamide adenine dinucleotide phosphate (NADPH) measurements, biomass estimation, and differentiation between aerobic and anaerobic metabolism. 2D fluorometry enables the simultaneous measurement of several analytes by scanning through a range of excitation and emission wavelengths, including proteins, vitamins, coenzymes, biomass, glucose, and metabolites (such as ethanol, adenosine-5'-triphosphate [ATP], and pyruvate). Thus, fluorometry can be used to characterize the upstream process. Generally, a fiber-optic light attached to the bioreactor shines light through a glass window in the bioreactor. One example of fluorometry detection is the BioView system (www.bioview.com). The BioView sensor is a multichannel fluorescence detection system for biotechnology, pharmaceutical, chemical, food production, and environmental monitoring. It detects not only specific compounds but also the state of microorganisms and their chemical environment without interfering with the sample. The BioView system measures fluorescence online directly in the process. Interference with the sample is eliminated, which reduces the risk of contamination. However, given the complexity of the spectra of multiple components, high-level resolution programming is required.

Many metabolic products present in a bioreactor can be readily detected by infrared (IR) spectroscopy. Yet, a water-absorbed IR beam for biomass analysis can be either near-IR (NIR) or Si-Rhodamine when used in the transmission mode. NIR transmission probes and attenuated total reflectance–IR probes for bioreactors are now commercially available. These probes are connected through silver halide fibers or radiofrequency connectors.

In addition to IR and fluorescence detection, optical methods based on photoluminescence, reflection, and absorption are also used. Optical electrodes or *optodes* can be attached to the bioreactors using glass fibers, leaving the measurement equipment outside of the bioreactor, similar to the setup for fluorescence detectors, allowing the use of these chemosensors in situ or online.

Oxygen sensors quench fluorescence by producing molecular oxygen; for quenching measurements, a fluorescent dye (metal complexes) is immobilized and attached to one end of an optical fiber, and the other end of the fiber is interfaced with an excitation light source. The duration and strength of fluorescence depend on the molecular oxygen concentration present around the dye in the environment. The emitted fluorescence is collected and transmitted for interpretation outside of the bioreactor. These electrodes work better than the traditional platinum probe electrodes to detect molecular oxygen, and they can be used in both liquid and gas phases. PreSens (www.presens.de) is an example of a noninvasive oxygen sensor that measures the partial pressure of DO and gaseous oxygen. Sensor spots are fixed on the inner surface of glassware or transparent plastic material (disposables). Therefore, molecular oxygen concentration can be measured in a noninvasive and nondestructive manner from outside through the vessel wall. Different coatings for different concentration ranges are available. It offers online monitoring of DO concentration, ranging from 1 ppb to 45 ppm, with dependence on flow velocity and oxygen measurement in the gas phase. These coatings can be autoclaved.

Ocean Optics (www.oceanoptics.com) offers the world's first miniature spectrometer with a wide array of sensors for oxygen and pH detection in the gas phase.

pH sensors act based on their absorption or fluorescence characteristics. For fiber-optic pH measurements are carried out based on both fluorescence- and absorbance-based pH indicators. The most common dyes for fluorescence-based measurements are 8-hydroxy-1,3,6-pyrene trisulfonic acid and fluorescein derivatives, while phenol red and cresol red are used for absorption-type measurements. Fluorescent dyes are sensitive to ionic strength, which limits their use for broad-range pH measurement (for pH beyond 3 U).

CO_2 sensors work on the principle of pH measurement for a carbonate buffer embedded in a CO_2-permeable membrane. The reaction time of the sensor is long, and quaternary ammonium hydroxide provides a faster response.

Fluorescence-based sensors are attractive because they facilitate the development of portable and low-cost systems that can be easily deployed outside of the laboratory environment. Such measurements are insensitive to changes in dye concentration, leaching, and photobleaching of the fluorophore and instrument fluctuations, unlike unreferenced fluorescence intensity measurements. The performance of the sensor system is characterized by a high degree of repeatability, reversibility, and stability.

4.3.5.2 Biomass Sensors

Information about the biomass concentration can be obtained using turbidity sensors. Generally, these sensors are based on the principle of scattered light. Most turbidity sensors have the disadvantage of a linear correlation only for low particle concentrations, but sensors that use backscattering light (180°) have linear properties for high particle concentrations. A translucent window is necessary in disposable bioreactors in order to check for the desired wavelength in the IR region. The S3 Mini-Remote Futura line of biomass detectors (www.applikonbio.com) incorporates sensors inside disposable bioreactors. This sensor system uses an ultra-lightweight pre-amplifier for connecting to the ABER disposable probe (www.bioprocess-eng.co.uk/product/aber-futura-pico/).

4.3.5.3 Electrochemical Sensors

Electrochemical sensors include potentiometric, conductometric, and voltammetry sensors. Thick- and thin-film sensors and chemically sensitive field-effect transistors (ChemFETs) possess the potential as potentiometric disposable sensors in bioprocess control because they can be produced inexpensively and in large quantities.

Many pH-sensing systems rely on amperometry methods, but they require constant calibration owing to instability or drift. The setups of most amperometry sensors are based on the pH-dependent selectivity of membranes or films on the electrode surface.

While turbidity sensors detect total biomass concentration, capacitance sensors provide information specifically about viable cell mass. Electrical capacitance and conductance generally characterize the electrical properties of cells in an alternating electrical field. Cell membrane integrity exerts a significant influence on the electrical impedance to estimate only viable cells. The Biodis Series by Hamilton (www.hamiltoncompany.com) and Aber (www.aberinstruments.com) for monitoring viable biomass in disposables applications is available. An integrated version is manufactured from Eppendorf (www.eppendorf.com).

4.3.5.4 Pressure Sensors

Pressure is another important process parameter frequently monitored during bioprocess unit operations such as filtration, chromatography, and many other procedures. A traditional stainless-steel pressure gauge can be used in conjunction with a single-use experimental setup, but this combined setup has the drawback that the pressure gauge must be sterilized separately. Furthermore, the connection of the sensor to the previously gamma-irradiated single-use assembly could raise problems.

Many bioprocess unit operations have in-built pressure-control systems to avoid significant pressure-related safety issues. In traditional stainless-steel reactors, pressure is monitored and tightly controlled, as pressure can influence mass transfer and prevent contamination. Moreover, a high-pressure event is a potentially hazardous situation. A clogged vent filter in a bioreactor can easily cause rupture of the bags, spillage of the reactor's contents, and exposure of the operators to unprocessed bulk.

Another application where pressure monitoring is central to process performance is depth and sterile filtration. A filter's ability is primarily measured by either flow decay or pressure increase. However, adding reusable traditional pressure transducers to a process train fails the purpose of using a single-use process setup. Depending on the process application, the contact surface of a traditional device's product requires either sanitization or moist heat sterilization.

Traditional devices are sterilized through SIP, where the product contact surface is exposed to steam sterilization in devices that can be placed in an autoclave, and the entire device is exposed to the steam. However, many single-use process components are not compatible with moist heat sterilization temperatures, which necessitates separate sterilization of the stainless-steel device and possibly less than that for an optimal connection to a pre-sterilized single-use assembly.

Single-use pressure sensing facilitates rapid changeover of product contact surfaces in both development applications and early-phase clinical manufacturing. For example, single-use pressure sensors from PendoTECH (www.pendotech.com) were designed to enable pressure measurement with single-use assemblies that have flexible tubing as the fluid path. These single-use pressure sensors are gamma-irradiation compatible (up to 50 KGy), and the fluid path materials meet United States Pharmacopoeia (USP) Class VI guidelines and are compliant with EMEA 410 Rev 2 guidelines.

The USP Class VI designation is considered the most stringent and, therefore, most useful for medical applications. It involves the following three evaluations for in vivo biological reactivity, generally performed on mice or rabbits to mimic use in humans:

- Acute systemic toxicity (systemic injection) test: This test measures toxicity and irritation when a sample of the compound is administered orally, applied to the skin, or inhaled.
- Intracutaneous test: This test measures toxicity and localized irritation when the sample is in contact with live subdermal tissue (specifically, the tissue intended to be in contact with the medical device).
- Implantation test: This test measures toxicity, infection, and irritation of intramuscular implantation of the compound into a test animal model over several days.

The compound will be assessed in these three tests in order to confirm that it has an extremely low toxicity level, and it will be subjected to several temperature assessments for set periods. Materials that meet USP Class VI standards generally have a high-level quality and better compliance with the US FDA because such materials will carry a substantially lower risk of causing harm to patients from reaction to a toxic material.

USP Class VI Testing is only one standard of biocompatibility. However, although not a limited series of tests, some biocompatibility requirements for medical devices may exceed the testing performed in USP Class VI. ISO-10993 is a more rigorous standard for the biological evaluation of medical devices.

ISO-10993 is a standard that involves systemic toxicity and intracutaneous reactivity testing. However, it also tests for additional cytotoxicity, genotoxicity, chronic toxicity, hemocompatibility, and, more importantly, systemic toxicity. A different level of ISO-10993 testing is primarily required for medical devices that will be permanently or semi-permanently implanted into a patient. Therefore, for devices that are not intended to be implanted or will have limited contact with patients, ISO-10993 testing may be more extensive than necessary.

In a single-use bioreactor, a sensor can be installed on a vent line to measure headspace pressure. Even though the sensors are qualified to be used up to 75 psi, the core sensor shows accurate values in the low-pressure range required for a single-use bioreactor.

4.3.5.5   Sampling Systems

Continuous sampling from a bioreactor can be accomplished using a sterile filter and a peristaltic pump to obtain a cell-free sample. A presterilized sampling container, which contains a needleless syringe that can be welded to the bag bioreactor's sampling module, is available for use. A sample is pumped into the container of these assemblies. The sampling containers can be removed when needed, and the tube is heat-sealed. Other sampling systems have a presterilized Leuer connection, including a one-way valve, which prevents the sample from flowing back into the reactor. The sample is withdrawn from the reactor using a syringe and directed to a reservoir through a sample line. For example, Cellexus Biosystems (https://cellexus.com) and Millipore (www.sigmaaldrich.com) use such sampling systems. The Cellexus system connected to the sample line can have up to six sealed sample pouches. The reservoir sample can then be pushed into the pouches, which are subsequently separated by a mechanical sealer, which results in sealed, sterile samples. Several sampling manifolds with a customizable option are offered by bioreactor manufacturers/suppliers.

The proprietary Millipore system comprises a port insert that can be fitted to several bioreactor side ports and several flexible conduits that can be opened and closed individually for sampling. These ports are connected to flexible, single-use sampling containers. Sampling is limited to the number of available conduits in each module.

These sampling systems allow aseptic sampling but are limited in terms of the number of samples collected per module and the lack of automation. While these methods help obtain good validation data, the risk of contamination is not completely removed because the bioreactor is breached every time a sample is withdrawn. Therefore, there is a need to develop or choose other methods that will not require contact with the media.

4.3.5.6   Connectors

The complexity of bioprocessing makes it difficult to design systems without any weaknesses; contamination is associated with a risk that requires all connectors, tubes, and implements to join various steps of a process and perform sampling in a sterile environment. Single-use components were first applied in connectors and lines, as cleaning was a challenging task. Unlike hard piping, the flexible tubing used in single-use transfer lines does not require costly and time-consuming cleaning and validation procedures. This allows manufacturers to quickly alter the process steps or convert the resultant over to a new product. This feature is a key advantage for multiple production facilities wherein process requirements change depending on the type of drug being produced. Innovative manufacturers now incorporate single-use tubing assemblies throughout the bioprocess, starting from seed trains to the final fill applications. Additional cost savings result from the need for reduced labor and the chemical, water, and energy demands associated with cleaning and validation.

Yet, in hard-walled systems, SIP systems are used only because steam is used for CIP/SIP operations. Even then, the risk of contamination persists. As much of the SUT systems in these applications are being used in the biomedical field, the device industry had always been ahead of the regulatory requirements. Biocompatibility issues have long been resolved, and vendors can provide detailed information on their devices that might be needed by regulatory agencies. As manufacturing of these devices is a complex process, it is unlikely for a user to request custom design devices; however, the diverse choices available today can adequately modify any system that would use an off-the-shelf item. As before, emphasis is being placed on the importance of an off-the-shelf item over custom designs. Tube connectors and sealers are newer entrants as single-use bags for mixing and bioreactors have become more popular; yet, there is a limited choice of suppliers, mainly Cytiva LifeSciences Sartorius Stedim Biotech. The cost of this equipment is still high, but then the alternative is to use expensive aseptic connectors. Generally, if a good choice of aseptic connectors is available, then such connectors should be preferred over tube connectors, as heat-activated systems always create issues related to poor connection. Additionally, the use of aseptic connectors allows connecting tubes that may not be thermolabile.

Modern bioprocessing facilities scale up inoculum from a few million cells in several milliliters of culture to production volumes of thousands of liters. This process requires an aseptic transfer at each point along the seed train. Traditional bioprocessing facilities accomplish the scale-up process using a dedicated series of stainless-steel bioreactors linked together with valves and rigid tubing. To prevent contamination between production runs, a CIP system is designed in each bioreactor, vessel, and piping line to remove any residual materials. Such CIP and SIP systems require extensive validation testing, and the valves and piping present in these systems can create additional validation-related challenges.

Advances in SUT systems have allowed bioprocess engineers to replace most storage vessels and fixed piping networks with single-use storage systems and tubing assemblies, respectively. Single-use systems eliminate the need for CIP validation for many components and reduce maintenance and capital costs by eliminating the need for expensive vessels, valves, and sanitary piping assemblies.

Single-use media storage systems are routinely used for volumes ranging from 20 L to 2,500 L. Media storage systems are generally sterilized by gamma irradiation by their manufacturers (before installation at the bioprocess facility) and are often fitted with integrated filters, sampling systems, and connectors. The use of single-use digital-to-analog connectors (DACs) or tube welders and sealers with compatible tubing allows operators to make sterile connections between the presterilized SUBs for aseptic transfer of media, cells, and any other liquid required to be added. The DACs can also be used for downstream applications. These aseptic connectors can be used for high flow and high-pressure applications.

Similarly, customized presterilized single-use tubing assemblies are used to transfer inoculum between bioreactors using a peristaltic pump or by applying headspace pressure. Flexible tubing with aseptic connectors is used as transfer lines between the bioreactors in the process. Such transfer lines reduce the number of reusable valves required for transfer and eliminate problem areas for CIP and SIP validation. Terminating each presterilized transfer line with a single-use SIP connector provides sterility assurance equal to the sterility in traditional fixed piping at lower capital costs.

In some instances, liquids are transferred from a higher to a lower ISO environment, and strong assurance for sterility (there should not be cross-contamination during the transfer) is needed; therefore, a conduit can be installed in the walls connecting the two areas, with the cleaner room having a higher pressure. A pre-sterilized tube is then inserted from the side of the lower ISO class to side of the higher ISO class, thereby forming a connection between the vessels, and the liquid is then transferred through a peristaltic pump. Upon completion of the transfer, the tube is pulled into the higher ISO class area and finally discarded. This method helps establish a connection between the downstream and upstream areas without the risk of contamination during transfer to a lower ISO class area, such as a downstream area.

4.3.5.7 Tubing

Flexible tubes are an essential part of all single-use systems and are subject to safety concerns described in an earlier chapter on leachables and extractables. Several attributes of flexible tubing require evaluation, namely heat resistance, operating temperature range, chemical resistance, color, density, shore hardness, flexibility, elasticity, surface smoothness, mechanical stability, abrasion resistance, gas permeability, sensitivity to visible and UV light, composition of layers, weldability, sealability, and sterilizability by gamma irradiation or in an autoclave.

All tubes used in bioprocessing conform to USP Class VI classification, FDA 21 CFR 177.2600, and EP 3A Sanitary Standard. In cGMP manufacturing, these are classified as bulk pharmaceuticals.

4.3.5.8 Pumps

Pumps are used for fluid transfer by generating hydrostatic pressure or differential pressure; the maximum allowable working pressure would be determined at the weakest part of the bioprocess component exposed to the pressure. In some unit operations such as harvesting, TFF, and chromatography, the molecule is highly sensitive to any changes in the pumping process. Pulsing of pressure can affect the fluid being pumped or even damage the pump parts. The pump must meet the following criteria for suitability with the intended use:

- Low volume and minimal surface area exposure.
- Low levels of leachables and extractables.
- Controlled flow and pressure.
- Low shear and pulsation.
- No mechanical spalling/shedding of contact materials.
- Self-priming.
- No heat buildup.
- Sterility.
- High volumetric efficiency.

Permanent stainless-steel process lines are not only expensive to install and are complex but also require extensive cleaning and validation. Some of the pumps use mechanical seals that cannot maintain constant flow or sterility, which makes them less suitable for handling biologics.

Currently, single-use pumping solutions include peristaltic pumps, syringe pumps, and diaphragm pumps. Single-use positive displacement quaternary diaphragm pumps are one of the best options for bioprocessing applications. These are volume displacement pumps, easy to use, and avoid contact with the product; however, they can exert stress on the tubing, especially when they are being operated for a prolonged period. The stress on the tube may lead to erosion of particles from the tube and contaminate the fluids being passed through. Many biological drugs are shear-sensitive, and peristaltic pumps can help preserve these drugs by applying low pressure and providing gentle handling. By contrast, a piston pump's valve system stimulates fast flow through small orifices, which potentially causes damage to the biological products. Even valveless piston pumps apply high pressures and high shear factors, ultimately harming a biological product.

High-end peristaltic dispensing pumps are advantageous in terms of an improved pulsation-free pump head design, precise drive motor, and state-of-the-art calibration algorithm. They are exceptionally accurate at microliter fill volumes. Peristaltic pumps with single-use tubing eliminate cross-contamination and do not require cleaning validation because the tubing is the only part that comes into contact with the product. Likewise, cleaning validation of peristaltic pumps with single-use tubing is significantly easier than that of piston pumps. On the contrary, viscous products can be a problematic issue for peristaltic pumps. Peristaltic pumps apply only approximately 1.3 bar of pressure, and their accuracy diminishes when they handle products with viscosity higher than 100 cP. Several improvements have been made to pumps intended for downstream processing, including HPLC, TFF, and virus filtration applications, which enable high process yields throughout the pressure range (e.g., quantum; www.watson-marlow.com/us-en/range/watson-marlow/single-use-pumps/quantum/). Single-use pumps usually consist of bags instead of stainless-steel vessels and use special agitators, single-use tubing, coupling aids, and valves. Single-use components reduce the cost of cleaning and eliminate extensive validation. Plug-and-play options are available for TFF applications. These pumps provide a linear flow across the pressure range required for the process; they induce ultra-low shear, thereby increasing the downstream process yield.

A diaphragm pump is a positive displacement pump that uses a combination of the reciprocating action of a rubber, thermoplastic, or Teflon diaphragm and suitable nonreturn check valves to pump a fluid. Quaternary diaphragm pumps are driven one after another by connector plates that move back and forth. These pumps are ideal for handling all liquid biologics, including viscous liquids. Some pumps have the ability to self-prime, run dry, be operated at a constant flow, involve only low shear and pulsation, and not involve any heat accumulation.

4.3.5.9 Tube Welder and Sealers

In scenarios where it is possible to use a thermoplastic tube, welding offers an easy, inexpensive, and very secure solution. Examples of thermoplastic tubes include C-Flex, PharMed, and Bioprene. Thermoplastic tubes must be aseptic, have the same dimensions (inner diameter and outer diameter), and have their ends capped. The thermoplastic tubes are placed in opposite directions, parallel to each other, and they can be simultaneously sealed by cutting across the tubes using a heated blade. The blade should be preheated to achieve the welding temperature, achieve sterility, and dehydrogenize the blade before the welding process. The dehydrogenization procedure normally lasts for 30 s at 250°C or for 3 s at 320°C. After the tubes are being cut across, they are moved against each other so that the ends of each tube connected to the aseptic systems are positioned directly opposite to each other on either side of the blade. A duration of a welding cycle can range from 1 to 4 min, depending on the material and tube diameter. The main welding systems available today include Sterile Tube Fuser (GE Healthcare), BioWelder (Sartorius Stedim), Aseptic Sterile Welder 3960 (SEBRA, www.sebra.com), TSCD (Terumo, www.terumotransfusion.com), and SCD 11B (Terumo—Terumo supplies its equipment mainly for blood transfusion purposes). Both GE Healthcare and Sartorius Stedim lead the installations in the bioprocessing industry.

When disconnecting an aseptic connection, the ends of the connection must be capped with aseptic caps, and this should be performed inside a laminar hood or by using tube sealers; some of the examples include products from PDC (www.pdcbiz.com), Saint-Gobain (www.saint-gobain.com), Sartorius Stedim (www.sartorius-stedim.com), Cytiva (www.cytivalifesciences.com/en/us), Terumo (www.terumotransfusion.com), and SEBRA (www.sebra.com). Most of these sealers can seal tubes with a diameter ranging from 0.25 inch to approximately 1.5 inch, and the sealing process can take 1–4 min. Most of the sealers operate on an electrical heating element, but radio-frequencies are also used for sealing tubes. There is no need to use a laminar flow hood for these procedures. In most instances, applying a crimper in two places and cutting the tube between the crimps offers the cheapest solution.

4.3.6 Sampling

During manufacturing, sampling is routinely performed to assure compliance by validating in-process parameters such as pH, DO, OD, pCO_2, and so on. Most of the single-use systems have one or more integrated sampling lines, partly equipped with special sampling valves, sampling manifolds, or special sampling systems. A popular single-use sampling valve is the Clave connector from ICU Medical (www.icumed.com), which is also used in intravascular catheters for medical applications. Through the sampling valve, it is easy to collect a sample using a Luer-Lok syringe. The dynamic seal present inside the valve guarantees that the sample can be collected only when the syringe is connected, thereby ensuring that the sample comes into contact with only the valve's inner aseptic parts. However, the samples drawn do not remain sterile.

Manifolds consisting of sampling bags, sampling flasks, or syringes are appropriate for collecting aseptic samples in single-use systems. These manifolds can be connected to the systems through aseptic connectors or tube welding. Sampling manifolds allow multiple sampling over a given period for quality purposes. The main feature of the manifold is that the number of manipulations in a process can be significantly reduced. The manifold systems are delivered ready for process use in a preassembled and sterile manner. Only one connection is sufficient to allow several bags to be filled.

Additionally, sampling can also be carried out using manifold systems, where sample containers of a manifold are arranged in parallel, and the last container is used as a waste container. The initial flow and the subsequent sample are guided to their respective containers using Y-, T-, or X-hose barbs and tube clamps. SIP connections, as expected, also allow the connection of manifold systems to conventional stainless-steel processing equipment.

4.3.7 Downstream Processing

SUT is an attractive solution for minimizing downtimes between batches, additional burden on cleaning, validation of these procedures, and, most importantly, risk of contamination between batches. SUTs also facilitate easy switching between product lines in a multiproduct facility. SUTs such as columns, certain disposable hardware systems, and single-use flow paths have been successfully used for upstream processing and have become an integral part of evolution with downstream processing.

Single-use liquid chromatography systems, such as ÄKTA ready XL chromatography systems, which have disposable flow paths and prepacked columns, can support large-scale commercial manufacturing and conveniently meet the capacity starting from single-use 2000 L upstream processes with a high titer. These systems are very useful in both technology transfer and process scale-up operations.

An increased emphasis is being placed on supporting therapeutic drugs to be more affordable. Single-use systems and CM operations are critical drivers for the decrease in the overall manufacturing and investment cost to make this a possibility.

The adoption of single-use components in downstream bioprocessing has been an evolutionary process with a few revolutionary peaks occasionally. Initially, buffer bags and devices were being used for normal flow filtration, including filtration of virus and guard filters in chromatographic columns. Yet, gradually, more complex concepts were introduced, including single-use devices for TFF and chromatography during downstream processing. Today, the industry has arrived at the consensus that, while many of the upstream operations can be converted to fully single-use systems, at least some elements of downstream processing will still be carried out in the traditional manner, and the reasons cited for this assertion are as follows: (1) columns and resins will always be too expensive to throw away, and (2) because columns can have a very large size, finding a suitable single-use substitution will be highly challenging. However, as pointed out by historical evidence, the same arguments were presented only 15 years ago, opposing bioreactors' conversion to single-use devices. Today, downstream processing science is developing more rapidly than upstream science; more recently, the use of membrane adsorbs has been recommended for large-scale purification of antibodies. These membranes are much cheaper than classical resins.

4.3.7.1 Cell Harvest

For cell harvesting and debris removal, filtration is an alternative approach to conventional centrifugation. Currently available single-use filtration systems offer flexibility and scalability of operations. They are advantageous in terms of the ease of scale-up and the availability of presterilized filter capsules that can be integrated directly into production lines. Although this stage is generally carried out by centrifugation or lenticular filtration, depth filter systems (e.g., Millipore Pod filters) have provided the first available alternative in single-use lenticular filters; these adsorptive depth filters combine two distinct separation technologies into one efficient operation to enhance filtration ability and retention while compressing multiple filtration steps. Depth filters use a porous filtration medium to retain particles throughout the medium, rather than just on the surface of the medium. Depth filters are made of fibers in the form of a mesh that is spread out on a substrate; special additives such as activated carbon, ceramic fibers, and other such specific components are embedded with a binder to form the filter. Depth filters use their entire depth to retain the particles based on sieving compounded by adsorption effects, unlike retentive filters where the filtered material is concentrated on the surface. These filters are commonly used when the fluid to be filtered has a high load of particles because, compared with other types of filters, they can retain a large mass of particles before clogging.

Scale-up is achieved by inserting multiple pods into a holder, with formats allowing 1–5 or 5–30 pods as required. Further single-use depth filter formats include the Stax-System from Pall Life Sciences, encapsulated Zetaplus from Cuno, and L-Drum from Sartorius Stedim, Millipore Clarisolve, double–open-end high capacity, and extended open-end high-capacity adsorptive depth filters for primary and secondary clarification. These filters allow efficient cell clarification by reducing the cell biomass, host cell protein (HCP), and host DNA and removing most of the cell debris to enable easy loading in the chromatographic column.

The performance of depth filters depends on the colloid content of the bioreactor offload and the cell debris removal ability of the upstream centrifuge. Usually, depth filters are operated at a constant flow of 100–200 L/(m^2 h) and up to 150 L feed/m^2 of filter depending on the composition of the feed stream. The Millipore Millistak+ Pod depth filter has a maximum filter area of 33 m^2, resulting in a batch capacity of 3–5,000 L. The Millipore Mobius FlexReady process equipment supports a larger filter area (55 m^2). As washing of these filters requires very large volumes of buffers, holding tanks of appropriate size can be lined with single-use PE liners.

In some instances, crossflow filtration of high volumes of clarified harvest is performed to reduce the volume for subsequent purification; however, debris buildup extends the total time taken for the filtration process. While this process is not sterile, the use of a single-use filter prevents the problem of cross-contamination.

Single-use continuous centrifugation devices such as Ksep® are available for processing recombinant proteins and vaccines. The Ksep is a closed continuous-flow centrifuge that works by creating centrifugal force and the feed-flow force. This system offers the benefit of efficient processing without affecting recovery because of its low shear, continuous operation.

Each technology has its advantages and drawbacks; therefore, testing each option, and choosing the appropriate one based on the specific method and cell type is recommended. The single-solution performance depends on the USP performance, cell density, viability, and the extent of the cell debris present in the bioreactor broth.

4.3.7.2 Purification

For protein isolation and purification, a steel column is packed with a resin (stationary phase) comprising porous beads made of a polysaccharide, mineral, or synthetic matrix conjugated to specific functional groups exploiting different separative principles. The protein mixed with other components is loaded onto the column slowly. Once the protein is bound to the resin, the resin is eluted with solutions of appropriate pH and containing required electrolytes to separate the target protein from the mixture. The resin is cleaned and sanitized for repeated use, and this process may involve dozens or, perhaps, hundreds of cycles.

Several vendors now offer columns (e.g., ReadyToProcess™ columns by GE Healthcare) for use in ÄKTA machines to overcome the time needed to pack the resin and operate a column. GE Healthcare offers a wide range of resins and custom resins. These are high-performance bioprocessing columns that are prepacked, prequalified, and presanitized. The ReadyToProcess™ chromatographic columns and the use of single-use or single-use flow paths eliminate the risk of cross-contamination. The ÄKTA ready system has a sanitary design and is well suited for use in a cGMP-regulated environment. The simple procedures and low downtime between products and batches of ÄKTA readily facilitate improved economy and productivity. Other prepacked columns such as the ReadyToProcess™ columns include Opus (Repligen), GoPure (Life Technologies).

The ÄKTA system is designed for seamless scalability, delivering the same performance level as that achieved with conventional processing columns such as AxiChrom™ and BPG™. The ÄKTA system is currently available with a range of BioProcess™ media in four different sizes (1, 2.5, 10, and 20 L), and these columns are designed to purify biopharmaceuticals for clinical phase I and II studies. Depending on the scale of operations, they can also be used for full-scale manufacturing and preclinical studies. The columns can be used in a wide range of chromatographic applications to separate various compounds such as proteins, endotoxins, DNA, plasmids, vaccines, and viruses.

Single-use chromatography solutions such as ÄKTA XL systems are available as prepacked columns, single-use flow paths, plug-and-play chromatography columns, and membranes, as well as presterilized filters and tubing to eliminate cleaning validation. ÄKTA ready chromatography systems are designed for process scale-up and manufacturing, and they operate through ready-to-use, single-use flow paths, thereby eliminating cleaning validation between products and batches.

Purification of proteins from complex mixtures is a key process in pharmaceutical research and production. However, protein purification using chromatography based on particulate matrices is a lengthy procedure and takes longer separation times. Several ligands are available (Table 4.2).

Membrane adsorbers are advantageous in removing high-molecular-weight contaminants such as DNA and viruses during monoclonal antibody manufacturing. Such contaminant molecules do not readily diffuse into traditional resins; thus, most of the purification steps relying on column chromatography require dramatically oversized columns. The hydrodynamic benefits of oversized columns provide the opportunity to operate membrane adsorbers at much greater flow rates than those for columns, thereby considerably reducing buffer consumption and shortening the overall process time by up to 100-fold. Commercially used membrane adsorbers are Mustang® (Pall), Sartobind®

TABLE 4.2
Different Types of Membranes and Ligands

Membrane Type	Description	Ligand	Pore Size (μm)
Sulfonic acid (S)	Strong acidic cation exchanger	$R\text{-}CH_2\text{-}SO_3\text{-}$	>3
Quaternary ammonium (Q)	Strong basic anion exchanger	$R\text{-}CH_2\text{-}N+(CH_3)_3$	>3
Carboxylic acid(C)	Weak acidic cation exchanger	$R\text{-}COO\text{-}$	>3
Diethylamine (D)	Weak basic anion exchanger	$R\text{-}CH_2\text{-}N(C_2H_5)_2$	>3
Phenyl	Hydrophobic interaction (HIC)	Phenyl	>3
IDA	Metal chelate	Iminodiacetic acid	>3
Protein A	Affinity	Protein A	0.45
Epoxy-activated	Coupling	Epoxy group	0.45
Aldehyde-activated	Coupling	Aldehyde group	0.45

Source: Sartorius Stedim

(Sartorius), ChromaSorb® (Millipore), and Adsept® (Natrix). These membranes are commonly used for removing process-related impurities such as DNA and endotoxin in the flow-through mode.

The accelerated seamless antibody purification process is an entirely single-use continuous downstream process for mAb production, based on ÄKTA periodic counter-current chromatography (PCC) Protein-A, mixed-mode, and anion exchange resin columns. In this process, all three columns are cycled simultaneously. These systems offer the advantage of both single-use and continuous processing in a single application while providing flexibility, ease of operation, and increased capacity.

When selecting single-use consumables, it is crucial to ensure that the supply chain is strong. Ensuring the right documentation and testing for extractables and leachables aligns with following regulatory compliance.

Single-use systems provide great flexibility to handle several products in a facility; the fast turnaround time between batches or products results in a quicker product release.

4.3.7.3 Virus Removal

Virus contamination is a risk to all biotechnology products derived from cell lines of human or animal origin. Contamination of a protein product with endogenous viruses from cell banks or adventitious viruses from personnel can have profound clinical implications. Three complementary approaches assure viral safety in licensed biological products:

- Thorough testing of the cell line and all raw materials for the presence of viral contaminants,
- Assessment of the ability of downstream processing to clear infectious viruses, and
- Testing of the product at appropriate steps for the presence of contaminating viruses.

A combination of methods based on inactivation, adsorption, and size exclusion are available. The FDA requires demonstration of virus clearance by two methods. Examples of inactivation procedures are the use of solvents and detergents, chemical treatments, low pH, or microwave heating. Adsorption-based methods include chromatography, and virus removal by mechanical or molecular size exclusion is executed by normal (forward) and TFF methods.

Ion exchange and protein A chromatography methods are widely used to remove viruses, and several key studies have been conducted in collaboration with the FDA. Yet, the developer is responsible for proving the suitability of any method for virus removal. Membrane filtration has been used for viral clearance in mAb production processes for many years. Hollow fiber membrane cartridges and even surface-modified, hydrophilic membranes with high void volume and minimal fouling capable of reducing high viral titers are some of the recent single-use options for viral clearance. Adsorptive filters can be used at the end of the purification process in line with the viral filtration step. These filters combine the principles of size exclusion and adsorption to retain aggregates by hydrophobic interactions while increasing viral filtration efficiency. Several manufacturers such as Sartorius, Pall, and Millipore offer single-use virus filtration solutions to remove large enveloped viruses and small nonenveloped viruses. Nano-sized filters are commonly used as viral removal filters. The most common virus retention of these filters is of the size 20 or 50 nm.

4.4 FILTRATION: ULTRAFILTRATION/DIAFILTRATION AND TANGENTIAL FLOW FILTRATION

Filtration applications are well suitable for single-use processing. Ultrafiltration and diafiltration are used to concentrate and change the buffer of a solution. During the final formulation, ultrafiltration and diafiltration are used to transfer the active pharmaceutical ingredient to a stabilizing environment and achieve the correct concentration of the product. A volume of up to 300–5,000 L may need to be processed, depending on whether the column eluates can be fractionated. Membranes with a 30-kDa molecular weight cutoff are often used to retain antibodies, and the process intermediate is concentrated and washed with 5× volumes. Membranes of up to 3 m² area that can process a volume of 200 L/(h m²) are available. Several single-use systems are available (SciLog, Millipore) for a limited filter area (area of up to 2.5 m²), but larger systems (such as single-use modules and pumps) might replace existing reusable systems with an area of 14 m², as it is logical to carry out filtration steps in a closed system.

Single-use TFF modules are available as ready-to-use cassettes to be used in TFF setups. These systems provide quick turnaround times and more flexibility. Single-use systems are available as preassembled units with gamma-irradiated flow paths and sensors, thus reducing setup time. Pre-sanitized pre-packaged cassettes are also another option as a single-use system. Cleaning a TFF system and the cassette is an important step in downstream processing, particularly for multiproduct use. It is essential to minimize cross-contamination risk while also ensuring that flux rates are well maintained. Cleaning procedures, including those in dedicated systems for each product, must be well validated to ensure no product carryover from previous batches. A completely single-use TFF system can be built together with off-the-shelf components (including valves, sensors, and 2D bags for liquids). Technology improvements and integration of single-use components can enable automated single-use systems to be applied conveniently for large-scale manufacturing.

4.4.1 General Filtration Applications

Generally, filters are rarely reused in the pharmaceutical industry, except for steel meshes in bulk manufacturing of nonsterile dosage forms. Single-use filter devices in biological manufacturing were the earliest forms that were used as single-use systems, mainly because of the problems related to cleaning them; the cost of their parts has always been reasonable.

Numerous filter designs and mechanisms are being utilized within the biopharmaceutical industry. Prefilters are commonly pleated, and wound filter fleeces are manufactured from melt-blown random fiber matrices. These filters are used to remove a higher amount of contaminant from the fluid. Prefilters have a large band of retention ratings and can be optimized for all necessary applications. The most common application for prefilters is to protect membrane filters, which are tighter and more selective than prefilters. Membrane filters are used to purify or sterilize fluids. These filters need to be integrity testable to assess whether they meet the performance criteria. Crossflow filtration can be performed with micro- or ultrafiltration membranes. The fluid sweeps over the membrane layer and therefore keeps it unblocked. This filtration method allows diafiltration or concentration of fluid streams.

Dead-end filtration is one of the simplest methods of filter operation. Dead-end filtration uses the principle of passing a fluid feed stream perpendicularly to a filter device at minimal pressure, which is usually applied using a pump or as compressed gas pressure above the filter device. All contaminants larger than the average pore size of the filter media are retained by the filter material, thereby leading to filter blockage by plugging its channels or pores. The setup of dead-end filtration uses minimum accessories such as tubing/piping, tanks, and controls. Dead-end filters involve microporous membranes made of synthetic polymers such as polyethersulfone, polyamide, cyano-acrylate, and polyvinylidene fluoride and are extensively used for sterile processing. They are used for media filtration into sterile bags and containers, bioburden reduction during cell harvest clarification, chromatography column protection, and final filtration of the purified bulk drug substance. These filters are often attached to single-use bags and are pre-sterilized by gamma irradiation.

4.4.2 Fill-Finish Operations

Fill-finish, which is the final processing step of drug substance and drug product, requires tight control of aseptic operations without compromising sterility and integrity while ensuring safety and efficiency. As such, fill-finish operations typically require sophisticated equipment and technology.

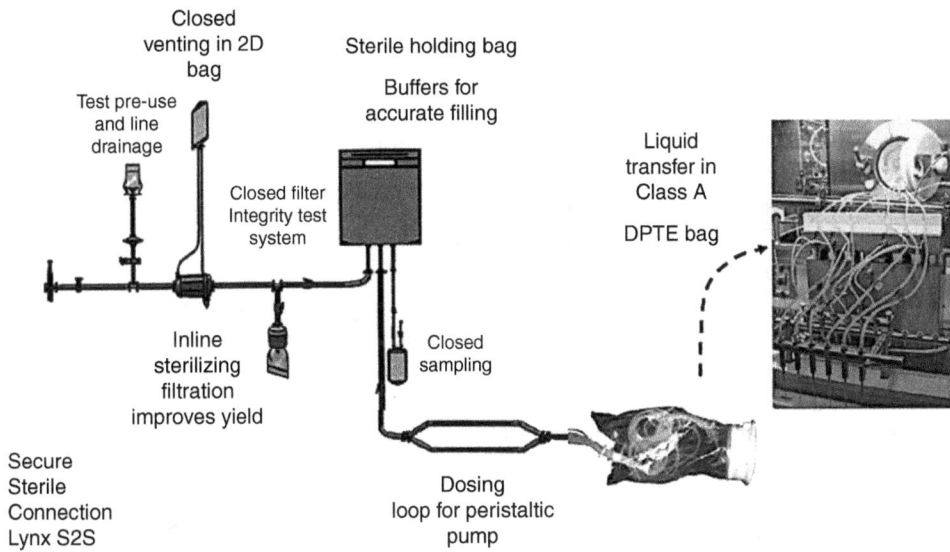

FIGURE 4.3   Closed-system filling transfer set to isolator

Source: www.emdmillipore.com

The traditional fill-finish setup uses fixed systems involving complex components that require extensive cleaning and sterilization, assembly, and disassembly. A time-pressure system and a piston pump are widely used for dosing and filling operations. However, these systems require assembly and validation of CIP and SIP to ensure the final product meets the sterility specifications. The use of single-use components for these critical processes is more likely to ensure that the final product is not compromised while reducing cross-contamination risk. Additionally, SUT in fill-finish operations can reduce the turnaround time between batches and increase flexibility, particularly for a multiple product facility.

A traditional, fixed system can adopt single-use solutions. Figure 4.3 presents a single-use fill-finish setup with installed hardware, hard-piped connections, and limited operational flexibility. This setup combined the expertise of Millipore in single-use fluid-path management to ensure sterility and integrity of the operation.

Successful implementation of a single-use system is beyond assembling single-use components. The use of suppliers with experience in validating such systems and understanding the manufacturer's requirements to integrate and offer customized solutions, ensure compatibility, and perform assessments will be critical to the success of single-use implementation and assurance of sterility. The flexibility of SUT makes its use more relevant for single- and multi-product filling facilities, thus increasing facility efficiency and utilization due to the ease of installation, operation, and elimination of CIP/SIP validation.

4.4.3   SAFETY

Biologics manufacturers must comply with regulatory requirements. This includes, for instance, ensuring that the supplier is reliable and can provide the necessary documentation supporting suitability (product contact material), qualification, and validation of the single-use systems to support audits by the end-user. The end-user must have a user requirement specification and perform technical evaluation with multiple vendors to determine suitability with their process. Single-use components must be qualified together with the equipment for intended use. Additionally, these components should be included in the process validation exercise.

Single-use devices make extensive use of plastic materials or elastomer systems, starting from filter housings to the lining of bioreactors. Today, perhaps the most significant impediment in the wider acceptance of single-use systems is the controversy surrounding the possibility of contamination of the product with chemicals from the plastic film. All final containers and closures should be made of a material that does not hasten the product's deterioration or otherwise render it less suitable for the intended use (Biologics *21CFR600.11(h)*).

Regulatory requirements pertain to the toxic effects of leachables, and risk to biological drugs arises based on the effect of leachables on the 3D and 4D structure of protein drugs. Such changes can render the drug more immunogenic if not less effective, and these side effects are, thus, of greater importance to the bioprocessing industry. Leachables refer to chemicals migrating from single-use processing equipment to various components of the drug product during manufacturing. Extractables are chemical entities (both organic and inorganic) extracted from single-use components using common laboratory solvents during controlled experiments. They represent the worst-case scenario and predict the types of leachables that may be encountered during biopharmaceutical production. Leaching is specific not only to plastics but also to chemicals from stainless steel. Stainless steel, commonly used in biopharmaceutical applications, is of grade 316L and is an alloy containing mainly iron, nickel, and chromium, with minor amounts of manganese and vanadium. Stainless steel is a significant source of metal leachables, especially if the surface of the equipment or tank is not properly treated. The main leachable components are iron, chromium, and nickel. Several fold higher concentrations of metals such as iron and nickel leach into the liquid formulation after storage at room temperature in un-passivated stainless-steel vessels compared with passivated stainless-steel vessels.

4.4.4 POLYMERS AND ADDITIVES

The materials used to fabricate single-use processing equipment for biopharmaceutical manufacturing are usually polymers, such as plastic or elastomers (rubber), rather than the traditional materials (metal or glass). Polymers offer more versatility because they are lightweight, flexible, and much more durable than their traditional counterparts. Plastic and rubber are single-use components, and their use eliminates cleaning validation. Additives can also be incorporated into polymers to clarify glass or to add color to labels or code parts. Polymer degradation can be controlled with the use of additives (stabilizers).

When a plastic resin is processed, it is often introduced into an extruder, wherein it is melted at high temperatures, and its stability is influenced by its molecular structure, the polymerization process, the presence of residual catalysts, and the finishing steps used in production. Processing conditions during extrusion (e.g., temperature, shear, and residence time in the extruder) can significantly affect polymer degradation. End-use conditions that expose a polymer to excessive heat or light (such as outdoor applications or sterilization techniques used in medical practices) can foster premature failure of polymer products, leading to loss of flexibility or strength. If left unchecked, the process can often result in total failure of the plastic component.

The complexity of chemical reactions involved in the manufacturing of plastics influences the presence of extractables and leachables, making the process very complex and challenging. When testing for extractables and leachables, lesser-known minor chemical species may be the ones that leach into a drug product, but this is not predictable, as it is, to a greater degree, a function of the product's characteristics. All byproducts of the polymer and additives (stabilizers, fillers, and elastomers) become available to leach from polymers into a drug product.

Despite the risk involved in using additives added to polymers, the utility of polymers in single-use bioprocess equipment (and in all medical or pharmaceutical applications) far outweigh the risks associated with their use. These risks can be managed well through three steps: material selection, implementing a proper testing program, and partnering with vendors.

TABLE 4.3
Summary of the Tests Carried Out and Results Obtained for a Plastic Film Used to Produce Bioreactor Bags

Biocompatibility

USP Acute Systemic Injection Test	Pass		USP<88>
USP Intracutaneous Injection Test	Pass		USP<88>
USP Intramuscular Implantation Test	Pass		USP<88>
USP MEM Elution Method	Non-cytotoxic		USP<87>
Physiochemical Test for Plastics	Pass		USP <661>

Extractables

	TOC after 90 days (ppm)		pH shift after 90 days
Purified Water (pH=7)	<2		–0.79
Acidic Water (pH<2)	<3		+0.01
Basic Water (pH>10)	<4		+0.87

Physical Data

Water Vapor Transmission Rate (g/100in²/24h)	0.017			ASTM F-1249
Carbon Dioxide Transmission Rate (cc/100in²/24h)	0.129			ASTM F-2476
Oxygen Transmission Rate (cc/100in²/24h)	0.023			ASTM F-1927
	Average Force	Average MOE	Average Elongation	
Tensile	32.73 lbs	25110 psi	1084%	ASTM D 882-02
	Min Force	Average Force	Max Force	
Tear Resistance	6.77 Ibs	7.21 Ibs	7.74 Ibs	ASTM D1004-03
Puncture Resistance	16.42 Ibs	18.16 Ibs	19.51 Ibs	FTMS 101C

4.4.5 Material Selection

The type of plastic used should match the required physical and chemical properties and compatibility of its additives. Ensuring compatibility with the drug product often reduces the amount of material leaching that can occur. It is also important to select polymers and additives approved for specific use by the regulatory authorities. Such compounds have already undergone a fair amount of analytical and toxicological testing, and adequate information of these compounds is often available. Thus, most manufacturers are likely to continue using these additives, and accordingly, the user does not alter the composition of these compounds at a later stage. The art of using polymers and additives is likely to survive, obviating the need for a change control step, as significant changes in the process need to be reported back to the FDA.

Commercially supplied plastic films are proprietary formulations and arrangements; for example, Advanced Scientific produces bags made of two films. The fluid contact film is made of 5.0-mm PE. The outer covering is a five-layer 7-mm co-extrusion film, which provides barrier and durability. A typical test report is presented in Table 4.3.

4.4.6 Testing

Polymers used in medical and pharmaceutical applications should comply with the appropriate USP guidelines, and it is recommended that these polymers meet USP Class VI testing, as documented in USP 88. Appropriate extractable and leachable testing programs must be implemented for all bioprocessing materials that directly come into contact with the drug.

Bio-Process Systems Alliance (https://bpsalliance.org/) provides the best-practice guidelines for conducting such testing as a two-part technical guideline for evaluating the risk associated with extractables and leachables, specifically for single-use processing equipment. This organization encourages the use of single-use systems and provides excellent support and assistance; the reader is highly encouraged to visit the website for newer information and participate in their seminars and conventions to stay abreast of the developments in this fast-changing field.

Testing for leachables does not end once the materials have been qualified. It is necessary to have a quality control program rather than testing the product or equipment alone. The level of quality control testing will depend on risk tolerance. Manufacturing of recombinant drugs involves extensive purification steps that are likely to remove most of these leachables. Additionally, the final medium used for protein solutions is aqueous, and many leachables are not soluble in water, further reducing the risk. A greater risk is also attributed to the final packaging components; for example, rubber stoppers used in packaging the final dosage form are more likely to cause risk to the protein formulation than any other component in the chain of a single-use drug that is exposed during the manufacturing process. Biologics manufacturers need to work in association with suppliers to ensure that regulatory requirements adhere to a product safety standpoint.

The DP of particulate matter should meet an important specification or testing requirement: visible and subvisible. Contamination of drug products with particulate matter is typically well controlled by filtration, and visual inspection is performed during filling. Single-use components must also be manufactured under controlled conditions that can reduce particulate matter and reduce them to a minimum in the final product.

4.4.6.1   Regulatory Standards

There are no specific standards or guidelines that reference extractables and leachables from single-use bioprocessing materials. Many references that do apply have been written to address processing materials and equipment without regard to construction materials.

The United States and Canada
The foundation for the requirement to assess extractables and leachables in the United States was introduced in Title 21 of the Code of Federal Regulations (CFR) Part 211.65, which states that: "Equipment shall be constructed to surface that contact components, in-process materials, or drug products shall not be reactive, additive, or absorptive to alter the safety, identity, strength, quality, or purity of the drug product beyond the official or other established requirements."

This regulation applies to all materials, including metals, glass, and plastics. Extractables and leachables would generally be considered an *additive*, although it is also possible for leachables to interact with a product to yield new contaminants.

The US FDA regulatory guideline for final container closure systems, although not written for process contact materials, provides directions regarding the type of final product testing that may be provided regarding extractables and leachables from single-use process components and systems. The guideline indicates the types of drug products and component dosage form interactions that the FDA considers to be at the highest risk for extractables. Generally, the likelihood of the packaging component interacting with the dosage form is highest in injectable dosage forms, mainly because of the low level of leachables that can be allowed in such drug delivery systems.

Drugs intended to be injectables or inhalants will have higher levels of regulatory concern than oral or topical drugs. Similarly, liquid dosage forms will have more serious regulatory concerns than tablets because the leachates migrate into liquids more easily than into solids.

Additionally, pharmaceutical-grade materials are expected to meet or exceed industry and regulatory standards and requirements, for example, those listed in USP <87> and <88>. The USP procedures test the biological reactivity of mammalian cell cultures following contact with polymeric materials. However, they are not considered sufficient regulatory documentation for extractables and leachables because many toxicological indicators are not evaluated, including subacute and chronic toxicity, especially an evaluation of carcinogenic, reproductive, developmental, neurological, and immunological effects.

The European Union
A statement related to the US 21 CFR 211.65 is found in the rules governing the manufacture of medicinal products in the European Union (EU). The EU, a useful manufacturing practice document, states, "Production equipment should not present any hazard to the products." "The parts of the production equipment that come into contact with the product must not be reactive, additive, or absorptive to such an extent that it will affect the quality of the product and thus present any hazard."

The EMEA published a guideline on immediate plastic packaging materials (www.ema.europa. eu/en/documents/scientific-guideline/guideline-plastic-immediate-packaging-materials_en.pdf) and addresses container closure systems; this guideline has been used to provide direction for contact materials in single-use processes. Data to be included relating to extractables and leachables are derived from extraction studies (*worst-case leachable*), interaction studies, and migration studies (similar to leachable information for those components). It also identifies what additional information or testing is required and then sets and executes a plan to fill the gaps.

4.5 ONLINE MONITORING

Online monitoring is widely used for upstream processes, such as temperature, pH, pCO_2 or pO_2, and other chemistry indicators. This allows adjustments to feed, pH modulation, and other changes continuously. However, online monitoring of downstream processes has not been possible because optimal parameters to monitor and optimize the observed properties and technology to alter downstream processing are not yet established.

However, in recent years, much emphasis has been placed on creating methodologies for online monitoring to alter the process to modify the yield, molecular structure, and safety elements of the product. Currently, online monitoring is now the fastest emerging technology, yet it is adopted slowly because of the technical and regulatory complexities of reliance on the data collected online. Table 4.4 shows how online monitoring can affect downstream processing, and Table 4.5 shows the status of available technology.

4.6 CONTINUOUS MANUFACTURING

CM is a form of highly intensified processing with short downtimes when compared with the typical time used for traditional batch production. Process intensification, therefore, becomes a prerequisite to CM technologies, as it can increase tier, manage high media volumes, buffers, and, overall, intensify the process to obtain a higher yield from the entire production process.

The advantages of intensification and continuous processing are mostly related to increasing productivity, reduced need to invest in conventional, highly expensive manufacturing facilities, mainly because businesses can synergistically use single-use and intensification facilities that lead to reduced facility footprints and costs. CM is a crucial step in promoting drug quality and enhancing production efficiency, resulting in lower drug prices.

One of the key drivers to the successful incorporation of CM is the principle of connected manufacturing, where unit processes are connected both physically and, most notably, even integrated digitally (automated). This helps in streamlining the process from start to finish using a fully integrated, connected system that can control and monitor product quality.

The benefit of improving product quality is that the product spends less time in some of the unit operations that can potentially cause degradation or generation of more variations, for instance, bioreactor processes and chromatography separation, which can effectively resolve the product and

TABLE 4.4
Potential Impact of Monitoring on Critical Properties, Factors, and Conditions in Downstream Processing

Critical Properties, Factors, and Conditions	Purpose/Motivation	Product Quality	Production Economy	Regulatory Compliance
Product-related properties				
Product activity	Immediate information on product activity during DSP	↗	↗	↗
Product variants	Evaluation and separation of different product variants	↗	↗	↗
Impurities	Assurance of sufficient removal of impurities (HCP, DNA)	↗	↗	↗
Contaminants	Detection of possible fungal, microbial, and yeast bioburden	↗	↗	↗
USP media components and introduced chemicals, resin leakage	Assurance of sufficient removal of USP media components and introduced chemicals	↗	↗	↗
Economic factors				
Investment costs of instrumentation	–	–	↘	–
Operational and maintenance costs	–	–	↘	–
Training costs of personnel	–	–	↘	–
Productivity	Productivity improvement based on monitoring	–	↗	–
Direct batch release after formulation	Batch release after the final DSP step, no storage	–	↗	↗
Process endpoint monitoring	Facilitation to determine the endpoint of each DSP step	↗	↗	↗
Lifetime of the instrument	Usage for an extended period	–	↗	↗
Monitoring of batch-to-batch variations	Determination of batch variations and comparison with previous results (batch trajectory)	↗	↗	↗
Conditions by regulatory demands				
Online monitoring and process control	Possibility to fine-tune each DSP step promptly and take corrective actions	↗	↗	↗
Robustness of the monitoring system	Adoption to changing process environment	↗	↗	↗
Identification of critical quality attributes	Increase process understanding and impact of CQAs in DSP steps	↗	↗	↗
Process automation	Improves process efficiency	–	↗	↗
Risk assessment	Evaluations of risks and risk-based product development	↗	↗	↗
Fulfillment of final product specifications	Ensuring quality criteria of each batch	↗	↗	↗

Source: After Patricia Roch and Carl-Fredrik Mandenius, Online monitoring of downstream bioprocesses, *Current Opinion in Chemical Engineering*, 2016. 14, pp.112–120. https://doi.org/10.1016/j.coche.2016.09.007

Note: ↗ indicates a positive impact, ↘ indicates a negative impact, and – denotes no influence

TABLE 4.5
Status of Technology to Implement Online Monitoring Downstream

Techniques	Biological Relevance	Sensitivity	Selectivity	Response Time	Precision	Reproducibility	Readiness for Implementation
Temperature and pressure sensors	•	•••	•	•••	•••	•••	•
pH sensor	•	•••	•	•••	•••	••	•
Optical density	•	••	•	•••	••	••	•
Mass flowmeters	•	•	•	•••	••	••	•
Dipsticks for antigens	•••	•	••	••	•	••	•
Flow injection analysis	••	••	••	••	••	••	••
HPLC online	••	••	••	••	•••	••	•••
Capacitive immunosensors	••	•••	•••	••	••	••	•••
Advanced mass spectrometry	•••	•••	•••	••	••	••	••
Multi-fluorescence spectroscopy	••	•••	•••	•••	•••	••	••
UV/Vis spectroscopy	••	••	•••	•••	•••	••	••
Near-infrared spectroscopy	••	••	••	•••	•••	••	••
Mid-infrared spectroscopy	••	••	•••	•••	•••	••	••
Raman spectroscopy	•••	••	•	•••	•••	••	••
Surface plasmon resonance	•••	•••	•••	••	••	•	•••
Capillary electrophoresis online	••	••	••	••	••		••
Flow cytometry online	••	••	••	••	••	••	••
NMR online	•••	••	•••	•	•••	••	••
Offline biosensors	•••	•••	•••	••	••	••	•••
Circular dichroism	•••	•••	•••	••	••	••	••
Light scattering	••	•••	•	••	••	••	••

Source: After Patricia Roch and Carl-Fredrik Mandenius, Online monitoring of downstream bioprocesses, *Current Opinion in Chemical Engineering*, 2016. 14, pp.112–120. https://doi.org/10.1016/j.coche.2016.09.007

its other variants (isoforms). An example of a continuous biomanufacturing process is a perfusion bioreactor coupled to a multi-column chromatography capture step, followed by flow-through virus inactivation, multi-column intermediate purification, a flow-through membrane adsorber polishing step, continuous virus filtration, and a final ultrafiltration step operated in continuous mode. Continuous capture steps gain a lot of traction, mostly because of modern multi-column chromatography ideal for commercial-scale manufacturing.

CM operations are a step toward reducing waste and streamlining operations to be more efficient. While the concept may be relatively new or more so underutilized in the biological medicine industry, other downstream operations such as ultrafiltration/diafiltration must also be adapted to this concept. Despite this being a challenge, using sterile ultrafiltration capsules, which allows for easy assembly and operation of closed systems with minimized contamination risks or reduced bioburden, is one solution. Additionally, incorporating automation for process monitoring and data acquisition combined with single-use technologies is considered to design ultrafiltration/diafiltration operations to a continuous approach. Single-pass TFF systems are gaining extensive attention and are indeed favorable single-use alternatives. Yet, there is undoubtedly more scope for improving these skids available for commercial-scale and formulations requiring high product concentration.

The first step toward adopting the concept starts with recognizing the need for continuous processing and sketching out specifics on how the batch process can be transformed or adapted into a continuous one. It may not be easy and straightforward to convert a batch operation into a continuous operation at the outset, for it must be understood that not all batch processes are designed to be continuous. Batch processing involves multiple steps, using online and offline analyses to define the control strategy and support the process. Hence, only a few steps may be initially easier to convert, but any changes made should only be carried out if it increases or maintains productivity and has no negative effect on product quality.

A hybrid approach to continuous biomanufacturing, such that only the upstream process or part of the downstream process is operated continuously, is a more logical and more sensible step toward adopting CM. This can be either operating upstream as a perfusion operation combined with batch mode purification or having a fed-batch process with a constant chromatography capture step.

CM is also gaining increasing support from the regulators. The FDA's recommendation for continuous unit operations is the confirmation that biological medicine processing is progressing toward a future that promotes emerging technologies. The need is driven to reduce product failure, increase quality, and improve efficiency. This aims to supplement further efforts toward automation, intensifying processes, and effectively utilizing resources (facility and equipment).

4.6.1 CONTINUOUS CHROMATOGRAPHY SYSTEMS

Continuous chromatography systems are designed for continuous processing, mainly when the purification stage is linked to upstream bioreactor perfusion or even a simple fed-batch process. In a batch chromatography mode, a single large column is used for each purification step. In a continuous multi-column setup, multiple smaller columns are operated in series over numerous cycles, thereby effectively and simultaneously managing activities across these columns. When product loading occurs on one column, the other column(s) can be prepped up or be placed in the wash, elution, and regeneration stages. Alternatively, the loading step can be split across two columns set up in series.

Continuous chromatography had garnered interest extensively in advancing the process toward clinical development and more likely for commercial-scale production, particularly with support and encouragement from regulators. Continuous chromatography operations can help minimize facility footprint by using smaller bioreactors (that can support high productivity), small- to mid-sized columns, and reduced buffer consumptions coupled with options to perform inline dilutions. Multi-column chromatography helps realize these potential benefits and provides an opportunity for better utilization of protein A resin capacity. A fed-batch process can be connected to a continuous chromatography capture step reducing time, costs, and, possibly, improving product quality. However, with greater sophistication of hardware systems and certain perceived regulatory complexities, obstacles that need to be addressed persist.

Nonetheless, before deciding whether continuous chromatography is the best alternative, a detailed review is performed for each project based on the protein's operational scale, properties, and other process requirements. Implementing a continuous end-to-end system may not be an immediate possibility, and an easy switch from batch processing to continuous processing is not always possible. However, emerging technologies such as straight-through processing (STP), simulated moving bed (SMB), and PCC can be used as alternatives to traditional batch processing, as a continuous or semi-continuous processing option.

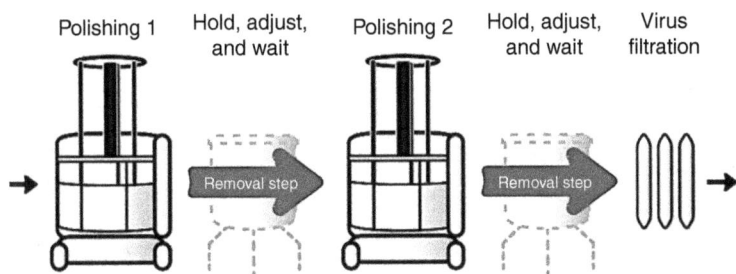

FIGURE 4.4 Total equipment footprint can be reduced by connecting the purification and filtration systems in a series and moving adjustments in line

Source: Cytiva Life Sciences

4.6.1.1 Straight-Through Processing

In STP, two or more chromatography steps are connected in series, with inline adjustment of process conditions between columns to ensure optimized loading conditions in the next step. This step eliminates the need for intermediate conditioning steps in conventional batch processes, requiring little to no intermediate hold-up tanks, improving efficiency, and minimal equipment requirements (Figure 4.4).

4.6.1.2 Periodic Countercurrent Chromatography

PCC is a multi-step approach to maximize the capacity utilization of chromatography resin (in turn, reducing resin volume) and minimize process time. PCC uses three or more column chromatography steps to complete capitalizing the resin capacity. Column 1 is loaded to 60%–80% breakthrough, after which it is disconnected for wash and elution and then for equilibration steps. The process is subsequently switched to Column 2, which is also loaded up to the breakthrough, after which it is disconnected for wash, elution, and equilibration steps. The same sequence of operations is performed with Column 3. At this point, Column 1 is ready to return back online to repeat these steps, thus creating continuous processing. This increases the utilization of available resin while allowing for a smaller equipment footprint and effective time management.

4.6.1.3 Simulated Moving Bed Chromatography

SMB chromatography has been in use in the petrochemical and food industries. It allows processes to achieve high productivity relative to batch methods owing to the efficient utilization of the solid and liquid phases required for separation.

The basic concept of simulated moving bed chromatography is to use multiple smaller columns containing the solid adsorbent (beds) and move the beds in the opposite direction of the fluid (feed, eluent, and product) to achieve a countercurrent flow. The "simulated movement" is typically executed through multiport valves interspersed between the columns, such that the input and output fluid streams (feed, eluent, and product) can be periodically switched from column to column in the direction of fluid flow. The arrangement and control of the valves help strategize the sample and solvent movement, thereby allowing various separation stages to be conducted simultaneously by different columns as a continuous cycle.

4.7 CONTINUOUS MANUFACTURING

Recombinant protein technology executed as a batch process meets the industry standards. However, proteins can also be produced in a vessel, from which the yield is continuously removed, provided

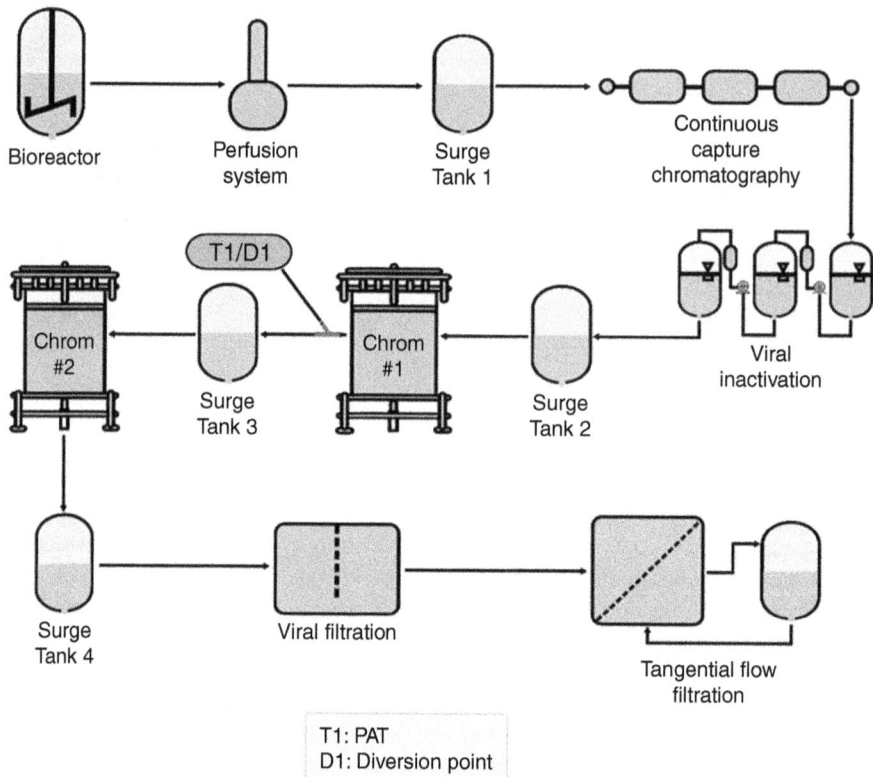

FIGURE 4.5 A continuous manufacturing system for the production of therapeutic proteins

Source: FDA

the protein is secreted into the culture medium. This process helps improve the yield of labile proteins and prevents inconsistent post-translational modifications while maintaining cells at higher viabilities, which is a critical factor. Apart from material costs, it reduces the need for testing, adding significant cost and time savings (Figures 4.4 and 4.5).

The quest for a CM process has been in research for several years[1]; however, it was in March 2023 when the FDA released its first guidance on CM addressing the scientific and legal issues that arise during the creation, installation, operation, and lifecycle management of CM for chemical and biological drugs. Figure 4.5 shows a flowchart for manufacturing in a CM for a therapeutic protein. The FDA also identifies other guidelines that control CM.

The setup consists of unit operations such as a bioreactor compatible with a perfusion culture system, continuous capture chromatography, virus filtration, virus inactivation, and buffer exchange and concentration through TFF chromatography columns. Each unit operation is integrated with adjacent unit operations, a surge line, or a tank connecting unit operations. Diversion points D1 and PAT (T1) are located after chromatography (Chrom #1). Using a surge line or tank allows continuous operations to accommodate differences in mass flow rates or process dynamics. Unit operations can be integrated as necessary.

The CM process continuously feeds input materials into, transforming in-process materials within, and simultaneously removing output materials from a manufacturing process in an integrated system involving two or more unit operations, regardless of their nature. The batch size produced by CM is defined as the quantity of the output material, the quantity of the input material, and run time (minimum or maximum) at a defined mass flow rate. In CM processes, a single thaw of one or multiple vials from the same cell bank may result in single or numerous harvests. The number or range of cell bank vials used to produce the specified drug substance batches should be defined. The cell bank vials should be traceable to the output drug substance batches. The FDA guidance also details how the electronic Common Technical Document (eCTD) filing should be managed for the CM process, making it possible for biosimilar developers to plan the process change properly. This technology can be applied to proteins that are secreted or made to secrete using *E. coli* (Table 4.6).

CM of chemical and biological products has long been a goal to optimize the cost of manufacturing; however, the cGMP compliance issues had pushed it back until March 2023, when the FDA released the first guideline to advise how to develop and adopt CM, particularly the biological products. CM requires a perfusion system, and it can be designed to use *E. coli*, which will be a better choice over CHO cells because of a much shorter batch cycle, generally a few hours than weeks for the CHO cells. In *E. coli*, the proteins can be directed to the cytoplasm, periplasm, or secreted directly into the culture media, offering several choices on routing the recombinant protein exploiting the features of each cellular compartment and the protein produced.

The quest for a CM process has been in research for several years.[2] While the FDA is yet to approve a biological product manufactured in a continuous system, it anticipates much interest. Consequently, in March 2023, the FDA released its first guidance on CM[3] addressing the scientific and regulatory issues, including the eCTD filing structure, which arose during the designing, installation, operation, and lifecycle management of CM for chemical and biological drugs. This guideline has opened the path to continuous systems over batch systems, which will significantly influence the development and production cost and the stability of proteins and cause a significant reduction in the size of the bioreactors. The FDA also identifies other guidelines that control CM. The recombinant protein technology executed as a batch process is the industry standard. However, proteins can also be produced in a vessel, from which the yield is continuously removed, provided the protein is secreted into the culture medium. It helps to improve the yield of labile proteins and prevents inconsistent post-translational modifications while maintaining cells at higher viabilities, which is a critical factor. Apart from material costs, it reduces the need for reduced testing, adding significant cost and time savings.

TABLE 4.6
Therapeutic Proteins Secreted in *Escherichia coli*

Adiponectin receptor
Adiponectin
Alpha-amylase
Amylase
Antibacterial peptides
Antibodies
Antithrombin III
Bone morphogenetic protein (BMP)
Chimeric antigen receptor (CAR)
Cholecystokinin (CCK)
Chymosin (rennin)
Ciliary neurotrophic factor (CNTF)
Coagulation factor VIII
Colony-stimulating factor 1 (CSF-1)
Connective tissue growth factor (CTGF)

(continued)

TABLE 4.6 (Continued)
Therapeutic Proteins Secreted in *Escherichia coli*

Epidermal growth factor (EGF)
Erythropoietin (EPO)
Erythropoietin receptor (EPOR)
Factor IX
Factor VII
Factor VIII
Fibrinolytic enzymes
Fibroblast growth factor (FGF)
Follicle-stimulating hormone (FSH)
Glucagon-like peptide-1 (GLP-1)
Glucagon
Glucocerebrosidase
Glucokinase
Glutathione S-transferase (GST)
Granulocyte colony-stimulating factor (G-CSF)
Granulocyte colony-stimulating factor receptor (G-CSF receptor)
Granulocyte-macrophage colony-stimulating factor (GM-CSF)
Green fluorescent protein (GFP)
Growth hormone (GH)
Hepatitis B surface antigen (HBsAg)
Hepatitis B surface antigen (HBsAg)
Human calcitonin
Human growth factor-1 (HGF-1)
Human growth hormone receptor antagonist (GHR antagonist)
Insulin-like growth factor 1 (IGF-1)
Insulin-like growth factor 2 (IGF-2)
Insulin-like growth factor-binding protein (IGFBP)
Insulin
Interferon alpha-2b
Interferon beta-1a
Interferon gamma (IFN-γ)
Interferon-alpha (IFN-α)
Interferon-beta (IFN-β)
Interferon-gamma (IFN-γ)
Interferon-lambda (IFN-λ)
Interleukin-1 receptor antagonist (IL-1RA)
Interleukin-10 (IL-10)
Interleukin-11 (IL-11)
Interleukin-12 (IL-12)
Interleukin-13 (IL-13)
Interleukin-15 (IL-15)
Interleukin-17 (IL-17)
Interleukin-18 (IL-18)
Interleukin-2 (IL-2)
Interleukin-2 (IL-2)
Interleukin-4 (IL-4)
Interleukin-5 (IL-5)
Interleukin-6 (IL-6)
Lactoferrin
Leptin

TABLE 4.6 (Continued)
Therapeutic Proteins Secreted in *Escherichia coli*

Lipase
Matrix metalloproteinases (MMPs)
Nerve growth factor (NGF)
Nerve growth factor beta (NGF-β)
Nerve growth factor receptor (NGF receptor)
Oncolytic viruses
Osteopontin
Parathyroid hormone (PTH)
Platelet-derived growth factor (PDGF)
Relaxin-2
Relaxin
Serine protease
Somatostatin receptor
Streptavidin
Streptococcal M protein
Streptokinase
Thrombopoietin (TPO)
Tissue plasminogen activator (tPA)
Transforming growth factor-beta (TGF-β)
Vascular endothelial growth factor (VEGF)

4.8 SUMMARY

Several regulatory advances include 3D printing of solid dosage forms, continuous batch manufacturing, and online in-process control in place of release testing. The role of artificial intelligence and machine learning will be heavily embedded in all manufacturing operations. SUT will eventually replace the hard-lined systems once the regulatory agencies begin approving products manufactured through SUT; more particularly, startups will adopt this approach.

NOTES

1 National Academies of Sciences, Engineering, and Medicine; Division on Earth and Life Studies; Board on Chemical Sciences and Technology. Continuous Manufacturing for the Modernization of Pharmaceutical Production: Proceedings of a Workshop. Washington (DC): National Academies Press (US); 2019 Jan 30. PMID: 30994997.
2 National Academies of Sciences, Engineering, and Medicine; Division on Earth and Life Studies; Board on Chemical Sciences and Technology. Continuous Manufacturing for the Modernization of Pharmaceutical Production: Proceedings of a Workshop. Washington (DC): National Academies Press (US); 2019 Jan 30. PMID: 30994997.
3 FDA. Q13 Continuous Manufacturing of Drug Substances and Drug Products www.fda.gov/media/165775/download

5 Analytical Assessment of a Biosimilar

5.1 INTRODUCTION

Analytical assessment of biosimilar candidates is the primary determinant of biosimilarity. Figure 5.1 shows the original Food and Drug Administration (FDA) pyramid that classified the tiers of development; in 2020, the FDA modified regulations to show a bigger role of analytical assessment, yet it became obsolete when, in 2023, the US Congress amended the BPCIA and removed the term "animal toxicology" and grouped it under nonclinical testing. Another major change was also established in 2023 when the FDA agreed that no efficacy testing in patients is needed for molecules that exhibit pharmacodynamic parameters (Figure 5.1).

Advancements in analytical instrumentation and a better understanding of proteins structure and functional relationships have established analytical assessment as the most robust tool for comparing critical quality attributes with the reference product.

These quality attributes stem from both the product and the process, identifiable and analyzable now with methods millions of times more sensitive. Product-related attributes pertain to the inherent expression property, often challenging or impossible to alter. Process-related attributes, on the other hand, are linked to the entire manufacturing process, spanning from upstream and downstream to fill and finish stages. These criteria, determined by the manufacturing process, become integral in the release specification, ensuring compliance. Defining acceptance criteria for these quality attributes can leverage requirements gleaned from testing the reference product. These criteria might be rooted in legacy values, established injectable product practices, or a blend of both. However, a limitation arises when using pharmacopeial specifications. The FDA prohibits their utilization for Drug Substance (DS) or Drug Product (DP), despite their applicability in pharmacopeial methods, which only necessitate verification without validation.

Proteins, in general, can manifest differences in three primary ways: (1) primary amino acid sequence; (2) modifications to amino acids, such as glycosylation or other side chain modifications; and (3) higher-order structure encompassing protein folding and interactions between proteins. Amino acid alterations can introduce heterogeneity, posing challenges for control. Environmental factors like light, temperature, moisture, packaging materials, container closure systems, and delivery device materials can influence protein modifications and higher-order structure. Moreover, process and product-related impurities might escalate the probability and severity of an immune response to a protein product. Certain excipients could hinder comprehensive characterization of the protein product.

Regulatory guidelines outline the assessment of analytical attributes required to demonstrate a proposed biosimilar product's eligibility for a marketing application submission. While these guidelines specifically target therapeutic protein products, the foundational scientific principles

DOI: 10.1201/9781003392026-5

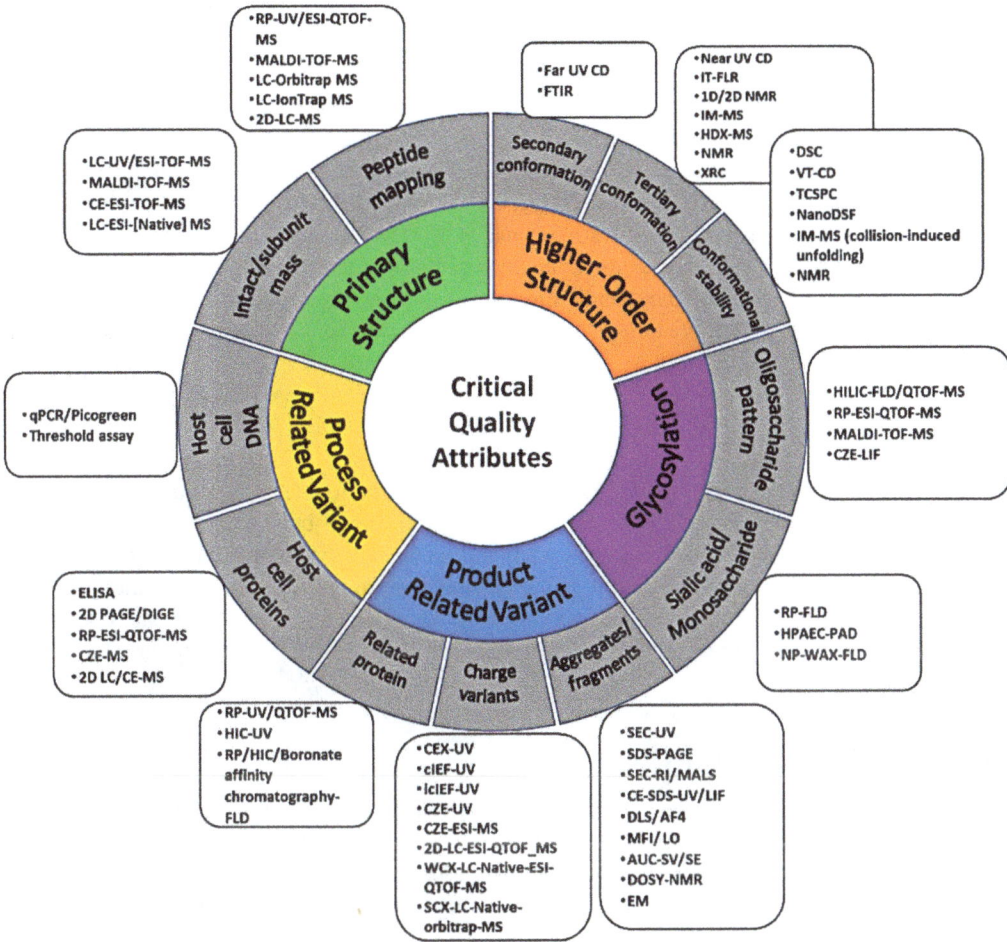

FIGURE 5.1 Methodologies for analytical assessment. Nupur N, Joshi S, Gulliarme D, Rathore AS. (2022) Analytical similarity assessment of biosimilars: global regulatory landscape, recent studies and major advancements in orthogonal platforms. *Front Bioeng Biotechnol.* 10: 832059. www.frontiersin.org/article/10.3389/fbioe.2022.832059. DOI: 10.3389/fbioe.2022.832059

could extend to the development of other protein products, including in vivo protein diagnostic products.

If the reference product lacks adequate characterization for pertinent analytical attributes, developers might be unable to file a marketing authorization application.

As part of a comprehensive CMC data submission, an application must include analytical studies showcasing the similarity of the proposed biosimilar product to the reference product. The rationale behind the comparative analytical assessment should be clearly articulated, considering the characteristics, known mechanism(s) of action, and function of the reference product.

The studies on physicochemical and functional characterization need to sufficiently establish the pertinent quality attributes, which encompass the defining elements of a product: its identity, quantity, safety, purity, and potency. By analyzing the outcomes of analytical studies that evaluate functional and physicochemical characteristics—such as higher-order structure, post-translational modifications, impurity, and degradation profiles—developers can establish a scientifically sound basis for a targeted approach in subsequent animal and clinical studies to validate biosimilarity.

Employing a meaningful fingerprint-like analysis algorithm that encompasses various product attributes and their combinations through highly sensitive orthogonal methods can aid in comparing differences in quality attributes between a proposed biosimilar product and the reference product.

According to the International Council for Harmonisation (ICH) Q8(R2), leveraging enhanced manufacturing science approaches can enable production processes that better align with the attributes of a reference product (RP). Refer to the ICH guidance documents for industry Q8(R2) Pharmaceutical Development (November 2009), Q9 Quality Risk Management (June 2006), Q10 Pharmaceutical Quality System (April 2009), and Q11 Development and Manufacture of Drug Substances (November 2012) for guidance on advanced manufacturing approaches. This strategic approach could further quantify the overall similarity between two molecules and potentially provide additional grounds for a more targeted and selective approach in subsequent animal and clinical studies.

5.2   TESTING PLAN

The description and discussion of any differences—whether intentional or observed through comprehensive analytical characterization of multiple manufacturing lots—between a proposed biosimilar product and the reference product must be clearly outlined. This discussion should encompass the identification and comparison of pertinent quality attributes from product characterization. If necessary, the potential clinical implications of observed structural and functional differences between a proposed biosimilar product and the reference product should be evaluated and supported by animal or clinical studies.

5.3   SOURCES OF VARIATION

Analyzing critical quality attributes requires a comprehensive understanding of the sources of variation between a proposed biosimilar product and the reference product. A primary goal in biosimilar development is to minimize differences between the proposed biosimilar product and the RP where feasible. Some efforts towards this end involve modifying the expression system, upstream and downstream processes, formulation, and manufacturing processes.

5.3.1   Expression System

Therapeutic protein products can be created in various systems: microbial cells (prokaryotic or eukaryotic), cell lines (such as mammalian, avian, insect, or plant), or tissues derived from animals or plants. It is anticipated that the expression constructs for a proposed biosimilar product will carry the same primary amino acid sequence as its reference product. Nevertheless, minor modifications, such as N- or C–terminal truncations (e.g., the heterogeneity of the C-terminal lysine of a monoclonal antibody), are not expected to alter the product performance. Such modifications might be justified and should be explained by the developer. Any potential differences between the selected expression system (i.e., host cell and the expression construct) of a proposed biosimilar product and that of the reference product should be carefully considered. This is because the chosen expression system will impact the types of process- and product-related substances, impurities, and contaminants (including possible adventitious agents) that might exist in the protein product. For instance, the expression system can significantly influence the types and degree of translational and post-translational modifications in a proposed biosimilar product, potentially introducing additional uncertainties into the demonstration that a proposed biosimilar product is proposed biosimilar to the reference product.

Minimizing disparities between the expression systems of a proposed biosimilar product and its reference product to the fullest extent possible can increase the likelihood of producing a biosimilar protein product. The use of different expression systems will be assessed case by case. However, developers should consider the extra testing burden required to validate an alternative expression system. In the market, surveillance should place more emphasis on demonstrating the product's safety.

5.3.2 Manufacturing Process

A comprehensive understanding of all stages in the manufacturing process for a proposed biosimilar product must be established during product development. As a scientific imperative, characterization tests, process controls, and specifications derived from information gathered during process development must be tailored to a proposed biosimilar product and its manufacturing process. Advanced pharmaceutical development approaches, combined with quality risk management and efficient quality systems, will facilitate the consistent manufacture of a high-quality product. For guidance on enhanced approaches in manufacturing science, refer to the ICH guidance for industry Q8(R2) Pharmaceutical Development (November 2009), Q9 Quality Risk Management (June 2006), Q10 Pharmaceutical Quality System (April 2009), and Q11 Development and Manufacture of Drug Substances (November 2012) for guidance on enhanced approaches in manufacturing science.

Developers contemplating manufacturing changes post-initial comparative analytical assessment or after concluding clinical studies intended to support an application must establish comparability between the pre- and post-change proposed biosimilar product. Depending on the nature and extent of the changes, additional studies may be necessary. Comparative analytical studies should encompass a sufficient quantity of a proposed biosimilar product used in clinical studies and a proposed commercial process if the process used for the clinical studies' material differs.

Manufacturing processes can modify a protein product, impacting its safety and effectiveness. For instance, variations in biological systems used for protein production can lead to diverse post-translational modifications, influencing the safety and effectiveness of the final product. Therefore, when altering the manufacturing process of a marketed protein product, the applicant must evaluate the effects of the change. This evaluation necessitates demonstrating, through suitable analytical testing, functional assays, and in some cases, animal and clinical studies, that the modification does not negatively affect the product's identity, potency, quality, purity, or strength concerning its safety or effectiveness.

The ICH guidance for industry Q5E, titled "Comparability of Biotechnological/Biological Products Subject to Changes in Their Manufacturing Process," outlines scientific principles for assessing manufacturing changes. Establishing the biosimilarity of a proposed biosimilar product to the reference product typically involves greater complexity compared to assessing the comparability of a product before and after manufacturing changes made by the same manufacturer. This complexity arises from the extensive knowledge a manufacturer possesses about its manufacturing process, including established controls and acceptance parameters. By contrast, the manufacturer of a proposed biosimilar product is likely to employ a different manufacturing process (e.g., distinct cell lines, raw materials, equipment, processes, controls, and criteria) from that of the reference product. Moreover, they lack direct knowledge of the reference product's manufacturing process. Consequently, although some scientific principles in ICH Q5E may apply to demonstrating biosimilarity, regulatory agencies expect a greater need for data and information to establish biosimilarity than to demonstrate comparability following a manufacturer's post-manufacturing change. Additionally, ICH Q5E does not mandate the use of the reference product, rendering it unsuitable for initially establishing biosimilarity.

5.3.3 Structural Attributes

Structural attributes such as primary, secondary, and tertiary structures are dictated by the nature of the recombinant expression engine. While a protein's gene sequence determines its amino acid sequence, post-translational modifications occurring during quality control in the endoplasmic reticulum (ER) and passage through the Golgi apparatus determine its final structure and function. These processes, specific to species and cells, present challenges to the biopharmaceutical industry when developing a production platform for generating recombinant biologic therapeutics. Proteins and glycoproteins (P/GPs) are susceptible to chemical modifications both in vivo and in vitro. The body tolerates molecular forms of self-molecules, but non-self-variants can trigger an immune response leading to the production of anti-drug antibodies (ADA). Aggregated forms may exhibit increased immunogenicity, prompting efforts to avoid or eliminate them. Monoclonal antibody therapeutics (mAbs) present a unique case because they aim to bind the target, forming immune complexes (ICs) which represent a specific aggregate form. Phagocytic cells possessing antigen-presenting capacity may eliminate such ICs. These factors make it challenging to mitigate mAbs' immunogenicity by strictly excluding aggregates from drug products.

Therapeutic antibodies possess various quality attributes, with FcRn binding and related structures known to significantly impact the product's pharmacokinetic profile. Other attributes, such as antigen binding, glycan structure, and isoelectric point, also potentially influence the pharmacokinetics.

Validation lots representing the commercial process should be compared for structural variants. If the primary structure mismatches, the cell line should be discarded, necessitating a fresh start. Achieving the primary structure often leads to corresponding secondary and tertiary structures. Do not use any public information data on structural attributes; only what is observed in a side-by-side comparison with the reference product. At this stage, the analytical methods need only be suitable and sensitive, not validated. Conducting testing simultaneously and side-by-side nullifies any potential impact of the test method. Given minor variations and stringent acceptance criteria, extensive testing with multiple lots is unnecessary.

If variability in post-translational and other modifications arises during testing, developers should refine the upstream and downstream processes to closely match the profile. However, achieving an exact match might be unfeasible due to modifications moving in opposite directions. The level of match required depends on the product's nature. For monoclonal antibodies, any differences should be justified through additional studies, potentially necessitating clinical efficacy testing. Post-translational modifications serve as release specification attributes and demand multiple lots to establish a reliable quality range.

5.3.4 FUNCTIONAL ATTRIBUTES

Among the critical quality attributes of therapeutic antibodies, FcRn binding and related structures significantly influence the product's pharmacokinetic profile. Additional attributes such as antigen binding, glycan structure, and isoelectric point potentially impact the pharmacokinetic profile as well. However, these attributes aren't included in release specifications; they are tested once to confirm similarity. As the testing is done alongside the reference product, the need for method validation is eliminated. An equivalence margin approach, requiring 6–10 lots (see below), is suggested to establish similarity.

5.3.5 PHYSICOCHEMICAL PROPERTIES

When developers design and conduct characterization studies, addressing the concept of the desired product (and its variants) as discussed in ICH Q6B becomes crucial. Understanding the heterogeneity between a proposed biosimilar and the reference product, including glycosylation levels, isoform variability, and post-translational modifications, is essential. Refer to the ICH guidance for industry Q6B Specifications: Test Procedures and Acceptance Criteria for Biotechnological/ Biological Products (August 1999).

Analytical methodologies assess specific physicochemical protein characteristics. These methods, outlined in published documents like scientific literature, regulatory guidelines, and pharmacopeial compendia, often provide multifaceted information. Selecting appropriate analytical test methods depends on the nature of the protein, knowledge about the structure, heterogeneity of the reference product, proposed biosimilar, and critical characteristics for product performance. Appendix 1 presents a representative example of test methods used by proposed biosimilar developers, provided for reference purposes in applications to the FDA and EMA.

5.3.5.1 Aggregates

Although aggregates are generally considered immunogenic, for monoclonal antibodies, establishing a range within which all lots must fall is necessary. An equivalence margin approach is recommended for this release specification attribute, requiring multiple lots for a reliable quality range. If a proposed biosimilar product exhibits lower aggregates, potential failure within the equivalence margin at the lower end is acceptable. However, it's crucial to note that reference product lots undergo time and transportation tests, potentially contributing to total aggregates. A proposed biosimilar product won't be considered a "biobetter" solely due to lower aggregates.

5.3.5.2 Impurities

Impurities are categorized as product-related or process-related. Active or inactive, product-related impurities must be classified based on available literature data. Any impurity not present in the reference product should be fully characterized regardless of its source due to potential immunogenicity. Developers should prioritize removing such impurities through process changes rather than justifying their safety, which may necessitate additional nonclinical or clinical studies.

Characterizing, identifying, and quantifying product-related impurities in both the proposed biosimilar and reference product, to the extent feasible, is essential. If a comparative analysis reveals similar levels of comparable product-related impurities between the proposed biosimilar and reference product, additional pharmacological and toxicological studies to characterize specific impurities' biological effects may be unnecessary. However, if the manufacturing process introduces different or higher levels of impurities in the proposed biosimilar than in the reference product, further pharmacological, toxicological, or other studies might be necessary. The terms "product-related" and "process-related" impurities align with their use and meaning in ICH Q6B.

Relying on purification processes to remove impurities is preferred over establishing a preclinical testing program for their qualification. (Refer to the ICH guidance for industry S6(R1) Preclinical Safety Evaluation of Biotechnology-Derived Pharmaceuticals, May 2012, page 2.)

Process-related impurities originating from cell substrates (such as host cell DNA and host cell proteins), cell culture components (like antibiotics and media components), and downstream processing steps (such as reagents, residual solvents, leachables, endotoxins, and bioburden) require evaluation. The anticipated process-related impurities in a proposed biosimilar product are not expected to match those found in the reference product and thus are not encompassed in the comparative analytical assessment. The selected analytical procedures must adequately detect, identify, and accurately quantify significant levels of impurities. For reference, consult the ICH guidance for industry Q2B Validation of Analytical Procedures: Methodology (May 1997). Specifically, immunological methods for detecting host cell proteins depend on assay reagents and cell substrates used. These assays need validation using the product cell-substrate and orthogonal methodologies to ensure precision and sensitivity.

As with any biological product, ensuring the safety of a proposed biosimilar product regarding adventitious agents or endogenous viral contamination necessitates screening critical raw materials and confirming robust virus removal and inactivation achieved during the manufacturing process. Refer to the ICH guidance for industry Q5A Viral Safety Evaluation of Biotechnology Products Derived from Cell Lines of Human or Animal Origin (September 1998).

5.3.5.3 Host Cell Protein and Residual DNA

When developing a new biological product, determining the acceptable limits of HCP (host cell proteins) and residual DNA involves demonstrating the feasibility of reducing this adverse attribute, evaluating the relative safety risk of the specific products, and monitoring these attributes. Both HCP and residual DNA are dependent on organism strain, so even if developers use the same expression system, replicating the originator's exact strain is impossible. Since HCP and residual DNA are strain-specific, directly comparing the relative safety of a proposed biosimilar product is only feasible through comprehensive safety studies assessing these attributes. Regulatory agencies necessitate a critical analysis of HCP and residual DNA, acknowledging that these might differ from those in the originator product. A 2D SDS resolution is also recommended to address these components for both the test and reference products. Claiming similarity between HCP and residual DNA in the test and originator product is challenging. While it is true that the HCP and residual DNA in a proposed biosimilar product may not match those in the reference product, if the same expression system (e.g., *E. coli*) is used, there is a high likelihood that safety will be proportional to the quantity of these components, despite any specific activity associated with a particular component. Consequently, it is plausible for the test product to demonstrate non-inferiority through an equivalence range approach.

5.3.6 Lot-to-Lot Variability

Observed lot-to-lot variability may stem from manufacturing conditions and analytical assay differences. Factors contributing to variability between lots in the production of a protein product include the origin of specific raw materials (such as growth medium, resins, or separation materials) and distinct manufacturing sites. Hence, it is crucial in the comparative analytical assessment to adequately characterize lot-to-lot variability of the reference product and a proposed biosimilar product.

In certain instances, modifications to the manufacturing process of a proposed biosimilar product may be necessary to address differences observed in the comparative analytical assessment. Data demonstrating resolution of observed differences through manufacturing changes should be provided, along with evidence that other quality attributes were not significantly impacted. If other attributes were affected by the manufacturing change, data should illustrate evaluation and mitigation of the change's impact.

5.3.7 Product- or Process-Related Substances

Advances in analytical sciences—both physicochemical and biological—have significantly enhanced the characterization of various protein products in terms of their physicochemical and biological properties. These analytical procedures have markedly improved the capability to identify and characterize the intended product, as well as product-related substances and impurities associated with the product and its manufacturing process.

The terminology "product-related substances" and "product-and process-related impurities" aligns with the usage and significance outlined in the ICH Q6B guidelines. A product-related substance refers to a variant of the targeted substance exhibiting at least 80% of the activity of the active target drug substance. Impurities can either be active or inactive.

It is imperative to identify, appropriately characterize, quantify, and compare the product-related impurities and substances using multiple lots of both the proposed biosimilar product and the reference product. This comparison, to the extent feasible and relevant, forms a crucial part of assessing potential impacts on the safety, purity, and potency of the product.

5.3.8 Method Sensitivity

Regulatory agencies advocate for the utilization of state-of-the-art technology. Developers should employ analytical methodologies with adequate sensitivity and specificity to discern differences between a proposed biosimilar product and the reference product.

Advancements in manufacturing science and production methods have increased the likelihood of demonstrating similarity between a proposed biosimilar product and the reference product, especially by targeting the physicochemical and functional properties of the reference product. However, despite advances in analytical sciences, some differences between protein products may be detected that might not be clinically relevant. Nevertheless, employing highly sensitive methods that demonstrate similarity provides increased confidence and reduces the need for additional studies.

Despite improvements in analytical techniques, the current methodology may not identify all relevant structural and functional differences between the two protein products. Understanding the limitations of each analytical method is crucial for developers to identify residual uncertainties and plan subsequent testing. Additionally, there might be an incomplete understanding of how a product's structural attributes correlate with its clinical performance.

Contrary to routine quality control assays, tests utilized for characterizing the product do not necessarily need validation. However, they should be scientifically sound, suitable for their intended purpose, and capable of producing reproducible and reliable results. Selection of these tests should consider the characteristics of the protein product, including known and potential impurities. Information on a method's ability to discern pertinent differences between a proposed biosimilar product and the reference product should be included in the comparison. The methods should demonstrate appropriate sensitivity and specificity to provide meaningful insights into the similarity between the two products.

5.3.9 Comparative Testing

In contrast to the standalone testing conducted for a new drug to establish its characteristics, the development of biosimilars doesn't necessitate such independent testing for safety or efficacy. Instead, all testing is carried out comparatively, emphasizing a pivotal difference in establishing test methods, protocols, and their scopes for comparison, not characterization.

Comparative analytical data serve as the cornerstone for developing a proposed biosimilar product, influencing decisions about the necessary type and quantity of animal and clinical data to support demonstrating biosimilarity. Comprehensive and robust comparative physicochemical and functional studies, which may include biological assays, binding assays, and enzyme kinetics, should be performed to evaluate a proposed biosimilar product against the reference product.

A comprehensive comparative analytical assessment relies significantly on the capabilities of state-of-the-art analytical assays. These assays determine various factors such as the protein's molecular weight, complexity (including higher-order structure and post-translational modifications), degree of heterogeneity, functional properties, impurity profiles, and degradation profiles, all of which indicate stability. Developers must detail the capabilities and limitations of the methods employed in these analytical assessments. Alternative analytical study methods offer distinct perspectives on quality attributes without redundantly testing the same attribute or utilizing a method that does not offer a unique viewpoint. It is imperative not to disregard a failed test based solely on orthogonal testing.

In conducting comparative analytical assessments, risk ranking and data analysis evaluate numerous attributes, often utilizing multiple orthogonal assays. Regulatory agencies assess the entirety of the analytical data. Failure to meet specific criteria in a particular assay alone does not necessarily negate the demonstration of similarity. If differences between products arise during the comparative analytical assessment (even within components not initially part of the risk ranking), developers may provide additional scientific information (such as risk assessment and supplementary data) along with justification for why these differences do not hinder demonstrating similarity between the products.

5.3.10   SIDE-BY-SIDE TESTING

For a proposed biosimilar product, developers should conduct comparative testing through side-by-side analyses of an appropriate number of lots of both the proposed biosimilar product and the reference product. Where available and suitable, comparison with an internal reference standard for relevant attributes (e.g., potency) should also be included. Evaluating multiple lots of both the reference and proposed biosimilar products allows for estimating variability across different lots. The required number of lots may vary case by case, and developers should provide a scientific rationale for their choice.

The emphasis on side-by-side testing is crucial in resolving variability in test methods, especially those that cannot be entirely validated. Conducting tests simultaneously helps resolve most, if not all, differences in test method reliability. Consequently, any published data concerning reference product quality attributes cannot be used for comparison with a proposed biosimilar product. Similarly, using a reference standard to match attributes between a proposed biosimilar product and the reference product is not valid. These limitations apply even to established attributes such as molecular weight, sequence, or other fixed attributes.

5.3.11   HETEROGENEITY

Therapeutic proteins, being produced in living systems, naturally exhibit variability in certain quality attributes. This variability can arise from various sources and significantly impact the anticipated clinical performance of a protein product. Errors during replication in the DNA encoding the protein sequence and misincorporation of amino acids might occur during translation, although these errors typically remain at low levels. Furthermore, most protein products undergo post-translational modifications that can modify the protein's functions by attaching additional biochemical groups like phosphate, lipids, carbohydrates, undergoing proteolytic cleavage after translation, changing the chemical nature of an amino acid (e.g., formylation), or through numerous other mechanisms. These modifications may result from intracellular activities during cell culture or intentional modifications of the protein (e.g., PEGylation). Additionally, manufacturing process operations might lead to other post-translational modifications; for instance, glycation may occur due to the product's exposure to reducing sugars. Certain storage conditions could also facilitate or impede specific degradation pathways like oxidation, deamidation, or aggregation. These various product-related variants have the potential to alter the biological properties of the expressed recombinant protein. Therefore, it's crucial to include the identification and determination of these variants' relative levels in comparative analytical characterization studies.

5.3.12   STRUCTURE CONFIRMATION

The three-dimensional conformation of a protein significantly influences its biological function. Proteins typically display intricate three-dimensional conformations (tertiary structure and, occasionally, quaternary structure) owing to their size and the rotational traits of protein alpha carbons, among other factors. This inherent flexibility allows for dynamic yet subtle changes in protein conformation over time, some of which may be necessary for functional activity. These rotations are frequently reliant on low-energy interactions, such as hydrogen bonds and van der Waals forces, which can be highly sensitive to environmental conditions. Present analytical technology is capable of assessing the three-dimensional structure of numerous proteins. Utilizing multiple, pertinent, cutting-edge methods can aid in defining tertiary protein structure and, to varying degrees, quaternary structure, thereby contributing to the information supporting biosimilarity. However, precisely defining a protein's three-dimensional conformation with current physicochemical analytical technology can pose challenges. Any disparities in higher-order structure between a proposed biosimilar product and the reference product should be scrutinized regarding potential impacts on protein function and stability. Consequently, functional assays are essential tools for evaluating the integrity of higher-order structures.

5.3.13 Acceptance Criteria

The acceptance criteria for each test are established by initially conducting exploratory tests on both the reference product and the proposed biosimilar product. This approach leads to defining specifications and acceptance criteria. A formal study, necessitating a specific number of lots determined by statistical calculations, compares the proposed biosimilar product with the reference product. Agencies encourage developers to consult with them to ensure the evaluation of an appropriate number of lots. Specific lots of the reference products used in comparative analytical studies, including expiration dates, analysis time frames, and their utilization in nonclinical or clinical studies, must be identified. This information substantiates acceptance criteria, ensuring product consistency, and supporting the comparative analytical assessment between the proposed biosimilar product and the reference product.

However, the acceptance criteria should not solely rely on the observed range of product attributes of the reference product. Instead, they should be based on comprehensive analytical data evidence. Certain product attributes interact, collectively influencing a product's safety, purity, and potency profile. Hence, their potential interactions should be considered when establishing specifications. For instance, in some glycoproteins, the content and distribution of tetra-antennary and N-acetylglucosamine repeats can collectively affect in vivo potency, and their evaluation should not occur independently.

Furthermore, data obtained from lots used in nonclinical and clinical studies, along with pertinent information on attribute-drug product performance relationships, can aid in establishing acceptance criteria. Refer to the ICH guidance for industry Q8(R2) Pharmaceutical Development (November 2009) for more details.

5.3.14 Orthogonal Testing

To comprehensively address physicochemical properties or biological activities, multiple analytical procedures are often necessary for evaluating the same quality attribute. Methods using diverse physicochemical or biological principles to assess the same attribute are particularly valuable as they offer independent data supporting that attribute (e.g., employing orthogonal methods to assess aggregation). Utilizing complementary analytical techniques in sequence, such as combining peptide mapping or capillary electrophoresis with mass spectrometry of separated molecules, offers a meaningful and sensitive approach to compare products.

Extensive analytical characterization may reveal differences between the reference product and a proposed biosimilar product, particularly when employing techniques capable of discerning qualitative or quantitative attribute variations. Prioritize the development of orthogonal quantitative methods to definitively identify any differences in product attributes. However, an orthogonal test should offer an alternative perspective on the quality attribute, or in cases where the validity of a test might be questioned. For instance, using both UV absorbance and HPLC to determine protein content could be considered. Nevertheless, the specification must always be definitive, leaving no ambiguity in the choice of testing method.

5.3.15 Accountability of Lots

The developer must ensure inclusion and characterization of all acquired reference product lots. The application should encompass data and information from all evaluated reference products and proposed biosimilar product lots across various studies: physicochemical, functional, animal, and clinical. Justification for the selection or exclusion of specific lots in analytical studies should be provided. The application should contain the dates of analytical testing and product expiration. Generally, expired reference product lots should not be included in the comparative analytical assessment due to potential deviations from typical observations in unexpired lots, leading to overestimated variability. Testing expired lots may be acceptable under certain storage conditions, such as long-term frozen storage at −80°C. The developer should submit data confirming that storage conditions do not compromise product quality.

Similar information and data gathered for reference product lots should also be provided for each manufactured drug substance and product lot of the proposed biosimilar.

All reference and proposed biosimilar product lots used in clinical studies (e.g., PK and PD studies, if applicable, similarity and comparative clinical study) must be included in the comparative analytical assessment.

Combining data from two reference products in testing is prohibited as it may lead to broader similarity acceptance criteria than relying solely on data from one reference product, potentially enlarging the range.

If the drug substance is extracted from the reference product for analytical studies, the developers should detail the extraction procedure. They must demonstrate that the procedure itself does not alter relevant product quality attributes, including impurities and product-related substances. Appropriate controls should ensure that the extraction procedure does not significantly modify the relevant characteristics of the protein.

5.3.16 Critical Quality Attributes

When conducting the comparative analytical assessment to establish biosimilarity, developers should consider all factors impacting the safety and efficacy of the proposed biosimilar product.

Critical quality attributes pertinent to analytical similarity can be categorized as inherent and legacy attributes. Inherent attributes include variable properties intrinsic to the manufacturing process, resulting in lot-to-lot variability. This classification covers both process- and product-related factors, such as post-translational modifications in cytokines and antibodies. Legacy attributes are fixed characteristics not subject to lot-to-lot variation, including the total mass of a protein (in some cytokines but not monoclonal antibodies), amino acid sequence, and other reported properties like disulfide bond positions. These characteristics are documented in protein databases, patents, publications, and pharmacopeias. Another category of legacy attributes encompasses labeled specifications of inactive ingredients and product characteristics such as pH, and osmolality.

While legacy attribute specifications significantly characterize the reference product, a proposed biosimilar product still requires testing against reference product lots. This is because the reference product isn't obligated to comply with any legacy attributes. Moreover, conducting side-by-side tests helps mitigate the impact of test method variability in identifying clinically meaningful differences between a proposed biosimilar product and the reference product. However, the release specifications for various quality attributes can be established independently based on established principles ensuring the product's efficacy. For example, protein content (e.g., ±3%), bioactivity (e.g., ±15%), post-translational modifications (e.g., ±10%), subvisible particles (USP specification), physical properties (e.g., pH, osmolality, density, etc., ±10%), aggregates (e.g., ±10% of the average from multiple lots of RP), fill volume (USP specification), impurities (e.g., no more than 3%, no single impurity more than 1%, and no unidentified impurity). Developers may propose other limits based on multiple analyses of reference product lots. The core principle in establishing analytical

TABLE 5.1
Common Critical Quality Attributes

Quality Attribute	Criticality	Potential Impact	Suggested Analytical Methods
Amino acid sequence	Very high	Efficacy, safety	Peptide mapping, MS, Edelman degradation
Glycan structure and content	Very high	Efficacy, safety	Glycan wnalysis
Biological activity	Very high	Efficacy, safety	Bioassay
Immunochemical identity	Very high	Efficacy, safety	SDS-PAGE+ immunoblotting, immunoassay
Higher-order structure	High	Efficacy, safety	Spectrophotometric, thermodynamic Methods
Isoform distribution	High	Efficacy	Isoelectric focusing
Insoluble aggregates	High	Safety	Light obscuration
High-molecular-weight aggregates	High	Safety	SE-HPLC, AUC, SDS-PAGE
Protein content	High	Efficacy	UV; use HPLC as an orthogonal method
Host cell proteins	High	Safety	SPR spectroscopy, cell-based assay
Receptor binding	High	Efficacy	SPR, cell-based assay
Truncated forms	Low	Efficacy	Reference product HPLC, other chromatography
Deamidation, oxidation	Low	Efficacy	Chromatography

Notes: AUC, analytical ultracentrifugation; HPLC, high-performance liquid chromatography; MS, mass spectroscopy; SDS-PAGE, sodium sulfate polyacrylamide gel electrophoresis; SE, sedimentation equilibrium; SPR, surface plasmon resonance; UV, ultraviolet

similarity and release specifications for drug substance and drug product is to eliminate uncertainties that could potentially impact safety and subsequently efficacy. For example, protein content (e.g., ±3%), bioactivity (e.g., ±15%), post-translational modifications (e.g., ±10%), subvisible particles (USP specification), physical properties (e.g., pH, osmolality, density, etc., ±10%), aggregates (e.g., ±10% of the average from multiple lots of RP), fill volume (USP specification), impurities (e.g., no more than 3%, no single impurity more than 1%, and no unidentified impurity). Developers may propose other limits based on multiple analyses of reference product lots. The core principle in establishing analytical similarity and release specifications for drug substance and drug product is to eliminate uncertainties that could potentially impact safety and subsequently efficacy.

Critical quality attributes are identified based on their impact on the product's safety and efficacy. Table 5.1 provides a non-exhaustive list of various attributes and their classification. The choice of the test method depends on the criticality of the attribute.

5.3.17 Reference Standard

Using a proposed biosimilar product in comparison with a publicly available standard, such as a pharmacopeia monograph or a reference standard, is not permitted for conducting comparative testing to establish biosimilarity. It is crucial to emphasize that any specifications from a pharmacopeia monograph or a reference standard provided by third parties are not deemed suitable to establish biosimilarity.

Pharmacopoeia reference standards are unsuitable for conducting comparative studies; their usage is restricted solely to test method qualification. A qualified reference standard should be internally developed by the developer, based on its thoroughly characterized batch.

While a physicochemical and functional comparison of a proposed biosimilar product with a suitable, publicly available, and well-established reference standard for the protein might offer valuable insights, studies with such a reference standard alone are insufficient to demonstrate the biosimilarity of the proposed biosimilar product to the reference product. For instance, if there exists an international standard for calibrating potency, it is necessary to compare the relative potency of a proposed biosimilar product with this potency standard. According to the recommendations outlined in ICH Q6B, in-house reference standard(s) must always be qualified and employed to control both the manufacturing process and the product.

Typically, an in-house reference standard is developed from early development lots or lots used in clinical studies. Additional reference standards may be qualified later in the development process and for submission. Ideally, developers will establish and properly qualify primary and working reference standards representative of proposed biosimilar product lots used in supporting clinical studies.

When developing a proposed biosimilar product, the reference product lot usually undergoes qualification as an initial reference standard. After manufacturing clinical lots of a proposed biosimilar product, one of these lots is expected to be appropriately qualified (including bridging to previous reference standards) for use as a reference standard for release, stability, and comparative analytical testing. Ideally, once an in-house reference standard is fully qualified, sufficient quantities should be available for use throughout the proposed biosimilar product's development. All reference standard lots used during the development should be suitably qualified. Additionally, the qualification protocol for reference standards should encompass all analytical methods reporting results relative to the reference standard.

For all methods reporting results relative to the reference standard, the assignment of potency at 100% should incorporate a narrow acceptable potency range to ensure control over product drift. For example, developers should consider utilizing a predetermined two-sided confidence interval (CI) of the mean of the replicates, where the mean relative potency and the 95% CI fall within a sufficiently narrow range (e.g., 90%–110%). An evaluation across multiple reference standard qualifications should be conducted to address potential drift over the history of qualification.

Developers should refrain from using a correction factor to compensate for differences in potency or biological activity between reference standards.

Using a proposed biosimilar product in comparison with a publicly available standard, such as a pharmacopeia monograph or a reference standard, is not permitted for conducting comparative testing to establish biosimilarity. It is crucial to emphasize that any specifications from a pharmacopeia monograph or a reference standard provided by third parties are not deemed suitable to establish biosimilarity.

5.4 FINISHED DRUG PRODUCT

Product characterization studies for a proposed biosimilar product should focus on the most downstream intermediate that best suits the analytical procedures. The assessed attributes should remain stable through subsequent processing steps. Consequently, characterization studies are typically conducted on the drug substance. However, if a drug substance undergoes reformulation and comes into contact with new materials in the finished dosage form, the effects of these changes must be considered. Whenever feasible, if the finished drug product is better suited for a particular analysis, developers should analyze the finished drug product. If an analytical method detects specific attributes in the drug substance more sensitively, but these attributes are critical and susceptible to change during the manufacture of the finished drug product, a comparative characterization may be necessary for both the extracted protein and the finished drug product.

Proteins are highly sensitive to their environment. Consequently, differences in excipients or primary packaging could impact product stability and clinical performance. Discrepancies in formulation and primary packaging between a proposed biosimilar product and the reference product are factors that could influence the selective and targeted approach of subsequent clinical studies. Referencing the ICH guidance for industry Q8(R2) Pharmaceutical Development (November 2009) is advisable. Developers should clearly identify excipients used in a proposed biosimilar product that differ from those in the reference product. The acceptability of differences in the type, nature, and extent of excipients between the finished proposed biosimilar product and the finished reference product should be evaluated and supported by appropriate data and rationale. Furthermore, the inclusion of different excipients in a proposed biosimilar product should be substantiated either by existing toxicology data for the excipient or by additional toxicity studies formulated specifically for the proposed biosimilar product.

After a drug substance has undergone purification through the downstream process, it's considered a chemical entity rather than a biological one. Consequently, it becomes subject to all cGMP requirements applicable to any other chemical drug's fill and finish process. Nevertheless, there are exceptional considerations such as proteins desorbing to the filling line, aggregate formation during filling, and concentration changes throughout the process. Cleaning validation of the fill and finish equipment poses a significant challenge. To mitigate risks associated with potential contamination of the protein solution by a chemical entity, albeit at a minimal concentration, a preferred method involves using a dedicated filling head for these operations. Further reduction in contamination risk is achieved by utilizing single-use heads.

5.4.1 EXCIPIENTS

Proposed biosimilar products may contain different inactive ingredients compared to those disclosed in the reference product's prescribing information. This allowance aids developers in overcoming potential patent protections related to formulations extending beyond the biological entity's gene patents. However, this alteration introduces additional challenges in demonstrating that the choice of inactive ingredients doesn't induce adverse responses in terms of toxicity, pharmacokinetics (including absorption), or product efficacy. Although incidents of toxicities are rare, notable examples such as pure red cell aplasia (PRCA) caused by changes in erythropoietin formulation and administration [McKay, J, et al., Epoetin-associated pure red cell aplasia: past, present, and future considerations. *Transfusion*, 48(8), July 2008] methods highlight the importance of careful consideration. Early biosimilars faced these challenges when the understanding of biosimilars was in its infancy. Today, such changes would not be permitted without a thorough investigation to identify associated risks.

Developers are advised to initially consider the formulation of the reference product as the preferred formulation, relying on the analysis of the reference product. They should establish release limits for any inactive substances solely based on the profile obtained for the RP. For instance, surfactants, commonly used in biological drug formulations, may exhibit concentration variations of 30%–50%. The purity of surfactants is crucial, and in some cases, it is recommended to discard any remaining surfactant in a new container to avoid potential safety risks to the product.

As a secondary option, developers can consider using a different formulation based on ingredients generally recognized as safe for parenteral products, avoiding the use of unusual components.

Opting for unique inactive ingredients as the final choice would necessitate more extensive safety studies, potentially leaving residual uncertainty about the formulation. Often, it's not feasible to infer the toxicity of proteins solely from analytical assessments. One must consider excipient interactions along with direct toxicities.

5.4.2 STABILITY

As part of an appropriate comparison of the stability profile between a proposed biosimilar product and the reference product, it's crucial to conduct accelerated and stress stability studies. Forced degradation studies should also be employed to establish degradation profiles and enable a direct stability comparison. These comparative studies should encompass multiple stress conditions (e.g., high temperature, freeze-thaw cycles, light exposure, and agitation), causing gradual product degradation over a defined period. The results from these studies may uncover product disparities requiring further evaluation and help identify conditions necessitating additional controls in manufacturing and storage. Refer to ICH guidance for industry Q5C Quality of Biotechnological Products: Stability Testing of Biotechnological/Biological Products (July 1996) and Q1A(R2) Stability Testing of New Drug Substances and Products (November 2003). Sufficient real-time, real-condition stability data from a proposed biosimilar product should validate the proposed shelf life.

Regulatory agencies expect a proposed biosimilar product to undergo side-by-side qualitative and quantitative testing for degradants' types and levels. However, challenges arise in sourcing reference products with production dates similar to those of proposed biosimilar products. Additionally, determining an acceptable deviation from theoretical degradation rates based on declared shelf-life remains a concern.

Developers must present data from at least three lots, potentially including development lots placed under stability testing. The stability study should extend for at least six months, aiming to obtain linear regression coefficients of degradation with high statistical significance (r2). These degradation rates' slopes are then compared with theoretical rates. For instance, if a product has a 36-month shelf-life with a stability limit of no more than 3% degradation, the theoretical slope of the regression line can be calculated. A proposed biosimilar product should not exhibit a higher degradation rate than predicted theoretically, even if the reference product demonstrates a higher rate that compromises the projected expiration dating.

Developers must recognize that stability data for proposed biosimilar products are instrumental in identifying structural differences in the protein structure, along with other factors contributing to degradation. Forced degradation studies hold particular significance as they highlight the stability of finer structures within the molecule.

5.4.3 INTERNATIONAL COUNCIL FOR HARMONISATION

The regulatory guidance describes considerations for Chemistry, Manufacturing, and Controls (CMC) information to assess the similarity of a proposed biosimilar product to the reference product. All product applications must include a complete CMC section providing necessary information (such as characterization, safety from adventitious agents, process controls, and specifications) to support the consistent delivery of a product with intended quality characteristics. Several ICH guidelines (Table 5.2) are relevant to presenting this guideline. However, Agencies are not obligated to accept recommendations from these guidelines.

5.4.4 EXAMPLES OF TESTING METHODS

Developers are advised to create a comprehensive testing protocol based on the product's nature. Below is a suggested test list for physicochemical and biological assessment of TNF alpha-blockers (Table 5.3) and oncology antibodies (Table 5.4).

ADCC: antibody-dependent cell-mediated cytotoxicity; AlphaScreen® and AlphaLISA® (amplified luminescent proximity homogeneous assay) are bead-based assay technologies used to study biomolecular interactions in a microplate format; CD: circular dichroism; CDC: complement-dependent cytotoxicity; CE-SDS: capillary electrophoresis–sodium dodecyl sulphate; CEX-HPLC: cation exchange–high-performance liquid chromatography; DSC: differential scanning calorimetry; FcRn: neonatal Fc receptors; FRET: fluorescence resonance energy transfer; Gal: galactosylated glycans; HDX-MS: hydrogen–deuterium mass spectrometry; HILIC-UPLC: hydrophilic interaction liquid chromatography–ultra-performance liquid chromatography; HMW: high molecular weight; icIEF: imaging capillary isoelectric focusing; ITF: intrinsic fluorescence spectroscopy; LC-ESIMS: liquid chromatography–electrospray ionization–mass spectrometry; LC/MS: liquid chromatography–mass spectrometry; LC-ESI-MS/MS: liquid chromatography–electrospray ionization–tandem mass spectrometry; PBMCs: peripheral blood mononuclear cells;

TABLE 5.2
Pertinent ICH Guidelines for Biosimilars

ICH guidance for industry M4: The CTD —Quality (ICH M4Q) (August 2001)

ICH guidance for industry Q1A(R2) Stability Testing of New Drug Substances and Products (ICH Q1A(R2)) (November 2003)

ICH guidance for industry Q2(R1) Validation of Analytical Procedures: Text and Methodology (ICH Q2(R1) (November 2005)

ICH guidance for industry Q2B Validation of Analytical Procedures: Methodology (ICH Q2B) (May 1997)

ICH guidance for industry Q3A(R) Impurities in New Drug Substances (ICH Q3A(R)) (June 2008)

ICH guidance for industry Q5A Viral Safety Evaluation of Biotechnology Products Derived from Cell Lines of Human or Animal Origin (ICH Q5A) (September 1998)

ICH guidance for industry Q5B Quality of Biotechnological Products: Analysis of the Expression Construct in Cells Used for Production of r-DNA-Derived Protein Products (ICH Q5B) (February 1996)

ICH guidance for industry Q5C Quality of Biotechnological Products: Stability Testing of Biotechnological/Biological Products (ICH Q5C) (July 1996)

ICH guidance for industry Q5D Quality of Biotechnological/ Biological Products: Derivation and Characterization of Cell Substrates Used for Production of Biotechnological/ Biological Products (ICH Q5D) (September 1998)

ICH guidance for industry Q5E Comparability of Biotechnological/Biological Products Subject to Changes in Their Manufacturing Process (ICH Q5E) (June 2005)

ICH guidance for industry Q6B Specifications: Test Procedures and Acceptance Criteria for Biotechnological/ Biological Products (ICH Q6B) (August 1999)

ICH guidance for industry Q7 Good Manufacturing Practice Guidance for Active Pharmaceutical Ingredients (ICH Q7) (September 2016)

ICH guidance for industry Q8(R2) Pharmaceutical Development (ICH Q8(R2)) (November 2009)

ICH guidance for industry Q9 Quality Risk Management (ICH Q9) (June 2006)

ICH guidance for industry Q10 Pharmaceutical Quality System (ICH Q10) (April 2009)

ICH guidance for industry Q11 Development and Manufacture of Drug Substances (ICH Q11) (November 2012)

ICH guidance for industry S6(R1) Preclinical Safety Evaluation of Biotechnology-Derived Pharmaceuticals (ICH S6(R1)) (May 2012)

SEC: size exclusion chromatography; SEC-MALLS/RI: size exclusion chromatography–multi-angle laser light scattering/refractive index; SPR: surface plasmon resonance; SV-AUC: sedimentation velocity analytical ultracentrifugation; UV: ultraviolet; UV/VIS: ultraviolet visible.

5.4.5 RISK ASSESSMENT

Developers are recommended to create a risk assessment tool to evaluate and rank the reference product's quality attributes concerning their potential impact on the mechanism(s) of action and product function. Certain quality evaluations of the reference product (e.g., degradation rates determined from stability or forced degradation studies) generally should not be part of the risk ranking. However, these evaluations should still be considered in the comparative analytical assessment of a proposed biosimilar product and the reference product.

The development of a risk assessment tool should take into account various pertinent factors, including:

- Potential Impact on Clinical Performance: It is advised that the developer carefully considers how an attribute may impact activity, PK/PD, safety, efficacy, and immunogenicity. This evaluation should draw from publicly available information and the developer's assessment of the reference product.

TABLE 5.3
Quality Attribute Testing for Monoclonal Antibodies (TNF-α Blockers)

Category	Product Quality Attributes	Analytical Attributes
Physicochemical characterization		
Primary structure	Molecular weight	Intact mass under reducing/non-reducing
	Amino acid sequence	conditions.
	Terminal sequence	Peptide mapping by LC-ESI-MS/MS using a
	Methionine oxidation	combination of digestion enzymes.
	Deamidation	Peptide mapping under non-reducing conditions
	C-terminal and N-terminal variants	
	Disulfide linkage mapping	
Higher-order structure	Protein secondary and tertiary	Far- and near-UV CD spectroscopy, ITF
	structures	HDX-MS, antibody conformational array
		DSC
Glycosylation	N-linked glycosylation site	LC-ESI-MS/MS
	determination	Procainamide-labeling and LC-ESI-MS/MS
	N-glycan identification	2-AB labeling and HILIC-UPLC
	N-glycan profile analysis	
Aggregation	Soluble aggregates	SEC-UV, SEC-MALLS/RI SV-AUC
Fragmentation	Low molecular weight	Non-reduced CE-SDS
		Reduced CE-SDS
Charge heterogeneity	Acidic variants	CEX-HPLC and icIEF
	Basic variants	
Biological characterization		
Fab-related biological	TNF-α neutralization activity	TNF-α neutralization assay by nuclear factor-κB
activity	TNF-α binding activity	reporter gene assay
	Apoptosis activity	FRET
	Transmembrane TNF-α binding assay	Cell-based assay
		FACS
Fc-related biological	FcRn binding	AlphaScreen®
activity	FcγRIIIa (V/V type) binding	SPR
	ADCC using healthy donor PBMCs	Cell-based assay
	CDC	Cell-based assay
	C1q binding	ELISA
	FcγRIa binding	FRET
	FcγRIIa binding	SPR
	FcγRIIb binding	SPR
	FcγRIIIb binding	SPR

Notes: 2-AB, 2-aminobenzamide; AUC, analytical ultracentrifugation; CD, circular dichroism; DSC, differential scanning calorimetry; ELISA, enzyme-linked immunosorbent assay; FACE, fluorescence-activated cell sorting; PBMC, peripheral blood mononuclear cell; SPR, surface plasmon resonance; SV, sedimentation velocity; TNF, tumor necrosis factor; UV, ultraviolet.

- The degree of uncertainty surrounding a certain quality attribute: When there is limited understanding regarding the correlation between changes in an attribute and its clinical implications, that attribute should be ranked with higher risk due to the associated uncertainties.
- Classification of high-risk attributes: Any attribute deemed high risk concerning performance categories (activity, PK/PD, safety, efficacy, and immunogenicity) should be classified accordingly. The risk assessment tool should ideally present a prioritized list of attributes based on patient risk. Risk scores for attributes should correspond to the level of patient risk. It is crucial

TABLE 5.4
Testing Methods for Oncology Monoclonal Antibodies

Category	Attribute (Method or Methods to Query That Attribute)
Primary structure	Primary sequence (e.g., UPLC peptide map, LC-MS/MS, amino acid analysis, Edman degradation, carboxypeptidase sequencing)
	Disulfide structure (e.g., LC-MS of nonreduced protein digest)
	Intact mass (e.g., LC-MS)
	Isoelectric point (e.g., IEF gels, cIEF, iCE)
	Extinction coefficient (e.g., UV/AAA or UV/RI)
Secondary and tertiary structures	Low-resolution secondary structure or indirect tertiary structure measurements (e.g., CD, DSC, FTIR, fluorescence)
	High-resolution measurements of higher-order structure (e.g., 2D-NMR, HDX-MS, X-ray crystallography)
Glycosylation	Glycosylation (e.g., HILIC, MS (MALDI, ESI), exoglycosidase sequencing, HPLC-FLD, HPAEC-PAD, CE-LIF)
	Glycosylation site mapping/site occupancy (e.g., peptide mapping by LC-MS)
Dose	Protein content (e.g., UV A280, RP-HPLC)
	Deliverable volume (extractable volume)
Particulates	Sub-visible particles (e.g., light obscuration, MFI, NTA)
Function	Biological activity (e.g., for mAb: proliferative bioassay, cytotoxicity assay, ADCC, and CDC; other assays may be appropriate for other proteins, e.g., enzyme kinetics for the proposed biosimilar enzyme)
	Receptor and ligand binding (e.g., SPR, ELISA)
Product variants (product-related substances and impurities)	High-molecular-weight species (e.g., SEC-MALS, AF4/HF5, AUC, DLS)
	Covalent dimers (e.g., SDS-PAGE, CE-SDS)
	Purity and impurities (oxidation, deamidation, glycation, isomerization, fragmentation, disulfide reduction, e.g., RP-HPLC, CEX, SEC, IEX, IEF, cIEF, LC-MS)
	Amino acid misincorporations (e.g., LC-MS/MS)
	Micro-sequence heterogeneity (e.g., LC-MS)
	C- and N-terminal modifications (e.g., LC-MS, Edman degradation)

Notes: AUC, analytical ultracentrifugation; CD, circular dichroism; DSC, differential scanning calorimetry; HPLC, high-performance liquid chromatography; LC, liquid chromatography; MS, mass spectroscopy; RP, reverse phase; SPR, surface plasmon resonance; SDS-PAGE, sodium sulfate polyacrylamide gel electrophoresis.

that the criteria used for scoring in the risk assessment are explicitly defined and justified. Justification for the risk ranking of each attribute should be supported with relevant citations from literature and data.

5.4.6 STATISTICAL CONSIDERATIONS

The evaluation of biosimilarity predominantly relies on statistical considerations. For clarity and to illustrate how regulatory bodies interpret data, Table 5.5 presents statistical concepts as they pertain to biosimilarity testing.

5.4.7 QUANTITATIVE AND QUALITATIVE DATA ANALYSES

Thorough analyses of comparative analytical data are essential to demonstrate the similarity between a proposed biosimilar and the reference product, accounting for minor differences in clinically

TABLE 5.5
Statistical Concepts Applied to Biosimilarity Determination

Subject	Definition and Concepts Applicable to Biosimilarity Testing
A stepwise Analytical Assessment	Evaluate quality attributes consistent with the risk assessment principles of the ICH Quality Guidelines Q8, Q9, Q10, and Q11. Consider criticality risk ranking of quality attributes concerning their potential impact on activity, PK/PD, safety, and immunogenicity. Use a selective approach for assessment: Equivalence interval testing for some critical attributes ($K*\sigma R+\Delta$) and the default value of Δ is zero. The equivalence margin can be determined by a proposed sample size/power adjusted method. Quality ranges (mean $\pm K*SD$) for other less critical attributes; X= ≤3 unless otherwise justified to be higher. The quality range can be determined by Mean $\pm K \times SD$, where $K = 2\text{-}3$ based on the targeted coverage; quality range tests will also assess all proposed biosimilar lots used in equivalence tests; 90% of proposed biosimilar lots need to be within the quality range. Raw/graphical comparisons for other least critical attributes. Graphic data displays are a useful tool to identify the potential issues with statistical methods listed above.
Significance level (also called "Size of a Test")	The size of a test, often called the significance level, is the probability of committing a Type I error. A Type I error occurs when a null hypothesis is rejected when it is true. This test size is denoted by α (alpha). The $1-\alpha$ is called the confidence level, which is used in the form of the $(1-\alpha)*100$ percent confidence interval of a parameter.

Reality of attribute	Conclusions about attribute	Description
Not similar	Similar	Type I error: patient (or regulatory) risk (α)
Similar	Not similar	Type II error: the developer's risk (β)
Similar	Similar	Power ($1\text{-}\beta$)

Confidence level	The confidence level refers to the percentage of all possible samples that can be expected to include the true population parameter. For example, suppose all available samples were selected from the same population, and a confidence interval was computed for each sample. A 90% confidence level implies that 90% of the confidence intervals would include the true population parameter. The confidence level can be lowered in some instances, and according to the literature reports, the lowest confidence level that it is recommended to evaluate analytical similarity is approximately 80%.
Confidence interval	The confidence interval expresses the degree of uncertainty associated with a sample statistic. A confidence interval is an interval estimate combined with a probability statement. For example, suppose an analysis allows the computation of an interval estimate; a confidence level will describe the uncertainty associated with the interval estimate. One may describe the interval estimate as a "90% confidence interval." This means that if we used the same sampling method to select different samples and computed an interval estimate for each sample, we would expect the true population parameter to fall within the interval estimates 90% of the time.
Statistical power	Statistical power is a function of the sample size, the effect size, and the probability level chosen:

Statistical Power

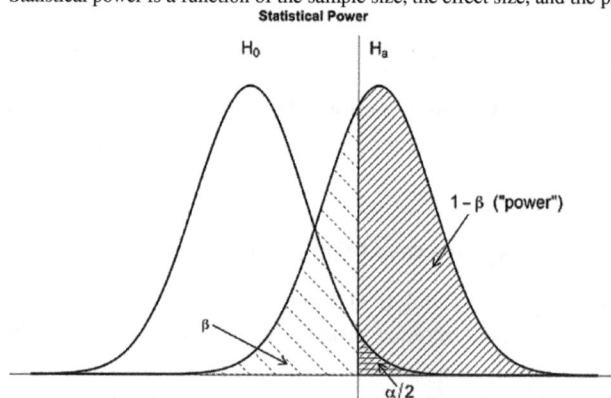

TABLE 5.5 (Continued)
Statistical Concepts Applied to Biosimilarity Determination

Subject	Definition and Concepts Applicable to Biosimilarity Testing
Equivalence interval model	To meet the "equivalence interval" most critical quality attributes, a two one-sided t-test (TOST) should be used for testing if the two-sided 90% confidence interval of the mean differences between a proposed biosimilar product and the reference product falls entirely within K*σR (σR is the population standard deviation of the lots of the reference product that is estimated by the sample standard deviation ($\widehat{\sigma}_R$) from the reference lots been tested.) Enough lots must be used to reach at least 80% statistical power. TOST for testing the hypothesis is represented as follows:

$H_0: \mu_B - \mu_R \leq -\delta$ or $\mu_B - \mu_R \geq \delta$
$H_a: -\delta < \mu_B - \mu_R < -\delta$

where μB and μR are the mean responses of a proposed biosimilar product and reference product lots, respectively, and δ > 0 is the equivalence margin. If the null hypothesis is accepted, the equivalence will be rejected.

$$H_0 \quad \mu_B - \mu_R \leq -\delta \text{ or } \mu_B - \mu_R \geq \delta$$
$$H_a \quad -\delta < \mu_B - \mu_R < \delta$$

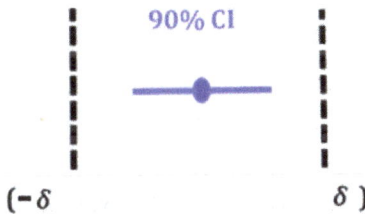

Statistical Equivalence Testing

Quality range model	The reference product data define the quality range for a specific quality attribute as $(\hat{\mu}_R - K * \hat{\sigma}_R, \hat{\mu}_R \hat{\sigma}_R)$ where r $\hat{\mu}_R$ Is the sample mean, a $\hat{\sigma}_R$ Is is the sample standard deviation based on the reference product lots. The standard deviation multiplier (K) should be scientifically justified for that attribute. The statistical analysis will generally support analytical similarity for the quality attribute if a sufficient percentage of test lot values (e.g., 90%) falls within the quality range. For establishing the scientific justification for the standard deviation multiplier (K), the two-sided tolerance intervals of the univariate normal distribution are used to calculate the multiplier K. The following equation estimates K with the given confidence (1–α) and a targeted portion (P) of the univariate normal distribution:

$$Pr_{\bar{X},S} \{ Pr_X (\bar{X} - kS < X < \bar{X} + kS \mid \bar{X}, s) > P \} = 1 - \alpha$$

For a sample size N=10 per product, the two-sided tolerance interval of 90% coverage for the distribution is 2.86 at the 95% confidence level. If the significant digit for an attribute reported at one decimal, set the tier multiplier as 2.9 (generally 3.0) in this study to cover 90% of the reference product distribution at N=10 per group. That is, the quality range is $(\hat{\mu}_R - 2.9 * \hat{\sigma}_R, \hat{\mu}_R \hat{\sigma}_R)$ if 90% lot values fall within the quality range.

The errors in mean ±3SD method for quality ranges

(μ-3σ, μ+3σ) = (-3, 3)	N = 6	N = 30	N = 100
Simulation 1	(−4.3, 4.4) too wide!	(−3.4, 3.6)	(−3.1, 3.3)
Simulation 2	(−1.4, 2.0) too tight!	(−3.2, 3.1)	(−3.0, 2.9)

(continued)

TABLE 5.5 (Continued)
Statistical Concepts Applied to Biosimilarity Determination

Subject	Definition and Concepts Applicable to Biosimilarity Testing
	It is possible that either the equivalence margin or and equivalence range may fail or vice versa. Products with similar standard deviation but different means may fail the equivalence range test but nor equivalence margin. For products where the means are the same, but the standard deviations are not, they may fail equivalence margin but not equivalence testing.
Fixed margin approach	The fixed margin approach used for bioequivalence testing used the fixed margin ($\delta 1$, $\delta 2$) = (0.80, 1.25) or (0.90, 1.11) for the ratio of means regardless of the variability of the tested CQAs. The testing requires a different number of lots for different CQA. However, this approach may lead to equivalence with the out-of-specification product. The margins are based on scientists' prior knowledge, which may require excessively large EAC by sponsors to assess the equivalence of a small number of the lot (e.g., a few lots) that may be highly variable. Note that after decades of scientific discussions, the 80%–125% limits of bioequivalence testing were adopted, admitting that there is not any real scientific rationale, except that it has been shown to work. Lately, there is a focus on the scaled average bioequivalence, wherein the standard deviation of the reference product determines the acceptance criteria.
Sample size and variance approach	The sample size and variance come from selecting an equivalence testing hypothesis:

$$H_o : \mu_T - \mu_R \leq \delta \text{ or } \mu_T - \mu_R > \delta$$

$$H_a : -\delta < \mu_T - \mu_R - < \delta$$

	Now we give lower power γ^* (for target equivalence) to small sample sizes and solve for (symmetric) Margin so that Power (Margin, Sample Sizes, True Mean Diff, Variability) = γ^*.
	The rationale for this approach is that it captures the product and quality attribute variability, allows an acceptable shift $\delta_0 \geq 0$, determined by scientists for each CQA, and rewards large sample sizes by controlling small samples' power.
Minimum to maximum approach	The quality criterion regarding coverage cannot be defined using this approach as it is unstable for small sample sizes and too wide for large sample sizes. For these reasons, Agencies reject this approach.
Raw and graphical comparisons	This testing method involves an approach that uses raw data/graphical comparisons for quality attributes with the lowest risk ranking. The examination of similarity for QAs using this method by no means is less stringent, which is acceptable because they have the least impact on clinical outcomes in the sense that a notable dissimilarity will not affect clinical outcomes. Depending on the nature of the testing output, if a numerical output is a result of graphical output, this method of testing must always be made; a fluorescence spectrum is tested on this basis, and the maximum emission wavelength or its ratio with 310 nm can be subjected to an equivalence range level testing.
	There is no guarantee that a given QA, which passes the equivalence margin or equivalence range test will pass this testing test and vice versa. Evaluation is based on raw data and graphical presentation; it is somewhat subjective and biased.
Number of lots	The number of lots tested side-by-side selected will depend on three factors:
	The power of testing is accepted; generally, like the bioequivalence testing, and 80% (0.80) power will be acceptance.
	Confidence level; generally, it is taken to be 5% giving CL of 0.90.
	Standard deviation: Large standard deviations can be reduced either by increasing the number of lots or by adjusting the analytical methods that are less variable.

TABLE 5.5 (Continued)
Statistical Concepts Applied to Biosimilarity Determination

Subject	Definition and Concepts Applicable to Biosimilarity Testing
	It is recommended that the developers include at least 6 to 10 lots of a proposed biosimilar product in the comparative analytical assessment to ensure 1) adequate characterization of a proposed biosimilar product and understanding of manufacturing variability, and 2) adequate comparison to the reference product should include lots manufactured with the investigational–and commercial-scale process and may include validation lots, as well as product lots manufactured at different scales, including engineering lots. These lots should be representative of the intended commercial manufacturing process. If there is a manufacturing process change pre-authorization, it may be possible, witan h adequate scientific justification, to use data generated from lots manufactured with a different process. However, data should be provided in the authorization application to support drug substance and drug products manufactured with different processes and scales. The extent of process development design (as described in guidelines ICH Q8 (R2) Pharmaceutical Development and ICH Q11 Development and Manufacture of Drug Substances) and process understanding should be used in support of the number of proposed biosimilar product lots proposed for inclusion in the comparative analytical assessment in the application. The ICH Q5 does not apply.
	The number of lots used is more critical when statistical modeling is used to compare a proposed biosimilar product with the RP; the statistical model may including using an equivalence interval or an equivalence range where applicable; in such instances, the power of the test is important as derived from the following equation: $Power(n_B) = 1 - \exp(-0.53948 - 0.14694n_B + 0.00205n^2{}_B)$ Equation 1 [Niazi, S. Biosimilarity—The FDA Perspective, CRC Press, Orlando, Florida 2018.] Using four lots will give a power of 65%, ten lots to give 85% power, and 20 lots allow the power of 92 percent. Generally, a power of 80% is recommended. Since not all testing is conducted using statistical approaches, fewer lots may be sufficient for some testing.
Types of lots	To the extent possible, proposed biosimilar lots included in the comparative analytical assessment should be derived from different drug substance lots to adequately represent the variability of attributes inherent to the drug substance manufacturing process. Drug product lots derived from the same drug substance batch(es) are not considered sufficiently representative of such variability, except for use in testing certain drug product attributes for which variability is mostly dependent on the drug product manufacturing process (e.g., protein concentration). Although it may be preferable to compare a proposed biosimilar product lots to the reference product lots, it may be acceptable also to include independent drug substance lots (if the drug substance was not used to make drug product), if needed, to attain enough of lots for the comparative analytical assessment.
	The comparative analytical assessment submitted with the marketing application to support the demonstration of biosimilarity of a proposed biosimilar product to the reference product should include lots of a proposed biosimilar product used in a principal clinical study, as well as a proposed commercial product. After completing the initial comparative analytical assessment or after completing clinical studies intended to support an application, the developers considering manufacturing changes may need to conduct additional comparative analytical studies of a proposed biosimilar product and the reference product. The nature and extent of the changes may determine the extent of these additional analytical studies.
Replicates	It is recommended that the same number of replicates be performed within each proposed biosimilar lot as within each reference product lot and that the same lots be used for equivalence testing, quality range testing, and visual assessment of graphical displays.

(*continued*)

TABLE 5.5 (Continued)
Statistical Concepts Applied to Biosimilarity Determination

Subject	Definition and Concepts Applicable to Biosimilarity Testing
Equal number side-by-side	There should be an equal number of lots when tested side-by-side. Suppose there are more lots available for reference. In that case, an unbiased selection should be made to select the equal number, and the rest can be used separately to develop the range acceptance criteria. This recommendation is challengeable once we demonstrate sufficient power of the test. If the number of samples of the reference product is higher, this will lead to a smaller standard deviation and a larger difference range that may cause the test to fail because of β error. The critical minimum number of lots tested side-by-side is approximately 8; however, if there is an unbalanced selection between test and reference, a higher number may be required.
Unbalanced samples	Samples of reference and test products are blinded before the testing of analytical similarity; if the reference samples to test out of specification, these are to be removed from the statistical calculation, creating an unbalanced design since Agencies requires an equal number of samples of test and reference product to be tested side by side. How can this be resolved?
	The developers should remove an equivalent number of test samples through a randomization process; this process must be presented in the analytical testing SOP and properly documented. It is important that if the reference product fails one attribute and is declared out of specification, other values drawn from that samples can not be used, even if they are not affected by the out of specification reading for one attribute. This exercise will create a situation where the test's power is reduced; to overcome this possibility, the developers should try to start with a larger number of samples, such as 11 instead of 10, if the target is ten samples. The developers may also adopt a procedure wherein the reference samples are tested before being blinded to avoid this situation. However, the selection and blinding of the reference product must still be made on a random basis.
Blinding	Before conducting the side-by-side analytical similarity testing, the developers would create a protocol that will include all acceptance criteria and blind the test and reference samples; where a larger number of samples are available, this will be preceded by a random selection of lots. However, when establishing EAC or other acceptance attributes using a separate set of lots, there is no need for blinding the reference samples.
Combining lots	Biosimilar, the developer, conducts several biosimilarity studies at different stages and accordingly conducts analytical and functional similarity testing; can these lots be combined to provide a composite description instead of one study?
Mixed graphic and numerical data	Some testing provides a graphical output, but the peak height and area under the peak curve can be quantitated. Whenever there is a graphical output, it should demonstrate no extraordinary peak, no extraordinary heights of the peaks, and no extraordinary baseline—this is an overall evaluation of the graphical output; however, where the peaks have known significance relating to potency, purity, and safety, and as a result, the quantifiable graphical attributes have clinical meaningfulness, these can be compared for equivalence margin and equivalence range analysis; for visual testing, there is no further need to perform any quantitative evaluation. However, if the numerical comparisons do not have any clinical relevance, a graphical representation alone would be sufficient, regardless of the attribute.
Significant figures	Before subjecting the data to statistical analysis, it must be rounded off to match the analytical method's sensitivity, instrument sensitivity, and other factors. For example, if a balance is sensitive to 0.1 gram, the weight, all weight values will be rounded off to one decimal point: 1.09 becomes 1.1 and 1.02 becomes 1.0; another approach is to express significance to a percentage of the value. For example, a method sensitive to giving $\pm 1\%$ will have the following values: 1.00; 10.0; 100.

inactive components. There exist multiple approaches to analyze the significance of analytical data. Regulatory bodies expect developers to possess comprehensive knowledge of statistical techniques and to provide justification for the chosen statistical modeling. Any observed differences in clinical response between the proposed biosimilar and the reference product are attributed to the variability in critical quality attributes (CQAs). This premise forms the basis for identifying CQAs, considering the wide dose-response relationship in biological products. Consequently, any modeling must factor in these possibilities.

One viable approach to data analysis involves employing descriptive quality ranges for evaluating quantitative quality attributes of high and moderate risk. For attributes ranked with lower risk or those that cannot be quantitatively measured (e.g., primary sequence), raw data and graphical comparisons could be used.

Acceptance criteria for the quality ranges (QR) method in comparative analytical assessments should be derived from the developer's analysis of the reference product for a specific quality attribute. The QR should be defined as the sample mean ( ), where is the sample standard deviation based on the reference product lots. The multiplier (X) must be scientifically justified and discussed with regulatory bodies. Tolerance intervals are discouraged for establishing similarity acceptance criteria due to the need for an extensive number of lots, as per our current experience. Developers can propose alternative data analysis methods, including equivalence testing.

The main objective of comparative analytical assessment is to confirm that each attribute observed in both the proposed biosimilar product and the reference product shares a similar population mean and standard deviation. Comparing a quality attribute typically supports the conclusion that a proposed biosimilar product is akin to the reference product when a substantial percentage of the proposed biosimilar lot values (e.g., 90%) fall within the defined QR for that attribute. It is advisable to apply narrower acceptance criteria in the (e.g., a lower X value) QR method for higher-risk quality attributes.

Apart from risk ranking, other considerations should influence the choice of quantitative data analysis for an attribute or assay. Additional factors to contemplate in determining the appropriate type of data evaluation and result analysis include

- Nature of the Attribute: Attributes identified as high risk should take precedence over attributes with unknown but potentially high risk due to uncertainties.
- Distribution of the Attribute: Generally, it is recommended that the manufacturing process aims to closely match the distribution centers of the reference product's quality attributes. Thus, the QR, assuming similar population means and standard deviation, serves as an appropriate approach to demonstrate similarity between the proposed biosimilar and the reference product. Any concerns about distribution may necessitate further information or analyses to support the QR method or alternative analysis approaches. For instance, if the distribution of an attribute in a proposed biosimilar product is skewed compared to the reference product, depending on the attribute's nature and role in the product's mechanism of action, it might raise concerns. In such cases, appropriate scientific justification would be necessary to support the comparative analytical assessment. When an attribute in the reference product has a non-normal distribution, developers should engage with regulatory bodies for guidance.
- Attribute abundance: The inherent variability within protein products means that attributes posing high risks in instances of high abundance (e.g., percent aggregation or oxidation) might present significantly lower or negligible risks when occurring in low abundance. It's essential to confirm the attribute's abundance in both the reference product (as determined by the proposed biosimilar product, developer's analysis of the RP) and the proposed biosimilar product. While limit assays don't always require QR evaluation, it is crucial to define and justify the selected limits for the attribute amount, considering its changes over time.

- Assay Sensitivity in Attribute Assessment: Although using multiple assays is encouraged, not all need the same evaluation approach. The most sensitive assay for detecting product differences should undergo QR evaluation, while others assessing the same attribute may use graphical comparisons. A rationale must be provided for each assay's chosen evaluation method.
- Attributes/Assays Types: Certain attributes or assays (e.g., protein sequence, certain higher-order structure evaluation assays, or solely qualitative assays) may not be suitable for quantitative analysis. The comparative analytical assessment plan should clearly identify these assays exempt from quantitative data analysis, along with the rationale for this exclusion.
- Utilizing Publicly Available Information: Publicly available information can influence the data analysis type and acceptance criteria in the comparative analytical assessment. Developers should seek guidance from Agencies regarding the inclusion of such information in their assessments.

Qualitative Analysis Recommendations: For lower-risk attributes, conducting qualitative analyses, presenting side-by-side data (e.g., spectra, thermograms, graphical data representations), is recommended. This method facilitates visual comparison between the proposed biosimilar product and the reference product. It is particularly useful for assays such as NMR, mass spectrometry, and biological activity, intended solely for analytical assessment and not product release validation.

5.4.7.1 Risk Ranking

The final comparative analytical assessment plan must include risk ranking for attributes, the type of data evaluation for each attribute/assay, and the final data analysis plan. It should specify the expected availability of proposed biosimilar and reference product lots for evaluating each attribute/assay and provide a rationale for why a specific number of lots is sufficient for evaluation. The comparative analytical assessment plan should be discussed with regulatory agencies as early as possible in the proposed biosimilar product development program to agree on the attributes/assays for evaluation. This final plan should be submitted to agencies before initiating the final analytical assessments, typically in a meeting with them. Developers must finalize and approve an analytical evaluation plan before commencing testing, which will include acceptance and rejection criteria.

5.4.7.2 Assay Variability

A high assay variability should not warrant a large σR. In such cases, optimizing the assay and increasing the number of replicates can help reduce variability. Also, when equivalence margins or quality ranges are excessively broad, it might be scientifically justified to narrow them. In instances where data do not adhere to a normal distribution, sponsors may opt for a non-parametric tolerance interval, but this generally requires a large sample size.

Determining an acceptable high variability is challenging, but several guiding principles can help. First, it involves assessing instrumentation variability—is there better equipment available? Second, understanding the limit of critical quality attribute (CQA) variability is essential. For instance, many pharmacodynamic responses inherently entail high variability in biological testing systems, similar to bioassays or binding assays (often tested for equivalence range). For example, if literature, especially the originator data reports, confirm a variability of ±30%, that could be considered the limit to achieve. Developers might consider using tests beyond those prescribed in the compendia or routine testing methods by adopting higher sensitivity and repeatability testing. Regulatory agencies do not make recommendations on the method to be used; it must be justified and shown to be appropriate and suitable. Later, it can be validated for release purposes. Replicate analysis of samples can reduce variability; however, agencies typically disallow multiple samples from the same lot.

5.4.8 Functional Assessments

Most biological products interact with the body in specific ways, such as binding to receptors, ligands, or substrates. The resulting effects are usually detectable at a molecular or cellular level. In vitro assays using human cells or receptors are commonly used to evaluate both the binding to the target and the subsequent functional effects, aiding in the characterization of structure and function. For monoclonal antibodies (mAbs), besides binding to the primary target's complementarity determining region (CDR), the Fc portion also contains binding sites for different receptors, potentially triggering various effector functions like complement activation, complement-dependent cytotoxicity (CDC), and antibody-dependent cell-mediated cytotoxicity (ADCC). Evaluating these Fc-related binding properties and effector functions can also be done in vitro.

5.4.9 Orthogonal Studies

Data from many comparative in vitro studies, some of which may already be available from quality-related assays, should normally be provided to assess the possible potential differences in biological activity between a proposed biosimilar product and the reference product.

These studies should cover relevant assays including:

- Binding to known target(s) (e.g., receptors, antigens, enzymes) involved in the pharmacological effects and pharmacokinetics of the reference product.
- Signal transduction, functional activity, or viability of cells relevant to the pharmacological effects of the reference product.
- These studies need to be comparative and not solely focused on assessing the response itself. To ensure clear results, appropriate methods suitable for their purpose should be used. These test methods do not need to be validated.

They should be sensitive, specific, and sufficiently discriminatory to demonstrate that observed differences in quality attributes are not clinically relevant. Comparing the concentration–activity/binding relationship of the proposed biosimilar product and the reference product at pharmacological targets is essential, particularly across a concentration range where potential differences are most sensitively detected.

5.4.9.1 Lots Tested

It is crucial to conduct testing using an adequate number of lots of both the reference and proposed biosimilar products, representing the intended material for clinical use. The number of lots tested should account for assay and batch-to-lot variability. It should be enough to draw meaningful conclusions regarding variability and similarity between the proposed biosimilar and the reference product. While it's generally recommended to use 6–10 lots to achieve suitable test power, assays providing non-quantitative data may be conducted on a smaller lot size. However, it is important to acknowledge that using fewer lots increases the risk of lot failure.

These assays should collectively cover the entire range of pharmacological and toxicological aspects relevant for both the reference product and the product class. In many cases, in vitro assays can detect differences between a proposed biosimilar product and the reference product more effectively than animal studies. Hence, these assays are crucial for the non-clinical comparative evaluation of proposed biosimilars.

Functional assays play a vital role in characterizing protein products, complementing physicochemical analyses, and quantifying the functional aspects of the protein.

If the reference product demonstrates multiple functional activities, developers must conduct a suitable set of assays to assess the spectrum of pertinent activities associated with that product.

For instance, proteins with various functional domains exhibiting enzymatic and receptor-mediated activities should have both activities evaluated if relevant to the product's performance. For products where functional activity can be measured by different parameters (e.g., enzyme kinetics or interactions with blood clotting factors), a comparative characterization of each parameter between products is essential.

Developers should acknowledge potential limitations in certain types of functional assays, such as high variability, which could hinder the detection of significant differences between a proposed biosimilar and the reference product. As highly variable assays may not meaningfully determine biosimilarity, developers are advised to create less variable assays that are sensitive to changes in product functional activities. Additionally, in vitro bioactivity assays might not fully predict the clinical activity of the protein. These assays typically do not forecast the product's bioavailability (pharmacokinetics and biodistribution), which can influence pharmacodynamics and clinical performance. Differences in glycoform distribution or other post-translational modifications can significantly alter bioavailability. Hence, these limitations should be considered while evaluating data quality supporting biosimilarity, potentially necessitating additional information to address uncertainties. Lastly, functional assays are crucial for detecting neutralizing antibodies in nonclinical and clinical studies.

When protein product activity involves binding, analytical tests should characterize a proposed biosimilar product based on its specific binding properties. For instance, if binding to a receptor is inherent to the protein's function, this property must be measured and utilized in comparative studies.

Several methods such as surface plasmon resonance, microcalorimetry, or classical Scatchard analysis can offer insights into the kinetics and thermodynamics of binding. This information can be correlated with the functional activity and characterization of a proposed biosimilar product's higher-order structure.

5.5   IN VIVO ASSESSMENT

It is a well-established scientific fact that biotechnology-derived proteins may induce in vivo effects that cannot be fully understood through in vitro studies alone. Consequently, non-clinical in vivo evaluations may be necessary to provide complementary information, contingent upon the availability of a pertinent in vivo model pertaining to species or design.

5.5.1   DETERMINATION OF THE NEEDS FOR IN VIVO STUDIES

Various factors should be taken into account when evaluating the need for non-clinical in vivo studies, including but not limited to:

- Identification of potentially relevant quality attributes that have not been identified in the reference product (e.g., new post-translational modification structures).
- Recognition of potentially significant quantitative disparities in quality attributes between a proposed biosimilar product and the reference product.
- Notable differences in formulation, such as the utilization of excipients uncommonly used for biotechnology-derived proteins.
- While the aforementioned factors may not inherently mandate in vivo testing, a holistic consideration of these issues is crucial to gauge the level of concern and ascertain the necessity for in vivo studies.
- If a proposed biosimilar product, following a comparative analysis of its physicochemical and biological characteristics alongside satisfactory non-clinical in vitro studies, assures human safety in testing, an in vivo animal study may be deemed unnecessary.

- In scenarios where product-inherent factors impacting pharmacokinetics (PK) and biodistribution—like extensive glycosylation—cannot be adequately characterized at the quality and in vitro level, in vivo studies might be indispensable. In such instances, developers should meticulously weigh the need for performing these studies in animals or as part of clinical testing, e.g., involving healthy volunteers.
- When additional in vivo information is required, the availability of a relevant animal species or other pertinent models (e.g., transgenic animals, transplant models) should be considered.
- Should a pertinent in vivo animal model not be accessible, developers may opt to progress to human studies, adhering to principles aimed at mitigating potential risks.

5.5.2 In Vivo Animal Studies

Animal toxicology studies have been omitted, but this doesn't entirely eliminate the potential need for animal testing, although such instances are rare. This stems from the understanding that animals might lack the receptors necessary to elicit a pharmacological response from therapeutic proteins, which is pivotal in determining toxicological and clinical responses. Nonetheless, several agencies, such as those in India, persist in requiring animal toxicology studies. For instance, in India, an excessively high dose, 4 to 5 times the human dose, is administered to establish safety, constituting a wholly wasteful exercise.

If an in vivo evaluation becomes necessary, the study's focus (pharmacokinetics, pharmacodynamics, and safety) hinges on the requirement for additional information. Animal studies should be meticulously structured to yield maximum information. The principles of the 3Rs (replacement, refinement, reduction) should be integrated into the design of any in vivo study. Depending on the endpoints used, sacrificing animals at the study's conclusion might not be essential. Justification for the study's duration (including the observation period) should be based on the reference product's pharmacokinetic behavior and its clinical utilization.

Where feasible and justifiable, a quantitative comparison between the pharmacokinetics and pharmacodynamics of a proposed biosimilar product and the reference product should be conducted, including a dose-concentration-response assessment resembling intended human exposure.

Regarding safety studies, an adaptable approach is advisable regardless of the species selected. Generally, conducting standard repeated dose toxicity studies in non-human primates is discouraged. If suitably justified, a refined design for a repeated dose toxicity study (e.g., utilizing only one dose level of the proposed biosimilar product and reference product, one gender, and no recovery animals) or an in-life assessment of safety parameters (e.g., clinical signs, body weight, vital functions) may be considered. For studies evaluating a single dose, it's usual to select the highest dose within the dosing range, requiring justification based on the expected toxicity of the reference product.

Conducting toxicity studies in species that aren't relevant (i.e., solely for assessing unspecific toxicity related to impurities) is not recommended. Due to potential differences in production processes between a proposed biosimilar product and the reference product manufacturers, there may be qualitative disparities in process-related impurities (e.g., host cell proteins). Efforts should be made to minimize these impurities, which is the most effective strategy for reducing associated risks.

Qualitative or quantitative differences in product-related variants (e.g., glycosylation patterns, charge variants) may influence the biological functions of biotechnology-derived proteins and should be evaluated using appropriate in vitro assays. These differences and impurities could impact immunogenic potential and hypersensitivity risk. Acknowledging the difficulty in predicting these effects through animal studies, further assessment in clinical studies is recommended.

While immunogenicity assessment in animals generally does not predict human immunogenicity, it might be necessary to interpret in vivo animal studies. Hence, blood samples should be collected and stored for potential future assessments of pharmacokinetic/toxicokinetic data if required.

Studies on local tolerance are typically unnecessary. However, if new excipients are introduced without prior experience in the intended clinical route of administration, evaluating local tolerance may become necessary. If other in vivo studies are conducted, assessing local tolerance might be integrated into the study's design rather than conducting separate local tolerance studies.

The results from animal studies can be utilized to bolster the safety assessment of a proposed biosimilar product. These studies can also contribute to demonstrating biosimilarity between a proposed biosimilar product and the reference product.

If there are limitations in the structural and functional data or concerns regarding the quality of a proposed biosimilar product, a general toxicology study cannot address these concerns adequately.

5.5.3 Animal Pharmacokinetics and Pharmacodynamics Measures

Under specific circumstances, a single-dose study in animals comparing a proposed biosimilar product and the reference product using PK and PD measures, if available, can contribute to the evidence supporting biosimilarity. The primary objective of evaluating PK and PD in animals is to identify structural differences between a proposed biosimilar product and the reference product. Nevertheless, animal PK and PD assessment cannot replace the need for human PK and PD studies. In most cases, PK/PD studies in primate animal species can be conducted with a small number of animals. The primary goal is not to establish statistical equivalence but to showcase an overall similarity among the tested animals.

5.5.4 Animal Immunogenicity Testing

Typically, animal immunogenicity assessments do not predict potential immune responses to protein products in humans. However, some regulatory agencies allow immunogenicity testing in animals as additional support for biosimilarity, even though some agencies assert that animal immunogenicity assessments might reveal potential structural or functional differences between a proposed biosimilar product and the reference product that are not detected by other analytical methods. There are limited examples of such studies:

- Detection of anti-Etanercept antibodies in Cynomolgus monkey serum in preclinical study 1 (under General Toxicology) using an ECL bridging immunogenicity assay. Subcutaneous administration of 1 or 15 mg/kg twice per week.
- Epoetin exhibited a higher incidence of A.D.A. (anti-drug antibodies) development in rats compared to the reference product. This occurrence is likely due to the route of administration (subcutaneous administration is more immunogenic than intravenous administration) and the presence of human serum albumin (HAS) in the reference product.
- Filgrastim was tested in rats for potentially associated immunogenicity. The study involved Sprague Dawley rats: 10 rats/sex/group + 5 rats/sex/group in control and HD for proposed biosimilar product or RP; TK Control: 6 rats/sex/group; TK 12 rats/sex/group, with doses tested at 0, 20, and 500 μg/kg administered subcutaneously daily for 29 days.
- Infliximab efficacy, pharmacokinetics, and immunogenicity were evaluated in the Tg197 transgenic mouse arthritis model. Ten treatment groups, 4/sex/group for efficacy study + 3 males/group for TK, were used, with dosages of 1, 3, or 10 mg/kg of a proposed biosimilar product and the RP administered twice weekly by intraperitoneal injection for seven weeks, beginning at 3 weeks of age. Additionally, a supplemental control group of two animals per sex was sacrificed at 3 weeks of age to initiate treatment.

6 Clinical Pharmacology Assessment of a Proposed Biosimilar

6.1 INTRODUCTION

The developers should realize that clinical studies do not aim to characterize the product (as this is already performed during the development of the reference product) but intend to compare the proposed biosimilar product with the reference product. This premise requires a different approach.

For further clarification, the developers are recommended to conduct a "classic" phase 1 study as a standalone study to characterize a drug's disposition characteristics. A "classic" phase 3 study has a placebo-controlled design and intends to establish drug safety and efficacy; neither of these "phases" apply to biosimilars—therefore, this term should be avoided. The correct terminologies to be used are "comparative clinical pharmacology" and "comparative efficacy testing."

In essence, clinical pharmacology studies are an extension of the analytical assessment, a biological tool used to identify the structural difference, which is, otherwise, not possible to study using any other testing method.

6.1.1 SCOPE OF STUDIES

Regulatory agencies expect the developers to conduct comparative studies of human pharmacokinetics (PK; if the route of administration allows such studies to be clinically meaningful) and pharmacodynamics (PD; if there are relevant PD measure(s)) and a clinical immunogenicity assessment, where required, to remove any residual uncertainty regarding the safety and efficacy of a proposed biosimilar product in a stepwise manner after the completion of all prior studies. In certain cases, the results of clinical pharmacology studies may provide adequate data supporting the conclusion that there is no clinically meaningful difference between a proposed biosimilar product and the reference product to allow marketing authorization of a proposed biosimilar product. (If a biological product is administered through a route that does not result in a definable blood concentration profile, then the developers may justify the waiver for PK studies. For well-characterized, less complex biological products, in cases where it is established that variations in immunogenicity do not affect the clinical efficacy of the biosimilar, the developers may justify waiver for clinical immunogenicity studies, more particularly in the case of insulin products.)

A human PK study revealing similar exposure (e.g., serum concentration over time) between a proposed biosimilar product and the reference product may support biosimilarity demonstration.

A human PD study demonstrating a similar effect between a proposed biosimilar product and the reference product in terms of relevant PD measure(s) related to effectiveness or specific safety concerns (except for immunogenicity, which is evaluated separately) represents even stronger support for biosimilarity demonstration. Even if relevant PD measures are not available, sensitive

DOI: 10.1201/9781003392026-6

PD endpoints may be assessed if such an assessment may reduce uncertainty regarding biosimilarity. The PK and PD studies may be combined into a single assessment.

Noteworthy, the PK and PD parameters are generally more sensitive than clinical efficacy endpoints in assessing the similarity between a proposed biosimilar product and the reference product. For example, determining the effect of the proposed biosimilar on thyroid-stimulating hormone levels would provide a more sensitive comparison of two different thyroxine products (two different proposed biosimilars) than a comparison of the effect of a proposed biosimilar on the clinical symptoms of euthyroid sick syndrome. The same holds true for evaluating filgrastim and erythropoietin products, where the endpoints of changes in the white blood cell counts and red blood cell counts serve as a more objective tool to evaluate the efficacy of these products.

Even in cases of residual uncertainty regarding biosimilarity, data from PK and PD studies prove useful in providing a scientific basis for applying a selective and targeted approach to subsequent comparative safety and efficacy testing.

6.1.2 Study Plan

Comparative studies of human PK and PD should use a population, dose(s), and route of administration (where the option is available) that are adequately sensitive to detect differences in the PK and PD profiles. However, there is one major difference in evaluating a proposed biosimilar product and a standalone biological product. Assessment of a proposed biosimilar product involves a comparative evaluation, not a characterization of the PK/PD profiles; therefore, the developers may choose a patient population that is least likely to produce highly variable results to minimize the population size as well as to enhance the ability and sensitivity of the study to differentiate a proposed biosimilar product and the reference product. This concept is different from the considerations when developing a new biosimilar product.

The developer should provide scientific justification for the selection of the population (e.g., patients versus healthy subjects) and parameters for human PK and PD studies, considering the relevance and sensitivity of the population and parameters, the population and parameters of the reference product studied for marketing authorization, and current knowledge of intra-subject and inter-subject variability of human PK and PD studies of the reference product.

The developer is recommended to consider the time duration required for the alteration of a PD parameter and the possibility of using nonlinear PK to design study protocols.

Regulatory agencies also recommend consideration of the importance of modeling and simulation when designing comparative human PK and PD studies. In silico modeling of PK/PD studies is a powerful tool to obviate the need for clinical efficacy testing.

The design of a PK study should consider various factors including clinical context, safety, PK characteristics of the reference product (target-mediated disposition, linear or nonlinear PK, time dependency, half-life, etc.). Furthermore, bioanalytical assays should be appropriate for their intended use and adequately validated.

6.1.2.1 Healthy Subjects versus Patients

Clinical PK and PD studies should be conducted in healthy subjects if the proposed biosimilar product can be safely administered. A study conducted in healthy subjects is considered more sensitive in evaluating product similarity because it is likely to produce less variability in PK and PD than a study in patients with potential confounding factors such as underlying and concomitant disease and concomitant medications. If safety or ethical considerations preclude the participation of healthy subjects in human PK and PD studies for certain products (e.g., immunogenicity or known toxicity from the reference product), or if PD biomarkers can be relevant only in patients with the relevant condition or disease, then clinical pharmacology studies should be conducted in such patients. A population that is representative of the patient population for the target drug will be desirable, but such population is not required if it can demonstrate the potential difference between a proposed biosimilar product and the reference product.

6.1.2.2 Study Size

The total number of subjects studied should provide adequate statistical power for PK, and, when relevant, PD biosimilarity assessments. Data analysis should be performed according to the pre-specified analysis plan, and a post hoc statistical analysis is exploratory only. The developers should realize that PK/PD studies aim to compare, not characterize, the PK/PD profiles; given the scientific argument that both types of studies provide a better assessment of the structural variations, a highly selected population to reduce intra- and inter-subject variability may be more suitable. In the past, several failed PK studies, such as those including subjects with a narrow range of body mass index, age, gender, and race, required retesting in a restricted population to demonstrate biosimilarity.

6.1.2.3 Study Design

To evaluate clinical biosimilarity through PK and PD studies for the development of the proposed biosimilar product, two study designs are of particular relevance: crossover design and parallel study design.

6.1.2.4 Crossover Design

For PK similarity assessments, a single-dose, randomized, crossover study design is generally preferred. A crossover study design is recommended for a product with a short half-life (e.g., shorter than 5 days), a rapid PD response (e.g., time of onset, maximal effect, and disappearance in conjunction with drug exposure), and a low anticipated incidence of immunogenicity. This design is considered most sensitive to assess PK biosimilarity and can provide reliable estimates of differences in exposure with a minimum number of subjects. For PD biosimilarity assessments, a multiple-dose design may be appropriate when the PD effect is delayed or otherwise not parallel to the single-dose drug PK profile. The time course of the appearance and disappearance of immunogenicity and its relationship with the washout period should be considered for studies that have a crossover design.

6.1.2.5 Parallel Design

Many biological products have a long half-life and elicit immunogenic responses. A parallel-group design is appropriate for studies assessing products with a long half-life or products wherein repeated exposures can lead to an immune response of high magnitude, which can affect the PK and PD biosimilarity assessments. This design is also appropriate for studying diseases exhibiting time-related changes associated with the drug exposure.

6.1.2.6 Multiple Studies Combined

The developers may conduct a smaller study labeled as a pilot study to determine the population size required to achieve at least 80% statistical power. In most instances, choosing a population with a narrow demographic will reduce the population size requirement, such as age, sex, body mass index, race, and other factors available. The PK/PD data for the reference product are unlikely to be available in the public domain data because that product would have been tested in a more diverse population. If a follow-up study is required and the developer can choose a relevant population that matches the study population and use the same lots of the proposed biosimilar product and the reference product, then data from additional study(ies) can be combined to conduct the final bioequivalence analysis. The developers are advised to secure approval from regulatory agencies before conducting a follow-up study.

6.1.2.7   Unified Study

The developers may consider a study design that combines both PK and PD studies with clinical immunogenicity testing to minimize drug exposure to the subjects. For example, a two-arm parallel-group study involving two dose levels and a follow-up after the second (higher) dose to study immunogenic attributes may suffice. However, to establish sufficient statistical power, the developers must provide scientific justification of the study size, criteria for the selection of subjects, and selection of doses.

6.1.2.8   Study Materials

All clinical pharmacology studies should be performed on the materials being used for the proposed biosimilar product sampled from the final manufacturing process expected to be used for the marketed product if marketing authorization is granted. All proposed biosimilar products must be manufactured at only one site. A study may include more than one comparator, but each comparator must be used throughout the study. The developers should know that the ICH Q5E considerations do not apply to biosimilars during the development of a proposed biosimilar product.

6.1.2.9   Dose Selection

As a general principle, a lower dose on the steep part of the exposure-response curve is generally appropriate when PK/PD is being measured or when healthy subjects are selected for evaluation. Doses higher than the clinical dose are not recommended because nonlinearity might obviate the assessment of true differences in the PK/PD parameters. For instance, if a study is conducted in a patient population, then the approved dose for the reference product can be the appropriate choice for the proposed biosimilar because this approved dose can best demonstrate the pharmacological effects in a clinical setting. Publicly available data for the dose (or exposure)–response relationship of the reference product can be analyzed using model-based simulations to justify the dose selected for the PK and PD study or studies.

A dose selected from a range of doses can be useful for a clinical PK and PD biosimilarity assessment in certain cases. For example, if the reference product's concentration–effect relationship is known to be highly variable or nonlinear, then a range of doses can be used to assess the dose–response relationship. Where multiple doses are tested, a lower dose, at least one dose, can be one-half the clinical dose.

Suppose the product can be administered only to patients. In that case, an alternative dosing regimen such as a single dose for a chronic indication or a lower dose than the approved dose may be preferable to increase the sensitivity for detecting differences if the approved dose results in nonlinear PK or exceeds the dose required for a maximal PD effect. The appropriateness of the alternative dosing regimen will depend on certain factors, for example, whether the lower dose is known to have the same effect as that of the approved dose and whether it is ethically appropriate to administer lower doses notwithstanding differences in the effect. Adequate justification for the selection of an alternative dosing regimen should be provided.

6.1.2.10   Route of Administration

A proposed biosimilar product must have the same route(s) of administration as that of the reference product. Suppose more than one route of administration (e.g., both intravenous and subcutaneous) is approved for the reference product. In that case, the route of administration selected for the PK and PD similarity assessments should be the one most sensitive in detecting clinical differences. In most cases, the most sensitive route is likely to be the subcutaneous or other extravascular routes of administration because extravascular routes can provide insights into potential differences in PK during the absorption phase in addition to the distribution and elimination phases. Moreover, extravascular routes may provide a more sensitive assessment for differences in immunogenicity.

6.1.3 PHARMACOKINETIC PARAMETERS

Bioequivalence studies are generally not required for generic chemical drug products administered through the subcutaneous or intravenous route because, by definition, they are considered 100% bioavailable. A bioequivalence test for generic drugs aims to compare the ability of a dosage form to release the drug at the target site. After a drug has been released, the remaining time-course of the drug from a generic product will be the same as that expected for molecules of the reference product because a proposed biosimilar product and the reference product are chemically identical. The study design for bioequivalence testing of a generic product is based on universal acceptance of variation (0.8, 1.25) because this testing is not intended to compare the product's safety or efficacy—both of which are already established.

Testing of the PK profile of the proposed biosimilar product against that of the reference product uses the same premise as that for testing for generic chemical drugs because, similar to generic chemical compounds, the purpose of PK profile testing is to establish efficacy based on overall exposure that depends on the disposition profile that may vary because of subtle differences in the chemical structure of the molecule, differences in clearance induced by differences in immunogenic response, and other factors that might alter the safety and efficacy of the proposed biosimilar product.

In instances where the products are administered through routes other than intravenous (such as the subcutaneous route), there may be differences in the absorption rates. Yet, in most cases, these differences will not be significant. However, where a delayed or prolonged absorption is anticipated, the PK profile will be appropriate for determining the differences, for example, long-acting insulin products.

The equivalence criteria (0.8, 1.25) can be challenged by the developers with appropriate scientific justification. The PK profile is used to detect possible differences in between the reference product and the proposed biosimilar product in terms of interaction with the body within a pre-specified acceptance dose range that may need modification. The location and width of the confidence interval (CI) should also be considered when interpreting biosimilarity. For example, statistically significant differences in 90% CIs within the justified acceptance range regarding relevant PK parameters should be explained and justified not to preclude biosimilarity. On the contrary, if the 90% CIs cross the prespecified boundaries, then the developers would need to explain such differences and explore the root causes of the differences. Correction for protein content may be acceptable on a case-by-case basis if pre-specified and adequately justified. The results from the assay of the proposed biosimilar and the reference product are included in the protocol.

All PK measures should be determined for both the proposed biosimilar product and the reference product. In a single-dose PK study, the primary parameters are area under the curve (AUC_{0-inf}) for intravenous administration and both AUC_{0-inf} and C_{max} for subcutaneous administration. Secondary parameters such as t_{max}, volume of distribution, and half-life should also be estimated. In a multiple-dose study, the primary parameters should be truncated AUC after the first administration until the second administration (AUC_{0-t}) and AUC over a steady-state dosage interval (AUC_{0-ss}). Secondary parameters are C_{max} and C_{trough} at a steady state. $AUC_{0-\infty} = AUC_{0-t} + Ct/K_{el}$ (or Ct [concentration at the last measurable time point] divided by K_{el} [elimination rate constant]) is calculated using an appropriate method. C_{max} should be determined from the data without interpolation.

For intravenous studies, $AUC_{0-\infty}$ will be considered the primary endpoint, whereas for subcutaneous studies, C_{max} and AUC will be considered co-primary endpoints. For multiple-dose studies, the total exposure measurement should be the AUC-time profile from time zero to the end of the dosing interval at steady state (AUC_{0-tau}) and is considered the primary endpoint. Both $C_{trough\ ss}$ (i.e., the concentration before the next dosing during multiple dosing) and C_{max} are considered secondary endpoints. Population PK data will not provide an adequate assessment for PK biosimilarity.

TABLE 6.1
Relevant Pharmacokinetics Parameters

Parameter	Significance
C_{max}	Rate of absorption, reaching minimum effective levels (dose and drug delivery system)
T_{max}	Rate of absorption with minimal impact of disposition because of faster absorption from parenteral administration (dose and delivery system)
$AUC_{0-inf, 0-ss, 0-t}$	Absorption, distribution, and elimination (structural difference, dose dependence)
Vd_{ss}	Distribution, receptor binding (structural differences)
dVd_{ss}/dt	Thermodynamic potential of molecules to interact with tissue receptors, distribute, and bind due to structural differences
$AUCV_d$	Distribution, receptor binding (structural differences, dose)
K_{el}	Metabolism (structural differences, dose dependence)

In any PK study, antidrug antibodies should be measured in parallel to PK assessments using appropriate sampling time points.

Table 6.1 lists the PK parameters and their significance.

6.1.3.1 New Approach to Pharmacokinetics Analysis

The PK parameters described above are most used for the comparison of PK profiles. However, an emerging approach for the analysis of PK parameters involves a thermodynamic assessment of the time-course of a drug in the body based on the distribution volume. The apparent volume of distribution (Vd) is an important PK parameter that relates drug plasma concentrations to the amount of drug in the body and is important for calculations drug loading dose and maintenance dose. Following an intravenous bolus of the drug, the volume of drug distribution varies with time. This redistribution occurs in two distinct phases with very different time scales: an avascular phase and a washout or dilution phase. During the avascular phase, the drug mixes throughout the plasma volume in the blood with a time scale of seconds or minutes. During the dilution phase, hydrophilic drugs are distributed in the interstitial fluid with a time scale of hours or days. While most drugs are actively redistributed from the plasma into the body tissues, the decrease in plasma concentrations of the drug is largely due to redistribution instead of actual drug elimination. We assume first-order kinetics, i.e., drug elimination is proportional to its concentration, which is the most common drug kinetic. The most calculated volume of distribution parameters are the apparent volume of drug distribution immediately after an intravenous bolus injection, i.e., at time zero (V_0); the apparent terminal volume of distribution following an intravenous bolus injection (V_{area}); and the expected volume of distribution (V_{ss}), i.e., the apparent terminal volume of distribution, analogous to V_{area} in a bolus model. For bolus experiments, V_{ss} is the expected physical volume of distribution of the drug, and unlike V_{ss}, it is invariant between the constant infusion and bolus experiments.

A thermodynamic approach to using the volume of distribution involves a temporally variable, apparent volume of distribution model for the sum of exponential functions based on conservation of mass. This variable volume model implies an explicit relationship between redistribution and the rate of volume of drug distribution expansion in time. Such a model specifies the duration required for the drug volume to reach a particular size relative to its apparent terminal distribution volume. In so doing, such a variable volume model could potentially provide unanticipated new information about time-based drugs effects on tissue metabolism and drug elimination. This model has implications for the effects of drugs on body tissues, i.e., therapeutic, toxic, or radiation exposure effects.

A variable volume model could be used to calculate the optimal instantaneous dose that will produce a desired concentration at the effector site without drug overload. A time-dependent apparent volume of distribution model based on mass conservation could be used with almost any concentration washout fit function. The distribution parameters can be sensitive to biological drugs that act by receptor binding, and the elimination constant can be more sensitive to structural variants, leading to differences in the drug degradation. Vd_{ss} is an appropriate parameter to be included as a function of time in a PK study apart from other Vd parameters.

The elimination rate constant, K_{el}, obtained from the terminal portion of the curve, or the half-life is sensitive to the mode of elimination of the molecules from the body; structural differences that are challenging to quantify using traditional methods may show differences in the metabolism of the administered drug, and this parameter should be considered a pivotal parameter.

6.1.3.2 Pharmacokinetic/Pharmacodynamic Waivers

Although a comparison of target-mediated clearance is of major importance in biosimilarity testing, it may not be feasible in patients because of major variability in target expression over time. However, because in vitro studies are expected to demonstrate comparable interaction between a proposed biosimilar product and its target(s) (including FcRn for a monoclonal antibody), the absence of a pivotal PK study in the target population is acceptable if additional PK data are collected during the efficacy, safety, and PD studies, as this allows further investigation of the clinical effect of variable pharmacokinetics and possible changes in PK over time. This can be achieved by determining the PK profile in a subset of patients or by population pharmacokinetics.

Comparative pharmacokinetic studies are a basic requirement for proposed biosimilar development and are usually more sensitive than clinical efficacy trials in detecting potential product-related differences. This may explain why a demonstration of equivalent efficacy does not overrule a finding of dissimilar pharmacokinetic profiles.

Comparative efficacy studies are no longer deemed necessary for several product categories (insulin, low-molecular-weight heparin, and (peg)filgrastim), for which pivotal evidence for similarity may be derived from physicochemical, functional, PK, and PD comparisons. Exceptions to this include complex, multifunctional biologicals, where comparative efficacy and safety clinical trials in patients are still viewed as a necessary component of proposed biosimilar development.

6.1.3.3 Route of Administration

If the reference product can be administered both intravenously and subcutaneously, then the evaluation of subcutaneous administration is usually sufficient to cover both the absorption and elimination aspects of the drug.

It is possible to waive the evaluation of intravenous administration if a proposed biosimilar product appears comparative in both absorption and elimination for the subcutaneous route. The omission of the PK study of intravenous administration needs to be justified, for example, in cases when the molecule has an absorption constant that is much lower than the elimination constant (flip-flop kinetics).

While most biological drugs are administered systemically, a special case situation arises for drugs such as ranibizumab, bevacizumab, and aflibercept, which are administered intravitreally. Given that the site of action of these drugs is aqueous humor, this is the most desirable sampling site. Systemic testing of these drugs suggests that the concentration of ranibizumab is the lowest. In terms of clearance rate, ranibizumab is cleared rapidly, followed by aflibercept and bevacizumab. Therefore, developers are encouraged to develop an appropriate animal testing model using in silico approach to suggest waiver for systemic PK/PD studies. Additionally, direct immune response cannot be tested because ocular immune privilege confers protection to the eye, thereby significantly lowering immunogenic response. However, as the drug is cleared through systemic fluids, antidrug antibody (ADA) response should be established.

6.1.3.4   Pharmacodynamics Parameters

A well-designed clinical PK and PD study in a proposed biosimilar development program aims to evaluate the similarities and differences in the PK and PD profiles between a proposed biosimilar product and the reference product. A well-designed clinical PK and PD study should include information about the exposure and, when possible, the exposure-response to the biological products, which are important aspects for assessing the presence of any potential clinically meaningful differences between the two products. Determining the exposure-response to a biological product can be particularly challenging because of the complex nature and heterogeneity of biological products. Thus, evaluation of clinical pharmacology similarity should include assessments of PK similarity and, if applicable, PD similarity.

To the extent possible, the developers should select PD measures that (1) are relevant to clinical outcomes (e.g., on a mechanistic path related to the mechanism of action or disease process related to drug effectiveness or safety); (2) are measurable for a sufficient period after dosing to ascertain the full PD response and with appropriate precision; and (3) have the sensitivity to detect clinically meaningful differences between a proposed biosimilar product and the reference product. The use of multiple PD measures that assess different domains of activities may also be of clinical significance.

The PD biomarker(s) used to measure PD response can be either a single biomarker or a composite of biomarkers that effectively demonstrate the effect characteristics of the product's target. The use of a scientifically appropriate PD biomarkers, either a single biomarker or a composite of more than one relevant PD biomarker, can reduce residual uncertainty regarding the presence of any clinically meaningful differences between products and can significantly add to the overall demonstration of biosimilarity. Using broader panels of PD biomarkers (e.g., by conducting a protein or mRNA microarray analysis) that capture the multiple pharmacological effects of the biosimilar product can be of additional value. When determining which biomarkers should be used to measure immunogenic responses, it is important to consider the following five characteristics:

- Time of onset of the changes in the PD biomarker relative to dosing and its return to baseline after discontinuation of the dosing.
- Dynamic range of the PD biomarker over the exposure range to the biological product.
- Sensitivity of the PD biomarker to differences between a proposed biosimilar product and the reference product.
- Relevance of the PD biomarker to the mechanism of action of the drug (to the extent that the mechanism of action is known for the reference product).
- Analytical validity of the PD biomarker assay.

In some instances, PD biomarkers with the aforementioned relevant characteristics are not identified. However, the developers are still recommended to incorporate PD biomarkers that achieve a large dynamic range over the concentration range in PK studies because these PD biomarkers represent potential orthogonal tests that can support biosimilarity.

When PD biomarkers are not sensitive or specific enough to detect clinically meaningful differences, the derived PK parameters should be used as the primary basis for evaluating biosimilarity from a clinical pharmacology perspective. The PD biomarkers can be used to obtain PK data. A combination of PK and PD similarity can be an important assessment in demonstrating the absence of a clinically meaningful difference between a proposed biosimilar product and the reference product.

The developers are recommended to add PD markers to the pharmacokinetic studies whenever feasible.

In certain cases, comparative PK/PD studies may be sufficient to demonstrate the clinical comparison between a proposed biosimilar product and the reference product, as enumerated in the testing requirements in the following section.

The selected PD marker/biomarker is an accepted surrogate marker and is associated with the patient outcome to the extent that demonstrating a similar effect on the PD marker will ensure a similar effect on the clinical outcome. Relevant examples of biomarkers include absolute neutrophil count, which is used to assess the effect of granulocyte–colony-stimulating factor; reduction in early viral load in chronic hepatitis C infection, which is used to assess the effect of interferon-alpha; plasma insulin concentration in the euglycemic clamp test, which is used to compare the effects of two types of insulin; and magnetic resonance imaging findings of disease lesions, which are used to compare two types of β-interferons in multiple sclerosis.

Some PD markers may have not been established surrogates for efficacy but are relevant for the pharmacological action of the active substance, and a clear dose-response or a concentration-response relationship has been demonstrated. In this case, a single or multiple dose-exposure-response study at two or more dose levels may be sufficient to waive a clinical efficacy study. This design would facilitate a comparison between the proposed biosimilar product and the reference product within the steep part of the dose-response curve.

When there are established dose-response or systemic exposure-response relationships (the response may be a PD measure or a clinical endpoint), it is important to select, whenever possible, and study a dose(s) on the steep part of the dose-response curve for a proposed biosimilar product. Studying doses on the plateau of the dose-response curve is unlikely to reveal differences between a proposed biosimilar product and the reference product.

When comparative PK studies provide evidence to establish the absence of a clinically meaningful difference, which is supported by evidence from studies on nonsurrogate PD/biomarkers, the plan should include a proposal describing the size of the equivalence margin(s) together with its clinical justification as well as the size of PK measures for the demonstration of a comparable safety profile.

The selection of appropriate time points and durations for the measure of PD biomarkers will depend on the characteristics of the PD biomarkers (e.g., PD response timing after the administration of the product based on the half-life of the product and the anticipated duration of the product's effect).

When a PD response lags after product administration, a study of multiple-dose and steady-state conditions can be critical, especially if a proposed therapy is intended for long-term use.

The PD biomarker(s) used for evaluating a proposed biosimilar product and the reference product should be compared by determining the area under the effect curve. If only one PD measure is available because of the characteristics of the PD biomarker, then the measure should be linked to a simultaneous drug concentration measurement. The relationship between drug concentration and the PD biomarker should then be used as a basis for comparison between products.

The use of scientifically appropriate PD biomarkers, either a single biomarker or a composite of more than one relevant PD biomarkers, can reduce any residual uncertainty regarding the presence of clinically meaningful differences between products and add significantly to the overall demonstration of biosimilarity. The use of broader panels of biomarkers (e.g., by conducting a protein or mRNA microarray analysis) capturing multiple pharmacological effects of the product can also add clinical significance.

A crossover design is appropriate, when feasible, for PD studies on products with a short half-life (e.g., shorter than 5 days), a rapid PD response, and a low incidence of immunogenicity. A parallel-group design is usually needed for products with a longer half-life (e.g., more than 5 days). The developers should provide scientific justification for the selection of the study dose (e.g., one dose or multiple doses) and route of administration.

The optimal sampling strategy used for determining PD measures can differ from that used for determining PK measures. For PK sampling, frequent sampling at early time points following product administration at a decreased frequency is generally most effective in characterizing the concentration-time profile. However, the PD-time profile might not mirror the PK-time profile; in such cases, PD sampling should be well justified. When both PK and PD data are obtained during a clinical pharmacology study, the sampling strategy should be optimized for both PK and PD measures.

In certain cases, the need for a confirmatory clinical study may be waived if physicochemical, structural, and in vitro biological analyses and human PK studies, together with a combination of PD markers that reflect pharmacological action and active substance concentration, can provide robust evidence for the safety and efficacy of the proposed biosimilar product.

6.2   STATISTICAL EVALUATION OF PHARMACOKINETICS AND PHARMACODYNAMICS RESULTS

Assessments of clinical pharmacology similarity of a proposed biosimilar product and the reference product in PK and PD studies are performed based on statistical evaluation. The recommended clinical pharmacology similarity assessment relies on (1) a criterion to allow the comparison, (2) a CI for the criterion, and (3) an acceptable limit for the biosimilarity assessment. A log-transformation of the exposure measures is recommended to be performed before the statistical analysis. The developers should use an average equivalence statistical approach to compare PK and PD parameters in replicate design studies and nonreplicate design studies. (See FDA's guidance for industry statistical approaches to establishing bioequivalence.) This average equivalence approach involves calculating 90% CIs for the ratio between the geometric means of the parameters of a proposed biosimilar product and the reference product. To establish PK and PD similarity, the calculated CI should fall within an acceptable limit. The selection of the CI and the acceptable limits can vary among products. An appropriate starting point for an acceptable CI limit for the ratio is 80%–125%; if other limits are proposed, then the developers should justify the selected limits for a proposed biosimilar product. There can be situations wherein the results of the PK and PD studies fall outside the pre-defined limits. Because such results can suggest the presence of underlying differences between a proposed biosimilar product and the reference product that can preclude development as a biosimilar, regulatory agencies encourage developers to analyze and explain such findings and discuss the results with the agencies before proceeding to the next step in the development program.

The developers should realize that differences in the PK/PD profiles of the proposed biosimilar product, when compared with the reference product, are generally not attributed to bioavailability but rather to bioactivity, referring mainly to the disposition profile that can be highly meaningful; it is for this reason that the PK/PD studies are more sensitive than any comparative efficacy study. The developers may not submit comparative clinical efficacy and safety testing without removing residual uncertainties regarding any failed PK/PD comparative studies.

Questions regarding the relevance of using the same equivalence intervals for all types of products as a "one size fits all" approach may arise; however, it is important to realize that each stepwise study of a proposed biosimilar product against the reference product is an approach for showing the lack of dissimilarity rather than establishing absolute similarity. It should be acknowledged that the dose-response of different biological products varies widely, and the equivalence interval may be too wide or too narrow with regard to the clinical response. Yet, PK/PD profiling is not directly related to clinical efficacy, which is only one of the many critical steps.

It is well known that differences in immunogenicity can cause significant changes in the clearance of therapeutic proteins—such differences may be associated with subtle structural differences that cannot be detected using available analytical methodologies.

6.2.1   UTILITY TOOLS

Modeling and simulation tools can be useful when designing PK and PD studies. For instance, these tools can contribute to selecting one or more optimally informative dose or for evaluating PD similarity. When a biomarker-based comparison is performed, it is preferable that the selected dose be on the steep portion of the dose-response curve of the reference product.

For instance, if the exposure-response data for the reference product are not available, then the developers can decide to generate this information through a small study to determine an optimally informative dose (e.g., a dose representing the effective dose to achieve 50% maximal response [ED_{50}] to the reference product). This small study can evaluate the PK/PD relationship at multiple dose levels (e.g., low, intermediate, and the highest approved doses) to obtain dose-response and exposure-response data.[16] Alternatively, when possible, the developers can conduct a PK/PD similarity study between the reference product and a proposed biosimilar product with low, intermediate, and the highest approved doses where a clear dose-response is observed. When multiple doses are studied, PK/PD parameters such as EC_{50}, maximum PD response (E_{max}), and slope of the concentration-effect relationship should be evaluated for similarity. Such studies should be useful for the demonstration of PK, PK/PD, and PD similarity when the clinical pharmacology evaluation is likely to be the major source of information to assess the presence of clinically meaningful differences. Publicly available information on biomarker–clinical endpoint relationships accompanied by modeling and simulation can also be used to define the appropriate limits for PD similarity.

6.2.2 ASSAY CONSIDERATIONS

When evaluating clinical pharmacology similarity, it is critical to use the appropriate bioanalytical methods to evaluate the PK and PD properties of a proposed biosimilar product and the reference product. Because of the complex molecular structure of the biological product, conventional analytical methods might not be suitable for assessing the biological products. The bioanalytical methods used for PK and PD evaluations should be accurate, precise, specific, sensitive, and reproducible.

The developers should design or choose an assay after gaining a thorough understanding of the mechanism of action (to the extent that the mechanism of action of the reference product is known) and structural elements of the proposed biosimilar product and the reference product that are critical for activity. An assay that yields concentration data correlating with pharmacological/PD activity is preferred. The same assay should be used for measuring the concentrations of the proposed biosimilar product and the reference product and validated for use with both products. Analytical assays should have design and performance parameters that are consistent with current industry best practices.

The developer should make every effort to use the most suitable assays and methodologies to obtain data that are meaningful and reflective of PK, biological activity, and PD effect of a proposed biosimilar product and the reference product. Furthermore, when submitting to regulatory agencies, the developers should provide a rationale for the choice of assay and the relevance of the assay to drug activity.

6.2.3 SPECIFIC ASSAYS

Three types of assays are of particular importance for the development of the proposed biosimilar product: ligand binding assays, concentration and activity assays, and PD assays.

6.2.3.1 Ligand Binding Assays

Currently, the concentration of most biological products in circulation is measured using ligand binding assays. These assays are analytical methods used for quantifying high-affinity and highly selective macromolecular interactions between assay reagents (e.g., antibodies, receptors, or ligands) and biological products. The ligand binding assay reagents chosen for detecting the biological product should be carefully evaluated to obtain product concentration data that are meaningful to, and reflective of, the pharmacological activity and PD effect of the biological product of interest. Assays that rely upon antibody reagents and epitopes involved in pharmacological/biochemical interactions with targets are most likely to produce concentration data that are meaningful for target binding activity.

Some biological products exert pharmacological effects only after multiple molecular interactions. For example, in some cases, the in vivo mechanism of action of monoclonal antibodies, bispecific antibodies, or fusion proteins involves binding mediated by different regions of the protein product (e.g., binding to both a ligand or receptor through a target antigen-binding epitope of the protein and to Fc gamma receptors with the fragment crystallizable (Fc) region of the protein). The developers should then choose the most appropriate interactions to measure. Generally, assays for monoclonal antibody product concentrations rely on molecular interactions involving the antigen-binding (Fab) region, particularly epitopes in the complementarity determining regions.

6.2.3.2 Concentration and Activity Assays

These refer to bioanalytical methods that are not based on ligand binding and can quantify a proposed biosimilar product and the reference product concentrations. For some biological products, such as those used to achieve enzyme replacement, the drug availability measurements may rely on activity and should be captured through an appropriate activity assay. Depending on the complexity of the structural features, some biological products should be evaluated using more than one assay to characterize the systemic exposure of a proposed biosimilar product and the reference product. If more than one assay is used, then mass spectrometry and other assays can help distinguish the structures of product variants, where relevant.

6.2.3.3 Pharmacodynamics Assays

Relevant PD assay biomarkers might not always be available to support the development of a proposed biosimilar product through clinical pharmacology studies. However, when PD assessment is a component of the biosimilarity evaluation, the developers should submit (1) a rationale for the selection of the PD endpoints and biomarkers and (2) data to demonstrate the quality of the assay. PD assays should be sensitive for a product or product class and designed to quantitatively evaluate the pharmacological effects of the biologic product. The use of multiple complementary PD assays that reflect different aspects of the pharmacological activity of the product might be particularly useful to reduce residual uncertainty regarding clinically meaningful differences between the products. Because the PD assay is highly dependent on the product's pharmacological activity, the assay validation approach and the assay performance characteristics might differ depending on the specific PD assay. However, the general guiding principles for choosing PD assays are the same as those for PK assays (i.e., demonstration of specificity, reliability, and robustness).

6.2.4 Reserve Samples

Reserve samples establish the identity of the products being tested in the actual study, allow confirmation and reliability of the results, and facilitate investigation of further follow-up questions that arise after completion of the studies. The developers of a proposed biosimilar product are recommended to retain reserve samples for at least 5 years since the date of approval of the application, or, if such application is not approved, for at least 5 years since the date of completion of a comparative clinical PK and PD study of the reference product and the proposed biosimilar product (or another clinical study wherein PK or PD assay samples are collected with the primary objective of assessing PK or PD similarity) that is intended to support submission. For a three-way PK similarity study, the developers are recommended to retain the samples of both comparator products, in addition to retaining the samples of a proposed biosimilar product.

For most protein therapeutics, the developers are recommended to retain the following quantities of product and dosage units, which are expected to be sufficient for evaluation using state-of-the-art analytical methods:

A minimum of 10 dosage units of each of a proposed biosimilar product, reference product, and, if applicable, another comparator product, depending on the amount of product within each unit, is required. In general, this should provide a total product mass of ≥200 mg in a volume of ≥10 mL.

The developers are recommended to contact regulatory agencies to discuss about the appropriate quantities of reserve samples in the following situations:

- A product mass of ≥200 mg in a volume of ≥10 mL requires many dosage units.
- Biological products other than a protein therapeutic product.

6.2.5 EXAMPLE PHARMACOKINETICS STUDIES

PK studies are emerging as a major gatekeeper in the clinical biosimilarity assessment, and this hurdle needs to be overcome. All results are fully justified before further clinical data can be deemed acceptable. The developers may submit in silico PK studies that might obviate the need for more extensive efficacy studies.

The European public assessment reports and the European Medicines Agency product-specific guidelines show that for the following molecules, P.K. studies in healthy volunteers are acceptable: Teriparatide, Low-molecular-weight heparin, Insulin, Interferon-β, Peg-filgrastim, Somatropin, Follitropin-α, Epoetin, Etanercept, Trastuzumab, Bevacizumab, Adalimumab, and Infliximab. Only for rituximab does the European Medicines Agency recommend a P.K. study in one therapeutic area plus efficacy/safety trial (plus P.K. data) in the other therapeutic area.

There were several failed studies documented in the European public assessment reports. Initial PK studies failed for Cyltezo (adalimumab), Hyrimoz (adalimumab), and Ziextenzo (pegfilgrastim). The 90% CIs of primary endpoints for Terrosa (teriparatide) and Grastofil (filgrastim) could not be met, and the study of Efgratin (pegfilgrastim) failed entirely.

6.2.5.1 ADALIMUMAB

Two PK studies on adalimumab biosimilars in healthy volunteers that initially failed but were subsequently successful have been published. In both studies, the differences in glycan structures known to affect PK (high mannose content) were too small to explain the initially observed PK differences, as only a high mannose content of at least 20% would have the potential to alter systemic exposure because of increased receptor-mediated elimination. In one of these cases, the initially failed PK study was performed with a clinical trial formulation, which exhibited differences in the buffering system when compared with the commercial formulation. Post hoc analyses correcting, for example, for body weight and protein content as covariates were performed but could not provide a satisfactory rationale for the observed differences. PK similarity was demonstrated in the second, improved PK study that used the formulation intended for commercialization, a larger sample size considering the high PK variability, a standard injection site, and the predefined covariates body weight and age.

In the other case, an extensive root cause investigation was performed on the following aspects: batch selection; investigational medicinal product (IMP) storage, transport, preparation, and administration; PK sampling, sample shipping, and testing; impact of body weight; ADA development; and other subject characteristics. However, no root cause driving the negative outcome of PK study could be identified by the developer.

Therefore, a second PK study was conducted with an adapted study design aiming to reduce intersubject variability (body mass index restriction, inclusion of only male subjects, and an increase in sample size). IMP handling and dosing were simplified by using prefilled syringes; therefore, they did not require IMP compounding, and this improved design, PK similarity could be shown.

6.2.5.2 Pegfilgrastim

Pegfilgrastim is associated with notably high PK variability. Two of six marketing authorization applications for the proposed biosimilar pegfilgrastim originally had failed PK clinical trials using traditional comparability margins of 80%–125%.

The dose-exposure relationship of pegfilgrastim is greatly disproportional; that is, in healthy subjects, a tenfold increase in dose leads to an approximately 75-fold increase in exposure, and correction for protein content using linear models is inappropriate; attention should also be paid to administering the same dose of the test drug and the reference product.

Interestingly, the high PK variability is not paralleled by the high PD variability. On the contrary, the exposure-response relationship appears rather flat, having led to highly similar PD responses (i.e., Absolute Neutrophil Count (ANCs) even in cases of high PK variability or failed PK similarity, thus rendering PD endpoints less sensitive than PK endpoints to detect potential differences between two pegfilgrastim-containing products.

One way to design pegfilgrastim pharmacokinetic studies is to select a population of highly selective volunteers; however, these studies are not phase 1 trials. The purpose of these studies is to compare, not characterize, a projected patient population. All failed studies missed to adhere to this feature.

6.2.5.3 Trastuzumab

For two trastuzumab biosimilars, a phase 3 study in patients with human epidermal receptor-2 (HER2)-positive early-stage breast cancer/locally advanced breast cancer did not formally meet the upper bound of the predefined equivalence margins for the primary endpoint (pathological complete response), confirming noninferiority but did not formally exclude the possibility of superior efficacy. The analytical assessment of some recent batches showed reduced ADCC activity; the overall contribution of ADCC activity versus antiproliferative effects through the inhibition of ligand-independent HER2 signaling to the therapeutic benefit of trastuzumab is unknown and was not concluded as the cause. There were no clinically meaningful differences in the safety profile, such as absence of differences in cardiac toxicity, measured by left ventricular ejection fraction, and no incidence of symptomatic heart failure, which allowed approval of trastuzumab.

6.2.5.4 Rituximab

Quality attributes (e.g., charge variants, glycan structures, ADCC) were noted for the European Union reference product and United States rituxan. Yet, as both versions of the reference product were on the market simultaneously, both were considered safe, effective, and appropriate for use in comparability studies.

7 Clinical Immunogenicity Assessment of the Biosimilar

7.1 INTRODUCTION

Immunogenicity to a therapeutic protein is associated with hypersensitivity-related responses. Type 1 hypersensitivity involves the production of antidrug antibodies (ADA) of the IgE isotype. However, the generation of both IgE ADA and high titers of IgG ADA may contribute to significant adverse effects including infusion reactions and/or anaphylaxis, although these types of adverse effects are uncommon. IgE ADA complexes can bind to Fcǫ receptors on basophils and mast cells and cross-link them, leading to IgE-mediated anaphylaxis. Additionally, IgG ADA can complex with the therapeutic protein, and the IgG ADA immune complexes can cross-link Fcγ receptors on neutrophils, thus releasing platelet-activating factors resembling histamine. Furthermore, large therapeutic protein–ADA complexes that fail to be cleared from the blood precipitate in tissues such as kidneys, synovial membrane, and choroid plexus, leading to tissue damage and organ failure.

The most significant adverse events occur when ADA demonstrate cross-reactivity with endogenous protein homologs. For instance, pure red cell aplasia (PRCA) developed unexpectedly after years of administration of recombinant erythropoietin (EPO) to patients, and this feature was attributed to the development of ADA without the development of any previous significant immunogenicity issue. The ADA led to the modification of the formulation and route of administration of EPO. A clinical trial of a generic EPO developed by Novartis demonstrated the occurrence of PRCA; in this case, PRCA occurrence was attributed to product aggregation induced by tungsten microparticles presently abundantly in the drug product. Other clinical scenarios wherein ADA showed cross-reactivity with endogenous proteins include neutralizing ADA caused by aggregates present in the human growth hormone formulation and ADA caused by the presence of residual host cell proteins (HCPs) in recombinant therapeutic products such as Factor VII.

Given that such serious outcomes result from cross-reactive ADA, a wide range of in vitro methods have been developed for measuring the presence of the developed ADA. Additionally, methods for identifying drivers of immune responses to monoclonal antibodies and HCPs are also available currently.

Considering these historical outcomes, regulatory agencies have recommended biotherapeutics developers to use a structured approach for measuring immunogenicity risk. For example, the European Medicines Agency (EMA) has published guidelines on immunogenicity assessment of biotechnology-derived therapeutic proteins, wherein factors influencing immunogenicity to therapeutic proteins were classified into helpful patient-, disease-, or product-related categories. In addition to the EMA guidelines, recent Food and Drug Administration (FDA) guidelines for new drug products and generic versions of existing products have also suggested immunogenicity risk assessment approaches, for example, the 2014 FDA guidelines—Guidance for Industry: Immunogenicity Assessment for Therapeutic Protein Products. This guidelines highlight

DOI: 10.1201/9781003392026-7

the contribution of T-cell epitopes to immunogenicity and mention immune modulation attributed to regulatory T cells. Furthermore, "critical quality attributes" documented in the FDA-sponsored Quality-by-Design initiative focused on manufacturing "process development" refers to factors that might predispose a therapeutic protein to be immunogenic.

A recently published guideline for synthetic peptide drugs continues to follow the regulatory guideline trend, insisting the importance of T-cell responses. Noteworthy, peptides smaller than 40 amino acids are not considered protein by the FDA, yet immunogenicity testing remains a consideration for these peptides, similar to the immunogenicity testing for proteins. The FDA has suggested that immunogenicity assessment should further extend to synthesis-related impurities and recommends peptide drug developers to determine the presence of T-cell epitopes in impurities that may be copurified with the active pharmaceutical ingredient.

For peptide or protein-based drugs, the primary amino acid sequence itself can be a strong determinant of immunogenic potential. Beyond the primary amino acid sequence, agency guidelines point to patient- and disease-related categories that may predispose a particular individual to an immune response. Some of the examples include immune deficiency and concomitant immunosuppressive treatments such as methotrexate, which may decrease immunogenicity and autoimmunity, which may increase risk due to ADA. By contrast, product-related factors, i.e., factors intrinsic to the final drug product itself that contribute to immunogenicity, may include modifications in the glycosylation profile, biophysical and biochemical attributes, peptide manufacturing impurities and/ or degradation products, or factors introduced during formulation preparation. Clearly, regulatory guidelines and updated preclinical immunogenicity risk assessment approaches are converging on a consensus, providing impetus for this review of the current state of the art.

7.2   FOCUS ON T-CELL DEPENDENT IMMUNOGENICITY ASSESSMENT AND MITIGATION

While immunogenicity testing involves ADA detection, the root cause is T-cell dependent (Td) immune response, whether the drivers are aggregates, HCPs, impurities, immune modulation due to target engagement, or the drug sequence itself. Thus, Td immunogenicity risk assessment focuses on peptides known as T-cell epitopes that may be derived from the sequence of the product (protein or peptide).

Certain drug-derived peptides/epitopes may bind to human leukocyte antigen (HLA)/major histocompatibility complex (MHC) class II molecules, and the peptide–MHC is then presented to T cells on the surface of antigen-presenting cells (APCs). More specifically, T-cell epitopes (T-helper cell epitopes) that are processed and derived from the drug substance are critically important for ADA development. The T-helper cell epitopes are presented by a subset of HLA class II molecules (predominantly HLA DR but also DP or DQ) to CD4+ T cells, which then release the essential cytokines for B-cell maturation and increase the binding affinity maturation of ADA. These interactions occur in the germinal center of lymphoid organs, where dendritic cells and B cells present T-cell epitopes to T follicular helper cells and T follicular regulatory cells, which regulate the maturation of humoral immune response.

Just as identification of T helper epitopes is central to immunogenicity risk assessment, removal of T-cell epitopes through de-immunization is key to Td immunogenicity risk mitigation. The de-immunization process is now entirely integrated into preclinical programs focused on mitigating Td immunogenicity risk. T-cell epitopes that have reduced immunogenicity (regulatory T-cell epitopes) are equally important for eliciting immune responses to protein drugs containing "human" components such as human-derived monoclonal antibodies, enzyme replacement therapies, and other human-origin biotherapeutics. Circulating regulatory T cells (Tregs), also known as natural Tregs (nTregs), contribute to the regulation of human immune responses and are known to be epitope-specific. The discovery of regulatory T-cell epitopes (Tregitopes) in IgG can improve risk assessment for monoclonal antibodies.

A Td immune response can drive an affinity-matured anti-idiotypic response. Such a mature response driven by long-term dosing can affect exposure, efficacy, and safety as evidenced in enzyme replacement therapies and clotting factor proteins, wherein the immune response not only can lead to loss of exposure and efficacy but can also have safety concerns owing to cross-reactivity to endogenous proteins or lack of other treatment alternatives. Some key examples of the formation of neutralizing antibodies associated with loss of response are antibodies to FVIII/FVII and tumor necrosis factor (TNF) inhibitors that cause loss of response. Key examples of safety concerns include the development of IgE antibodies to cetuximab associated with anaphylaxis, antibodies to EPO associated with PRCA, and antibodies to megakaryocyte growth and development factor/thrombopoietin leading to thrombocytopenia.

7.2.1 DEFINITIONS: T-CELL–DEPENDENT IMMUNE RESPONSES TO BIOTHERAPEUTICS

Immune responses to biotherapeutics can be divided into two broad categories. In the first category of biotherapeutics, immune response to "foreign" proteins (foreign agent to the patient) is typical of responses elicited against pathogens, vaccines, or allotype antigens. Blood factors such as Factor VIII fall in this category because they develop in individuals who lack, in entirety or partly, the endogenous counterpart. This is also true for replacement enzymes such as acid alpha glucosidase for Pompe disease. In the second category of biotherapeutics, immunogenicity to autologous proteins ("self" proteins) suggests a breach of B- and/or T-cell tolerance, similar to the response elicited to autologous self-proteins in certain autoimmune diseases.

Self-tolerance is actively regulated by circulating regulatory T cells. These T cells respond to epitope sequences in self-proteins (such as immunoglobulin) that may be identical to those in non-self-proteins in terms of HLA binding features, but they respond differently to the activation of their T-cell receptor (TCR). For example, regulatory T cells secreting IL-10 in response to HLA DR-restricted T-cell epitopes in IgG have been identified by Franco and Sette in immunoglobulin-treated patients with Kawasaki disease. IL-10 responses (probably due to Treg activation) to specific T-cell epitopes derived from infliximab have also been recorded in infliximab-treated patients.

Given that many self-proteins such as monoclonal antibodies contain regulatory T cell epitopes, the mechanisms underlying the breach of immune tolerance are not well defined, similar to the mechanisms for immune response to foreign proteins, but they may include epitope mimicry, cross-reactivity of T cells, presence of trace levels of innate immune activators such as Toll-like receptor agonists, and/or aggregated proteins. Genetic variations in Toll-like receptors, polymorphisms in co-stimulatory molecules, and modifications to cytokine receptors, among others are likely to be involved in the breach of tolerance. Patients who have autoimmune diseases may have some of these genetic anomalies and can be considered being at higher risk of developing ADA.

7.2.2 T-CELL–INDEPENDENT VS. T-CELL–DEPENDENT RESPONSES

Beyond regulation by T-cell responses, humoral immune responses such as ADA production can be thymus independent (T-cell independent [Ti]) rather than Td in origin. For instance, B cells may be activated in a Ti manner when structural patterns such as polymeric repeats or carbohydrate molecules directly activate B cells through the B-cell receptor (BCR). Ti activation of B cells can be distinguished from Td activation. Antibodies resulting from Ti activation are limited in both isotype and affinity, and if memory B cells are generated, then the antibody responses are not long-lived. By contrast, Td activation of B cells is characterized by class switching (IgM to IgG), and if memory B cells are generated, then the antibody responses have higher affinity, are more robust, and more long-lived. The development of IgG antibodies following the administration of a biotherapeutic generally indicates that the therapeutic is driving a Td immune response.

Td responses, by definition, are contingent upon T-cell recognition of therapeutic protein–derived epitopes through antigen processing and presentation of the protein. As human populations express different types of HLA class II alleles, the interaction between antigenic epitopes and HLA may exhibit varying binding stabilities across the spectrum of HLA alleles expressed in the human population. This HLA genetic polymorphism and its consequent effect on the binding of specific peptides (HLA restriction) is the primary mechanism by which patient genetics (HLA haplotype) becomes a major determinant of immune responses to particular protein therapeutics.

7.2.3 INNATE IMMUNE RESPONSE

The innate immune system controls the initiation of Td immunity. When innate immune cells, known as APCs, are activated in the periphery, they migrate to the local lymph node where they can present drug-derived peptide antigens to antigen-specific T helper cells in the presence of the proper co-stimulatory signals. Unlike the specific nature of the TCR and BCR, cells of the innate immune system express germline-encoded invariant receptors, termed pattern recognition receptors (PRRs), that recognize common microbial motifs (pathogen-associated molecular patterns). PRRs include several families of receptors, such as Toll-like receptors, RIG-1 helicases, and C-type lectin receptors.

PRRs recognize not only microbial patterns but also a class of alarm signals called alarmins or danger-associated molecular patterns (DAMPs) that are released in large quantities by stressed and dying cells to promote a localized inflammatory response. DAMPs help combat pathogens, tissue damage, and stress that occurs in DAMP-mediated inflammation during the administration of a therapeutic protein and promotion of the adaptive immune response. Additionally, host cell and process–derived impurities, termed innate immune response–modifying impurities (IIRMIs), can stimulate the innate immune system by interacting with PRRs promoting adaptive immunity. In vitro and in vivo studies have shown that IIRMIs, even at trace levels, can break tolerance to therapeutic proteins and promote an unwanted immune response.

Newer understanding of Td immunogenicity includes disease state, for example, treatments targeting patients with cardiovascular disease are generally less likely associated with increased production of ADA, whereas patients with autoimmune disease may present with a spectrum of immune dysfunctions that can lead to increased propensity for antitherapeutic response. Alternatively, some patient populations may have unusual HLA distributions that are linked to greater presentation of T effector epitopes derived from the drug sequence, leading to higher or lower levels of immunogenicity. Lastly, the mechanism of action of the drug itself may interfere with, or promote, the activation of the immune system, leading to higher or lower risk of immunogenicity.

It is not uncommon to see one or two individuals (per 100 people) having higher baseline immune responses than others; these higher risk individuals may also have exaggerated immune responses to the delivery vehicle. The baseline immune status of a subject (including B- and T-cell repertoire as well as HLA haplotype) can influence their ability to mount an immune response to a biologic. Moreover, as described above, biotherapeutics may be more immunogenic in patients with autoimmune disease because of the underlying inflammatory status of the recipient patient's immune system.

In past years, drugs specific for patients with autoimmune diseases included anti-TNF agents, which had remarkably different immune profiles in selected patient populations.

Explanations for the increased titers of ADA in patients with rheumatoid arthritis (RA) and autoimmune diseases vary; however, such patients may have defective regulatory T cells or lack functional regulatory T-cell cytokine receptors (interleukin [IL]-2 and IL-10). Perturbation in the function of regulatory T cells or regulatory cytokines that are critical for Treg function may remarkably decrease Treg response to drugs containing Tregitopes, which include many of the monoclonal antibodies that are used to treat autoimmune diseases. Drugs such as methotrexate and TNF inhibitors restore Treg function, potentially reducing ADA titers when the drug reaches therapeutic levels. This is one potential explanation for the high titers of ADA in patients with active, flaring RA, and this may also explain why ADA may disappear after treatment with an effective anti-inflammatory drug.

Clearly, the immune system can be modulated by anti-inflammatory treatments (see also Tolerance induction section). Clinicians and drug developers may benefit from collaboration so as to improve the proactive assessment of immunogenicity in the context of autoimmune disease. Collaboration will enable providing personalized treatments and making better clinical decisions based on improved awareness and detection of immunogenicity risk factors.

7.2.4 Drug Function as a Determinant of Immunogenicity

The emergence of immune-system-targeting biotherapeutics has made it evident that the drug action, by itself, can also contribute to, or modulate, immunogenicity and postulated to play an important role in the activity of anti-TNF agents because of the effect of TNF on regulatory T cells, as described above. Improved Treg function after anti-TNF therapy may lead to reduced titers of ADA to anti-TNF agents over the clinical course. Similarly, IL-2, a cytokine required for the function of regulatory T cells may not only induce a pro-regulatory environment but also reduce the likelihood of the production of ADA to the drug. This mechanism may contribute to the effectiveness of low-dose IL-2 therapy in autoimmune diseases. Conversely, IL-2 can also enhance the function of effector T cell responses and has been used at high doses in the treatment of viral and oncological diseases.

7.2.5 Drug Target and Immunogenicity: Checkpoint Inhibitors

Some drugs such as checkpoint inhibitors (CPIs) enhance immune responses; therefore, CPIs have been proven successful in the treatment of aggressive cancers. However, some CPIs are more immunogenic than expected, potentially leading to loss of efficacy with continued treatments. One hypothesis is that their action reduces the tolerizing effect of natural Tregitopes that may be present in the sequence of the CPIs and/or enhances effector T cell responses to foreign epitopes in the drug sequence.

7.2.6 Drug Target and Immunogenicity: Inhibition of Anti-inflammatory Cytokines

In contrast with CPIs, certain anticytokine agents are much less immunogenic than expected. One such drug is tocilizumab, an anti-IL-6 biologic currently widely used for the treatment of RA and other autoimmune diseases. Notably, as IL-6 is required for T-cell activation, interference with IL-6 may reduce T cell engagement and thereby reduce ADA titers. Rituximab is another example of a drug that may directly interfere with immunogenicity; this drug targets CD20 on developing B cells and reduces the formation of antibody-secreting plasma cells, which may explain why ADA are generally not detected during rituximab treatment.

7.2.7 Peptide Drugs

Over the past several decades, important advances in peptide synthesis have contributed to a major shift in the manufacturing of therapeutic peptide drugs and an expansion in the number of novel peptides entering clinical pipelines. As for monoclonal antibodies, blood factors, and recombinant enzymes, HLA-binding sequences present in peptide drugs may activate regulatory or effector T cells, and therefore, such peptides can demonstrate immunogenicity in clinical use. The transition from fully recombinant to synthetic peptide drugs has raised regulatory concerns about synthesis-related impurities that may induce unwanted immune responses including production of ADA.

Regulatory experience with selected generic peptides has led to the development of draft guidelines for generic peptide products recently introduced by the Office of Generic Drugs at the FDA.

Immunogenicity to peptide drugs is primarily related to methods used for peptide synthesis because of the possibility of the introduction of peptide impurities that may be difficult to remove from the final drug formulation. These impurities may contain novel T-cell epitopes that could contribute to T-cell activation (and, subsequently, ADA). In some cases, the presence of impurities is associated with anaphylaxis. Several classes of peptide impurities may inadvertently be generated at each step of the peptide synthesis process such as amino acid insertions and deletions, incorporation of diastereomeric amino acids, and oxidation of amino acid R groups. Impurities can also arise during storage.

Relative to Td immunogenicity, new T cell epitopes may be introduced when unintended modifications to the amino acid sequence of the drug result in impurities that contain new HLA-binding ligands or changes to the TCR-facing contours of existing epitopes.

7.2.8 In Silico Screening

Current practice of immunogenicity screening generally starts with an in silico screening assessment and then proceeds to HLA binding assays, T cell assays, and MHC-associated peptide proteomics (MAPPs) as needed. Some groups start with MAPPs and do not use in silico tools; however, MAPPs are resource-consuming and costly. Greater experience and familiarity with available in silico tools can likely facilitate greater adaptation of these tools as the first step in immunogenicity assessment in the future. This section briefly describes available tools for in silico screening and highlights improvements to these tools.

7.2.9 T-Cell Epitope Prediction

ADA-mediated responses develop due to adaptive immune responses, supported by T cells responding to linear peptide epitopes displayed by HLA binding onto the surface of APCs. For biotherapeutics delivered through conventional routes (exogenous, i.e., intravenous, subcutaneous, and topical), presentation to CD4+ helper T cells through the class II pathway is most relevant; however, as also discussed above, biotherapeutics involving CD8+ T cell response delivered by viral vectors and cell therapies is an emerging concern. Fortunately, T-cell epitopes can now be predicted with a high degree of confidence.

The core residues of a T-cell epitope sequence (comprising nine amino acids) define the binding affinity and stability to pockets of HLA DR, DP and DQ alleles.

Various methods to assess the immunogenic potential of a complete protein are available on several public and academic platforms, and in some cases, these methods are paired with mathematical models based on hypothetical binding affinities and T-cell precursor frequencies or with MAPPs-determined peptidomes.

Publicly available websites for epitope scanning may appear and disappear and can also be modified, often without notification, which lead to changes in immunogenicity interpretations over time. For this reason, many mid- to large-pharmaceutical companies import online algorithms and operate them within their firewalls to reduce the risk of intellectual property disclosure. Other companies or institutions use web-based tools such as the secure-access commercial-grade ISPRI toolkit or outsource immunogenicity interpretations to commercial research organizations. Some tools such as the commercial ISPRI platform use unique algorithms and codes to identify Treg epitopes in monoclonal antibody sequences and perform a statistical assessment of the epitope content relative to random expectations and adjusted for selfness (i.e., tolerogenic potential). Direct ranking of new biologic drug products against other known nonimmunogenic and immunogenic products is possible using a normalized "immunogenicity scale." The toolkit also features not only novel algorithms to search for epitopes that are "human-like" (see the next section) and therefore less likely to engage activated T cells but also methods for deimmunization and tolerization for direct in silico analysis.

7.2.10 Screening for Selfness (Tolerogenic Potential)

T cells recognize not only peptide sequences but also the peptide complex bound in the cleft of an HLA molecule. In any HLA ligand, certain amino acids are in contact with the HLA molecule itself, while others are accessible to the TCR. If TCR-facing residues from a given epitope are conserved among multiple HLA-binding sequences from the human proteome, then the epitope in question may activate T cells specific to these human proteins. This may lead to a regulatory response generated by natural Tregs or to a limited or null response resulting from T cell anergy or deletion during thymic selection.

For many HLA alleles, the peptide positions for anchorage in the HLA binding cleft are known, and other residues interact with the TCR. Algorithms such as JanusMatrix can be employed to screen predicted epitopes derived from candidate therapeutics against the human proteome to distinguish peptides that are more self-like, and thereby likely to be tolerated, from those peptides that have limited human cross-conservation, and thereby are more likely to be recognized as "foreign" by the human immune system. Therapeutic-derived "foreign" epitopes are most likely targets of antitherapeutic T-cell response.

7.2.11 Screening Against Relevant Peptide Libraries

If the T-cell epitopes are identified, then it is also possible to determine whether the epitope has been tested in vitro or in vivo. The Immune Epitope Database (www.iedb.org), a contracted endeavor from the United States National Institute of Allergy and Infectious Diseases, has now curated 20,860 journal articles and direct submissions, cataloging nearly 622,105 peptide epitopes. By screening novel sequences against this database, researchers can determine whether peptides present in the epitopes of products in development have been reported as MHC ligands and whether the phenotype of T-cell response is known, which allows for the triage of well-understood sequences from unknown sequences of greater immunogenic risk. Furthermore, when risk signals are identified, proteomics databases that contain sequences derived from APCs can reveal important relationships across tissues and disease states to inform careful monitoring during clinical studies.

7.2.12 Ranking Biologic Candidates by Immunogenic Potential

With all other factors being equal, the greater the burden of T-cell epitopes contained in a given protein, the more likely it is that the protein will induce an immune response. It is possible to accomplish a comparison of one biologic to another by normalizing epitope content scores across HLA alleles and adjusting for sequence lengths, as performed on the ISPRI toolkit. Regional epitope density can also drive immune responses.

7.3 IN VITRO METHODS FOR ASSESSING IMMUNOGENICITY RISK

Extensive validation in vitro assays may be cost-prohibitive; thus, in current clinical practice, analysis with advanced in silico tools is being performed. Following in silico analysis, HLA binding and T-cell assays can be performed or outsourced to commercial research organizations. These assays can be applied (i) at the very early stages of drug development to design de novo therapeutics with low predicted immunogenicity, (ii) at a later stage to deimmunize a clinical asset exhibiting high immunogenicity in first-in-human studies, or (iii) retrospectively after program termination, to decipher the mechanisms and risk factors for immunogenicity underlying the high observed clinical immunogenicity. Clearly, for new (and generic versions of older) biologic drugs to be successful, immunogenicity risk assessment is most cost-effective if performed in the preclinical phase of development.

7.3.1 HUMAN LEUKOCYTE ANTIGEN BINDING ASSAY

The first step in generating a T-cell response is recognition of a peptide antigen presented on a HLA class II/MHC class II molecule to a T cell by an APC. Once a potential epitope is identified by in silico analysis, the prediction can be first validated through HLA binding assays, according to the method described by Steere et al., to assess the ability of a peptide to bind to one or more HLA supertype alleles. Supertype alleles refer to families of HLA-DR alleles that share epitope binding motifs. By taking advantage of these supertype families, it is possible to perform binding assays on a relatively small number of alleles while covering >95% of the human population worldwide.

A key factor in the generation of meaningful binding assay data is the design of the peptide sequence to be tested and source of the test peptide. The core binding region in a class II peptide contains nine amino acids that sit within the peptide-binding groove of an HLA molecule. This interaction is stabilized by flanking residues on either side of the core binding region and extend outside of the binding groove. When designing peptides for binding assays, it is important to properly center the binding motif within the HLA binding assays and have an optimal peptide design. Briefly, the peptide of interest is incubated with an allele-specific labeled tracer peptide and a soluble HLA supertype monomer to equilibrium. The following day, the binding reaction is halted and the mixture is transferred to assay plates precoated with a pan anti-HLA-DR antibody, and the plates are incubated overnight. Following this incubation, the plates are developed and peptide binding is indirectly measured by time-resolved fluorescence spectroscopy. Using a fixed concentration of the labeled tracer peptide and a range of concentrations for the test peptide, it is feasible to generate a multipoint dose ranging curve that enables the calculation of the IC_{50} value, which provides information not only about the binding ability of the peptide to HLA (yes/no) but also about the relative affinity of the peptide to a given HLA-DR supertype. The IC_{50} values can be utilized to divide peptides into categories based on their affinity for a given HLA allele, such as high, moderate, low, and nonbinding. As new technology becomes available and accessible, investigating the kinetics of the binding reaction will provide more details.

Peptide purity can also affect the outcome of a binding assay. Purity of peptides from some manufacturers can be as low as 60% because of the manufacturing process and the purity of the raw materials. Impurities within the peptides can lead to false-positive results and, consequently, faulty conclusions. Peptides for binding assays should have a minimum purity of 85% and should be ordered as a net peptide. Spurious results can also be attributed to faulty synthesis. For example, nonbinding peptides may have been synthesized on the same machine as earlier runs used to synthesize HLA-binding peptides. Such contamination can derail a drug development program; an example is provided in the reference.

7.3.2 PERIPHERAL BLOOD MONONUCLEAR CELL ASSAYS

Peripheral blood mononuclear cells (PBMCs) isolated from whole blood are the most widely used source of responder cells for in vitro cell-based assays for immunogenicity prediction. The PBMCs used in experiments can be freshly isolated from healthy volunteers' or affected patients' samples or thawed from a cryopreserved bank of material potentially covering an appropriate representation of disease relevant or common well-documented HLA alleles. Because of the high throughput and ease of execution, PBMC assays using whole-blood PBMCs or CD8+ T-cell–depleted PBMCs are still the most commonly performed in vitro cell-based assay for measuring the immunogenicity potential.

In addition to typical biological products such as proteins and antibodies, co-impurities in the product, including such as HCP components, protein aggregates, synthesized peptide fragments, and others can also be evaluated in these assays. Multiple rounds of stimulation can be performed by replacing cell supernatants with fresh media spiked with the desired stimulant during extended culturing so as to expand populations of antigen-specific T cells for further characterization. Schultz et al. recently reported a variation of the PBMC-based assay that allows enrichment of the number of CD4+ T cells before co-culture with irradiated syngeneic PBMCs in an effort to increase the throughput and sensitivity of the assay.

The biological outcomes of T-cell activation can be measured in these in vitro assays (both PBMC-based and dendritic cell (DC)-T cell-based [see the following sections]) using a number of readouts. Thymidine incorporation and carboxyfluorescein diacetate succinimidyl ester (CFSE) dye dilution are frequently used methods to assess T-cell proliferation. Activation-induced cytokine secretion may be measured using focused (IL-2, IL-4, interferon-γ) or large multiplexed cytokine immunoassay panels and ELISPOT and are used as markers for T-cell activation and immunogenicity, and compared with in silico predictions.

7.3.3 Dendritic Cell–T-Cell Assays

In vitro co-cultures of monocyte-derived DCs (moDCs) and autologous CD4+ T cells are increasingly used to evaluate the immunogenicity potential of drug candidates and product critical quality attributes (CQAs). The DC-T cell or DC-PBMC methods pare the system down to the basic components of cell-mediated immunity: CD4+ T cells interacting with APCs at relevant cell ratios, which enhances sensitivity as the total number of potential responder cells in the experimental system, are much greater than the whole-PBMC method. However, this method is time consuming and requires the isolation and differentiation of monocytes into DCs followed by an antigen-loading/pulsing step that may be reagent, operator, and material dependent.

Monocytes may be isolated from PBMCs as the starting material by utilizing plastic adherence or isolation steps using magnetic bead separation methods. Differentiation and maturation of moDCs using cytokines or other factors are then performed, concurrently with the addition of the desired biotherapeutic, peptide fragments, or aggregates. The matured, pulsed moDCs are then typically combined in a co-culture with autologous, purified CD4+ T cells to allow for antigen presentation and T-cell activation depending on the immunogenicity potential. The responses are measured as is performed for PBMC assays, which is described above. An advanced variation of the moDC-T cell system is the modular immune in vitro construct (MIMIC R) model, which is capable of reproducibly generating both antigen-specific innate and adaptive immune responses against biologics such as proteins, peptides, monoclonal antibodies, and novel modalities including nucleic acids, has also been described for these purposes.

7.3.4 Flow Cytometry Analysis of T-Cell Phenotype

Flow cytometry has become a valuable tool for immunogenicity testing that allows for the characterization of an immune response down to the single-cell level. As more sophisticated instruments involving more laser and filter combinations are being used as well as with advances in staining and detection methods, a wealth of information can be obtained from a patient's blood sample.

T-cell epitopes have the ability to be either immunogenic or tolerogenic. While measuring the expansion of Tregs in cell culture may be challenging, the presence of Treg epitopes can be confirmed by co-incubation with effector T cells in the presence of immunogenic peptides. In this bystander assay, activated Tregs inhibit antigen-specific T effector responses to the immunogenic peptides.

A standard bystander assay makes use of the immunologic memory toward antigens such as tetanus toxin, to which the majority of the cell population has had previous exposure through vaccination or natural exposure. PBMCs are cultured for 10 days in the presence of inactivated tetanus toxoid and the Tregitope at varying concentrations. Cells are subjected to staining analysis and then counted by flow cytometry (Teff cells are defined as CD3+CD4+CD25+FoxP3low, Treg cells are defined as CD3+CD4+CD127lowCD25+FoxP3hi). Cell proliferation can then be measured by CFSE dilution. The proliferation of T effector cells is reduced in the presence of Tregitope and tetanus toxoid when compared with that in the presence of tetanus toxoid alone.

7.3.5 MAJOR HISTOCOMPATIBILITY COMPLEX–ASSOCIATED PEPTIDE PROTEOMICS ASSAYS

In the early 1990s, an additional method called MAPPs was first described. This assay has proved valuable in identifying processed peptides presented on the surface of APCs by relevant HLA. Additionally, this approach provides detailed information of the variability in antigen processing contributed by enzyme cleavages in healthy subjects and patients with disease, and sequencing of the peptide associated with HLA can provide confirmation/validation to the sequences identified using algorithms.

Recent advancements in liquid chromatography–mass spectrometry sensitivity and proteomics analysis have enabled HLA-bound mapping assays to be utilized pre-clinically to map potential antigenic sequences present within a biological therapeutic. Not all potential HLA-binding peptides are processed and presented by APCs because of a combination of partial unfolding HLA binding and cathepsin trimming. Additionally, editing functions of HLA DM and HLA DO further enhance the selectivity of the peptides to be presented.

In these assays, APCs are produced in vitro and incubated with the therapeutic protein of interest for 24 h, after which they undergo a cytokine/mitogen-induced maturation step to upregulate HLA expression. After cell lysis, HLA receptor–peptide complexes are subjected to immune precipitation, where the complexes are isolated, and then an acid elution step, wherein the peptide dissociates from the HLA complex, after which the peptide is sequenced by liquid chromatography–mass spectrometry. Subtraction of endogenous peptides and mapping of the peptides to the therapeutic can be performed using proteomics protein database algorithms. These assays are likely to identify antigenic peptides that can be targeted for deimmunizing protein engineering. Furthermore, whole-blood analysis from a patient with disease can provide insights into alterations in the presentation as well as tolerance for recombinant replacement therapeutics. Algorithms, innate and adaptive phase outputs, and MAPPs, all of which were used in a case study, were applied to anti-IL-21 receptor ATR-107. In silico analysis of the primary sequence predicted two overlapping CD4+ T-cell epitopes in the heavy chain complementarity-determining region (CDR) 2, and one single epitope in the light chain CDR2. The MAPPs confirmed the presence of the epitope in LC CDR2 as a dominant peptide presented by DCs. ATR-107 induced DC activation as evident by an upregulated expression of cell surface activation markers, increased cytokine production, and specific proliferation of autologous CD4 T cells under co-culture conditions. Validation of in silico predicted results using MAPPS can be reassuring for developers.

However, elution of a peptide in a MAPPs assay does not confirm whether the peptide drives Td immune response. T-cell responses may differ depending on the phenotype of the T cells responding to the sequence. Immunogenicity may be overpredicted when MAPPs are used without additional tools that explore the phenotype of T cells responding to the eluted peptides.

The importance of individual epitopes driving immunogenicity was reinforced in a recent demonstration by Cassotta et al., who conducted a MAPPs analysis of natalizumab immunogenicity, a humanized antibody directed against alpha4 integrins. Taking advantage of the combination of in silico and cellular in vitro assays, such as a MAPPs assay performed with B cells isolated from patients' peripheral blood, the authors established that two patients with multiple sclerosis treated with natalizumab who developed neutralizing ADA demonstrated a T-cell response against a CD4+ T-cell epitope located in the V region of the light chain.

7.4 MITIGATION BY DEIMMUNIZATION AND TOLERIZATION

7.4.1 DEIMMUNIZATION

Mitigation of immunogenicity ideally starts with the engineering of molecules designed to exhibit a low risk of provoking unwanted immune responses in patients. This can be achieved by combining the deimmunization and tolerization processes. In the case of monoclonal antibodies, the deimmunization process encompasses two non–mutually exclusive approaches: ultrahumanization, wherein murine CDRs are grafted into antibody frameworks of human origin, and removal of T-cell epitope sequences, wherein the sequences are identified using a combination of epitope prediction logarithms and in vitro confirmatory assays.

Grafting of murine CDRs into V regions in humans often leads to a decrease or loss of affinity, which can be restored by the introduction of murine amino acids (so-called "back-mutations") in the human framework at positions critical for drug–target interactions. These back-mutations have the potential to introduce additional T-cell epitopes; hence, there is a need to apply an iterative and timely deimmunization strategy to exhaust the possibilities of epitope removal as the molecule sequence is refined to reach the desired predicted efficacy. In this context, the augmented binary substitution technology could prove an effective combinatory approach but needs further exploration.

7.4.2 TOLERIZATION

Complementary to the removal of deleterious CD4+ T-cell epitopes is the introduction of T regulatory sequences, a process known as tolerization. Tolerization is of particular interest in replacement therapies, wherein removal of T-cell epitopes might affect drug function, or in gene therapy to counterbalance the activation of the cytotoxic response induced by capsid antigenic determinants. Indeed, prophylactic administration of an Adeno-Associated Virus AAV-derived capsid protein fused to Tregitopes can reduce viral capsid–specific CD8+ T-cell responses together with a concomitant increase in Treg cell counts. To date, the demonstration of the expected reduced immunogenicity of deimmunized and/or tolerized molecules relies on in vitro and ex vivo assays or preclinical models. Deimmunized forms of highly immunogenic monoclonal antibodies are yet to be fully applicable in the clinical setting, as biotherapeutics developers have focused on developing novel, less immunogenic molecules that have a longer patent life and greater freedom to operate.

7.4.3 TREATMENT-INDUCED TOLERANCE

Efforts to mitigate the risk of ADA development often focus on reducing the intrinsic immunogenicity of a therapeutic protein, except for the well-established immune tolerance induction protocols for patients with hemophilia A and B who develop inhibitory molecules to recombinant clotting factors. The development of ADA against monoclonal antibody–based drugs can also lead to loss of response and switching of the drug, even in the case of fully humanized molecules. In this context, various approaches to induce immune tolerance to biotherapeutics have been envisaged and reviewed elsewhere. ADA responses to other lifesaving therapeutic proteins, such as enzyme replacement therapies, have compromised treatment efficacy, sometimes leading to death. As for gene therapy, the development of ADA to the transgene and the viral vector remains a major obstacle to successful treatment: patients who have a pre-existing neutralizing antibody response to the viral capsid are not eligible for receiving treatment, and patients who develop treatment-induced humoral immunity will not be eligible for re-dosing.

"Deimmunization" refers to the removal of T helper epitopes driving T helper–mediated immune responses may reduce T helper immune responses, whereas "immune engineering" or "tolerization" refers to the identification and augmentation of Treg responses by preservation or introduction of

Treg epitopes (Tregitopes) into the protein sequence. This in silico approach enables the introduction of regulatory T-cell epitopes to reduce the potential for immunogenicity.

Alternatively, regimens associated with immune tolerance induction can be formulated using available drugs that target the major players of the immune cascade associated with ADA development by either inhibiting deleterious effector T-cell responses or activating tolerogenic pathways. The former can be realized by interfering with mechanisms related to T- and B-cell activation or by depleting immune cells with immunosuppressive agents such as cyclophosphamide or methotrexate, anti-CD3 or anti-CD20 antibodies, proteasome inhibitors, or a combination of multiple depleting agents. Several such approaches are already being applied, including concomitant treatment with methotrexate to diminish T-cell–mediated immunogenicity.

In Pompe disease and in tolerance induction to inhibitors to FVIII therapy, currently used regimens involve a combination of multiple agents such as rituximab (to eliminate antibody-secreting B cells) and intravenous immunoglobulin (to bind and remove antibodies or to induce tolerance). Methotrexate is added to the regimen used for Pompe disease, and this modified regimen has been successful in establishing tolerance to alglucosidase alfa in infants with high-risk Pompe disease.

Other methods under consideration include concomitant administration of a regimen of rapamycin in the nanoparticle form or co-administration with Tregitopes. Under in vitro conditions, infusion of expanded Tregs and B regs engineered to express antigen-specific receptors can control the development of inhibitors in a preclinical model of hemophilia A.

Most of the immune tolerance induction approaches are still at an early stage of development, and the long-term effect of these interventions remains unknown. However, the value of the tolerizing regimen that has reached the clinical setting is an incentive to pursue the evaluation of immune tolerance induction as a mean to mitigate unwanted immunogenicity of biotherapeutics.

7.4.4 ANTIDRUG ANTIBODY ASSAY STANDARDIZATION

A comparison of the immunogenicity of therapeutic proteins across clinical studies has been challenging because of the lack of standardization and harmonization of the ADA assay. For a given therapeutic protein, variability in critical assay parameters such as sensitivity and drug tolerance can lead to dissimilar estimation of clinical incidence across various laboratories. In this context, the Innovative Medicines Initiative(IMI)-funded ABIRISK consortium (anti-biopharmaceutical immunization: prediction and analysis of clinical relevance to minimize the risk) generated monoclonal antibodies to serve as standards in ADA assays. Such universal standards could be used to benchmark assay sensitivity and drug tolerance, routinely monitor assay performance, and validate antigenicity equivalence of comparator products in ADA assays for biosimilars. Additionally, immunogenicity assessments based on such standards can help inform the clinician about dosing strategies if loss of efficacy is observed. Monoclonal neutralizing antibodies of various isotypes and affinity specific for rituximab, natalizumab, infliximab, adalimumab, or interferon-beta were generated from B cells isolated from patients immunized with the respective therapeutic proteins according to the method described previously. Production scale-up and further characterization analyses using ABIRISK to validate ADA assays are ongoing. Ultimately, all antibodies will be openly available at the National Institute for Biological Standards and Control.

7.5 NEW MODALITIES AND IMMUNOGENICITY RISK ASSESSMENT

As discussed in the section "New Modalities," new modalities such as cellular and gene therapies have shown immunogenicity in the clinical setting. The mechanisms by which these modalities can stimulate immune responses are complex because of the high level of engineering, intracellular expression, introduction of engineered gene products, and complex delivery systems. Modified immunogenicity risk assessment tools and assays developed primarily for protein therapeutics can be used to minimize immunogenicity risk in these novel therapeutics.

7.5.1 Specific Cell Lines/Soluble T-Cell Receptors

Novel in vitro assays relying on the ability of APCs displaying the processed peptides in the context of HLA class I/II to interact with T-cell repertoires are proving to be useful for further defining antigen specificity and immune response propagation. Additionally, the use of engineered B-cell lines expressing class I and class II HLA facilitates the high-throughput prediction of intracellular processing and presentation of potential antigenic epitopes. For example, a in a competitive approach, soluble TCRs recognizing the HLA-reference peptide complex are used to detect the presentation of potential immunogenic epitopes by mono-allelic APC lines (Merck, unpublished data).

7.5.2 Modeling

As described above, a variety of in silico and in vitro tools can be deployed at the early stage of development to guide protein engineering and design drug candidates with predicted low immunogenicity. However, the tools can be used to assess product-related risks, in particular sequence-based risk, but they may not reveal factors pertaining to immunogenicity such as patient- and treatment-related factors. The overall risk of immunogenicity relies on the weighting and integration of the different risk factors, some of which are either empirical or theoretical. Immunogenicity quantitative systems pharmacology (QSP) simulators could help simplify and homogenize this integration. They incorporate biotherapeutics, physiologically based pharmacokinetic (PK), and mechanistic models of immune responses to simulate large-scale clinical trials and predict the incidence of immunogenicity. The impact of critical variables such as HLA genotype, combination therapies, dosing regimens, and route of administration on ADA incidence as well as the impact of ADA on drug PK can be modeled. QSP simulators are still in development, and they require a greater set of empiric input data and refinement of parameters related to the immune system, such as kinetics of antibody development. After validation, QSP simulators could facilitate personalized management and mitigation of immunogenicity.

7.5.3 Immunogenicity-Focused Organizations

Owing to challenges in accurately performing immunogenicity risk assessments and in measuring and determining the clinical relevance of ADA, pharmaceutical companies, biotechnology institutes, and contract research organizations joined forces to make progress in the field by addressing the existing gaps. Scientific nonprofit associations were created, such as the European Immunogenicity Platform (www.e-i-p.eu/). This platform aims to facilitate exchanges among immunogenicity experts, encourage, and lead interactions with regulatory agencies as well as share knowledge and state-of-the-art in the immunogenicity field with the broader scientific community and training courses on the practical and regulatory aspects of immunogenicity.

The ABIRISK consortium is another collaborative approach toward contributing to the advancement of immunogenicity sciences. Clinical and basic research academic centers worked with industrial partners on a 6-year research project and addressed some of the main questions and practical hurdles related to unwanted immunogenicity, such as the value of existing predictive tools, ADA assays, harmonization and standardization, clinical relevance of the detected ADA, identification of patients' risk factors, and predictive markers.

A spin-off initiative emerged from this extensive collaboration across laboratories in Europe, the United States, and Israel. BIOPIA (https://ki.se/en/cns/biopia) is a nonprofit effort of European laboratories with expertise in biopharmaceutical PK and immunogenicity in many diseases, and this initiative aims to raise awareness about immunogenicity and advocate integration of drug levels and ADA testing to improve patient management. The website provides information about ADA and drug level testing, mainly to help clinicians with the implementation of routine, clinical testing for immunogenicity and drug levels. Similar efforts are underway in the United States, under the umbrella of the Therapeutic Protein Immunogenicity Community as part of the AAPS (American Association of Pharmaceutical Scientists). The Immunogenicity Risk Assessment and Mitigation working group conducted a survey to characterize performance and harmonize methods for risk assessments including algorithms and in vitro assays through member surveys. The future focus is on adapting the current tools and developing innovative assays to answer questions around novel modalities and next-generation therapies.

7.5.4 Regulatory Perspective on Immunogenicity

The recent FDA guideline proposes a risk-based approach to assess the induction of immune responses to a therapeutic protein and its impact on safety and efficacy on a case-by-case basis. There is also a recommendation that the risk-based strategy should be developed at an early stage during biosimilar development, preferably after humanization and in parallel with other developability efforts. Early assessment would enable a more robust understanding of the liabilities due to structure and sequence. Continuous evaluation of the risk through different stages of drug development can guide the bioanalytical strategy for clinical application, which is described in the following sections. Risk assessment includes risks due to changes in process development, manufacturing, formulation, and device.

7.5.5 Integration of Risk Assessment Into the Preclinical Pipeline

Briefly, immunogenicity risk assessment should consider potential therapeutic benefits and weigh those against the potential impact of immunogenicity considered the type of patient population and indication as well as previous experience with the therapeutic target.

Early assessment of biologic candidates allows ranking based on the least probability of the identified risk. There is also room for deimmunization/sequence optimization, wherein a few amino acids are removed so as to remove the epitope or regulatory sequences are inserted to drive a suppressive T-cell response. Furthermore, the risk-based strategy should include any liabilities due to post-translational modifications that are a consequence of process-related changes associated with protein expression and purification as well as formulation-/excipient-induced aggregation or degradation.

Knowledge of early pharmacology of the therapeutic protein, including on and off–target engagement and consequent activation of the immune pathways should also be considered during the development of the risk-based strategy. This is particularly relevant for therapeutic proteins targeting immune modulatory pathways. Preclinical toxicology studies provide insights into the safety of the biosimilar.

Tools and assays that can be utilized at different stages of lead candidate selection to minimize immunogenicity risk. For example, in in silico screening, computer-based algorithms can be used to evaluate not only the amino acid sequence for potential HLA class I and II binding and residues that are likely to undergo chemical modification but also assess the protein structure of the aggregate. In vitro assays can be performed to assess the potential of biological therapeutics to activate T cells in diverse donor sets. These assays can be performed with whole protein to potentially include target engagement or with overlapping peptides to exclude target engagement. MAPPs and HLA binding assays aim to identify the antigens within the molecule. Ex vivo and in vivo models encompassing additional compartments of the immune system can be used when specific questions arise during drug development. Innate immune system activation assay, which evaluates the impact of nonsequence biophysical parameters, can be used to optimize process development and formulation or process changes. Clinical immunogenicity data and patient characterization are critical components to validate, evaluate, and improve the effectiveness of preclinical tools and assay-associated concerns related to on- and off-target liabilities, especially when the preclinical and clinical targets have homology. The risk-based strategy can also become a benefit when there is previous clinical experience, such as clinical experience with proteins with similar targets that are already in the commercial phase. Additionally, if there is enough clinical experience around the therapeutic proteins for one disease indication, then the outcome of the studies related to safety and efficacy can also be summarized for the application of the investigational new drug (IND) being developed for the new IND.

7.6 FIVE-YEAR VIEW

Because of advances in immunogenicity risk assessment methods as well as de-risking efforts pertaining to both the product (primary sequence and formulation) and improved understanding of the patient factors that may contribute to the development of ADA, most biotherapeutics developers integrating the assessments into PK/pharmacodynamics (PD), and safety and clinical efficacy outcomes to better understand the risk of a new product or biosimilar. Ongoing consideration should be given to the use of emerging technologies (novel in silico, in vitro, and in vivo assays) during drug development (designing new sequences, selecting lead compounds, de-risking the identified liabilities, or comparing biosimilar prioritization). These methodologies also provide an estimation of risk, including prior knowledge of individual risk (HLA type) disposition for clinical immunogenicity. In vivo studies in animal models are not currently recommended for immunogenicity testing because of the differences between HLA in an animal model and the HLA in humans. Instead, in vitro assays are preferred for evaluating the risk of cell-mediated immune responses. Variation in MHC-related immune responses can be expected when transitioning from one model species to another, or to humans. T-cell epitopes bound by MHCs in mice, nonhuman primates, and other model species are frequently different from those bound by human MHCs. Most preclinical studies on biologics circumvent this concern by testing for immunogenicity under in vitro conditions, wherein human PBMC samples are selected to provide a broad coverage of human MHCs.

Within 5 years, it is expected that most part of the risk assessment will be performed first in silico before moving to (limited) in vitro and in vivo models. This is because most drug companies performing comprehensive preclinical development actually generate thousands of potential candidates for a single target. In silico analysis is a good first-pass approach to immunogenicity, enabling detailed inspection of certain molecular features using in vitro methods, where required. The accuracy of computational tools will increase as more results become available to public review.

Machine-to-machine interfaces, which enables integrated and high-throughput screening of multiple candidates for the same target, will simultaneously improve preclinical selection of candidates for clinical development. Drug developers should become familiar with available tools because the sheer volume of candidate compounds that are expected to be screened will make it impossible to manage without automated in silico analysis pipelines. It is also likely that the breadth of in silico analysis (and in vitro validation) will include HLA class I immunogenicity assessment and in vitro assays in the future. This is due to the introduction of novel modalities and viral vectors, which interface with the MHC class I pathway.

The field of immunogenicity risk assessment has matured and will continue to evolve as new modalities are introduced in the clinical setting.

Immunogenicity or adverse immune response is defined as the propensity of the therapeutic biologics to generate immune responses to itself and related proteins or induce immunologically related nonclinical effect or adverse clinical events. There are two types of immunogenicity in the therapeutic biologics development process:

- Wanted immunogenicity is typically related to the administration of vaccines. The injection of an antigen (the vaccine) stimulates an immune response against the pathogen (virus, bacteria, cancer cell, etc.), with an aim toward protecting the host.
- Unwanted immune responses to therapeutic biologics may also neutralize their biological activities and induce adverse events not only by inhibiting the efficacy of the therapeutic biologics but also by cross-reacting to an endogenous protein counterpart, leading to loss of its physiological function (e.g., neutralizing antibodies to therapeutic EPO cause PRCA by neutralizing the endogenous protein). This overview of immunogenicity is the latter adverse immune response in the discovery and development of therapeutic biologics.

Antigenic processing is performed by professional APCs such as DCs, macrophages, and B cells. This process involves two steps: first, the antigen capture, wherein antigens are delivered to the cellular antigen processing machinery; and second, antigen processing and presentation, wherein antigenic peptides bound to MHC molecules are generated for presentation to adaptive immune cells. Extracellular antigens are captured by the APCs through phagocytosis, macropinocytosis, and receptor-mediated endocytosis. In the acidic environment of endosomes or lysosomes, antigens are degraded into many immunogenic peptides containing T-cell epitopes. Following the uptake of antigens, MHC class II molecules are first synthesized in the endoplasmic reticulum and then transported by the Golgi apparatus to combine with antigen peptides to form peptide-MHC II complexes, after which these complexes are presented to the surface of APCs. TCRs can then recognize the peptide-MHC-II complexes to activate T cells to initiate an immunogenic response. The quality of antigen presentation depends on the affinity of the peptide-MHC complexes, and a direct relationship exists between peptide-MHC complex stability and immunogenic response. The binding ability between APCs and CD4+ T cells is determined through DC-T-cell assay.

Immune responses to therapeutic biologics can significantly affect both therapeutic biologics efficacy and patient safety. First-generation therapeutic monoclonal antibodies are of murine origin, and drugs based on these antibodies cause highly adverse immune responses when administered in patients because of the antibodies; much of these immunogenic responses are subdued in humanized monoclonal antibodies, yet there remains a definite concern.

Adverse immune responses lead to the production of ADA, which result in many clinically relevant effects (Table 7.1), leading to anaphylaxis, cytokine release syndrome, and cross-reactive neutralization of endogenous proteins that mediate critical functions.

TABLE 7.1
Clinically Relevant Effects of Immunogenicity

Effects on bioavailability
Effect on safety and efficacy
Effect on pharmacokinetics including potential cross-reactivity to endogenous proteins
Inhibition of the function of endogenous protein
Injection-site reactions
Mild or life-threatening systemic reactions
Formation of antidrug antibodies (HAMA, HACA, and HAHA)
Formation of neutralizing antibodies
Formation of immune complexes
Formation of anti-idiotypic antibodies

TABLE 7.2
Immunogenicity-Associated Factors

Category	Example
Treatment-associated factors	Mechanism of action
	Route of administration
	Frequency of administration, Duration of therapy
Patient-associated factors	Disease type
	Disease status
	Immune system function
	Genetic factors
	Concomitant disease
	Concomitant medications
	Prior exposure
	Prior sensitization
Drug property–associated factors	Recombinant expression system
	Post-translational protein modifications
	Impurities
	Contaminants
	Aggregates

When the presence of ADAs has been confirmed, further characterization beyond the titer and analysis of the neutralizing ability of the antibodies may be useful, for example, immunoglobulin class in case of acute hypersensitivity. It may also be possible to perform further typing of clinically important ADAs or determine the "threshold" level of ADAs beyond which there is a significant impact on drug efficacy and safety.

Fundamentally, given that many therapeutic biologics are being developed today, the most important factor concerning immunogenicity is that it is a covariate of PK; when immunogenicity occurs against a therapeutic biologic, it increases drug clearance from the body and decreases exposure to that therapeutic. Both patient-related and product-related factors may affect the immunogenicity of therapeutic biologics. These factors are critical elements in immunogenicity risk assessment (Table 7.2) and require consideration in immunogenicity testing protocols.

7.7 IMMUNOGENICITY INVESTIGATION

Immunogenicity should be investigated in the target population, as animal testing and in vitro models cannot always predict immune response in humans. Immunogenicity plays an important role in demonstrating product comparability following manufacturing changes and similarities in the context of changes in the manufacturing process after a product has been approved. Yet, this protocol is unsuitable for testing the proposed biosimilar products during development. Even minor differences can potentially affect bioactivity, efficacy, or safety, including the immunogenicity of a proposed biosimilar product.

Assessment of physicochemical or formulation-based attributes in the therapeutic biologics, such as impurities, heterogeneity, aggregate formation, oxidation, and deamidation, can guide the prediction of immunogenicity and development of less immunogenic therapeutic agents. Moreover, predicting potential immunogenic epitopes in therapeutic biologics is an important and effective strategy to improve drug safety and efficacy. A variety of preclinical immunogenicity assessment strategies are available during therapeutic biologics development, as listed in Table 7.3.

TABLE 7.3
Strategies for Managing the Immunogenicity of Therapeutic Biologics

Prediction	Reduction
Physiochemical characterization	Deimmunization (epitope modifications)
In silico immunogenicity assessment	Humanization
T-cell epitope predictions	
B-cell epitope predictions	
In vitro immunogenicity assessment	Purity and formulations
Ex vivo immunogenicity assessment	Purity and formulations
T-cell response modifications	
Human leukocyte antigen binding assays	Fusion proteins
In vivo immunogenicity assessment	Combination biologics or combination therapy

7.7.1 ASSAY

Biosimilar developers should evaluate the following antibody-related parameters in clinical immunogenicity assessment:

- Titer, specificity, relevant isotype distribution, time course of drug development, persistence, disappearance, impact on PK, and association with clinical sequelae.
- Neutralization of product activity: Neutralizing ability to all relevant functions (e.g., uptake and catalytic activity, neutralization for enzyme replacement therapeutics).
- The developer should consult with regulatory agencies on the sufficiency of assays before initiating any clinical immunogenicity assessment.

The developers should develop assays that can sensitively detect immune responses, even in the circulating drug product (proposed biosimilar product and reference product). The proposed biosimilar product and the reference product should be assessed using the same assay and using the same patient sera whenever possible. It is recommended that immunogenicity assays be developed and validated at an early stage of biosimilar development, and the validation should be carried out on both the proposed biosimilar product and the reference product.

It is recommended to adopt a multi-tiered testing approach involving the development and validation of screening assays, confirmatory assays, titration assays, and neutralization assays. Screening assays, also known as binding antibody assays, are used to detect antibodies that bind to the therapeutic protein product. Confirmatory assays establish the specificity of ADA to the therapeutic protein. Titration assays characterize the magnitude of the ADA response. Neutralization assays assess the neutralizing activity of ADA. Setting the appropriate cutoff point in assays is critical to minimizing the risk of false-negative results.

Independent ADA binding assays incorporating the proposed biosimilar product or the reference product as the capture ligand should be developed in parallel. Each assay should be validated and have demonstrated the ability to sensitively detect ADA in the presence of the drug. Samples from both treatment arms should be tested for the presence of ADA using both assays to demonstrate ADA cross-reactivity against the proposed biosimilar product and the reference product. Deviation from this approach should be scientifically justified.

7.7.2 SENSITIVITY

It is recommended that screening and confirmatory IgG and IgM ADA assays achieve a sensitivity of at least 100 ng/mL, and a limit of sensitivity of more significant than 100 ng/mL may be acceptable depending on the risk and prior knowledge of the biosimilar.

7.7.3 SPECIFICITY

Lack of assay specificity can lead to false-positive results; there are challenges in demonstrating the specificity of antibody responses to monoclonal antibody, Fc-fusion proteins, and Ig-fusion protein and providing guidance on managing such challenges.

7.7.4 SELECTIVITY

The assay results may be affected by interference from the matrix or onboard therapeutic protein products. Failure to establish assay selectivity can contribute to a nonspecific signal, obscuring a positive result.

7.7.5 PRECISION

The results should be reproducible within and between assay runs; assay precision is critical to the assessment of ADA because assay variability is the basis for determining the cutoff points and ensuring that weakly positive samples are detected as positive.

7.7.6 REPRODUCIBILITY

The developers should establish data comparability, including assay sensitivity, drug tolerance, and assay precision, if multiple laboratories are running an assay in a study.

7.7.7 ROBUSTNESS AND SAMPLE STABILITY

The complexity of bioassays makes them susceptible to variations in assay conditions. It is therefore essential to evaluate and optimize parameters such as cell passage number, incubation times, and culture media components. Additionally, a plan for managing short- and long-term stability is required to preserve antibody reactivity.

7.7.8 FORMAT

The developers should consider the pros and cons of each type of assay format, including throughput, sensitivity, selectivity, dynamic range, ability to detect various Ig isotypes, ability to detect rapidly dissociating antibodies, and availability of reagents. The number and vigor of washes, which can influence assay sensitivity and epitope exposure, are should also be considered.

7.7.9 REAGENTS

If positive control antibodies, negative controls, and system suitability controls are generated specifically for the assay, then it is important for the developers to ensure consistent assay performance with critical reagents.

7.7.10 Reporting Results

Assay methods should be evaluated for appropriateness, the most common one being qualitative assays.

Table 7.4 presents common screening assays, and Table 7.5 presents assay methods for antibody testing.

7.7.11 Lifecycle Management

Differences in immune responses between a proposed biosimilar product and the reference product in the absence of observed clinical sequelae may be concerning. Such assays may warrant further evaluation (e.g., an extended period of follow-up evaluation).

TABLE 7.4
Commonly Used Screening Assays

Type of Assay	Advantages	Disadvantages
Direct/indirect enzyme-linked immunosorbent assay	High throughput, inexpensive, easy to use, and automated High therapeutic tolerance in the solution phase Generic reagents and instruments	May bind nonspecifically, potential for a high background Antigen immobilization may alter antigen conformation and mask epitopes May fail to detect low-affinity antibodies Low therapeutic tolerance in the solid phase Requires a species-specific secondary reagent
Bridging enzyme-linked immunosorbent assay	High throughput, inexpensive easy to use, and automated Low background High specificity (dual-arm binding), can be used cross-species generic reagents and instruments	Antigen labeling may alter antigen. May fail to detect low-affinity antibodies. Highly susceptible to interference by therapeutic serum components, e.g., anti-human Ig molecules, multivalent targets May not detect IgG4 and IgM
Electrochemiluminescence (with direct/indirect bridging format)	High throughput, large dynamic range Minimally affected by matrix, high tolerance to therapeutics Detection signal consistent during the life of a thioctic acid glycerol) (TAG) conjugate	May require two antigen conjugates (indirect) Antigen labeling may alter antigen susceptibility to interference by therapeutic serum components, e.g., antihuman Ig molecules, multivalent targets May not detect IgG4 Vendor-specific equipment and reagents
Radioimmunoprecipitation assay	Moderate throughput, high sensitivity, can be specific, inexpensive	Can be isotype specific May not detect low-affinity antibodies Requires a radiolabeled antigen Decay of radiolabel may affect antigen stability
Surface plasmon resonance	Moderate throughput Determines specificity, isotype, relative binding affinity Enables the detection of both low-affinity and high-affinity antibodies High tolerance to therapeutic detection reagent not required	Antigen immobilization may alter the therapeutic activity The regeneration step may degrade the antigen Sensitivity may be less than that of the binding assay Expensive Vendor-specific equipment and reagents

TABLE 7.5
Methods for the Detection of Neutralizing Antibodies

Type of Assay	Advantages	Disadvantages
Cell-based bioassay	Functional assay reflecting the mechanism of action of the therapeutic effect May correlate with the clinical response	Relatively time-consuming Can have a complex protocol design Often variable. Affected by serum (matrix) effects and interfering factors Susceptible to interference by therapeutic Validation can be difficult, e.g., cell lines, reagents, etc.
Competitive ligand binding assay	Rapid simple assay design Relatively easy to use Does not require cell lines Easy to develop and validate	Antigen labeling may alter antigen. Susceptible to interference by the therapeutic. May not represent true functional read out. May not correlate with the clinical response

The duration of follow-up evaluation should be decided based on (1) the time course for the generation of immune responses (such as the development of neutralizing antibodies, cell-mediated immune responses) and the expected clinical sequelae (informed by experience with the reference product), (2) the time course of the disappearance of the immune responses and the expected clinical sequelae following treatment cessation, and (3) the length of administration of the product. For example, for agents administered for a long term, the follow-up period is recommended to be 1 year unless a shorter duration can be scientifically justified based on the totality of the evidence to support biosimilarity.

The developer should then obtain a lifecycle management report, which includes the following sections, as the product moves through various stages:

- Immunogenicity risk assessment: This assessment should be specific to the therapeutic protein and include information on product quality and subjective factors.
- Tiered bioanalytical strategy and assay validation summary: The developers should summarize the assessment strategies for each clinical development phase.
- Clinical study design and detailed immunogenicity sampling plans: The developers should include sampling plans for all clinical studies wherein an assessment was performed.
- Clinical immunogenicity data analysis: The developers should include a summary of immunogenicity analyses for all clinical studies having an immunogenicity component.
- Conclusions, risk evaluation, and mitigation strategies: The developers should discuss how immunogenicity affects the safety and efficacy of the protein product for the patient population, including how the product will be monitored in the postmarketing phase.

7.7.12 IMMUNOGENICITY TESTING METHODS

Minor differences in immunogenicity without correlation at the quality level and without any negative impact on clinical efficacy (reduced or loss of efficacy) and safety might be acceptable. Evaluating the clinical impact of an observed difference in immunogenicity may be challenging because of the limited sample size and follow-up duration. If the clinical impact of the observed difference is uncertain, for example, because of the rarity of the potentially severe adverse effect or the slow evolution of an immune response, then a specific risk management strategy and an update of the risk management plan may be required through postmarketing surveillance, or studies particularly for monoclonal antibodies are available at the EMA.

Immunogenicity studies aim to detect and characterize an immune response to the product and investigate correlations of ADA with PK and PD and with efficacy and safety. Therefore, immunogenicity assessment should be included in the planning of pivotal clinical studies, including synchronization of sampling for ADA and relevant biomarkers, if available, evaluation of biosimilar efficacy and safety.

7.7.12.1 Population

It is important to select a suitable population to compare immunogenicity. For selecting an appropriate population, factors such as immunocompetence, prior or concomitant use of immunosuppressant therapies, and historical data concerning the immunogenicity of the reference product should be considered. Because the immunogenicity testing is usually undertaken as part of the pivotal comparative safety and efficacy study, the aforementioned factors must be considered during the design of the program's clinical portion to demonstrate biosimilarity.

The type of immunogenicity studies, if required, should be justified based on the observed difference(s), route of administration, dose-response curve, therapeutic window, and the potential clinical impact. The target population of for efficacy, safety, and immunogenicity testing needs to be sensitive to differences in immunogenicity and its consequences and representative of the population(s) for whom the product is indicated. In high-risk situations, the samples should be analyzed on a postapproval basis.

In several instances, a healthy population will be the preferred choice if the drug treatment, either previous or concomitant, can suppress the immune response; a good case in point is the evaluation of filgrastim products preferred in a healthy population.

7.7.12.2 Side-by-Side Assessment

A comparative immunogenicity study aims to rule out clinically meaningful differences in immunogenicity between a proposed biosimilar product and the reference product. The presence of antibodies that can impact biosimilar safety and efficacy is highly concerning; for example, this issue can be overcome by altering PK, inducing anaphylaxis, or neutralizing the product and its endogenous protein counterpart. For each treatment arm, the comparative study(s) should characterize the incidence and magnitude of the ADA response, time-course of ADA development, ADA persistence, and impact of ADA on biosimilar safety, efficacy, and PK.

Side-by-side comparative immunogenicity studies are required during the development of the proposed biosimilar product. If the initial physicochemical and in vitro testing indicates a difference, then there is a higher likelihood of detecting differences in immunogenicity, especially in cases where the molecules are known to be highly immunogenic.

Immunogenicity testing should be integrated with PK, safety, and efficacy testing. Patient samples that test positive for binding ADA in confirmatory binding assays should also be tested for their ability to neutralize the drug unless a strong rationale exists for not doing so. The selection of an appropriate format for neutralizing antibody testing is essential and should consider the mechanism of action of the drug. Depending on the mechanism of action, competitive ligand binding assays or cell-based assays may be appropriate.

7.7.12.3 Endpoints

The selection of clinical immunogenicity endpoints or PD measures associated with immune responses to therapeutic protein products (e.g., antibody formation and cytokine levels) should consider immunogenicity issues reported for the reference product. The developers should prospectively define the clinical immune response criteria (e.g., definitions of significant clinical events such as anaphylaxis), using established criteria where available, for each type of potential immune response. They should obtain agreement from regulatory agencies on these criteria before study initiation.

7.7.12.4 Sampling Schedule

The frequency of sampling and the timing and extent of analyses will depend on the risk assessment for a particular drug. Sampling schedules should be designed to distinguish patients who are transiently positive from patients who have developed a persistent antibody response. The post-treatment sampling period should be long enough so as to draw conclusions on the persistence of the immune response triggered by the therapeutic protein and uncover an immune reaction suppressed by the therapeutic protein itself. The timing of post-treatment sample(s) collection is determined by the protein's half-life and the drug tolerance in ADA assay.

More frequent sampling is necessary for testing in the earlier phase of treatment, where patients are generally at the highest risk of ADA development. Long-term follow-up of immunogenicity with less frequent sampling yields additional information on the occurrence and consequences of immunogenicity. In the case of continuous long-term treatment, immunogenicity data for 1 year of treatment should generally be available during the pre-authorization period, but shorter follow-up is possible with proper scientific justification.

Immunogenicity should be systematically tested in patients routinely as scheduled, involving repetitive sampling, in a symptom-driven manner, and an additional sample should be collected when the occurrence of an unwanted immune response is suspected.

Several product-related factors will influence the development of an immune response against a therapeutic protein. Therefore, the sampling schedule for detecting an immune response should be adapted and applied individually for each product, considering its PK (e.g., elimination half-life) and ADA assay drug tolerance. Baseline samples should always be collected.

The developer should use generally accepted terminologies when describing the kinetics of the ADA response and potential immune-mediated adverse effects, considering the experience of comparable products and relevant regulatory and scientific publications. During treatment, samples should be collected before administering the product because residual levels of the active substance in the sample can interfere with the assay.

If the product can be administered through different routes, then developers should justify their approach regarding immunogenicity assessment for each route of administration in the Marketing Authorization Application.

7.7.12.5 Dependence on Pharmacokinetics

ADA can influence PK, especially the elimination phase. Non-neutralizing "binding" antibodies may sometimes modulate, rather than just decrease, the efficacy of a product, for example, by prolonging the half-life. Changes in PK may be an early indication of antibody formation. Thus, developers are encouraged to incorporate concomitant sampling for both PK and immunogenicity into all repeat dose studies.

7.7.13 Safety and Efficacy Relationship

The immunogenicity associated with intermittent treatment should be considered based on immunogenicity risk assessment, for example, experience from other similar products, risks associated with potential immunogenicity, boosting effect, and persistence or appearance of antibodies after exposure to the biosimilar.

The presence of ADA may or may not have clinical consequences. Therefore, clinical development should be based on an analysis of potential risks and possibilities to detect and mitigate them. Planning of the analysis of immune-mediated adverse effects should be based on risk analysis, including previous experience of the product (class), potentially immunogenic structures in the protein, and type of patient population. Patients with pre-existing ADA may exhibit a different efficacy and safety profile and should be analyzed as a subgroup when feasible. The analysis plan should define symptom complexes associated with acute or delayed hypersensitivity, autoimmunity, and loss of efficacy. Potential immunological adverse effects should be addressed in the risk management plan.

7.7.13.1 Management of Immunogenicity Testing

A harmful immune reaction to a therapeutic protein cannot always be avoided despite the developers' efforts to select compounds with a low immunogenic potential. In such cases, the developers should, if feasible, explore possibilities to reduce the adverse effect of immunogenicity observed during clinical development. In some cases, immunosuppressive or anti-inflammatory co-medication may significantly prevent or reduce adverse immunological effects. In some cases, as observed with coagulation factors, it may be possible to re-establish the immunological tolerance with tolerization regimens, for example, by administering larger doses of a therapeutic protein. Clinical studies should document such therapeutic regimens.

7.7.14 EXAMPLE STUDIES

Appendix 3 provides the details of a few study protocols used to secure biosimilar approval from the EMA and FDA.

7.7.14.1 Infliximab

While the primary efficacy analysis demonstrated equivalent ACR_{20} response rates at week 30 with the proposed biosimilar (Flixabi) and the reference product, the ADA rate measured in a highly sensitive assay was approximately 5%–12% higher in a proposed biosimilar cohort at the individual time points of determination (with nearly 50% of patients in the proposed biosimilar cohort being ADA positive at any time in the trial). However, no meaningful effect on any of the efficacy parameters analyzed was observed, as the primary endpoints were within the predefined comparability margins.

7.7.14.2 Etanercept

While the product (Benepali) met all biosimilarity tests, a significant difference in overall ADA formation was observed at week 24. The clinical effect of the difference in ADA seemed negligible, and the difference largely vanished after 8 weeks of treatment.

The notion that PK studies are generally more sensitive in detecting potential product-related differences than clinical trials may explain why a finding of similar efficacy could not overrule the differences in PK. This may be perceived as overly strict. Yet, the outcome of efficacy trials depends not only on drug exposure but also on the effective pharmacological action of the biological substance in vivo. Therefore, the objectives of both types of studies differ.

8 Clinical Efficacy Assessment of the Proposed Biosimilar

8.1 RESIDUAL UNCERTAINTY

A comparative clinical study will be necessary to support biosimilarity through scientific evidence if there is residual uncertainty regarding clinically meaningful differences between a proposed biosimilar product and the reference product based on structural and functional characterization, animal testing, human pharmacokinetics (PK) and pharmacodynamics (PD) data, and clinical immunogenicity assessment. The developers should provide scientific justification if they believe that a comparative clinical study is not necessary.

A proposed biosimilar product undergoes testing in a stepwise manner for the detection and removal of residual uncertainty at each step before moving to another testing. The steps involved in the testing are as follows (in the same order): analytical, functional, in vitro, in vivo, clinical pharmacology, and immunogenicity. While the developers of most of the biosimilars routinely conduct clinical efficacy testing as listed in Appendix 3, agencies consider unnecessary patient exposure as being inappropriate and encourage them to meet up with agencies to understand what the agencies consider as the remaining residual uncertainty.

In most cases, at this stage of development, a failed PK/PD/immunogenicity testing will reject a proposed biosimilar product for a proposed biosimilar status. The developer may choose to refile the applications as a new biological drug. The residual uncertainties persisting at this stage are identified through structural, functional, or nonclinical testing, where the variation may not be evaluated fully for its effect on the safety and efficacy of the product.

8.2 WAIVERS

When appropriate PD endpoints are achieved and when the mechanism of action is clearly understood, a PK/PD study may be an adequate clinical workup for marketing authorization. However, for complex, multifunctional biologicals, comparative efficacy and safety clinical trials conducted in patients are still considered necessary components in the development of a proposed biosimilar product. The need for testing in patients is driven by the often-unresolvable complexity of interactions resulting from the molecule size, diverse moieties with different functions (e.g., Fab/Fc-parts), multiple mechanisms of action, the effect of glycosylation pattern, and potential for immunogenicity and life-threatening adverse effects.

As more proposed biosimilar products are approved globally and safety and efficacy data are becoming available to regulatory agencies, there is a trend of questioning the relevance of any comparative efficacy testing. When clinical efficacy testing does not show a meaningful comparison, exposes patients to avoidable risks, and does not establish relevance to multiple indications approved

DOI: 10.1201/9781003392026-8

for the reference product, then agencies will expect the developers to adduce arguments supporting the avoidance of such clinical efficacy testing.

In most cases, a comparative clinical study is essential to rule out clinically meaningful differences in efficacy and safety between a proposed biosimilar product and the reference product. A clinical efficacy trial may not always be necessary, for instance, when a clinically relevant PD endpoint is available. In such cases, scientific justification is needed to conduct an efficacy study, yet safety and comparative immunogenicity data are still required.

8.3 TYPES OF STUDY DESIGN

Comparative safety and efficacy testing is conducted using three types of study design.

Generally, an equivalence design should be used. A noninferiority design may be acceptable if justified based on a strong scientific rationale and considering the characteristics of the reference product, for example, safety profile/tolerability, dose range, and dose-response relationship. A noninferiority trial may be accepted only where the possibility of a significant and clinically relevant increase in efficacy can be excluded based on scientific and mechanistic evidence. However, as in equivalence trials, assay sensitivity has to be considered in a noninferiority trial.

The correlation between the "hard" clinical endpoints recommended by the guidelines for new active substances and other clinical/pharmacodynamic endpoints that are more sensitive in detecting clinically meaningful differences may have been demonstrated in previous clinical studies assessing the reference product. In this case, it is unnecessary to use the same primary efficacy endpoints as those used in the reference product's registration application. However, it is recommended to include some common endpoints (as secondary endpoints) to facilitate comparison with the clinical studies assessing the reference product.

The developers are advised to consult the European Medicines Agence (EMA) European Public Agency Reports (EPARs) and the FDA Biological Licensing Application (BLA) review documents relating to the proposed biosimilar product to choose the testing model for establishing clinical safety and efficacy; in the absence of such data, the developers should suggest a testing model to the agencies for marketing authorization by agencies before study initiation. However, neither the agencies nor the developers are bound or required to use any testing model that is published or submitted/accepted by any regulatory agency.

8.3.1 STUDY DESIGNS FOR COMPARATIVE SAFETY AND EFFICACY TESTING

8.3.1.1 Traditional Comparative (Two-Sided) Study

In a traditional comparative study, the null hypothesis states that the proposed biosimilar and the reference product do not have any difference. The burden of proof rests on the research hypothesis of the difference between the two products in terms of efficacy. If the evidence is not strong enough in favor of a difference, then equality cannot be ruled out. This model is not suitable for the assessment of biosimilars.

8.3.1.2 Equivalence Testing

In an equivalence testing, the null hypothesis states that the proposed biosimilar is not equivalent to the reference product in terms of equivalency, and the burden of proof rests in the research hypothesis. If the evidence in favor of equivalence is not strong enough, then nonequivalence cannot be ruled out. The null and research hypotheses in an equivalence testing are simply the converse of those of a traditional comparative study. This is the most common model used in testing except that the margin of difference, M2, is based on the clinical judgment that can be questioned. The term "equivalent" means that the efficacy of the two therapies is close enough to not be considered superior or inferior to the other. This concept is formalized in defining a constant, called the "equivalence margin," defining a range of values for which the efficacies are "close enough" to be considered equivalent. Practically, the margin is the maximum clinically acceptable difference that one is willing to accept in return for the secondary benefits of the new therapy.

An inherent disadvantage in using the equivalence model lies in the choice of difference (M2) considered acceptable; this difference is established mainly based on clinical judgment, as objective studies will not be available for reference. The total response (M1) is deduced from the reference product data.

The choice of equivalence margins in comparative efficacy studies is more complicated. Prespecified margins include the largest differences that would not be clinically relevant. The margins need not be symmetric if dose-related toxicities occur or if the dose used is closer to the plateau of the dose-response curve. There is a small likelihood of dose-related effects. In most studies, a margin of 15% is suggested, such as in the testing of Remsima for American College of Rheumatology 20 at 30 weeks and Samsung Bioepis' infliximab biosimilar. However, the adalimumab "similar biologic," approved in India (Exemptia) (www.ncbi.nlm.nih.gov/pmc/articles/PMC5215647/), is used at an equivalence margin of 28.5%, allowing for a much smaller sample size and a margin of 23% for an infliximab biosimilar biologic in India. The choice of margin becomes more complicated, for instance, when comparing anticancer drugs, where the outcome is binomial and often difficult to predict.

8.3.1.3 Noninferiority Testing

In a noninferiority testing, the null hypothesis states that the proposed biosimilar product is inferior to the reference product. The research hypothesis is that the new therapy is either equivalent or superior to the current therapy. Only one margin (the lower or upper limit, depending on what is appropriate for the specific study or endpoint) is used in a noninferiority model. The noninferiority testing requires a smaller sample size than that required in an equivalence model. The confidence interval expresses the degree of uncertainty associated with a statistical parameter, such as the difference between two treatment effects (e.g., risk difference) or the ratio. For example, if the objective response rate is the primary endpoint, then the risk ratio would serve as a primary efficacy parameter. The confidence interval is different from the point estimate for a population parameter. For example, the sample mean, objective response rate, and median survival duration are some examples of point estimates of unknown population parameters. Noninferiority trials do not rule out the possibility of increased activity of a proposed biosimilar product associated with more adverse events.

Comparability margins in applying statistical modeling are established based on the effect size of the reference product and clinical judgment. They should represent the largest difference in efficacy that would be negligible in clinical practice; treatment differences within this range would then be acceptable because they have no clinical relevance. The acceptable equivalence margins depend on the patient population, endpoints, backbone therapy, and estimated treatment effect, and slight differences may occur depending on the selection of publicly available reference studies.

Relying on noninferiority studies to establish biosimilarity is remarkably criticized for the very nature of the need for such studies that includes the overall rationality of these studies.

When noninferiority testing is conducted, a response (M1) and an acceptable difference that can only be arbitrary should be established, given the observed high variability of biological responses.

Agencies are open to suggestions on in silico PK studies and other modeling studies, possibly obviating the need for comparative efficacy studies; the developers are encouraged to minimize testing in patients to secure faster and low-cost marketing authorization of biosimilars. In our opinion, such studies will be limited only to a few highly complex drugs with mixed mechanisms of action and where other assessments cannot be matched well.

8.3.2 Justification of Extrapolation

All indications approved for the reference product as of the marketing authorization date are extrapolated for the proposed biosimilar product. However, suppose a proposed biosimilar product is tested in a comparative efficacy trial, in a single study in one of the many available indications where the mechanisms of action can differ among the indications, a question arises regarding the suitability of a single comparative efficacy testing to allow such extrapolation.

8.3.3 Ethics and Practicality

In most cases, recruiting a suitable patient population is very difficult, such as in the case of anticancer drug testing, where the patients have inevitably been exposed to many drugs, and it is unethical to expose patients to treatment regimens of monotherapy that are not in the best interest of the patient. In several instances, the patients may not survive until study completion, which creates a dilemma for both the developer and the patients.

8.4 SELECTION OF STUDY PROTOCOLS

A comparative clinical study should be adequately sensitive to rule out clinically meaningful differences within predefined comparability margins. The developers should consider the following factors when designing an adequately sensitive clinical study:

- Characteristics of the study population(s) (e.g., underlying disease, immune competence).
- Clinical studies' characteristics, such as study duration, route of administration, dosage regimen, clinical endpoint(s), and assessment duration.
- Risk and effects of immunogenicity.
- Effects of concomitant therapies (e.g., monotherapy vs. combination therapy).
- Use of appropriate comparability margins.
- In some instances, the evaluation of more than one sensitive population may be necessary.

The following are examples of factors that may influence the type and extent of the comparative clinical study data needed:

- The nature and complexity of the reference product; extensiveness of structural and functional characterization; and findings and limitations of comparative structural, functional, and non-clinical testing, including the extent of the observed differences.
- The extent to which differences in structure, function, and nonclinical pharmacology and toxicology predict differences in clinical outcomes, in conjunction with the degree of understanding of the mechanism of action of the reference product and disease pathology.
- The extent to which PK or PD in humans is known to predict clinical outcomes (e.g., PD measures known to be relevant to effectiveness or safety).
- The extent of clinical experience with the reference product and its therapeutic class, including the product's safety and risk-benefit profile (e.g., whether there is a low potential for off-target adverse events), and appropriate endpoints and biomarkers for safety and effectiveness (e.g., availability of established and sensitive clinical endpoints).
- The extent of any other clinical experience with a proposed biosimilar product.

The developers should provide scientific justification for how they intend to use these factors to determine the clinical study type(s) that is needed and whether any necessary study design was needed. For example, suppose a comparative clinical study is needed, then the developers should explain how these factors were considered in determining a study design, including the endpoint(s), population, similarity margin, and statistical analyses.

Additionally, specific concerns related to safety or effectiveness regarding the reference product and its class (including the history of manufacturing- or source-related adverse events) may yield more comparative clinical data. Alternatively, suppose there is information regarding other biological products that could support a biosimilarity determination (with marketing histories that demonstrate no apparent differences in clinical safety and effectiveness profiles), then such information may serve as an additional factor for supporting a selective and targeted approach to the clinical program.

In the absence of surrogate markers for efficacy, it is usually necessary to demonstrate comparable clinical efficacy between a proposed biosimilar product and the reference product in an adequately powered, randomized, parallel-group comparative clinical study(s), preferably with a double-blind design, using efficacy endpoints. Generally, the study population should represent approved therapeutic indication(s) of the reference product and be sensitive in detecting potential differences between a proposed biosimilar product and the reference product. Occasionally, changes in clinical practice may require a deviation from the approved therapeutic indication, for instance, a concomitant medication used in combination treatment, line of therapy, or severity of the disease. Deviations need to be justified and discussed with regulatory authorities.

8.5 STUDY DESIGN

Careful consideration should be given to the study design, including the choice of primary efficacy endpoints and comparative clinical margins. Each of these aspects is important and should be justified on based on clinical evidence. The study should be conducted using a clinically relevant and sensitive endpoint to show the absence of a clinically meaningful difference between the proposed biosimilar product and the reference product. The chosen endpoint could be different from that set in the original study for the reference product (e.g., a well-established surrogate or a more sensitive endpoint). An acceptable comparability margin should be defined in all cases, considering the smallest effect size that the reference product would reliably be expected to have based on publicly available historical data. If multiple endpoints are used, then the principles described above should be applied.

In line with the principle of similarity, equivalence trials are generally preferred. If noninferiority trials are considered, then they should be justified, and the developer is advised to consult with regulatory agencies before study initiation. The developers should be aware that such trials' results could suggest the statistical superiority of a proposed biosimilar product relative to the reference product. In such instances, the superiority observed should be assessed for clinical relevance, including its effect on safety. If the superiority observed is considered clinically meaningful and is associated with increased adverse drug reactions over those seen with the reference product, the product would no longer be considered a biosimilar. Moreover, demonstration of noninferiority of a proposed biosimilar product to the reference product might not provide strong supporting evidence for the authorization of other indications, particularly if the other indications include different dosages than those tested in the clinical study.

8.5.1 EFFICACY ENDPOINTS

Using a comparative clinical study, the developers should set endpoints to assess clinically meaningful differences between a proposed biosimilar product and the reference product. The endpoints may differ from those used as primary endpoints in clinical studies of the reference product if they are scientifically supported. Certain endpoints (such as PD measures) are more sensitive than clinical endpoints and, therefore, may enable more precise comparisons of the relevant therapeutic effects.

TABLE 8.1
Clinical Endpoints in Testing of the Proposed Biosimilar

Absolute neutrophil count for granulocyte–colony-stimulating factor
Blood glucose concentrations in clamp studies for detecting insulin
Complete pathological response in breast cancer
Disease Activity Score-28 versus American College of Rheumatology-20 in rheumatoid arthritis disease
Objective response rate in solid tumors and lymphoma
Factor X and anti-factor II activity, magnetic resonance imaging–related endpoints for interferon-β,
Use of serum calcium levels for teriparatide
Bone mineral density together with serum C-terminal crosslinks, a bone resorption marker, as co-primary efficacy
    endpoints for denosumab to treat and prevent osteoporosis
α4-integrin receptor saturation for natalizumab as the binding is directly linked to clinical outcomes
Serum lactate dehydrogenase levels and for eculizumab

In some situations, assessing many PD measures using a comparative clinical study will enhance the sensitivity of the study. The adequacy of the endpoints depends on the extent to which PD measures correlate with the clinical outcome, the extent of structural and functional data supporting biosimilarity, the extent of understanding of the mechanism of action, and the nature or severity of the outcome affected.

While the "hard" clinical outcome remains the most desirable endpoint, other clinical endpoints that require shorter study durations have been widely used (Table 8.1).

The developers should justify that the chosen model is relevant and sensitive to detect potential differences in efficacy and safety. Differences detected between the efficacy of a proposed biosimilar product and that of the reference product should always be discussed as to whether they are clinically relevant. Generally, clinical data help in addressing slight differences observed in the previous steps and confirm the comparable clinical performance of the proposed biosimilar product and the reference product. Clinical data cannot be used to justify substantial differences in quality attributes.

Comparative margins should be prespecified and justified based on both statistical and clinical evidence by using the reference product's data as well as all comparative clinical study designs and assay sensitivity (see ICH topic E9 Statistical principles for clinical studies and CHMP guideline CPMP/EWP/2158/99 on the choice of the noninferiority margin).

8.6 CLINICAL SAFETY

Clinical safety is important throughout the clinical development program and is assessed during the initial PK and PD evaluations and in any comparative clinical efficacy study. Comparative safety data should generally be collected during pre-authorization, depending on the type and severity of safety issues known for the reference product. The duration of safety follow-up pre-authorization should be justified. More attention should be paid to comparing the type, severity, and frequency of the adverse reactions between a proposed biosimilar product and the reference product, as reported in literature. The developers should evaluate the specific risks anticipated for a proposed biosimilar product in the application dossier. This includes, in particular, a description of possible safety concerns that may result from a manufacturing process different from that of the reference product, especially those related to infusion-related reactions and immunogenicity.

Immunogenicity testing of a proposed biosimilar product and the reference product should be conducted during comparative efficacy testing of a proposed biosimilar product in the same assay format and sampling schedule as those for the reference product, which must meet all current standards. Analytical assays should be performed in parallel with the reference product and the proposed biosimilar product (in a blinded manner) to measure the immune response against the product received by each patient. The analytical assays should preferably detect antibodies against both the proposed biosimilar product and the reference product. Yet, they should, at minimum, detect all antibodies developed against a proposed biosimilar product. Generally, the incidence and nature (e.g., cross-reactivity, target epitopes, and neutralizing activity) of antibodies and antibody titers should be measured and presented. They should be assessed and interpreted about their potential effect on clinical efficacy and safety parameters.

The duration of immunogenicity studies should be justified on a case-by-case basis depending on the duration of the treatment course, the disappearance of the product from the circulation (to avoid antigen interference in the assays), and the time for the emergence of the humoral immune response (at least 4 weeks when an immunosuppressive agent is used). Follow-up duration should be justified based on the time course and characteristics of unwanted immune responses described for the reference product, for instance, a low risk of clinically significant immunogenicity or no significant trend for increased immunogenicity over time. For long-term administration, 1-year follow-up data will usually be required pre-authorization. Shorter follow-up data pre-authorization (e.g., 6 months) might be justified based on the reference product's immunogenicity profile. If needed, immunogenicity data for an additional period, that is, for up to 1 year, could then be submitted post-authorization. For the individual, refer to product-specific proposed biosimilar guidelines.

Increased immunogenicity when compared with the reference product may become concerning for the benefit/risk analysis and may question biosimilarity. However, lower immunogenicity for a proposed biosimilar product is a possible scenario that would not preclude authorization as a biosimilar. In case of defective development of neutralizing antibodies against the biosimilar, then efficacy analysis of the entire population could erroneously suggest that the proposed biosimilar product is more efficacious than the reference product. Therefore, it is recommended to pre-specify an additional exploratory subgroup analysis of efficacy and safety in patients who did not mount an antidrug antibody response during the clinical study. This subgroup analysis could help establish that the efficacy of a proposed biosimilar product and the reference product is, in principle, similar if not affected by an immune response.

8.6.1 STUDY POPULATION

The choice of the study population should enable the assessment of clinically meaningful differences between the proposed biosimilar product and the reference product. Often, the study population used for testing a biosimilar will have characteristics consistent with those of the population studied for the reference product's marketing authorization for the same indication. However, there are cases where a study population could be different from that used in clinical studies supporting the reference product's marketing authorization. For example, if a genetic predictor of response was developed following the reference product's marketing authorization, then it may be possible to use patients with the response marker as the study population.

8.6.2 SAMPLE SIZE AND STUDY DURATION

The sample size for and duration of a comparative clinical study should be adequate in order to detect clinically meaningful differences between a proposed biosimilar product and the reference product. Certain endpoints, such as PD measures, may be more sensitive than clinical endpoints and facilitate a smaller sample size in a study of limited duration. In cases where the sample size and duration of the comparative clinical study may not be adequate for detecting relevant safety signals, a separate assessment of safety and immunogenicity may be needed.

8.6.2.1　Study Design and Analyses

A comparative clinical study for a proposed biosimilar development program should be designed to investigate whether a proposed biosimilar product and the reference product exhibit clinically meaningful differences. The design should consider the nature and extent of residual uncertainty about biosimilarity based on data generated from comparative structural and functional characterization, animal testing, human PK and PD studies, and clinical immunogenicity assessment.

Generally, agencies expect a clinical study or studies designed to establish statistical evidence that a proposed biosimilar product is neither inferior nor superior to the reference product by more than a (possibly different) specified margin. Typically, an equivalence design with symmetric inferiority and superiority margins would be used. Symmetric margins would be reasonable when, for example, there are dose-related toxicities.

In some cases, it would be appropriate to use an asymmetric interval with a larger upper bound to rule out superiority than a lower bound to rule out inferiority. An asymmetric interval could be reasonable; for example, in cases where the dose used in the clinical study is near the dose-response curve plateau. There is a small likelihood of dose-related effects (e.g., toxicity). In most cases, the use of an asymmetric interval would generally allow for a smaller sample size than would be needed with symmetric margins. However, if there is a demonstration of clear superiority, then further consideration should be given as to whether a proposed biosimilar product can be considered a proposed biosimilar to the reference product.

In some cases, depending on the study population and endpoint(s), ruling out only inferiority may be adequate to establish that the proposed biosimilar product and the reference product have no clinically meaningful difference. For example, if it is well established that doses of the reference product pharmacodynamically saturate the target at the clinical dose level, then it would be unethical to use lower than clinically approved doses; in such cases, a noninferiority design may be sufficient. The developers should provide adequate scientific justification for the choice of study design, study population, study endpoint(s), estimated effect size for the reference product, and margin(s) (how much difference to rule out). The developers should discuss their study proposal(s) and the overall clinical development plan with regulatory agencies before initiating the comparative clinical study.

8.6.3　Clinical Endpoints

One or more clinical studies are sufficient to demonstrate the safety, purity, and potency of a proposed biosimilar product in one or more of the indications for which the reference product is licensed. This typically includes assessing immunogenicity, PK, and, in some cases, PD, and it may also include a comparative clinical efficacy study. The European Medicines Agency (EMA) guidelines state that clinical data help in addressing any slight differences observed in analytical similarity, nonclinical pharmacology, and PK and PD (where possible in healthy subjects) to confirm the comparable clinical performance between a proposed biosimilar and the reference product. However, clinical data cannot be used to justify substantial differences in quality attributes. The developers may choose to withdraw their proposed biosimilar application and file it as a new biologic, a strategy that worked for Teva for its filgrastim product, which was ultimately approved as a new biologic (Granix); noteworthy, when exploiting this path, the developer is not required to provide any comparative data with the reference product, but the literature data can be used to justify safety and efficacy claim to some extent.

The outcome of efficacy trials depends not only on drug exposure (PK profile) but also on the proper pharmacological action of the biological substance in vivo. Therefore, the objectives of both types of studies differ. Efficacy trials are usually designed as equivalence trials (or noninferiority trials) to ensure that the efficacy of a proposed biosimilar decreases or increases when compared with that of the reference product. However, some residual uncertainty regarding the potentially

TABLE 8.2
Suggested Comparative Clinical Study Endpoints

Pathological complete response in breast cancer

Disease Activity Score-28 versus American College of Rheumatology-20 in rheumatoid arthritis disease

Objective response rate in solid tumors and lymphoma

Absolute neutrophil count for granulocyte–colony-stimulating factor

Blood glucose concentrations in clamp studies for insulin detection

Low-molecular-weight heparin. Factor X and anti-factor II activity

Magnetic resonance imaging–related endpoints for interferon-β

Serum calcium levels for teriparatide

Anti-factor X and anti-factor II activity

Bone mineral density together with serum C-terminal crosslinks, a bone resorption marker, as co-primary efficacy
    endpoints for denosumab, a monoclonal antibody used to treat and prevent osteoporosis

For natalizumab, α4-integrin receptor saturation as the binding is directly linked to clinical outcomes

For eculizumab, a potential pharmacodynamics marker to study biosimilarity is serum lactate dehydrogenase because of the
    sustained reduction observed in intravascular hemolysis for the treatment period owing to the reduced need for red blood
    cell transfusions and less fatigue

increased efficacy of a proposed biosimilar may be acceptable in exceptional cases. The data from other evaluation exercises support the conclusion of biosimilarity and safety.

Clinical endpoints (Table 8.2) used in comparability studies of the proposed biosimilar should enable the measurement of any unconfounded pharmacological effects and be sensitive in detecting potential clinically relevant differences between the proposed biosimilar candidate and its reference product. However, the clinical endpoints need not be the same as those approved in the development of the reference product; if the endpoints are sensitive in demonstrating any clinically meaningful difference, then these should be acceptable.

Clinical endpoints used in clinical efficacy comparability studies should ideally measure unconfounded pharmacological effects and be sensitive in detecting potential clinically relevant differences between the proposed biosimilar candidate and its reference product. In this regard, hard clinical endpoints such as overall survival are relatively insensitive and are often influenced by disease- and patient-related factors. Regulatory agencies encourage the developers to suggest novel validated clinical markers as a better choice than patients' responses (Table 8.2).

8.6.4 EXTRAPOLATION OF CLINICAL DATA ACROSS INDICATIONS

Suppose a proposed biosimilar product meets the biosimilarity and other regulatory requirements for marketing authorization as a proposed biosimilar product based on, among other things, data derived from one or more clinical studies sufficient to demonstrate safety, purity, and potency in an appropriate condition of use. In that case, the developers must seek marketing authorization of the proposed biosimilar product for one or more additional conditions of use for which the reference product is authorized.

However, the developers would need to provide sufficient scientific justification for extrapolating clinical data to determine biosimilarity for each condition of use for which marketing authorization is sought.

Such scientific justification for extrapolation should address, for example, the following issues for the tested and extrapolated conditions of use:

- Mechanisms of action of the proposed biosimilar in each condition of use for which marketing authorization is sought; this may include

- • Target/receptor(s) for each relevant activity/function of the product
- • B, dose/concentration-response, and pattern of molecular signaling upon engagement of the target/receptor(s)
- • Relationships between the product structure and target/receptor interactions
- • Location and expression of the target/receptor(s).
- PK and biodistribution of the product in different patient populations (relevant PD measures may also provide important information on the mechanism of action).
- Immunogenicity of the product in different patient populations.
- Differences in the expected toxicities in each condition of use and patient population (including whether expected toxicities are related to the pharmacological activity of the product or off-target activities).
- Any other factor that may affect the safety or efficacy of the product in each condition of use and each patient population for which marketing authorization is sought.
- Differences between conditions of use concerning the factors described above do not necessarily preclude extrapolation. Scientific justification is needed to address the differences in the totality-of-the-evidence context, supporting the demonstration of biosimilarity.
- When choosing which condition of use to study that would permit subsequent extrapolation of clinical data to other conditions of use, it is recommended that the developers consider choosing a condition of use that would be adequately sensitive to detect clinically meaningful differences between the proposed biosimilar product and the reference product.

The developers of the proposed biosimilar product are required to obtain marketing authorization for all conditions of use that have been previously approved for the reference product at the time of applying. If the reference product receives marketing authorization for additional indications, then the developers must add those indications before or after the marketing authorization. However, if an indication is protected under intellectual property laws, then the developers may request fewer indications and then add more indications as the intellectual property expiration allows them.

8.6.5 Extrapolation Across Indications

The reference product may have more than one therapeutic indication. When biosimilarity in a comparative study has been demonstrated for one indication, extrapolation of clinical data to other indications of the reference product could be acceptable, but this needs to be scientifically justified. In case it is unclear whether the safety and efficacy confirmed in one indication would be relevant for another indication, then additional data will be required for confirmation. Extrapolation should be considered in the light of the totality of data, that is, quality, nonclinical, and clinical data. It is expected that the safety and efficacy can be extrapolated when thorough physicochemical and structural analyses have demonstrated that the proposed biosimilar's comparative and in vitro functional tests complemented with clinical data (efficacy and safety and PK/PD data) in one therapeutic indication. Additional data are required in certain situations, some of which are as follows:

- The active substance of the reference product interacts with several receptors, leading to a possibly a different effect on the tested and nontested therapeutic indications.
- The active substance itself has more than one active site, and the sites may have a different effect on different therapeutic indications.
- The studied therapeutic indication is not relevant for the others in terms of efficacy or safety, that is, it is not sensitive to differences in all relevant aspects of efficacy and safety.

Immunogenicity is related to multiple factors, including the route of administration, dosing regimen, patient-related factors, and disease-related factors (e.g., co-medication, disease type, and immune status). Thus, immunogenicity could differ among indications. Extrapolation of immunogenicity from the studied indication/route of administration to other uses of the reference product should be justified.

8.6.6 ADDITIONAL CONDITIONS OF USE

Agencies recognize that the application holder of a proposed biosimilar product may be interested in seeking marketing authorization for an additional condition(s) of use after market authorization of the product. While this option is generally available in many jurisdictions, regulatory agencies allow a proposed biosimilar product to add any new indications allowed to the reference product in the future, provided there are no changes to the reference product. If an indication is protected under a patent, then it is the developers' discretion to judge whether the patent is applicable in its region and they are solely responsible for the litigation. Marketing authorization by the agencies does not constitute an opinion regarding intellectual property associated with the reference product.

9 Recombinant Manufacturing System for Biopharmaceuticals

9.1 OVERVIEW

A robust biopharmaceutical production process is governed by several elements: integrated process design and critical process elements; the quality of starting materials; and the quality systems to confirm that the manufacturing process is reproducible, consistent, and robust. The process design has its own set of challenges both upstream and downstream. However, an upstream process and an efficient purification process capable of providing maximal recovery can yield a highly pure product, which are the most desirable features of any production process.

As biopharmaceuticals have complex chemical structures, it is impossible to synthesize them with currently available technology. Furthermore, even if it becomes possible to synthesize these macromolecules, it would be difficult to produce a molecule that does not have a fixed structure. Therefore, the production of biopharmaceuticals relies on recombinant systems where DNA produces these molecules; DNA portions containing genes of interest are relatively easy to construct, allowing their use as an engine to make the target molecules in living entities. Thus, the starting material for manufacturing biopharmaceuticals is a genetically modified bacterial, yeast, insect, or mammalian cell culture system expressing the target therapeutic protein of interest.

The technology for recombinant manufacturing is widely protected by patents, inclusive of the critical steps and methods, such as isolation of the target gene sequence (coding for the desired protein), its amplification, generation of recombinant DNA, transformation of host cells, screening, and subsequent selection of the expression cell line. For example, the US Patent No. 4,237,224 (Cohen et al.), which is now expired, details the transformation process in microorganisms such as *Escherichia coli* to generate recombinant plasmid DNA. The patent also describes the procedures for the manufacture of the first transformation vector. Cohen's patent is now expired, and the technology is available in the public domain.

The recombinant expression is carried out in a variety of living systems such as

- Prokaryotes such as archaea and bacteria are unicellular organisms with an outer cell membrane but do not have any membrane-bound cellular components, including a nucleus or mitochondria. Thus, the transcription and translation processes are carried out simultaneously, and mRNA translation occurs before the complete synthesis of a mature mRNA transcript.
- Eukaryotes such as animals and plants are multicellular organisms with a nucleus, mitochondria, and Golgi apparatus; these are also. The transcription and translation processes occur sequentially. Transcription, that is, DNA to RNA, occurs in the nucleus, and translation, that is, RNA to protein, occurs in the cytoplasm. Post-translational modifications (PTMs), which are chemical modifications required for a protein's functionality, occurs in the endoplasmic reticulum and the Golgi apparatus following protein synthesis (at different stages, e.g., before

DOI: 10.1201/9781003392026-9

protein folding, post-localization, etc.). The most common PTMs include glycosylation, phosphorylation, acetylation, proteolysis, specific conformation, and oligomerization reactions. The degree and the complexity of these PTMs vary in eukaryotes. As such, depending on the desired protein to be expressed, the choice of the expression system varies. For example,

- Glycosylation and phosphorylation are crucial PTMs occurring in simple eukaryotes such as yeasts and fungi. However, yeasts produce mannose residues that have extensively undergone N-glycosylation, and these residues can be highly immunogenic for humans. As such, the choice of this expression organism is limited to the production of simple proteins.
- Complex proteins requiring a high degree of glycosylation or other PTMs are best produced using eukaryotes such as mammalian cells (e.g., Chinese hamster ovary [CHO], human cells, etc.), insect cells, and plant cells. Among them, mammalian cells, notably CHO cells, have been the most extensively used expression systems for a wide range of complicated proteins (monoclonal antibodies).

For more than 90% of the currently approved products, *E. coli*, CHO cells, and *Saccharomyces cerevisiae* are the most utilized expression systems (hosts). Other cell lines include baby hamster kidney (BHK) cells, mouse C127, African monkey kidney cells, lymphocyte activated, mouse myeloma, myeloma NS0, and prostate epithelium cells, in addition to these cell hosts.

Examples of approved biotherapeutic proteins and their corresponding host cell systems used for protein production are summarized in Table 9.1.

DNA is responsible for producing proteins required by the cells for survival and physiological functions. Recombinant protein expression differs widely—from in vivo use for structural studies to large-scale development for biotherapeutic drugs.

Transcription and translation are the underlying mechanisms for gene regulation and protein expression, respectively. The information contained in the genetic code (DNA) is transcribed into mRNA. The mRNA-coded message is then translated into specific amino acid sequences, leading to formation of the desired protein (Figure 9.1). R DNA is produced by a process wherein the gene of interest is first inserted into a plasmid (e.g., a virus) introduced into a living cell (such as a bacterium or mammalian cell). The plasmid modifies the cellular DNA and forces it to start producing the target protein.

In prokaryotes, transcription and translation occur simultaneously, whereas in eukaryotes, these processes occur sequentially, followed by PTMs that further alter the protein structure or functionality, which are critical for complex therapeutic proteins. These processes are key to harnessing living cells, including microbial systems, animal cells, and plant cells, to construct the desired protein of interest using recombinant DNA technology.

The DNA sequence according to the code of the desired protein is constructed and inserted into a host system (also referred to as a production system or expression system). Chapter 3 discusses cell line development in detail for microbial and mammalian expression systems.

The process of gene insertion starts from choosing a host plasmid that holds the gene of interest in the entity designated to produce a recombinant protein (Figure 9.2). Cloning involves transferring a gene of interest of a DNA fragment to an expression vector.

Expression vectors must possess the following four basic key features: (i) presence of the gene-of-interest cassette, (ii) antibiotic selection cassette, (iii) bacterial origin of expression (*ori*), (iv) multiple cloning site linkers, epitope tags, protease recognition sites, internal ribosome entry sites, and secretion signals. However, not all elements are required.

In the figure, the arrows denote the direction in which the genes are transcribed. The *ori* denotes the origin of DNA replication. The regions marked as "*amp*" and "*tet*" denote the antibiotic resistance genes ampicillin and tetracycline, respectively. The regions marked in blue at the specific sequence (nucleotide) numbers represent the restriction sites for enzymes to recognize and cut out a specific region in the DNA plasmid.

TABLE 9.1
Host Cells Used for Approved Biotherapeutic Products

Pichia pastoris	Collagenase Santyl	N/A
Escherichia coli	Interferon-Alpha-2b Intron A	1986
Escherichia coli	Epoetin Alfa Epogen/Procrit	1989
Pichia pastoris	Interferon Gamma-1b Actimmune	1990
Escherichia coli	Filgrastim Neupogen	1991
CHO cells	Abciximab Reopro	1994
Pichia pastoris	L-Asparaginase Oncaspar	1994
Escherichia coli	Insulin Lispro Humalog	1996
Trichoplusia ni High Five cells	Platelet-Derived Growth Factor Regranex	1997
CHO cells	Rituximab Rituxan	1997
CHO cells	Etanercept Enbrel	1998
CHO cells	Infliximab Remicade	1998
CHO cells	Palivizumab Synagis	1998
CHO cells	Trastuzumab Herceptin	1998
Escherichia coli	Insulin Aspart Novolog	2000
Escherichia coli	Insulin Glargine Lantus	2000
CHO cells	Alemtuzumab Campath	2001
CHO cells	Darbepoetin Alfa Aranesp	2001
CHO cells	Adalimumab Humira	2002
Sf9 cells	Alpha-1 Antitrypsin Prolastin-C	2002
Escherichia coli	Pegfilgrastim Neulasta	2002
Escherichia coli	Teriparatide Forteo	2002
Pichia pastoris	Laronidase Aldurazyme	2003
CHO cells	Omalizumab Xolair	2003
CHO cells	Bevacizumab Avastin	2004
CHO cells	Cetuximab Erbitux	2004
Escherichia coli	Insulin Glulisine Apidra	2004
CHO cells	Natalizumab Tysabri	2004
Sf9 cells	Fibroblast Growth Factor Eperisone Hydrochloride	2005
CHO cells	Ranibizumab Lucentis	2006
CHO cells	Eculizumab Soliris	2007
CHO cells	Golimumab Simponi	2009
Hansenula polymorpha	Prucalopride Resolor	2009
CHO cells	Ustekinumab Stelara	2009
HEK 293 cells	Belimumab Benlysta	2011
CHO cells	Brentuximab Vedotin Adcetris	2011
CHO cells	Insulin Degludec Tresiba	2012
Nicotiana benthamiana tobacco plant	Taliglucerase Alfa Elelyso	2012
CHO cells	Vedolizumab Entyvio	2014
CHO cells	Daratumumab Darzalex	2015
CHO cells	Secukinumab Cosentyx	2015
HEK 293 cells	Atezolizumab Tecentriq	2016
HEK cells	Eftrenonacog Alfa Alprolix	2016
PER.C6 cells	Follitropin Delta Rekovelle	2016
Sp2/0 cells	Infliximab-Dyyb Inflectra	2016
Escherichia coli	Insulin Glargine/Lixisenatide Soliqua	2016
CHO cells	Ixekizumab Taltz	2016
BHK cells	Octocog Alfa Kovaltry	2016
NS0 cells	Olaratumab Lartruvo	2016
HEK 293 cells	Avelumab Bavencio	2017

TABLE 9.1 (Continued)
Host Cells Used for Approved Biotherapeutic Products

HEK 293 cells	Axicabtagene Ciloleucel Yescarta	2017
CHO cells	Brodalumab Siliq	2017
Escherichia coli	Cenegermin-Bkbj Oxervate	2017
CHO cells	Durvalumab Imfinzi	2017
CHO cells	Emicizumab Hemlibra	2017
CHO cells	Guselkumab Tremfya	2017
HEK 293 cells	Inotuzumab Ozogamicin Besponsa	2017
Saccharomyces cerevisiae	Insulin Aspart Injection Fiasp	2017
CHO cells	Non-Acog Beta Pegol Refixia	2017
CHO cells	Rh Coagulation Factor IX Rebinyn	2017
CHO cells	Sarilumab Kevzara	2017
HEK cells	Simoctocog Alfa Vihuma	2017
HEK 293 cells	Tisagenlecleucel Kymriah	2017
CHO cells	Adynovi Rurioctocog Alfa Pegol	2018
CHO cells	Aimovig Erenumab-Aooe	2018
CHO cells	Benralizumab Fasenra	2018
CHO cells	Coagulation Factor Xa Zhzo Andexxa	2018
NS0 cells	Ibalizumab-Uiyk Trogarzo	2018
Pichia pastoris	Insulin Glargine Semglee	2018
Escherichia coli	Metreleptin Myalepta	2018
CHO cells	Mogamulizumab Poteligeo	2018
Escherichia coli	Pegvaliase-Pqpz Palynziq	2018
CHO cells	Velmanase Alfa Lamzede	2018
CHO cells	Aducanumab Aduhelm	2021

Source: www.accessdata.fda.gov/scripts/cder/daf/0

9.2 EXPRESSION SYSTEMS

The choice of the organism and the cell line type as the host organism are the primary and most important aspects that govern a biotherapeutic production process. The starting material for manufacturing recombinant drugs, which is the primary focus of today's biopharmaceuticals, is genetically modified prokaryotes (bacteria) or eukaryotes (e.g., mammalian cells such as CHO, yeast, insects, or cells) expressing the target therapeutic protein product or monoclonal antibody of interest. Biosimilar developers do not have to use the same expression system as that used for the reference product, but it is not advisable, particularly if PTMs are involved.

Well-organized management for a systemic cell bank, with controlled monitoring and testing, is key to assuring a cell line's integrity and biological characteristics. A controlled environment is likely to prevail with a reputable repository or commercial cell line developer. Upon acquiring a new cell line, a collection center will generally characterize the cell line to establish and verify its identity and ensure the purity of the culture—for animal cells, it is essential to demonstrate that the cell line is free from microbial contamination and mycoplasma. The possibility of inadvertently introducing errors (e.g., cross-contamination, contamination with an adventitious virus, etc.) in a cell line is infinite and quite common. Therefore, care must be taken when handling all material to ensure the safest possible working environment. This applies to both cells and to the individuals handling this. Cell culture is considered a biohazard, and the degree of hazard depends on the cells and experimental protocol. Primary cultures have a high risk of harboring undetected viruses.

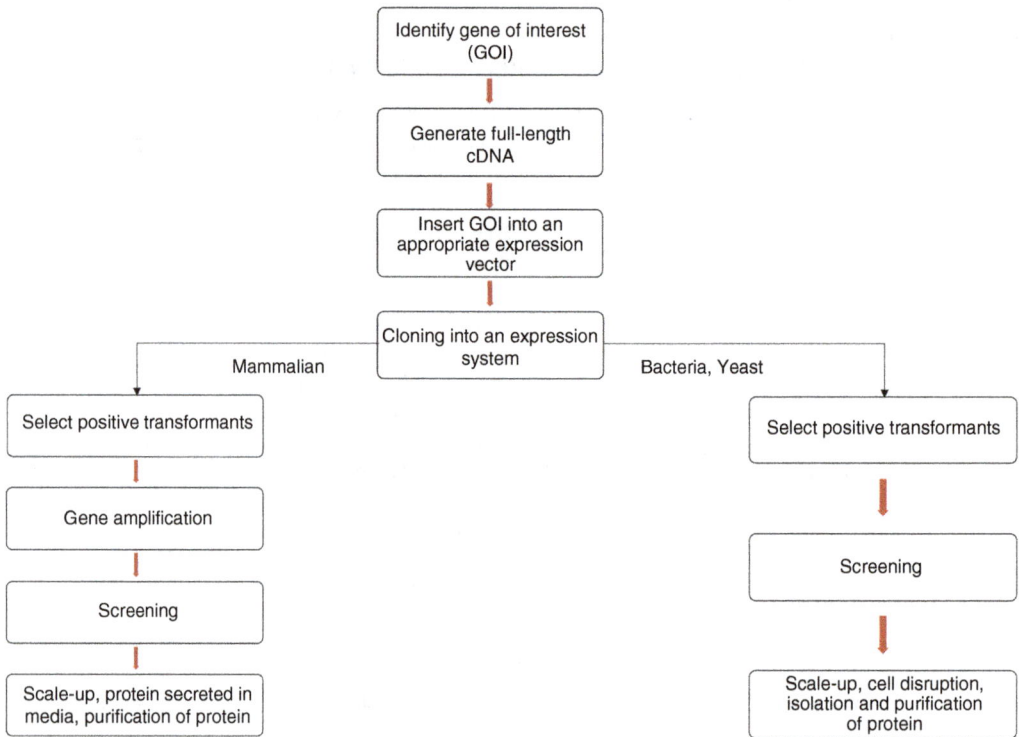

FIGURE 9.1 Flowchart of the development of expression and manufacturing system for recombinant proteins

The robustness of the organism is critical to the success of the biomanufacturing process and dictates commercial manufacturing scalability. It is essential to provide evidence of the organism's history, starting from the first stage of creation to establishing a cell line for future production. Given the high cost of biopharmaceuticals, there has been a significantly continuous improvement in product titer, cell densities, and even enhanced product quality. For example, in the early years, antibody production using mammalian culture processes had relatively low yields of <0.8–1.0 g/L, and in recent years, the productivity of commercial processes has increased to >3 g/L.

9.3   BACTERIAL CELLS

However, bacterial expression systems (such as *E. coli*, *Bacillus*, *Streptococcus*) enable intracellular and extracellular protein expression without any PTMs. The key benefits of using a bacterial expression system for the production of simple target drugs are their relatively short doubling time, easy manipulation, simplified handling, high productivity, and cost-effectiveness, particularly for large-scale production.

The protein production process, which involve gene expression, cloning, and small-scale protein production, it can take approximately 5–7 days to produce adequate protein (ranging from a few hundred milligrams per liter to grams per liter). The nutritional and aeration demands for bacterial production systems are simple, allowing relatively straightforward scale-up operations in fermenters. Additionally, bacterial systems are robust in their ability to withstand the shear forces occurring when increasing operational scales and volumes. These fermentation processes can be operated in both batch and fed-batch modes.

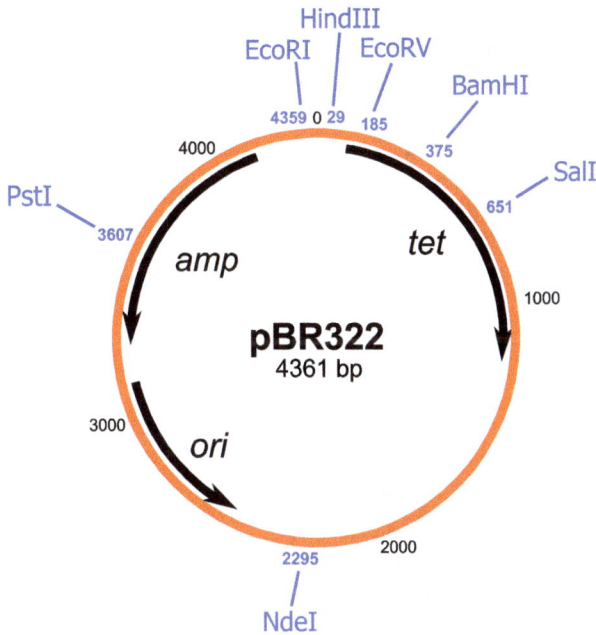

FIGURE 9.2 Schematic representation of the pBR322 plasmid, one of the first plasmids widely used as a cloning vector

Source: By Ayacop (+Yikrazuul)-Own work, Public Domain, commons.wikimedia.org/w/index.php?curid= 11840365

E. coli is the most widely used expression system since the approval of Humulin (insulin) in 1982, specifically for small proteins and peptides, and most recently, it has been used to produce antibody fragments and derivatives such as Fab fragments single-chain variable fragment antibody that does not require any PTMs. Some of the recombinant proteins that have been successfully manufactured using *E. coli* are human growth hormone, interferon-alpha 2a, and 2b, interleukin, granulocyte–colony-stimulating factor, parathyroid hormone, and somatostatin. Of the biopharmaceuticals approved in Europe and the US, approximately 39% are manufactured using *E. coli*. Table 9.1 lists examples of proteins produced using *E. coli* production systems.

A schematic detailing the process of gene expression, cloning, and generation of recombinant bacterial cells is presented in Figure 9.3.

The rapid growth rates and basic nutrient requirements while not compromising titer are the critical features of the *E. coli* expression system for the production of nonglycosylated molecules. Therefore, optimal conditions including temperature, pH, dissolved oxygen, aeration, and agitation, as well as convenient nutrient feeds, are essential parameters that determine the productivity of fermentation.

The expression and production of recombinant proteins in *E. coli* occur intracellularly (e.g., cytoplasm, periplasm) and extracellularly (extracellular space). Typically, the protein expression targeted in the cytoplasm or periplasm often leads to aggregates called inclusion bodies, which harbor the protein. These inclusion bodies are isolated from the rest of the cellular components after fermentation to extract and purify the protein. The protein present in the inclusion bodies exists in the inactive state and requires conversion to the active state. This is typically accomplished through solubilization and refolding to enable the movement of the protein into its native conformation. The *E. coli* expression system lacks the ability and mechanism to carry out PTMs such as glycosylation,

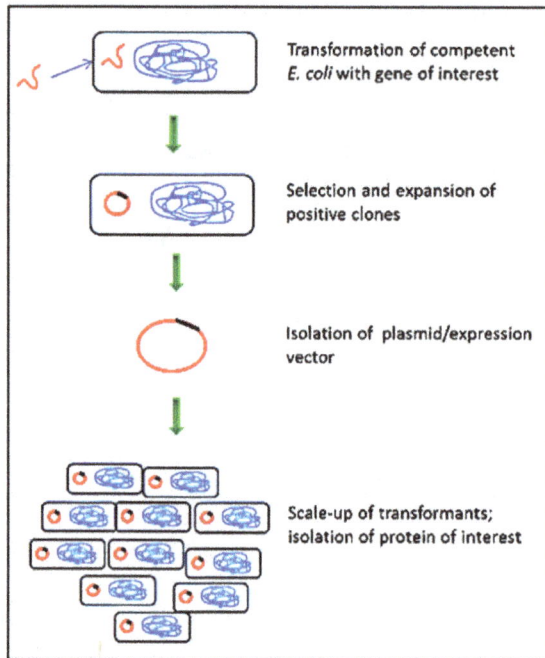

FIGURE 9.3   Bacterial expression system

disulfide bond formation, and phosphorylation, among others. Therefore, only relatively simple protein molecules that do not need any PTMs are often produced using bacterial cells. The formation of inclusion bodies can be considered advantageous, particularly in cases where the protein produced is susceptible to degradation or loss in its activity and function. The product, in its inactive state, is safely harbored within these inclusion bodies. Inclusion bodies are generally recovered by centrifugation and are subjected to additional washing with various chemicals to obtain inclusion bodies of high purity. To promote disulfide bond formation, typically during protein refolding, an appropriate redox pair (e.g., GSH/GSSG) or reducing agents such as dithiothreitol or mercaptoethanol may be added during and/or after solubilization to reduce the formation of any undesirable intermolecular and intramolecular disulfide bridges. During refolding, controlling the product/protein aggregation is key to ensuring that aggregates are limited. This is typically accomplished by diluting the medium to relatively low concentrations of the protein and a controlled rate. Additional processing steps—solubilization and refolding, although it is crucial to regain the correct protein configuration and activity during these steps—are considered disadvantageous, adding to the increase in liquid handling volumes (due to refolding at low protein concentrations) which increases overall costs and likely decreases the yield.

Another significant drawback often encountered with bacterial production systems is the generation/presence of cell-substrate impurities including endotoxins and host cell proteins (HCPs). This requires various process controls to be monitored to ensure that endotoxins and HCPs are within acceptable limits and meet regulatory requirements for permissible amounts in doses. Some of the common processing steps that may require additional in-process controls or monitoring include the cell lysis steps, body solubilization, and refolding. Thus, downstream operations must be highly robust and capable of minimizing these impurities. Other alternatives such as in vitro folding and N-terminal cleavage can be considered as overall process improvements. Despite these limitations, *E. coli* cells are still popular and are the preferred choice for producing simple protein molecules.

TABLE 9.2
Key Characteristics of Commonly Used *Escherichia coli* Expression Strains

Parent *E. coli* Strain	Strain	Resistance	Key Features	Protein Expression
B	BL21 (DE3)	Ampicillin	IPTG-inducible strain containing T7 RNAP (DE3)	Best suited for general protein expression
	BL21 (DE3) pLysS	Chloramphenicol (pLysS)	pLysS expresses T7 lysozyme Has lower basal expression levels	Used for the expression of toxic proteins
	BL21 (DE3) pLysE	Chloramphenicol (pLysE)	pLysE has higher T7 lysozyme expression than pLysS	Most suitable for the expression of toxic proteins
	BL21 Star (DE3)	Ampicillin	T7 based, has high mRNA stability, capable of high yields	Best suited for a high level of expression and for the expression of nontoxic proteins
	BL21-AI	Tetracycline/ kanamycin	Arabinose-induced T7 expression	Best suited for general protein expression but can also be used for the expression of toxic proteins
	BLR (DE3)	Tetracycline	Rec-A-deficient derivative of BL21 Suitable for stabilizing plasmids with repetitive sequences	Suitable for the expression of unstable proteins
	Tuner (DE3)	Chloramphenicol	Contains mutated lac permease (lac ZY deleted) Derivative of BL21	Suitable for the expression of toxic or insoluble proteins Can be used for low levels of expression
	Rosetta 2 (DE3)	Chloramphenicol (pRARE)	Derivative of BL21 Contains seven additional tRNAs for rare codons that can support the expression of eukaryotic proteins	Expression of eukaryotic proteins
	T7 express	Ampicillin, kanamycin	IPTG-inducible T7 RNAP expression Protease deficient	Best suited for general protein expression
K12	HMS174 (DE3)	Rifampicin	Rec-A deficient	Suitable for the expression of unstable proteins
	Origami2 (DE3)	Streptomycin, tetracycline	Mutated K12 strain for thioredoxin reductase and glutathione reductase genes	Best suited for the expression of proteins that require disulfide bond formation for proper protein folding
	M15 pREP4	Kanamycin (pREP4)	Cis-repression of the *E. coli* T5 promoter	Suitable for the expression of toxic proteins

The two most commonly used *E. coli* strains are K12 and B. Table 9.2 details the commonly used strains derived from the *E. coli* B strain and K12 strain. The growth characteristics of the B and K12 strains are completely different. Therefore, the features and characteristics of these strains must be carefully considered and evaluated for determining the appropriate strain for use as the expression system for the desired protein. Additionally, the strains vary in terms of their coding of the disulfide bonds in the protein or even encoding toxic proteins.

In recent years, various new strains with significant improvements are being used to manufacture biopharmaceuticals (e.g., bacilli, *Ralstonia eutropha*, *Staphylococcus carnosus*).

TABLE 9.3
Industrial Attributes of Expression Systems for Commercial Manufacturing (Fewer Stars Are Desirable)

Platform	High Cost	Long Cycle Time	Low Capacity	Difficult Propagation	Low Yield	Low Quality	Contamination Risk	High Purification Cost
Transgenic plants	****	**	*	***	*	*	***	*
Plant cell	**	**	**	***	*	*	****	**
Plant virus	***	***	*	**	*	**	****	*
Microalgae	***	*	*	***	*	*	****	**
Yeast	**	**	*	***	*	**	***	**
Bacteria	***	***	*	***	**	***	**	*
Mammalian cell	*	*	****	*	**	*	*	*
Transgenic animals	*	*	***	**	*	*	*	*
Insect cell	**	**	*	**	*	**	***	**
Filamentous fungi	***	*	*	***	*	**	***	***

9.4 YEAST

S. cerevisiae and *Pichia pastoris* are two yeast species that are increasingly used as an expression system (Table 9.3). They have high efficiency (short doubling time, high cell density, high yield owing to better mass transfer of nutrients in unicellular growth morphology), and low fermentation costs. In 1991, the Food and Drug Administration (FDA) authorized Novo's human insulin as the first product made from the yeast strain *S. cerevisiae*. This yeast has since been utilized to express and synthesize more than 40 distinct recombinant proteins such as insulin peptides, human serum albumin, and hepatitis vaccines. The full genome sequence of *S. cerevisiae* is known, and the FDA has designated it as "Generally Recognized As Safe." Unlike bacteria, yeast cells can express or secrete the protein directly into the medium, and the expressed protein can undergo PTMs.

Yeast cells have the characteristic rigid cell wall. Because yeast cells secrete the expressed protein into the culture medium, unlike bacterial cells, the possibility of host-cell-related impurities is less with yeast cells but more predominant in bacterial cells. The purification process with the yeast expression system is also relatively simple compared with that of the bacterial system (owing to product secretion) and eliminating the need for additional processing such as the recovery of inclusion bodies, their solubilization, and refolding to allow for native protein folding. Despite these advantages, one of the disadvantages with yeast systems is the lack of PTMs and unexpected mono- and di-glycosylated forms of the target proteins that may be difficult to remove.

While *S. cerevisiae* is the most commonly used yeast, *Schizosaccharomyces pombe*, *Kluyveromyces lactis*, and *Yarrowia lipolytica* have been used. The main reason for the popularity of using *S. cerevisiae* is attributed to its high cell densities and fast-growing characteristic that can be easily achieved in the fermenters without affecting the costs and production timelines. Table 9.3 details all the recombinant proteins that have been produced using *S. cerevisiae*.

Another yeast strain commonly used for biomanufacturing is *Pichia pastoris*. Like *S. cerevisiae*, the methylotrophic *Pichia pastoris* can grow to very high cell densities with a tightly regulated expression system. Like *S. cerevisiae*, the *Pichia pastoris* strain has the ability to either secrete the recombinant protein into the culture medium or express it intracellularly. *Pichia*, a methylotrophic microorganism, metabolizes methanol as its primary energy source (carbon), and this characteristic is used in preparation of the expression system. The alcohol oxidase gene 1 (AOX1) promoter is used for cloning the gene of interest. Methanol is fed during the fermentation process to induce protein expression. Additional protective measures must be followed when handling large volumes of methanol, as it is a volatile solvent. Some of the recombinant proteins produced in *Pichia pastoris* include human serum albumin, human insulin, kallikrein inhibitor protein, interferon-alpha 2b, and microplasmin heparin-binding epidermal growth factor–like growth factor, to name a few. The N-linked glycosylation pattern for this system is different from that in higher eukaryotes, and this observation can be generalized for the other yeast strains. One of the major disadvantages with *P. pastoris* is proteolytic degradation, which is a major issue particularly with high-cell density cultures. This results in loss of yield and biological activity. Various strategies, including the addition of protease inhibitors (e.g., phenylmethylsulfonyl fluoride, ethylenediaminetetraacetic acid, benzamidine, and other protease inhibitor cocktails), yeast peptone; optimization of the fermentation culture conditions (e.g., pH); use of certain specific components in the culture medium, feed, or supplements (e.g., casamino acid); use of other alternative carbon sources; and optimization of the induction strategy, have been proposed and are being evaluated to overcome this challenge.

Yeast is considered a perfect choice for large-scale production of recombinant proteins that can mostly be produced in highly complex eukaryotes owing to its highly evolved, yet well-defined, genetic system, high productivity, rapid growth, ease of scale-up, ability to support certain PTMs, and decreased manufacturing time and cost. However, management of proteases present in the yeast is challenging, as these enzymes can degrade the recombinant protein.

The expression vector is the core of the yeast production system. Vectors that can integrate into and establish themselves in the host cell because of their mitotic stability are commonly used for expression studies. An alternative to genomic integration is episomal vectors (extrachromosomal DNA, which can replicate autonomously in the host cell) for some yeast systems. Expression vectors comprise a yeast promoter/terminator and a selectable marker cassette, and they enable cloning a gene insert downstream of a secretion leader. This ability of expression vectors allows the secretion of heterologous proteins from the cells into the medium. The three most common vectors used for protein expression in *Saccharomyces cerevisiae* are

- Yeast integrating plasmid (YIp): This is a single-copy plasmid and can be integrated into the host genome.
- Yeast centromeric plasmid (YCp): This is a replicating single-copy plasmid and is used for complementation studies.
- Yeast episomal plasmid (Yep): This is a replicating multicopy plasmid and is used for recombinant protein production.

Figure 9.4 shows the creation of a target protein expression system using *S. cerevisiae*.

A typical process of creating a target protein expression system using *S. cerevisiae* starts with identifying the gene of interest that encodes the protein of interest. The gene of interest is then used to generate the cDNA cloned into a bacterial system (competent *E. coli* cells). Positive clones harboring the modified plasmid are identified using a selection marker, after which the clones are isolated, transformed into yeast cells for integration of the plasmid into the yeast chromosome, and screened for positive transformants. Finally, a high expressing clone is selected and scaled up to create the cell line to further produce the protein of interest. The commonly used methods for transformation into yeast are spheroplast transformation, whole-cell transformation using lithium acetate, and electroporation. A combination of lithium acetate and polyethylene glycol is also a widely used transformation method, mainly for single-stranded DNA. Typically, the transformants are selected by applying a selectable marker so that they can be detected while screening for positive clones (Figure 9.4).

- Using dominant selection markers such as resistance to G418, formaldehyde, cupric ions, or cycloheximide.

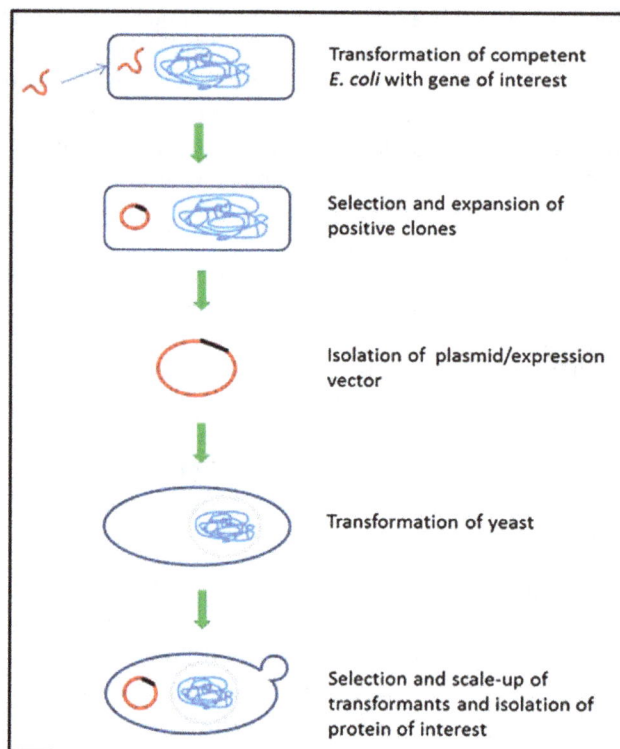

FIGURE 9.4 Yeast protein expression system: *Saccharomyces cerevisiae*

- By complementation, wherein the plasmid contains the functional gene that is not present (mutated) in the host strain (e.g., trp1, his3, and ura3).

There is an increase in the number of engineered yeast strains targeted toward either increasing the yield, altering the composition of N-glycans, and improving the performance of affinity tags.

Despite the several advantages of yeast cells, including quick growth, simple medium requirements, and PTMs, one of the major drawbacks is the possibility of hyperglycosylation, which can significantly affect immunogenicity, as previously discussed; given that the protein is expressed and secreted into the culture medium, the chances of protein degradation remains a major concern. Additionally, the low redox potential of the culture medium can also often lead to disulfide bond cleavage.

Overexpression of the recombinant protein, which leads to intracellular accumulation and low product yield, is another common problem with yeast systems, often leading to increased cellular stress. Several novel systems are being developed to facilitate easy expression of recombinant proteins in yeast cells. For improved processing of recombinant biopharmaceuticals, CRISPR/Cas9 has been successfully used in yeast engineering to insert a site-specific gene or knockout specific unwanted genes.

9.5 MAMMALIAN CELLS

The impact of cell culture on mankind and the progress achieved in biology have been enormous. The advancements made in biopharmaceuticals, for example, vaccines, new drug entities, or modalities such as antibody-drug conjugates, bispecific antibodies, cell therapy, and gene therapy, have depended mainly on cell culture. There has been an increasing shift toward the use of mammalian systems (human and nonhuman [animal cell lines]) for production purposes, specifically for complex proteins that require PTMs. All cell types vary in their growth profile, optimum conditions, and nutritional requirements.

A diverse variety of nutrients are required for the dynamic metabolism of animal cells. Hence, fetal bovine serum, a byproduct of the dairy and cattle industries, is now widely used in cell culture media. Recent concerns about transmissible spongiform encephalopathies (TSEs) and blood-borne infections, as well as severe regulatory requirements for TSEs and bovine spongiform encephalopathy (BSEs), have led to a slew of serum-free, animal-product–free, and even protein-free media formulations. Recently, recombinant insulin, transferrin, and bovine serum albumin (produced by bacterial fermentation), as well as human serum albumin produced by yeast fermentation, have replaced animal origin serum in a variety of modern cell culture processes without significantly affecting process performance or product quality.

Mammalian cells are extremely sensitive to culture conditions, and they frequently overreact to even small changes in temperature, pH, aeration, and agitation speed. During the log phase, animal cells proliferate more slowly than bacterial cells, within a doubling time of 15–48 hours.

Animal cells are naturally more delicate than microbial cells, as their cell wall lacks strength. Therefore, they are unable to tolerate most of the fermentation conditions that microbial cells tolerate, necessitating the use of specially built fermenters. For a culture-friendly approach of animal cells, several newer "airlift" and "fermenter" designs have pumps as a substitute for impellers.

During agitation, there is a considerable risk that traditional impellers break fragile cells suspended in the culture medium. Although impellers with round blades (such as the three-blade impeller used to drive motorboats) are used for generating reduced shear stresses, the sheer force with which they come in contact with the cells can be equally harmful.

Forced air sparging or other methods of introducing air into the mixture are used in bioreactors for the growth and culture of animal cells. In suspension culture, several animal cell lines multiply by floating around in their liquid media, whereas others require a solid substrate to adhere to the inner walls of roller bottles, gas-permeable polymer tubes in "hollow-fiber" bioreactors, or microcarrier beads or flat disks attached to plastic microcarrier beads or flat disks.

For animal cell culture operations, forced air sparging is one way of infusing air into the bioreactor culture medium. A robust substrate bonded to the inner walls of roller bottles, gas-permeable polymer tubes in "hollow-fiber" bioreactors, or plastic microcarrier beads or flat disks is required for culturing some animal cells (anchorage-dependent). Certain animal cell lines multiply by floating in their liquid medium as a suspension.

Traditionally, anchorage-dependent cells (mainly primary cell lines) have shown high levels of expression. To achieve high expression levels, streamlined cell lines such as NS0, CHO, human cervix (HeLa), and HEK-293 are successfully used in suspension culture. Suspension cell lines, on the contrary, have proven to be more useful and advantageous, especially for greater volume protein production procedures.

It is crucial to be aware that some bioreactor cultivation conditions can cause apoptosis (cell death), and such culture conditions can collect undesired products and cell debris, which will slow down the downstream processes.

9.5.1 Nonhuman Cell Lines

9.5.1.1 Chinese Hamster Ovary Cells

Monoclonal antibodies and complex eukaryotic proteins that have undergoing PTMs are commonly produced in mammalian cells such as CHO cells, HeLa cells, African green monkey kidney cells (COS), BHK cells, and hybridomas. These mammalian cells have been used to produce biopharmaceuticals such as monoclonal antibodies and other sophisticated eukaryotic proteins that have undergone PTMs.

In most cases, the target protein is produced in its original form and secreted directly into the culture medium. Establishing a small-scale process capable of producing proteins ranging from a few milligrams per liter to grams per liter may take approximately 4–5 months, commencing with gene assembly, clone generation, and selection. Because the protein is expressed in the medium, the downstream processing is straightforward. The downstream procedures should be robust and capable of eliminating or minimizing HCPs, cell debris, nucleic acid, and other components that are commonly produced during the fermentation process. As the possibility of viral contamination is substantial, steps involving viral inactivation and removal must be included during downstream processing. To verify viral clearance, extensive control measures (e.g., end-of-production testing, validation of the presence of virus) must be applied. After the N-1 or final purification stage, it is usual practice to incorporate a viral inactivation step by decreasing pH of the medium and a viral elimination step by filtration.

Animal cells are more delicate than microbial cells and grow very slowly, which makes them particularly vulnerable to shear forces; batch or fed-batch cultures are commonly used for antibody synthesis, while other recombinant proteins can be produced in cultures for 4–8 weeks constantly. Animal cells have slower growth and more complications concerning their growth characteristics than microbial cells. In addition, the fragile nature of these animal cells makes them highly vulnerable to shear forces. The most operated fermentation modes are batch or fed-batch cultures, but recent advancements have made continuous culture and perfusion equally successful, particularly for high yields.

The type of nutritional requirements from the culture media makes it extremely expensive relative to those used for microbial and yeast protein expression. This, combined with the low expression levels, makes the overall production process prohibitively costly. However, given that complex proteins cannot be expressed in microbial or yeast cells, mammalian cells are preferred over transgenic plants or animals.

In cell genetics research, T. Puck created the first CHO cell line in 1957. Activase, a tissue-plasminogen activator created by Genentech, was originally manufactured using CHO cells in 1987. Ever since the CHO cell line has dominated the biopharmaceutical industry as the preferred system for recombinant protein manufacturing, all the currently approved recombinant products are produced using CHO cell lines. The initial CHO cell line has been subcloned many times, resulting in a plethora of variants. The most commonly used cell lines in biomanufacturing are CHO-K1, CHO DG44, and CHO-S cells, which are derived from a different CHO lineage (Figure 9.5). This figure shows an illustration from several published papers documenting the history and evolution of the CHO cell lines widely used today.

CHO-K1 was the first cell line produced from a single clone of the original CHO cells (ovary tissue isolate). Later, these cells were modified for industrial use in both suspension and serum-free media. Several expression systems have been developed using this customized CHO-K1 cell line. They are utilized in association with the glutamine synthetase (GS) selection strategy, wherein the gene of interest is introduced into the host cell alongside a copy of the GS gene, which allows stable cells to be selected solely in glutamine-free media. Furthermore, the CHO-K1 cell line was mutagenized using ethyl methanesulfonate to form the CHO-DXB11 (also known as CHO-DUKX) cell line, which is deficient in dihydrofolate reductase (DHFR) activity.

The original CHO cells were mutagenized by gamma radiation, which resulted in the loss of both DHFR alleles and the emergence of the DHFR-deficient CHO-DG44 cell line. The de novo synthesis of purine, thymidine, and other amino acids, as well as the proliferation of CHO cells, requires DHFR. Therefore, CHO-DG44 cells must grow on a medium containing glycine, hypoxanthine, and thymidine (GHT). This feature is used in the same manner as that of the GS selection system when screening for transformants (selection marker) in a thymidine or GHT-deficient medium. If

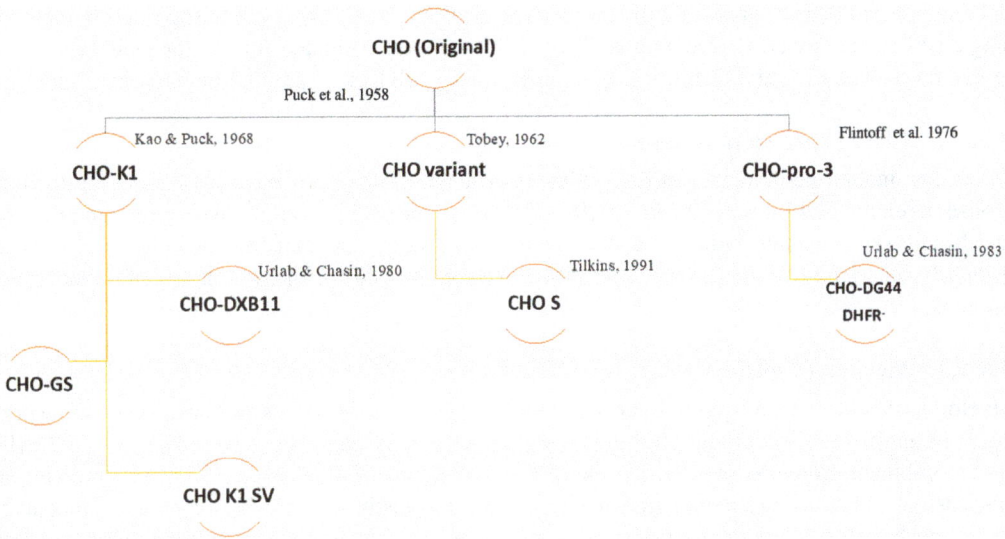

FIGURE 9.5 CHO cell lineage

the transformed clones (recombinant plasmid DNA expressing the gene of interest and the replacement DHFR gene) have effectively taken up the recombinant plasmid DNA, then they will grow in a GHT-deficient medium.

Methotrexate (MTX) as a selection pressure for screening transformed DHFR-deficient cells encoding the gene of interest is another approach extensively used for screening transformants. CHO cells lacking DHFR will amplify a transgene when transfected with MTX-treated cells. MTX binds to the catalytic site of the DHFR enzyme, preventing dihydrofolate from being converted to the active form tetrahydrofolate, which is required for DNA synthesis. Selection pressure is induced by increasing MTX concentration of in the culture media of the transformed DHFR-deficient CHO cells (encoding the gene of interest, DHFR, and vector). This causes both DHFR and the gene of interest to be amplified in the genome, allowing cells to produce a higher amount of recombinant protein. However, MTX-mediated gene amplification might cause clone instability resulting from chromosomal abnormalities, which is an important concern in biomanufacturing.

CHO-S is a subset of CHO cells that can grow as suspensions without the need for anchoring or an adhering surface (originating from the CHO pro-5 cell line). The ability of CHO cells to grow in suspension was a game-changer, paving the way for large-scale recombinant synthesis in stirred tank reactors. Commercially available CHO-S cells with cGMP storage are available.

The diversity of CHO cells dictates different growth conditions, selection pressure, and media used for protein expression to achieve functional attributes, including PTMs and high cell density, and specific productivity from the process. Of particular interest with CHO processes is the glycan distribution, given that variations in glycan patterns can affect product quality, functionality, and possibly even safety. To a large extent, PTMs are a combination of both the choice of cell line and the process conditions, including media, feed, supplements, temperature, pH, and dissolved oxygen. Therefore, optimizing these parameters is key to producing the desired product that meets its critical quality attributes.

CHO cells are commonly used for expressing recombinant proteins and generating a stable cell line. A standard approach for this recombinant protein expression using CHO cells lacking the DHFR enzyme. The target gene and the DHFR gene are both cloned into a single mammalian expression system. The recombinant DNA plasmid (carrying the two genes) is then transfected into the host cell (DHFR-deficient CHO cells). The DHFR gene serves as a selection marker that allows only transfected cells to grow in a thymidine-free medium. Next, using a limiting dilution method, single-cell stable clone(s) are obtained. The clones are then evaluated further for their expression levels, product quality, and stability to generate the final cell line expressing the protein of interest.

9.5.1.2 CHO Expression System

Other mammalian nonhuman cell lines utilized for large-scale pharmaceutical processing include mouse myeloma cell lines NS0 and Sp2/0, BHK cells, Vero cells from the African green monkey, and Madin-Darby canine kidney (MDCK) cells from a dog. Vero and MDCK cells were utilized primarily for vaccine research, while the others were employed for the production of recombinant proteins.

9.5.1.3 Myeloma Cells

Myeloma cells have been used in hybridoma technology since the 1970s and have become a workhorse in antibody development, and only very recently, they have been overtaken by CHO cells for recombinant protein expression. Some of the advantages of myeloma cells include growing in suspension culture, using a serum-free medium, and being easily scalable. However, given that myeloma cells have the ability to produce nonhuman glycoforms that cause immunogenicity and adverse effects, they are viewed as a potential risk. Endogenous retroviruses are abundant in mouse cells, which make viral clearance very burdensome. The most commonly used myeloma cell lines are NS0 and Sp2/0, which have been used successfully for manufacturing biopharmaceuticals. For example, Sp2/0 cell line was used for manufacturing Remicade (infliximab) and Erbitux (cetuximab), and NS0 was used for Zenapax (daclizumab) and Soliris (eculizumab) in addition to other blockbuster products. NS0 cells have a deficient endogenic expression of GS and require exogenous cholesterol added to the medium for growth and protein production. The risks of using animal-derived components and the price of synthetic cholesterol have led to the development of cholesterol-independent NS0 clones. The lack of a fully functional GS is used as a selection pressure to identify transfectants.

To effectively use myeloma cells, it is essential to recognize clones that produce low levels of these nonhuman glycan structures.

9.5.1.4 Human Cells

The first human cell line, HeLa, was established in 1951. Human diploid cells were used for vaccine manufacture in the 1960s, but concerns regarding oncogenic viruses at that time discouraged the widespread use of human cells. Instead, nonhuman cells, namely CHO and mouse myeloma cell lines, have been successfully used to manufacture approved recombinant therapeutics. As for human cell lines, HEK293, fibrosarcoma HT-1080 cell line, and Namalwa lymphoma cells have been used for approved products. More recently, Per.C6 and CAP are being used for products under development.

HEK293 cell line was established in 1977, and since then, it has been a versatile system for manufacturing recombinant therapeutics, viral vectors (adenovirus, retrovirus, and lentivirus), and other proteins for research use. HEK cells can be used as a suspension culture in a serum-free medium. Four recombinant products (Xigris, Alprolix, Eloctate, and Nuwiq) that are produced in HEK cells have been approved.

Per.C6 was established in 1998 from nontumorigenic human embryonic retinoblastoma cells and has been used for adenovirus vector and recombinant protein production. This cell line can also be grown in suspension culture in a serum-free medium and can reach high cell densities.

The low productivity and low process efficiency are commonly encountered challenges with mammalian cells during recombinant protein production. Both stable and transient expression processes are being evaluated to improve productivity and ease of scalability.

9.6 ALGAE

Green microalgae, such as *Chlamydomonas reinhardtii*, have been used to produce products such as full-length human antibodies, signaling molecules such as vascular endothelial growth factor, and structural proteins such as fibronectin, particularly those with strong disulfide bonds. Algae chloroplasts have the same ability to express genes as that of other eukaryotic species such as yeast. While the algal nuclear genome can also be transformed owing to reduced gene silencing and higher protein accumulation, the chloroplast genome has been the source in most cases of transgene expression to date.

More than 100 antibodies, subunit vaccines, immunotoxins, subunit oral vaccines, and growth factors are produced using the algae platform.

While filamentous fungi are widely used to produce enzymes, their effective utilization in the production of recombinant therapeutic proteins is not widely made because of the low yield and variability in the protein produced or morphological defects introduced. The common fungi used for manufacturing recombinant proteins include *Aspergillus nidulans*, *Aspergillus niger*, *Neurospora crassa*, and *Trichoderma reesei*.

9.7 INSECT CELLS

In the 1990s, the insect cell baculovirus expression system was created as an alternative to the mammalian expression system. The baculovirus system has quickly gained acceptance, given its potential to convert the lepidopteran insect cells into a high-level expression system. Additionally, these systems have better glycosylation abilities than yeast and bacterial expression systems. The most common mechanism of expression for insect cells is transient.

To create expression systems, an insect host cell and a virus vector, such as baculovirus *Autographa californica* multiple nuclear polyhedrosis virus, known as AcMNPV, are required. Baculovirus is a lytic, double-stranded DNA virus frequently amplified in Lepidoptera insects.

It is noninfectious in vertebrates and has inactive promoters in mammalian cells, which makes it safe for use in humans. *Spodoptera frugiperda* (Sf9 and Sf21) and *Trichoplusia ni* are the most commonly used insect host cell lines. For academic and industrial research and development, MultiBac, a sophisticated baculovirus/insect cell system, has been designed and used to generate multiprotein complexes containing hitherto inaccessible components. Since its launch, many MultiBac vector derivatives have been produced to express proteins with cleavable N-terminal signal peptides.

The FDA approved GSK's groundbreaking insect cell product Cervarix, a human papilloma virus vaccine, in 2009.

The recombinant DNA plasmid expression (encoding the gene of interest) is co-transfected with a second plasmid (containing viral genes required for the formation and multiplication of viral particles) into the host insect cells. The gene of interest is inserted behind a strong promoter, and transduction of the baculovirus genome into the insect cell leads to the expression of both the viral gene and the gene of interest. The recombinant viral stock is then purified and amplified. The host cells are grown to a specific cell density before adding the virus stock at a predetermined time point (time of infection) with a given number of viruses per cell. The protein production is carried out until cell lysis occurs, which is typically 48 hours post-infection. Insect cells can be grown in cell suspension in both serum-free and protein-free media as either single cells or as clumps. The optimum temperature suitable for growth is approximately 27°C–28°C, but insect cells are more susceptible to shear stress than mammalian cells. Insect cells are ideal for the production of both cytoplasmic and secreted proteins.

9.7.1 INSECT CELL EXPRESSION SYSTEMS: SF9 AND SF21

The entire production cycle is faster in insect cells than in mammalian cells, especially with regard to the generation of recombinant virus and ending with the purification of the protein of interest. This cycle takes nearly 4 weeks to complete. Fermentation is carried out only in single or semi-continuous batches owing to the vulnerability of the cells to shear strain. During the fermentation cycle, the insect cell counts increase by nearly 50-fold within approximately a week but only in single or semi-continuous batches owing to their sensitivity to shear forces.

Culture media expenses range from moderate (serum-free media) to expensive (bacteria and yeast media). Because the cells can be cultured in a healthy state before infection, the technique is well adapted for producing hazardous cell products. Despite this, scaling up is problematic because of the need for special aeration and the type of plasmid infection required for a high expression level.

Baculoviruses do not infect vertebrates and hence represent no health danger, while the risk of adventitious viruses remains unknown, necessitating virus inactivation and active filtration. Recurrent death and the subsequent lysis of the host cell causes the release of intracellular proteins and nucleic acids into the media, putting downstream purification processes under extreme pressure (such as for bacterial cells with inclusion bodies). Insect cells have a major regulatory track record, with no FDA-approved products yet.

Insect cell culture is advantageous in terms of lower cost and easier cultivation than mammalian cell culture. The levels of heterologous protein expression achieved with this technique are often varied, ranging from 1 to 600 mg/L culture media. At a protein expression level of 10–40 mg/L, certain collagens are synthesized in insect cells. One issue with insect cells is that they rarely produce recombinant proteins, as they prefer to keep the synthesized proteins in the cytoplasm. This feature is attributed to the transfection method used, and it can make downstream processing more difficult. Baculovirus expression vectors (noninfectious to humans) are commonly employed as an expression system for heterologous proteins in cultivated insect cells. Production of multi-subunit protein complexes, co-expression of protein-modifying enzymes to increase heterologous protein production, and new baculovirus display technology applications are some of the recent advancements.

Insect cell–based expression systems have several drawbacks, including nonmammalian glycosylation patterns and low productivity. Insect cells are unable to digest proteins that are initially produced as larger inactive precursor proteins (e.g., peptide hormones, neuropeptides, growth factors, and matrix metalloproteases). Several approaches for circumventing this issue have, however, been studied. One approach is to co-express these enzymes with the gene of interest in baculoviruses, while another approach is to introduce mammalian glycosyltransferases into insect cells.

9.8 COMPARATIVE ANALYSIS

Table 9.3 compares the industrial attributes for the commercial manufacturing of recombinant products, pointing out the negative attributes (therefore, a low rating is preferred).

The type of target protein, PTMs, expression level, intellectual property rights, and manufacturing cost influence the choice of the expression system. Each of the current expression systems has its own set of benefits and drawbacks (Table 9.4).

TABLE 9.4
Comparison of Various Expression Systems, Advantages, and Disadvantages

Host	Advantages	Disadvantages
Bacteria, e.g., *Escherichia coli*	A well-characterized system wide choice of cloning vectors controlled gene expression quick doubling times easy to grow with relatively high yields, the product constitutes up to 50% of total cell protein can be tailored for secretion into growth media allowing for the elimination of undesirable N-terminal methionine groups low cost, short production time, and virus-free	There is no post-translational modification Biological activity and immunogenicity may differ from those of the native proteins The gram-negative bacteria have a high endotoxin level, which can burden the downstream purification processes for the removal/reduction of these endotoxin levels to acceptable limits The produced protein product may be harmful to the cells Inclusion bodies require additional processing steps to induce the protein into its native conformation There is a high chance of proteolysis of target protein during cell disruption, and additionally, the cells carry the risk of phage infections
Bacteria, e.g., *Staphylococcus aureus*	Secretes fusion proteins into the growth media	Does not express such high levels as *E. coli*; pathogenic
Mammalian cells, e.g., Chinese hamster ovary cells	Mammalian cells secrete product (extracellular) into the media, thus eliminating cell lysis and other extensive steps to recover the protein The proteins expressed have the same biologic activity as that of native proteins Mammalian cells can perform advanced post-translational modifications that can closely mimic even human glycosylation patterns It can be easily scaled up to significantly large volumes	Mammalian cells are more susceptible to virus contamination, thus requiring additional processing to demonstrate viral clearance and removal Cell lines are expensive Cells exhibit slow growth with longer doubling times Fermentation and seed generation are time-consuming and lengthen the production time significantly (1–2 months depending on production scale)
Yeasts, e.g., *Saccharomyces cerevisiae*	Yeast has been classified under the generally regarded as safe (GRAS) category They are suitable for both intracellular expression and extracellular expression (i.e., secretion into the medium) Yeast cells do not have any detectable levels of endotoxin or release any The fermentation process costs are relatively low Yeasts can support both disulfide bond formation and post-translational modifications such as glycosylation	Gene expression is more difficult to regulate The glycosylated product is not like that in the human/mammalian systems (N-linked glycan structures are different from mammalian proteins) This can have a great impact on both bioactivity and immunogenicity

(continued)

TABLE 9.4 (Continued)
Comparison of Various Expression Systems, Advantages, and Disadvantages

Host	Advantages	Disadvantages
Cultured insect cells (Baculovirus vector)	The FDA has approved the baculovirus vector for the clinical trial High levels of protein expression can be achieved. Additionally, the virus can inhibit host protein amplification Insect cell systems can support both glycosylation and disulfide bond formation The system is considered safe for both humans and vertebrates. The gene construct integrated into the host is stable	Insect cells are difficult to cultivate mostly due to their slow growth as well the scale-up issues There is a high risk of virus infection The glycosylation is likely to be different from that of mammalian proteins– possibly impacting activity There is no clear understanding or information on the glycosylation mechanism The final product expressed is not always entirely functional–there are variations in functional attributes between the expressed protein and its native form Any proteases that may be present can cause degradation of the target protein
Fungi, e.g., *Aspergillus* sp.	A well-established system for the fermentation of filamentous fungi; growth is inexpensive	Lack of high expression levels The system still not thoroughly studied with regard to its genetic mechanism
Fungi, e.g., *Aspergillus niger* sp.	Classified as generally regarded as safe (GRAS) The cells can express high levels of product into the media Widely used as a source for many industrial enzymes	No cloning vectors are available
Transgenic animals	Capable of protein folding and glycosylation	High production costs low scale-up capacity high risk of contamination and purification is cumbersome and expensive
Transgenic plants	Recently developing acceptance by regulatory agencies unlimited opportunities of expressing a wide range of molecules capable of protein folding and glycosylation low cost and easy to propagate	Low transformation efficiency long generation time often commercially not viable and significantly high purification costs

10 Upstream Processes Involved in Protein Production

10.1 OVERVIEW

Both traditional and modern biotechnology procedures utilize living cells (microbial, mammalian, or plant), organelles, or enzymes as biocatalysts to induce chemical and physical changes in biochemical components obtained from the media. To be viable in an industrial setting, bioprocessing must offer advantages over competing manufacturing methods, such as chemical technology. Many bioprocessing technologies are the only viable options for producing certain products, like vaccines and antibiotics. Biological engineering involves designing vessels and equipment for conducting biochemical processes and transformations.

The use of microorganisms to produce various foods, including cheeses, yogurts, sauerkraut, fermented pickles, sausages, soy sauce, and other Oriental products, as well as beverages like beer, wine, and spirits, has its roots in fermentation technology, now commonly referred to as bioprocess technology. Today's manufacturing procedures for such products share striking similarities in some aspects. While these bioprocessing techniques were historically considered crafts or arts, they are increasingly being integrated into modern science and technology. Researchers have recognized the role of microbes in eliminating harmful waste materials, leading to advancements in water purification, effluent disposal, and solid waste management worldwide.

Bioprocesses are typically classified into upstream and downstream processes. The upstream process involves the synthesis stage of production, while the downstream process focuses on isolating and purifying the product. Commercialization of recombinant therapeutic proteins, such as monoclonal antibodies (mAbs), has made significant progress in recent decades, thanks to innovative technologies. Platform procedures have gained traction for reducing development time, costs, and meeting regulatory standards. From an upstream process perspective, advancements in host cell line engineering, clone screening, culture media, feed optimization, and process intensification have significantly improved process efficiency. Additionally, the shift from traditional systems to single-use systems has streamlined manufacturing operations.

Extensive development efforts are necessary to manufacture a specific protein and optimize process conditions. Further optimization of protein properties can be achieved in the process design.

Upstream processing comprises several unit operations. Common tasks in the upstream phase include preparing the growth medium, sterilizing raw ingredients, and inoculum preparation. Additionally, factors like nutrient composition, fermentation variables (such as temperature, pH, and other parameters affecting proteolytic activity, secretion, and production levels, as elaborated in Chapters 2 and 3 for specific host expression systems and cell line development), play crucial roles. These variables contribute to the synthesis of the desired substance. Following clone selection, the development of the cell culture process represents the subsequent step in bioproduction. This chapter focuses on industrial upstream processes utilizing the two most prevalent processing systems: CHO and *E. coli.*

10.2   CULTURE MEDIA

Culture media are integral to the upstream process, supporting and sustaining cell growth for protein production. The choice of culture media depends on factors like cell type, bioreactor operation mode, and target protein characteristics. It is imperative that the culture media components remain free from substances hazardous to the cells or detrimental to the product's stability. This precaution is especially significant as impurities can traverse the fermentation and purification processes, ultimately affecting the final product.

The composition of the culture medium carries substantial significance, influencing both cellular growth and protein expression. Alterations in the culture medium, including its physical properties, can impact the translation of distinct mRNAs. Changes in nutrient composition directly influence the quantity of protein released into the medium and product quality. In industrial fermentation methods employing bacterial and mammalian cells, product yields play a vital role in assessing economic feasibility.

Culture media can be categorized into the following types:

- Rich broth, comprising a complex and undefined mixture of carbon sources (e.g., glucose, glycerol, methanol) and yeast extract or yeast nitrogen base. Additional components like peptones or biotin may be added if needed. Potassium phosphate commonly serves as a buffer.
- A culture medium that includes carbon and nitrogen sources, along with trace elements, salts, and amino acids. Supplements such as vitamins and casein hydrolysates are often incorporated. Hydrolysates play a role in preventing proteolytic degradation of the final product by inhibiting extracellular proteases and anti-foam agents.

10.2.1   CULTURE MEDIA FOR MICROBIAL CELLS

Culture media for microorganism growth must provide essential elements to support cellular components and metabolic products. In *E. coli* and yeast production processes, various carbon and nitrogen sources constitute the primary components of culture media. The composition is critical for products whose expression relies on growth (primary metabolites) and those that are growth-dependent but emphasize formation (e.g., secondary metabolites).

Microbial culture media can be classified based on the following criteria:

- Physical State: Culture media supporting microorganism growth can be solid, liquid broth, or semi-solid. Nutrient broth, a liquid culture medium, consists of essential nutrients dissolved in water and is primarily used for large-scale fermentation. Solid and semi-solid culture media are typically used for isolating microorganisms and estimating viable populations. Agar is often added to liquid culture media and poured into Petri dishes to solidify it, providing a solid medium for microbial growth, as most microorganisms cannot metabolize agar.
- Chemical Nature: Culture media with a known chemical composition are referred to as chemically defined culture media, which can be either synthetic or semi-synthetic. Complex culture media, also known as undefined culture media, contain components with unknown exact compositions, including carbon sources, salts, and nitrogen sources.
- Functionality: Culture media serve various purposes, including enumeration, isolation, or cultivation. Based on functionality, culture media can be categorized as follows:

TABLE 10.1
Key Culture Media Components

Type	Common Substrate	Sources
Carbon	Glucose	Glucose, Dextrose
	Molasses	Sugar cane molasses, sugar beet molasses, high sucrose content and also contains nitrogen, vitamins, and trace elements
	Malt	Malted barley contains glucose, fructose sucrose, and maltose, also contains nitrogen
	Starch, dextrin, and cellulose	Quickly metabolized by microorganisms, commonly used for alcohol production
	Whey	A byproduct of dairy and a good source of carbon but mostly used in vitamin production, lactic acid, etc.
	Methanol and ethanol	Certain types of bacteria and yeast can only use the cheapest substrate. Commonly used in single-cell protein and acetic acid production
Nitrogen	Inorganic nitrogen	Ammonium salts, free ammonia
	Organic nitrogen	Urea
	Yeast extract	Nitrogen source and rich in amino acids, peptides, vitamin
	Soy meal	Protein and carbohydrates
	Peptones	Casein, gelatin, keratin, plant-based
Growth factors	Vitamins	Plant and animal sources with moderate mineral content, yeast extract

- Selective Culture Media: These provide nutrients that promote the growth and dominance of specific organisms while inhibiting others. Examples include MacConkey Agar and culture media with specific antibiotics like eosin methylene blue.
- Differential Culture Media: These allow differentiation of microorganisms based on indicators, distinguishing one type from another. Examples include eosin methylene blue, blood agar, and X-gal plates.
- Transport Culture Media: Designed for interim storage during transportation while maintaining microbial viability, e.g., thioglycolate broth.
- Enriched Culture Media: Selectively enhance the growth of particular bacterial types in mixed populations.

Table 10.1 provides a list of culture media components.

10.2.2 Cell Culture Media

Cell culture refers to the in vitro proliferation of cells, tissues, or organs from animal or human sources. Creating an environment (example: growth media, a substrate for attachment, temperature) conducive to their growth and survival, including growth media, substrate for attachment, and temperature control, is essential for cell culture processes. Common components of culture media include essential nutrients, vitamins, and elements, with their ratios and functions varying among different cell lines. A standard culture medium typically contains amino acids, vitamins, inorganic salts, glucose, and serum containing growth factors, hormones, and attachment factors. Additionally, the medium helps maintain pH and osmolality (Figure 10.1).

In many mammalian cell culture processes, serum is necessary for growth and serves as a source of growth factors, micronutrients, attachment factors, and trace elements. However, concerns about viral contamination associated with serum have led to the development of serum-free culture media. This shift is primarily driven by stringent regulatory requirements and the potential risks. Serum can be a source of contamination by adventitious organisms and bovine spongiform encephalopathy

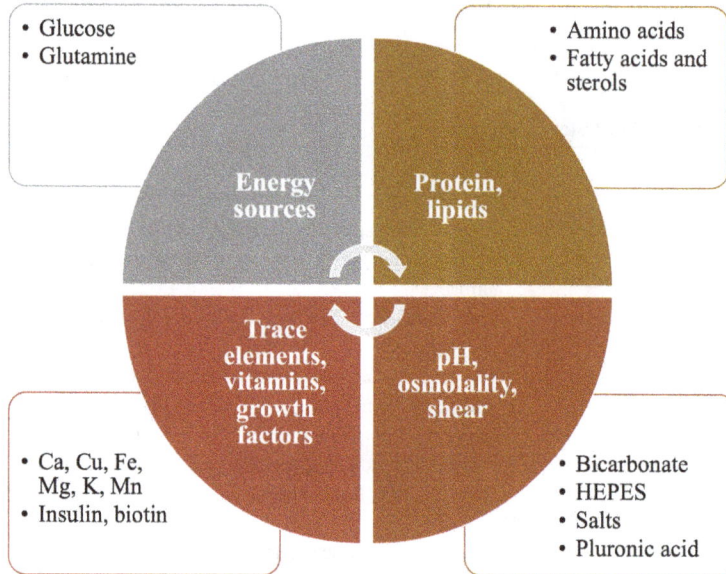

FIGURE 10.1 Components of culture media to control media properties

(BSE). Hence, for processes requiring serum, it is crucial to identify and trace its origin and conduct a risk assessment as mandated by the Food and Drug Administration and other regulatory agencies.

The inclusion of serum in culture media is commonly related to the following disadvantages, including

- Batch to batch variation leading to growth inconsistencies.
- A potential source of contaminants such as viruses, mycoplasma, and prions.
- Risk of transmission of these contaminants to the finished product (e.g., BSE).
- High cost.

Serum-free formulations are highly sought after due to their undesirable characteristics. Various substitutes mimic the actions and benefits of serum. Several hormones and growth factor combinations, including animal and plant hydrolysates, have been successfully used to support cell culture processes. The key components of cell culture media are briefly summarized in the figure.

Today, most cell culture media used in bioproduction processes are serum-free, chemically defined, and devoid of animal proteins (Table 10.2).

- Classic Culture Media: This is the traditional serum-dependent culture media that can support a wide range of cell types and applications. Glucose, amino acids, metals, and buffering agents are included in this culture media mix. Serum is an excellent source of essential fatty acids, growth hormones, lipids, and vitamins. The challenge here is lot-to-lot variability, especially from the serum component, which leads to inconsistent outcomes in cell culture processes. Examples of standard classic culture media include MEM, RPMI 1640, and DMEM.
- Chemically Defined (CD) Culture Media: CD Culture Media consist of identified components in known quantities. They do not contain any animal-derived components, including serum. A chemically defined medium includes basal culture media (amino acids, vitamins, glucose, inorganic salts, buffer agents) and is generally supplemented with recombinant proteins and growth factors such as albumin and insulin. Suitable surfactants like Pluronic or other

TABLE 10.2

Media Type		Example
Natural media	Biological fluid	Plasma, serum, human placental cord serum
	Tissue extracts	Extract of liver, spleen, leucocytes, bovine embryo, rat tail collagen
Artificial media	Basal Media	MEM, DMEM, Medium 5A, F12, RPMI-1640
	Chemically defined media	CD CHO (Known chemical components (generally animal origin free)
	Protein-free media	RPMI-1640, No protein but may contain synthetic peptides/hormones (e.g., plant hydrolysates)
	Serum-free media	Similar to chemically defined media without serum but may contain proteins
	Serum-containing media	Fetal bovine serum-containing media

Source: Adapted from M. Arora, Cell Culture Media: A Review, *Materials and Methods*, 2013; 3; 175, doi.org/10.13070/mm.en.3.175

poloxamers may also be used to support suspension cultures and minimize shear stress caused by agitation.

- Animal Component-Free (ACF) Culture Media: This culture media must derive its components from non-animal sources. Plant-based or microbial-based production techniques, for example, recombinant methods, are used to synthesize or process nutrients. The goal is to eliminate all risks and concerns related to contamination by adventitious agents.
- Protein-Free Culture Media: This type of culture media lacks any protein sources but may not always be chemically defined. Instead, other culture media components must provide the functionalities of the protein sources being replaced.

MEM is typically recommended for adherent cell lines and RPMI-1640 for suspension cells.

Some of the common components included in cell culture media and their function are detailed in Table 10.3.

Culture media supplementation is common during the cell culture process. It can occur at the time of culture media preparation, after culture media hydration, or even during the cell culture fermentation stage to ensure optimal cell growth quality (feed-forward strategy). Examples of routine supplements include glutamine, cholesterol, anti-foaming agents, and trace elements. The supplementation requirements depend on the base culture media composition, cell line, component compatibility, and intended application (e.g., cryopreservation, protein production, expression). Table 10.4 provides details on commonly studied cell lines and recommended growth media. Note that these recommendations serve as a basis for selection, and commercial-scale fermentation processes may use different growth media (Table 10.4).

10.2.2.1   Culture Media Preparation

Culture media forms commonly used in the biopharmaceutical process are available in either powder or liquid forms. For large-scale production, culture media in powder form is prepared by dissolving a bulk powder with fixed component proportions in water. Sometimes, additional pH adjustments using recommended acid and base solutions (in specific concentrations) may be necessary to dissolve the powder. Dry powder culture media have a longer shelf life, are easier to transport, and are cost-effective. However, they may have drawbacks like caking, poor solubility, powder dust, and handling difficulties. Compacting dry powder can improve dissolution and minimize dust formation, making it easier and safer to handle, with less caking. Different technologies such as pin milling and granulation are also employed to create dry culture media powder.

Preparing culture media from powder requires significant volumes of high-quality water and large mixing tanks. In contrast, liquid culture media offers the convenience of being ready-to-use

TABLE 10.3
List of Culture Media Components and Their Function

Component	Examples	Function
Amino acids: essential and nonessential	Arginine, asparagine, cystine, glutamic, glutamine, histidine, hydroxyproline, isoleucine, leucine, methionine, serine, tryptophan, tyrosine, valine	Growth, cell viability, productivity
Animal proteins/ carrier proteins	Bovine serum albumin, transferrin	Used as a carrier for lipids and to solubilize iron
Antibiotics	Penicillin, streptomycin	Inhibit the growth of other microorganisms (generally preferable to avoid incorporating these)
Buffer	Sodium bicarbonate, HEPES	pH maintenance and buffering
Carbohydrates	Glucose, sucrose, malic acid, glutamine, galactose	Energy source
Cytokines	Interleukin-3, Interleukin 6	Support various cellular activities,
Growth factors, hormones, and peptides	EGF, fibroblast growth factor, Insulin, IGF-1, IGF-2, transferrin, hydrocortisone, ethanolamine	including differentiation, proliferation, morphogenesis, activation
GS components	Methionine sulfoximine	Selection agents and gene amplification
HAT components	Hypoxanthine, thymidine	
Hydrolysates	Soy, yeast	Source of peptides, amino acids, vitamins, metals, carbohydrates
Inorganic salts	Calcium chloride, magnesium sulfate, magnesium chloride, potassium chloride, sodium chloride, sodium bicarbonate, sodium biphosphate, calcium chloride, magnesium sulfate, magnesium chloride, potassium chloride, sodium chloride, potassium chloride, sodium chloride, sodium bicarbonate, sodium biphosphate	Osmotic balance, transmembrane potential
Lipids	Inositol, glutathione, cholesterol, lipoic acid, phospholipids, ethanolamine, linoleic acid, oleic acid	Metabolism, structural components for cell membrane, important to signal transduction pathway necessary for growth
Serum	Fetal calf serum, bovine, equine	Source of some critical components necessary for cell growth and survival
Shear protectants	Pluronic	Antifoaming and reduce any shear due to agitation during growth
Trace elements	Manganese, copper, zinc, magnesium, calcium, valium, iron, selenium	Support cell growth, enzyme activity
Vitamins	Biotin, choline (e.g., choline chloride), nicotinamide, thiamine, riboflavin, vitamin B12, folic, polyoxometalate calcium, inositol, pyroxidine	Growth and proliferation of cells
Water		

(single-use packaging), eliminating the need for additional labor, infrastructure, and resources. The main disadvantage of liquid culture media is its higher cost compared to dry powder. Regardless of the format chosen, drug manufacturers can collaborate with culture media manufacturers to stream-line operations and explore customizable culture media solutions.

TABLE 10.4
Common Cell Lines and Recommended Media

Cell Line	Medium
3T3 clone A31	DMEM with FBS
Chick embryo	199/109 media
CHO	HamF10/HamF12, F12K Medium (Modified Ham's F12 media)
COS-7	DMEM with FBS
HEK 293	EMEM with FBS
HeLa	Eagle's MEM with nonessential amino acids and FBS, RPMI-1640
HepG2	McCoy 5A, Eagle's MEM with FBS
HL60	RPMI 1640, IMDM with FBS
MSCs	D-PBS mesenchymal stem cell basal medium for adipose, umbilical, and bone marrow-derived MSCs DMEM, alpha MEM with FBS and L-glutamine, D-PBS mesenchymal stem cell basal medium for adipose, umbilical, and bone marrow-derived MSCs mesenchymal stem cell basal medium for MSCs derived from adipose, umbilical, and bone marrow
NRK	DMEM with bovine calf serum
NS0	ProNS0, Ex-Cell NS0 (serum-free media)
PC12	RPMI-1640 with FBS
VERO	EMEM with FBS

Commercial culture media manufacturers also provide culture media tailored to specific cell types and, more recently, to support various manufacturing methods such as batch mode or perfusion mode. Consequently, selecting a culture media manufacturer and supplier constitutes a crucial step in the manufacturing process. This selection process begins with an evaluation of the culture media components, assessing their regulatory compliance, conducting facility audits, considering lot-to-lot variations, pricing, and ensuring traceability, all while adhering to Good Manufacturing Practice (GMP) standards.

Before utilization, culture media must be either sterile for liquid culture media or prepared from dry powder in a sterile state for other culture media. Hydrated culture media must undergo sterilization through methods such as in-place sterilization or continuous sterilization. Furthermore, any nutrients or additives, such as trace element solutions and buffers, added after this stage must also be sterile. Proper storage of culture media is critical to maintaining its optimal performance throughout the manufacturing process.

Manufacturers face the challenge of avoiding patent infringement when using specific culture media in their processes, as the exact specifications of commercial media are often closely guarded trade secrets. In some instances, producers may need to develop their own media formulations to ensure they do not violate existing intellectual property.

10.2.2.2 Culture Media Optimization

Culture media optimization plays a pivotal role in bioproduction processes. What works as the optimal culture media for one cell type or clone may not be suitable for another. Culture media optimization is necessary to foster cell growth and enhance productivity. While various heuristic and industry-standard approaches exist, there is no universally applicable method. Techniques like Design of Experiments (DoE) can range from simple to highly complex, depending on the number of components and interaction effects. Response Surface Methodology (RSM) is used to investigate the relationship between multiple explanatory variables and one or more response variables, aiming to attain optimal results through a series of well-planned experiments. RSM, coupled with DoE, has gained popularity for formulation optimization in recent times.

In contrast to traditional approaches, statistical techniques can help assess the relationship between process variables. Simple factorial or fractional factorial designs approximate first-degree polynomial models, identifying critical explanatory variables affecting the desired outcomes. For more complex situations, central composite designs can approximate second-degree polynomial models, allowing optimization of the response variables, whether it's maximizing, minimizing, or hitting specific targets. Response Surface Methodology (RSM) and Design of Experiments (DoE) are frequently employed in formulating culture media for bacteria, fungi, and mammalian cells.

The current trend in selecting culture media for cell culture processes emphasizes serum-free, animal component-free, chemically defined formulations with low protein content, whenever feasible. Even if the primary manufacturing platform has been established, multiple culture media (different types and manufacturers) are often tested due to variations in individual clones or entities produced, impacting culture media requirements.

Nutrient and growth factor requirements in culture media optimization vary depending on the product and process. Balancing objectives such as maximizing cell densities, achieving recombinant expression rates, and maintaining product quality is crucial. For example, promoting high cell densities can sometimes hinder protein expression in certain cell culture processes, while adding specific additives may enhance the release of periplasmic protein without causing cell lysis in microbial fermentation. Tailoring the medium to a specific clone and production process type (batch, fed batch, or perfusion) can significantly boost production yield. Additionally, culture media composition can have a profound impact on post-translational effects, such as glycosylation, which affects product quality attributes and overall effectiveness.

Following culture media optimization, the selected trial culture media is used, and the clone is adapted to it. A performance study is conducted on a small-scale model that mirrors commercial-scale production conditions to assess the impact of culture media on culture growth characteristics, product quality, productivity, and downstream purification processes.

An essential tool in culture media development and optimization is spent culture media analysis, which helps identify the need for additional titrations to the culture media components to support cell growth, product yield, and product quality. This analysis provides insights into the consumption and accumulation of components in the culture broth. In *E. coli* and yeast cultures, carbon sources can significantly influence cell metabolism, protein expression, and yield. Similarly, this tool is valuable for analyzing its impact on product quality and enhancing specific productivity in mammalian cell culture. Components commonly measured, depending on the cell type, include glucose, lactate, glutamine, ions (Na^+, K^+, Ca^{2+}), trace elements, growth factors, lipids, and vitamins.

10.3   CELL CULTURE FERMENTATION

The target protein, its characteristics, fermentation, and cell cultures can all be operated in batch, fed-batch, or continuous mode, depending on the expression system. Each operation has its advantages and limitations. The primary considerations in bioreactor processes include:

- Supporting Cell Growth and Minimizing Cell Death: Proper feeding strategies are crucial to counteract nutrient depletion and reduce cell death. In a fed-batch process, dead cells may persist in culture, leading to potential leakage of intracellular components into the culture media. This poses challenges for downstream purification and product stability. Factors such as cell culture medium formulation, feeding strategy, and bioreactor parameter settings must be carefully considered.
- Ensuring Product Quality: While high productivity is desirable in microbial and cell culture processes, it doesn't necessarily guarantee product quality. Additional procedures may be

necessary to ensure product quality meets essential standards. Product quality significantly impacts total yield and recovery rates. Controlling factors like cell line engineering, clone selection, culture media composition, and bioreactor process parameters can enhance product quality.

- Managing Overall Process Time: *E. coli* processes offer a substantial advantage with their relatively short processing time, typically taking 2–3 days from vial to harvest. In contrast, animal cell processes from vial to harvest can take up to 2 months to complete. This can impact the overall number of batches that can be manufactured annually. Shortening this time can enhance facility productivity, and steps targeting process intensification and continuous manufacturing can help achieve this goal.

The bioreactor operation plays a central role in enabling product synthesis as part of the upstream process. It involves closely monitoring and controlling process parameters conducive to cell growth and efficient protein expression. Critical process parameters that affect these outcomes must be identified and closely monitored, including cell growth, pH, dissolved oxygen (DO), mixing efficiency, byproduct levels, foaming, and feeding strategies. Validating computer programs for fermentation control, data logging, and data analysis is also crucial.

All upstream activities, including cell handling, bioreactor inoculation, transfer, and harvesting, must be performed aseptically. Steam-sterilized lines and steam-lock assemblies are typically used to add supplements and sample from industrial bioreactors. Care must be taken to prevent steam from damaging the culture within the bioreactor. Single-use devices have advantages over traditional stainless-steel bioreactors in this regard. In bioreactor systems for recombinant microorganisms, maintaining a pure culture and containment are essential. A host-vector system that is less likely to survive outside the lab can achieve containment, following NIH Guidelines for Environment Control.

The composition of culture media can significantly influence protein production. In the case of mammalian cells, nutrient-deficient culture media are often used as selection mechanisms (e.g., HAT and GS systems). However, there are certain drawbacks to this approach. Substitutions caused by insufficient culture media components can negatively impact product quality. For example, when *E. coli* is deprived of methionine and leucine during development, it produces norleucine instead of methionine, resulting in a wild-type protein analog. This can lead to problems in downstream processing, particularly in chromatography stages, where separating closely related compounds becomes challenging and affects product functionality.

Similarly, for CHO-derived recombinant proteins, the composition of culture media can influence the distribution of galactosylated glycoforms (e.g., G0F, G1F, and G2F). Several interrelated variables contribute to this cause-and-effect relationship. For instance, the concentration of asparagine in the culture media affects ammonia metabolism, which in turn impacts pH and the distribution of glycoforms. These changes are not solely dependent on culture media but also on process parameters such as temperature and pH, which can introduce variations in the product profile.

Temperature and pH shifts may intentionally be incorporated into the process design to enhance product quality and biological safety. Temperature shifts can promote initial rapid cell growth and maintain cells in the dividing stage when the temperature is lowered.

10.4   BASIC CONCEPTS

A robust process delivers at the upstream stage high yield and the desired product quality, and the downstream process optimizes the product a pre-defined specification. Therefore, a good understanding of the fundamentals that dictate the biological approach towards product synthesis is required for optimizing the bioproduction stages. Given the underlying nature of microorganisms and cells, the behavioral pattern is not always expected to make the upstream process challenging since variations can lead to significant process outcomes. However, a thorough understanding of these concepts and their relationship with each other can help minimize these differences and design a process that can operate within an established range for a robust and consistent process.

All organisms share a basic metabolic pathway involving both degradation and biosynthesis. Cellular energy is generated through carbon consumption, driving overall metabolism.

A mass balance for aerobic culture can be represented by a generic equation:

Rate of accumulation = Rate of inflow + Rate of outflow + rate of generation

Understanding substrate utilization and cell growth is essential in determining optimal conditions for product formation.

Cells + Substrate = Product Formation + Cell Growth

The exponential growth of cells can be represented by

$$r = \mu X,$$ Equation 10.1

where r is the cell growth rate (g/Ls), X is the cell concentration, and r μ denotes the specific growth rate.

10.4.1 CELL GROWTH

Cell growth or reproduction, also known as proliferation, occurs through regulated events that vary depending on the organisms. In a fast-growing *E. coli* culture, the doubling time is typically 15–20 minutes, whereas eukaryotes like mammalian CHO cells can take 12–24 hours to double. These times are highly dependent on the available conditions required to maintain the cell in a dividing state, including the right nutrient supply, oxygen source, and temperature, among others. A production cell line with a short doubling time, ease of scale-up, and the ability to mimic suitable conditions across all stages while reducing batch time in the production bioreactor is always desirable. A fast-growing cell line shortens the time needed to produce seeds, allowing for a quicker turnaround. The four stages of cell growth kinetics are the lag phase, exponential growth phase, stationary phase, and death phase (Figure 10.2).

During the lag phase, cells adapt to the bioreactor vessel's environment before proliferation begins. Subsequently, when the cells have adjusted to the environment, they enter the exponential growth phase. In this stage, cells reach the maximum cell division rate under favorable nutrient and environmental conditions. The length of this phase can vary greatly depending on the cell type and specific growth conditions. Following the exponential growth phase, cells enter a stationary phase, where the cell population reaches its maximum, and the rate of cell growth becomes equal to the rate of cell death. This ultimately leads to the death phase due to a decline in the growth rate caused by nutrient depletion and the accumulation of toxic by-products.

The primary goal of any biomanufacturing process is to maintain cells in a state where productivity or product formation is maximized. This can involve increasing the number of cells (as in the case of *E. coli* processes) or enhancing the secretion of proteins (e.g., CHO cells) for a growth-associated process. In non-growth-associated processes, productivity is increased by prolonging the stationary phase.

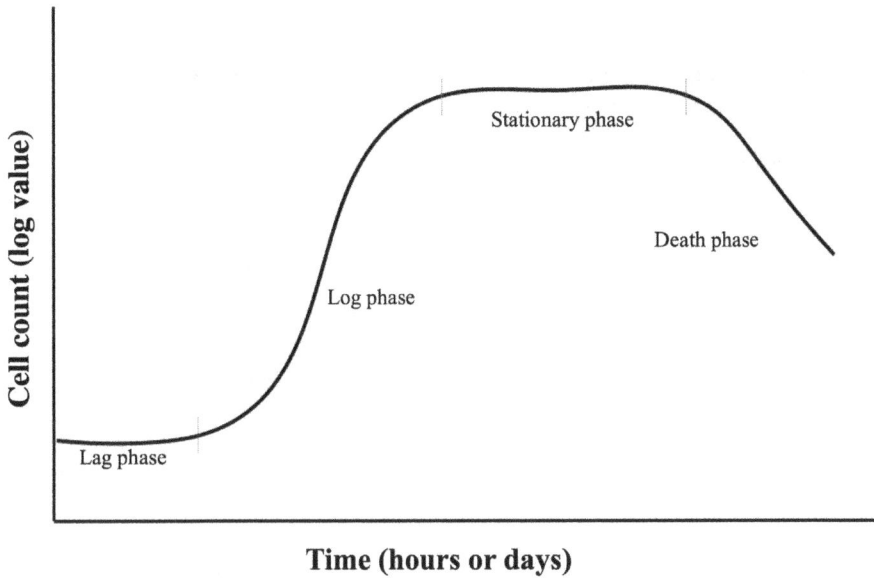

FIGURE 10.2   Phases of cell growth

10.4.2   CELL DEATH

While cell death is a natural part of the culture process cycle, it can lead to processing problems, such as decreased overall product yield and increased impurities like DNA, HCP, and other cell debris. Animal cell death can occur through necrosis or apoptosis. Necrosis results from unfavorable conditions like shear stress and extreme pH levels, causing cells to swell and eventually burst due to osmotic pressure, releasing their intracellular components. Apoptosis, on the other hand, is a genetically controlled process induced by certain environmental conditions such as nutrient depletion and oxygen limitation. Therefore, delaying the onset of cell death and maintaining the culture in a highly viable state is essential to minimize cell debris generation, which is critical for downstream process purification.

10.4.3   METABOLIC CONTROL

The upstream fermentation process depends on physicochemical parameters and culture media composition that can impact cell metabolism. The metabolic demands differ between growing cultures in a dividing state and those in a non-dividing state. Accumulation of by-products and imbalances in nutrient uptake can obstruct cellular metabolism. For instance, in CHO cell culture processes, glucose consumption can result in lactate accumulation, affecting culture osmolality and pH and potentially causing apoptosis. Similarly, in *E. coli* cultures, the consumption of carbon sources can lead to an acetic acid build-up, lowering the culture's pH and impacting cell growth (Table 10.5).

Oxygen supply is essential for supporting cell growth, especially in aerobic cultures. Oxygen can be a limiting factor for microbial processes and animal cell cultures, particularly during scale-up. The oxygen transfer ratio should exceed the oxygen uptake ratio for a culture process. The concentration of dissolved oxygen in the culture is expressed as a percentage and calculated as follows:

TABLE 10.5
Operational Parameters of the Cell Culture Process have an Impact on the Process Performance and Product Quality

Process Parameters (Bioreactor Control)	Control Strategy	Impact
pH	CO$_2$ or base addition	Cell Growth,
DO	Airflow rate, oxygen flow rate, agitation rate, sparger	Viability Product concentration
Temperature	RTD	Product quality
Pressure	Gauge	

$$\%DO = \frac{C_L}{C_L^*} \times 100$$ Equation 10.2

where C$_L$ is the actual oxygen concentration in the medium, and C$_L^*$ is when the medium is saturated with air.

The difference between C$_L^*$ and C$_L$ drives oxygen transfer in the culture. Glucose consumption can lead to lactate production in mammalian cells and acetic acid in microbial cultures. Tight control of pH is maintained by adding CO$_2$ or base. The pH dead band and pH set point together form the pH control strategy.

Microbial cultures have a higher oxygen demand that depletes rapidly. Oxygen is added through headspace aeration and sparging using a microsparger. Variations in these parameters, as well as other culture operating parameters such as temperature, agitation speed, carbon dioxide, pH, osmolality, and metabolite levels (including by-products such as lactate, acetic acid, and amino acids), significantly impact culture performance, yield, and product quality. pH can also have a significant impact on culture development and metabolism.

Process performance parameters are established, and the controls achieved in a small-scale process are used for final scale-up. These variables are either volume-dependent (e.g., agitation, aeration, feed volume) or volume-independent (e.g., pH, temperature, DO set point).

10.5   CULTURE PRODUCTION PROCESS

This section presents the sequence of operations, timing, and precise control of process parameters for fed-batch fermentation with *E. coli* and CHO mammalian cells. In a fed-batch process, cells progressively grow to high cell densities by increasing the quantity of ingredients in a time-dependent manner to match exponential growth and minimize the accumulation of harmful by-products. Typically, this growth is carbon-source limited to maintain low residual carbon concentration and maximize productivity. Feeding can be both growth-dependent and time-dependent, with feeding strategies often following a pre-set time profile using a pump integrated into the bioreactor's control system. It is common to time feeding with an expected DO spike in microbial cultures, primarily due to carbon source depletion. However, during process development, careful evaluation and balance are required to ensure that the depletion of the carbon energy source does not shift the cells' growth phase and metabolism, reducing overall biomass yield.

A sample growth curve and glucose consumption pattern are illustrated in Figure 10.3. Initiating feeding before depletion can support exponential growth, although it is typical for the carbon source to be entirely depleted as the culture reaches maximum cell concentration, leading to an accumulation of carbon source as cells enter the death phase.

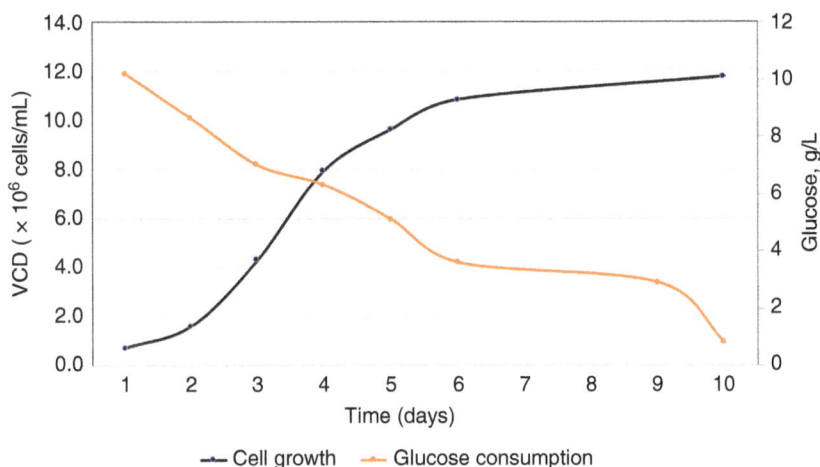

FIGURE 10.3   Cell growth and glucose consumption

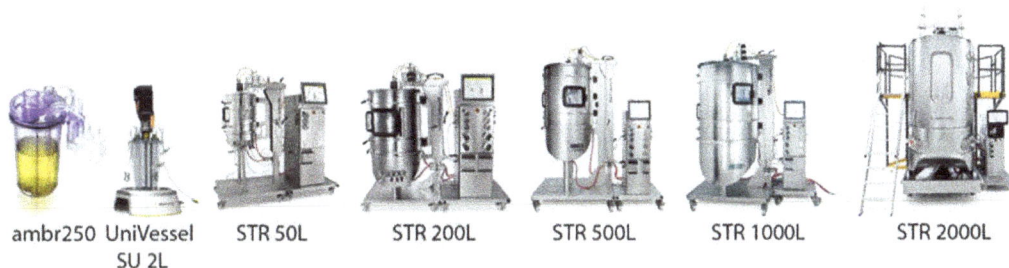

FIGURE 10.4   Conventional culture process from vial to production bioreactor process

Source: Copyright Cetiva

10.5.1   SEED TRAIN

A traditional fed-batch process involves multiple stages of seed expansion, starting from a vial or vials, progressing to a large-scale production bioreactor. This is necessary to cultivate a sufficient number of cells for inoculating the production bioreactor. The seed train begins by thawing cells (one or multiple frozen vials) from a qualified cell bank, typically a WCB, into a shake flask containing suitable growth culture media. Subsequently, the culture in the shake flask is incrementally expanded in volume using bioreactors of increasing size, ultimately leading to the production bioreactor. A typical outline of this culture process is shown in Figure 10.4.

In microbial cultures, seed train generation usually lasts for 24 to 48 hours until the production bioreactor can be inoculated. However, in mammalian cell culture processes, the combined seed train and inoculum train can take up to a month to generate a sufficient cell volume for inoculation into the production vessel.

For mammalian cells, regular sub-culturing (also known as passage) is essential to keep the cells in a dividing state and prevent them from entering the stationary phase before reaching the production stage. Subculturing can be based on a split ratio (volume) or a target starting (seeding) density for the next stepwise expansion. It is crucial to minimize the number of passages (the number of times the cells have been split) to prevent potential genetic drift or instability. The impact of passage

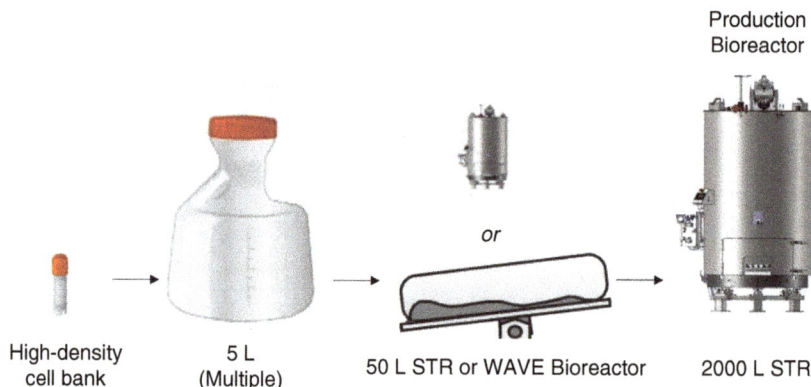

FIGURE 10.5 Illustration of an intensified seed generation process

Source: Copyright: Cytiva

number on the overall production process must be carefully evaluated and validated. In contrast to the conventional method, which takes around 30 days for seed generation, process intensification can significantly reduce the seed generation time by at least half (Figure 10.5).

The volume factor or scale-up factor indicates the increase in volume from one inoculum preparation step to the next. It determines how much fresh culture media can be added to the cells and whether the entire cell volume is required or just a portion. For example, a scale-up factor of ten means that one seed reactor's volume is ten times that of the previous seed reactor. Unlike mammalian cell cultures, microbial cultures can sustain higher volume factors, which may require a relatively lower volume factor. A significant scale-up factor can greatly reduce the seed train generation process. This scale-up factor is crucial in determining the number and sizes of bioreactors needed to support a specific commercial-scale operation. Additionally, when designing the seed train, one must consider the recommended or maximum working volume, as it can impact the optimal performance and maintenance of process parameters supporting cell growth.

Seed generation is a critical process in ensuring the overall success of a bioproduction process. The quality of the cell bank is paramount throughout the journey from vial to production fermenter, ensuring that the upstream process remains robust and consistently productive and of high quality.

Glass shake flasks and stainless-steel bioreactors have been long-used for small volume and expansion of seed culture stages, respectively. However, they have now been successfully replaced with single-use disposable shake flasks and single-use bioreactors available in various sizes for the seed train stage. These are employed for small volume cultures (< 10 L). The increased use of disposables at these stages enables a faster turnaround by eliminating cleaning steps and reducing the risk of contamination. For cultures in the range of 10–50 L and higher, a rocking bioreactor, such as WAVE™, is more suitable than a stirred tank reactor. Shake flask cultures are maintained in an incubator shaker under controlled humidity, carbon dioxide (for mammalian cells), temperature, and agitation, which is adequate for microbial cultures.

10.5.1.1 Vial Thaw

The process of thawing the vial(s) should be swift and performed under controlled temperature conditions using a water bath at approximately 37°C. This helps prevent damage to the cells from ice crystal formation. Then, inside a laminar flow hood or biosafety cabinet, the cells are added to fresh culture media in a shake flask and allowed to incubate until the next process step.

10.5.1.2 Fermenter Setup

The bioreactor vessel, whether for seed generation or production, is set up following the outlined instructions. The vessel is filled with culture media (except for heat-sensitive ingredients) and then sterilized. Any heat-sensitive components are added later through filter sterilization. In single-use systems, culture media and other essential components are added to the bioreactor bag via a 0.2-μm filter. It is standard practice to perform this operation at least 24–48 hours before adding cells. This allows the culture media to equilibrate to the process conditions, perform calibration checks, and, most importantly, ensure sterility before inoculation. The composition of culture media and process conditions for seed generation may differ from those used for the production stage. Various procedures, including sterilization (SIP), sanitization, tube welding, tube sealing, and autoclaving, are used to support sterile processing.

10.5.1.3 Inoculation of Production Vessel and Sampling

In the production bioreactor, cells are introduced (i.e., inoculated) under positive air pressure to prevent contamination. Sterile air is used to pressurize the production bioreactor, and the inoculum is delivered through sterile tubing equipped with a dedicated port. Establishing sterile connections, for example, using pre-sterilized aseptic connectors such as AspetiQuik tubing assemblies, simplifies the process and eliminates the need for on-site sterilization of parts such as piping and valves.

Production vessels are equipped with dedicated sampling ports to facilitate the collection of culture samples according to process requirements. These samples are utilized for determining cell density, either by using a spectrophotometer for *E. coli* cultures or a trypan blue-based method, or automated cell measurement systems such as Vicell, in addition to other metabolite measurements. In traditional stainless-steel fermenters, the sampling ports are positioned away from the vessel and sterilized with steam before sample withdrawal. Bioreactors typically come equipped with sensors or probes for continuous monitoring of pH and dissolved oxygen (DO), at the very least. They may also feature more advanced capabilities, such as integrated cell density monitoring sensors and metabolite measurement. The pH is initially calibrated using standardized buffers. After the culture media is added and equilibrated, a one-point standardization is performed using an offline pH meter. This adjustment is then incorporated into the control unit to enhance accuracy for subsequent measurements. In some cases, processes may continue to use offline pH measurements to intermittently adjust the pH drift.

DO calibration involves creating conditions of 100% saturation and 0% oxygen (achieved by sparging nitrogen to remove air). Periodic offline measurements are conducted to assess the cellular environment conditions and determine appropriate feeding strategies. These offline measurements can employ various techniques, such as enzyme-linked membrane technology (e.g., NOVA Bioprofile Flex), photometric methods (e.g., Opto Cell, Cedex, spectrophotometer), or ion-selective approaches utilizing a reference electrode. For gas analysis and glucose measurement, on-line measurements can be integrated using advanced technologies like soft sensors and integrated HPLC systems.

10.5.1.4 Fed-Batch Process Outline

10.5.1.4.1 Escherichia coli

1. Prepare culture media, feed, and other necessary supplementary solutions for the batch.
2. Sterilize liquid components using either filtration or autoclaving.
3. Assemble the bioreactor components, transfer lines, containers, pH and DO probes, sensors, agitators, and gas lines required for the fermentation process.
4. Retrieve a vial from a −70°C freezer and thaw it in a water bath set to a temperature between 34°C and 37°C.

5. Under a biosafety cabinet, transfer the cells into a flask(s) containing the required amount of medium (e.g., LB culture media, TB culture media, etc.) with the appropriate antibiotic (e.g., kanamycin) if the plasmid carries a resistance gene. Ensure that the flask is filled to approximately 0.25–0.3 of its capacity to ensure proper aeration of the culture.

6. Incubate the shake flask culture(s) in an incubator shaker set to a specific temperature and agitation speed. Measure the optical density (OD), which assesses cell growth, using a spectrophotometer at a wavelength of 600 nm. The incubation time can vary from 12 to 20 hours, depending on the target OD600 to be achieved.

7. Depending on the final commercial scale, one or two seed generation stages may be required. Use the shake flask culture as the inoculum for a 10 L fermenter vessel. Multiple shake flasks may be used to generate a sufficient volume of cells to inoculate larger or multiple fermenters simultaneously. This 10 L inoculum can, in turn, be used to inoculate a higher volume seed bioreactor.

8. Calibrate pH and DO sensors, probes, pressure gauges, and pumps. Add an appropriate amount of culture media to the production vessel and allow the system to equilibrate to the process conditions (DO, temperature, pH, agitation) for at least 24 hours before adding the inoculum. Conduct a sterility check to confirm that the culture media is free of contamination.

9. Sparge air at the designated flow rate (e.g., 0.5–1.0 vvm), which is expressed as volume gas/volume culture/min, throughout the fermentation process.

10. Aseptically add the inoculum into the production vessel through a septum port for stainless steel or a dedicated inoculation port for single-use systems. Perform a final system check to ensure that DO, pH, temperature, and agitation set points align with the process requirements.

11. Periodically monitor the culture's progress (e.g., every hour) by measuring OD600. If at any point during the process, the DO or pH deviates from its set point, the sensors, through a control strategy, work to correct it. For instance, the mass flow meter may open to aerate the culture in case of low DO, or CO_2 may be sparged to lower the pH or a base added to increase the pH.

12. Implement an induction procedure for protein expression when the target cell concentration is reached by adding an inducing agent. Induction can be performed either earlier in the production process or later at a higher cell density. Similarly, based on nutrient consumption, a bolus feed consisting of a concentrated solution of key nutrients (e.g., glucose and other trace elements) is added to the production bioreactor, depending on fermentation time or optical density.
    • Induction for lac and tac promoters and T7: Add a specific concentration of IPTG solution.
    • Induction for pBAD promoter: a certain concentration of Arabinose solution.

13. Optionally, collect samples before and after induction for SDS-PAGE analysis to determine yield and monitor protein expression progression during fermentation.

14. Terminate the fermentation process at a specified time once the target OD600 is achieved. Proceed with harvesting the batch to recover the cell pellet for further downstream processing.

10.5.1.4.2 CHO Cells

1. Prepare all the cultutre media, feed, and other necessary supplementary solutions for the batch.

2. Sterilize the liquid components, either through filtration or autoclaving. Assemble the bioreactor components, transfer lines, containers, pH and DO probes, sensors, agitators, and gas lines required for the fermentation process.

3. Retrieve a vial from the liquid nitrogen cryo unit and thaw in a water bath set to the thawing temperature (~37°C).
4. Under a biosafety cabinet, transfer the cells into a flask containing the required growth medium supplemented with glutamine. Typically, use no more than 25–30 mL of culture in a 125 mL shake flask to ensure proper aeration.
5. Incubate the shake flask culture(s) in a humidified CO2 incubator (5% CO2) at a specific temperature and agitation. Measure the viable cell density daily until the target cell density is achieved.
6. Subculture the cells by gradually increasing the volume for subsequent passages until the target inoculum volume is achieved. This may involve multiple shake flask steps (or spinner flasks) followed by small-scale/pilot-scale bioreactors (rocking or stirred tank).
7. Calibrate pH and DO sensors/probes, as well as pressure gauges and pumps. Add an appropriate amount of culture media into the production vessel and equilibrate it to the process conditions (DO, temperature, pH, agitation) for at least 24 hours before adding the inoculum. Perform a sterility check to confirm that the culture media is free of contamination.
8. Pump the initial amount of culture media into the production vessel and equilibrate the system with air (headspace and sparger) and the process temperature setpoint.
9. Calculate the initial amount of culture media needed based on the target volume at harvest, the expected amount of inoculum to be added for a starting density, and any feed/supplement solutions required during the fermentation process.
10. Establish the air sparging flow rate and DO setpoint before adding the inoculum. The feedback mechanism of the sensor and control unit allows the mass flow meters to respond and sparge air and oxygen as needed. The agitation speed can either be kept constant or adjusted to meet the process's aeration requirements.
11. Add the inoculum to the production vessel, either using sterile connectors and pre-sterilized transfer lines for single-use systems or following the traditional procedure for stainless-steel systems.
12. Monitor the culture growth by measuring cell density daily, either once or multiple times a day. Conduct offline analysis of the culture sample for pH and metabolite measurements.
13. Start feeding or adding supplements as determined from process development studies. This can be based on achieving the desired cell density or done periodically (e.g., adding 1 L of feed per day from Day 2 to Day 10 of the fermentation process).
14. Temperature and pH set points as the process progresses.
15. Proceed to harvest and clarify the culture to recover the secreted protein.

The upstream processes have advanced to the point where yields are no longer a limiting factor. The integration of hardware and software components has enhanced our understanding of the key parameters that can influence the outcome of cell culture processes. Manufacturers are continually seeking improved yields through an integrated approach, from cell line engineering to enhanced process control, and more recently, through continuous manufacturing and process intensification. The adoption of Quality by Design (QbD) principles and the integration of Process Analytical Technology (PAT) tools have become increasingly common to ensure compliance with every batch.

10.6   CELL SEPARATION AND HARVESTING

After completing the synthesis phase, the subsequent process stages include product isolation, recovery, and purification. Product isolation, also known as separation, marks the beginning of downstream operations. For the sake of continuity in concluding the production culture operations, we include the separation process, i.e., isolating the product from the production system, in this chapter on upstream processing.

Once the desired product is produced, whether intracellularly in the cytoplasm, periplasm, or secreted into the culture media by the respective production system (e.g., *E. coli* cells, mammalian cells such as CHO), it must be separated and recovered from the host system. Cell harvesting, which involve,.es extracting or separating the host cells from the culture broth, is employed for this purpose. In *E. coli* processes, the protein is held within the cells as inclusion bodies, requiring the isolation and further processing of the cells for product recovery. In the case of mammalian cells, the protein is secreted into the culture media. Therefore, removing the cells from the product stream and clarifying it for further purification forms the general outline for mammalian-based production processes.

Understanding the advantages, evaluating the success of these methods at the commercial scale, and considering the limitations, including cost, are crucial for optimizing the process. It has become common to follow a platform approach used for one product to apply for every product being manufactured in the facility.

While this may be advantageous in some cases, it may not be suitable for all products. The selection of the primary clarification step can significantly impact subsequent filtration and purification operations. Variables such as the solid-to-liquid ratio, culture viability, cell debris, and other impurities can affect the outcome of the recovery.

The most widely used separation strategies for both *E. coli* and CHO systems are detailed below.

10.6.1 CENTRIFUGATION

Centrifugation relies on differences in density between solid particles, such as cells and cell debris, suspended in a feed stream, typically a culture broth. As a result, processing volumes in commercial-scale operations can be quite high, making continuous centrifugation the preferred choice. While the basic principles of centrifugation have remained largely unchanged for over 50 years, recent advances in membrane technologies have improved process purity, control, efficiency, speed, yield, and cost (Figures 10.6 and 10.7).

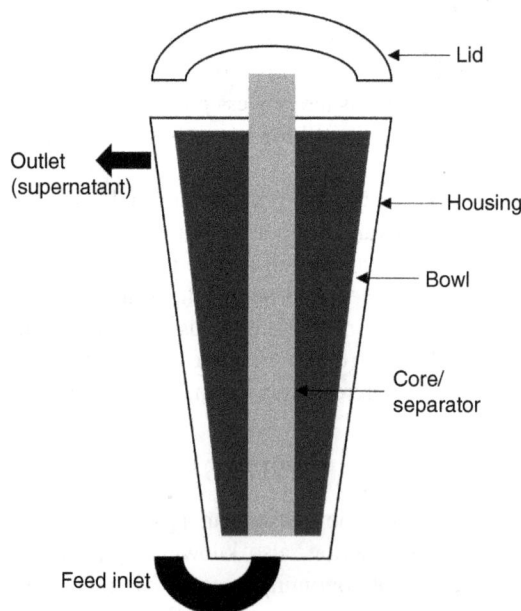

FIGURE 10.6   Schematic of a continuous flow centrifuge

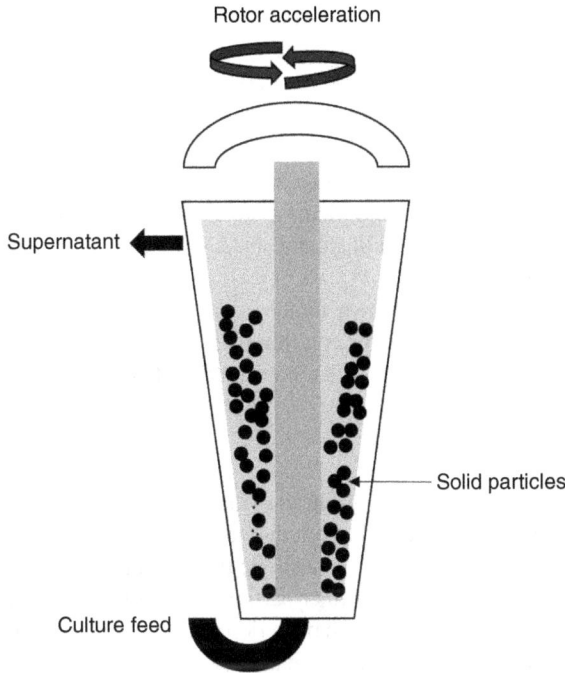

FIGURE 10.7 Mechanism of continuous separation

A continuous flow centrifuge is capable of processing large volumes at high centrifugal forces. The culture feed is introduced through the inlet at the bottom of the centrifuge bowl. The combination of centrifugal speed and feed flow rate causes solid particles, such as cells and debris, to become trapped in the gradient as they move from the bottom to the top of the vessel. These solids settle against the bowl's walls under the centrifugal force, while the clarified liquid, also known as supernatant, moves up the channel and exits through the outlet. If the product of interest is present in the supernatant, a collection tank is used for further processing. Alternatively, if the product is within the solid particles, these settled solids can be continuously removed through nozzles or at specified time intervals.

This process eliminates the need for filling and decanting centrifuge bottles or stopping and starting the system multiple times, which is often required with conventional centrifuges or benchtop models primarily suited for smaller volumes.

Continuous flow centrifugation offers several advantages, including high volumetric throughput, strong centrifugal forces, and the ability to handle high solids feed streams, reducing the time spent on sample handling. These attributes make it a preferred choice for large-scale operations involving bacterial cultures, viruses, and as an initial step in mammalian cell clarification.

Factors that can affect the efficiency of this process include

- Centrifugal force (g-force): Excessive centrifugal force can sometimes lead to shear that may damage cells, releasing impurities such as DNA, host cell proteins, and additional debris. In contrast, low centrifugal force may result in uneven settling of solids, leading to less clarified supernatant.
- Residence time: Extended residence time can reduce throughput and potentially harm product quality (possible degradation).
- Flow rate: Solid particles' sedimentation depends on both centrifugal force and flow rate. Smaller particles require higher centrifugal force and more sedimentation time than larger

particles. Choosing a lower flow rate can provide sufficient time for smaller particles to settle before leaving the rotor or bowl, and optimizing flow rate can enhance process efficiency.

• Cell density, viability, and cell type are other variables to consider when choosing centrifugation as a separation choice. The solid to liquid ratio will determine how soon the pellets (solid's settling) accumulate and fill the bowl leading to a possibility of packing up into the clarified stream. As such, the pellet may need to be intermittently or continuously removed. Turbidity measurements of the supernatant/clarified liquid can be useful in such scenarios, which will increase as the bowl reaches its holding capacity. A balance is critical to minimize loss.

Assessing these variables on scale-down models can be challenging due to the limited availability of suitable representative models for continuous flow centrifuges. Benchtop or conventional centrifuges cannot replicate the dynamics of a continuous centrifuge.

10.6.2 DEPTH FILTRATION

Unlike surface or membrane filtration, depth filtration employs the depth of the filtering medium and its absorptive properties (porous substrate) to retain particles from the feed stream. The structure of depth filters consists of multiple layers or even a single thick layer of culture media. Larger particles are captured at the surface, while smaller or finer particles are entrapped within the various layers or structures. Depth filters are not identified to have a defined pore structure like other filters do. In a membrane filter, particles larger than the pore size are trapped on the membrane's surface. Thus, the depth filter leverages the depth of the membrane media and surface-based sieving for applications such as cell culture harvest and intermediates (e.g., precipitated solutions, refolded protein processing before chromatography steps; Figure 10.8).

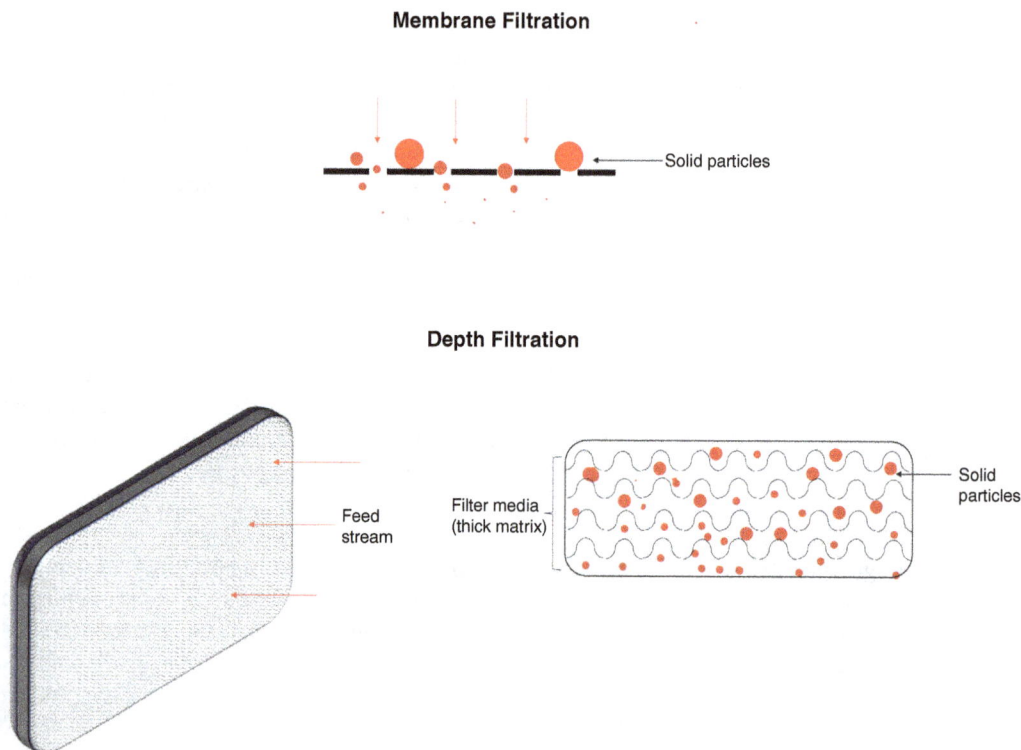

FIGURE 10.8   Comparison of membrane and depth filter functionality

Depth filters are constructed using cellulose or polypropylene fibers combined with filter aids like diatomaceous earth (DE) or perlite. These fibers are bound together with a polymeric resin using the wet-laid process, forming the matrix of the filters. The fiber matrix provides rigidity and structure, while filter aids increase surface area to enhance retention properties. Additionally, the resin imparts wet strength and a positive charge to the filter surface. Some filters may incorporate an additional filter membrane layer with different pore sizes (e.g., 0.2 μm). When selecting a suitable depth filtration system for primary or secondary clarification of the feed, consider variables such as filter selection, format, and surface area. The choice of depth filtration for cell culture applications depends on culture conditions and the physical properties of the product, particularly if it involves proteins present in the feed for mammalian cultures.

Depth filtration offers several advantages, including ease of implementation, single-use capability, faster turnaround times, reduced or no cleaning requirements, scalability, and low investment. In single-use systems, filter units can be stacked together to increase surface area, allowing for easy scaling to handle large volumes (greater than 5,000 L of harvest). These filter units, or capsules, consist of filter culture media, along with inlet and outlet single-use manifolds equipped with vents positioned between filters. These capsules are arranged into stainless steel holders, although the stainless steel parts do not come into contact with the product. Commercially available single-use systems, such as 3M Encapsulated Zeta Plus and Millistak+ Pod filter systems by Millipore, are widely used in various industries. Depth filters are well-suited for a range of clarification applications, including cell culture, yeast, *E. coli* lysates (after centrifugation), refolded proteins (after *E. coli* IB solubilization), vaccines, and plasma proteins.

The setup for depth filtration is straightforward (Figure 10.9). Before starting the harvest process, it's essential to flush the depth filters with water or a recommended buffer to remove any loose particulates and extractives that may have been trapped during the manufacturing process. Subsequently, the unclarified culture is introduced into the filter setup through the inlet. A pump is then used to drive the feed from the outside, passing through the filter culture media and traveling through its depth to achieve clarification. After completing the harvest process, the filter culture media is once again flushed with water buffer to recover the unit's volume and minimize product loss.

The void volume of depth filters varies depending on pore structures, with more open pore structures having a high void volume (around 90 percent) and tighter pore structures having lower void volumes (around 30–40 percent). To ensure successful clarity, it is crucial to select the appropriate filter grade based on the particle size distribution. In many cases, multiple filter grades are arranged in series to improve overall clarification performance. Following clarification, the harvested material is filtered through a 0.2 μm filter. Single-use bags are advantageous in this application for easy storage and maintaining sterility until further processing. Properly sizing the depth filtration process is essential for tight process control, preventing batch losses, or processing delays. Depth filtration also offers benefits in reducing shear stress, limiting cell damage, and removing impurities such as HCP, DNA, and endotoxins, compared to centrifugation.

10.6.3 Ultrafiltration and Microfiltration Tangential Flow Filtration

Membrane filtration techniques, such as ultrafiltration and microfiltration, can be effectively used in the recovery and separation process post-fermentation. Hollow fiber filters have enabled

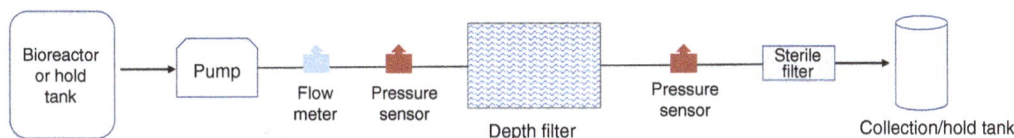

FIGURE 10.9   Schematic of a depth filtration setup (primary or secondary clarification)

the application of ultrafiltration and microfiltration TFF (tangential flow filtration) in large-scale operations, including clarification and cell retention in perfusion processes. The choice between microfiltration and ultrafiltration depends on membrane pore size, with microfiltration typically having pores around 0.1 μm and ultrafiltration membranes having even smaller pores categorized by molecular weight cutoff. While microfiltration and ultrafiltration are commonly used in downstream processing, recent advances have positioned these methods as suitable alternatives to traditional centrifugation. TFF is successful in cell harvest and cell lysate processing, relying on size exclusion for filtering separation and utilizing crossflow to remove cells and detritus from the membrane's surface. The retentate pool containing cells is concentrated while the cell culture is treated. A frequently encountered issue with this system is filter fouling, which drops the performance and recovery. This can be overcome by incorporating diafiltration or cell washing, which is beneficial for buffer exchange in chromatography applications and cell lysis.

The selection of the appropriate membrane pore size is crucial for process efficiency. Hence, identifying the membrane with the appropriate pore size is key to developing an effective clarification or cell harvesting process. Smaller pore size membranes provide higher permeate flux under steady-state conditions, so choosing a larger pore size ultrafiltration membrane for *E. coli*, even with relatively small pores compared to the cells, may be advantageous. For applications where proteins are secreted in the medium, open pore size microfiltration membranes in the range of 0.2 to 0.65 μm are preferred, especially for larger recombinant proteins like monoclonal antibodies. Selecting a membrane pore size at least ten times larger than the target material ensures proper passage through the membrane.

In the case of hollow fiber filters, the cartridge's length and the inner diameter of the fibers influence the process. Shorter path lengths are suitable for processing cultures. Other variables affecting the clarification process include permeate flow rate, recirculation flow rate, and timing of diafiltration (cell washing) to facilitate particle passage (cells or proteins).

10.6.3.1   Choosing the Appropriate Method

The primary goals for clarification include

- consistent removal or separation of cells,
- removal of insoluble debris,
- reproducibility and scalability

In addition to these goals, increasing throughput to reduce processing time, minimize product degradation, product loss, and downstream operation burden are essential considerations when selecting a clarification method.

The choice of clarification method should be based on the cell type. *E. coli* is primarily used for producing simple proteins and antibody fragments that do not require glycosylation. Most bacterial expression systems involve a centrifugation step to recover the pellet from which the protein is purified. Subsequently, cell lysis is performed to release the recombinant protein. During the cell lysis and inclusion body (IB) recovery process steps, alternatives to centrifugation such as microfiltration and ultrafiltration, can be considered for processing cell lysates and recovering IBs. For refolded proteins, particularly on an industrial scale, depth filtration is often the preferred choice of clarification. Microfiltration membranes can concentrate cells and disrupt them using a homogenizer to separate the inclusion bodies. Cell debris and IBs can be separated using either microfiltration membranes (0.2 μm) or ultrafiltration membranes.

Harvesting methods for *E. coli* secreting soluble proteins are similar to those used in mammalian production systems, such as centrifugation, depth filtration, and sterile filtration. While process modifications may be necessary to accommodate the more intensive fermentation characteristics of *E. coli* cultures, like high cell density and short cell culture time, similar process equipment and

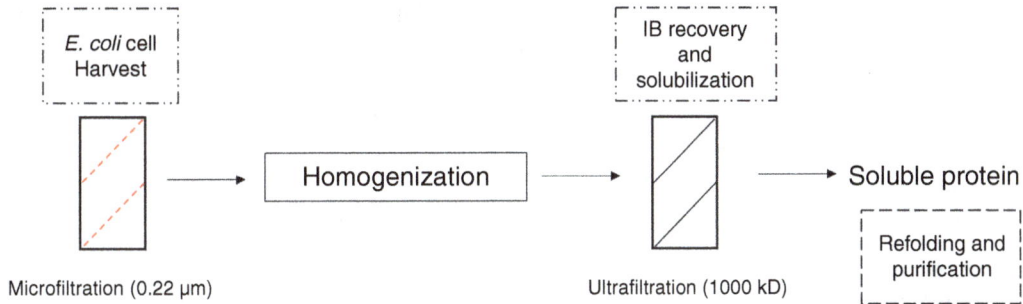

FIGURE 10.10   Alternate filtration system for processing *E. coli* products

optimization strategies should be expected. In processes where cells are engineered (e.g., using secretion tags and other changes to the *E. coli* construct) to release the product from the periplasm or into the extracellular space, it's crucial to avoid shear stress on the cells. Precipitation and floc-culation (e.g., with polyionic polymers like PEI and dextran) in conjunction with centrifugation can assist in rapid processing, stabilizing the product, and efficiently removing cell debris, colloidal proteins, and nucleic acids.

CHO cells are another common expression system. In most mammalian systems, proteins are secreted from these cells into the culture medium. Therefore, the clarifying process involves removing cells and soluble debris. Centrifugation, depth filtration, or tangential flow microfiltration are commonly used for primary clarification. To eliminate smaller particles and protect the chro-matography column, a final filtration step is included. For this purpose, a 0.2 μm rated sterilizing grade filter is used. To preserve the more sensitive sterilizing grade filter layer, a dual-layer sterile filter, such as a 0.45 μm over a 0.2 μm filter, is commercially employed. Recent techniques, such as intensification and cell engineering, have led to higher cell densities, necessitating improved impurity removal to facilitate downstream operations. The clarification process is critical to min-imize particle content (cells, debris, impurities like DNA, endotoxin, HCP) in the load for the subse-quent chromatography step (e.g., Protein A) and reduce fouling of the stationary phase.

The solid content per unit volume, often referred to as cell density and viability, plays a crucial role in determining the choice of clarification method, performance efficiency (yield), and overall effectiveness. High cell density can lead to increased levels of DNA, HCP, and other cell debris. Centrifugation is effective for handling high cell concentrations and processing large volumes, rendering depth filtration or microfiltration less effective at such high cell densities. However, cen-trifugation can have drawbacks due to the shear stress it imparts on cells, increasing the risk of cell lysis and impurities. To address this concern, flocculation or precipitation techniques may be employed. Figure 10.10 illustrates the available options for establishing a robust harvest system tailored to the specific cell line and target protein.

The modernization of existing harvesting methods to accommodate high cell density, increased biomass, and improved impurity removal can significantly enhance the purification process. Therefore, it may be beneficial to explore additional techniques and strategies, if necessary, to achieve the highest level of clarification efficiency.

10.7   ANALYTICAL TOOLS

Qualitative and quantitative analytical tools play a pivotal role in validating the process across various scales. Analytical methods must be precise, accurate, and robust. The data obtained from these analyses inform decision-making throughout the entire process, from early-stage cell line development to the final product. In-process testing is a crucial component in enabling Process

Analytical Technologies (PAT), which involves understanding process parameters, conditions, and materials to develop an effective control strategy. According to the ICH Q10 guideline, a control strategy is defined as "a planned collection of controls derived from current product and process understanding that guarantees process efficiency and product quality." Here, we summarize some of the critical upstream analytical tools frequently used.

10.7.1 CELL CULTURE/FERMENTATION

Growth monitoring is the primary analysis in the culture process, determining whether the existing conditions favor cell growth. Various offline methods are available for monitoring bacterial cells, with spectrophotometry being the most widely used due to its simplicity, speed, and reliability. Microscope counting is an alternative, albeit cumbersome and less reliable method. For mammalian cell cultures, the trypan blue method (using a microscope and hemocytometer) is common. Several automated cell-counter instruments, such as the Vicell Cell Viability Analyzer and Cedex Cell Analyzer, offer pre-programmed and customizable solutions, estimate cell sizes, and handle various animal cells.

While these methods remain popular for cell density measurements, recent years have seen the emergence of online cell density measurements, similar to the monitoring of pH and dissolved oxygen (DO). Microfluidic mass sensors and in-situ sensors now allow for continuous measurements. For example, the Incyte Arc sensors by Hamilton utilize capacitance to measure the polarization of viable cells. Another example is the Dencytee Total cell density sensors, also by Hamilton, which rely on optical density or turbidity measurements at near-infrared (NIR) wavelengths.

Measurement of parameters such as pH, pCO_2, osmolality, and various metabolites (e.g., glucose, lactate, glutamine, sodium, potassium) is typically carried out using offline blood gas analyzers such as the YSI analyzer and NOVA Biochemical Analyzer.

Productivity estimation is commonly performed through periodic sampling during the fermentation process. Common quantitation methods include ELISA, Protein A HPLC, and protein biosensor systems (e.g., ForteBio Octet). AlphaLISA, a high-throughput immunoassay with high sensitivity, reduces testing time and eliminates some steps involved in traditional ELISA. In the case of bacterial cells, SDS-PAGE is the most frequently used method for culture analysis and inclusion body (IB) separation.

Glycosylation patterns depend significantly on cell culture conditions and media/feed composition, which can have a substantial impact on downstream purification strategies. Glycan mapping using the UHPLC method is commonly employed for analyzing glycan profiles (O-linked and N-linked). Additionally, high-resolution mass spectrometry aids in determining glycosylation patterns and degrees (glycoprotein profiling). While several orthogonal methods are used for glycan analysis of the drug substance (Critical Quality Attributes testing), these methods may not be necessary in the early stages of the manufacturing process.

Both offline and in-line product monitoring offer several advantages, including the identification of optimal feeding strategies and culture conditions that can enhance product quality and potentially reduce the need for additional testing until the final drug substance preparation (e.g., glycan analysis).

10.7.2 CELL HARVEST

Turbidity serves as a valuable tool for assessing clarification efficiency. It measures the extent of light scattering when passed through a sample containing suspended particles. This measurement is expressed as Nephelometric Turbidity Units (NTUs), with lower NTU values indicating better clarification. This method is used to effectively compare different clarification techniques.

The step yield is determined based on the amount of product recovered at the end of the harvest process. Additionally, for certain processes, estimating the levels of HCP and DNA, predominantly achieved in downstream purification processes, can offer valuable insights into the achieved level of purification.

10.8 UPSTREAM EQUIPMENT

The technology for upstream unit processes has evolved significantly over the past few decades. Originally developed for fermentation, these systems now enable the growth of various cell cultures capable of yielding a target protein molecule. The biological process of cell growth and expression becomes more sensitive when genetically modified organisms are involved. To address these challenges, bioreactors are now designed with advanced technology to ensure reproducible batch yields. This chapter provides an overview of the equipment and operational processes that play a central role in biopharmaceutical production. While the science of bioprocessing involves a deeper understanding of the physics and chemistry of bioprocesses, this chapter focuses on the equipment commonly used in commercial settings.

One of the key criteria for biomanufacturing processes is creating an optimal environment for all unit operations that support cell growth, isolation/clarification, and purification to produce the desired product. Consequently, the facility and equipment are critical components in defining the process, its performance, and its robustness.

Upstream processing includes cell growth, cell isolation, and harvest, which require equipment and systems such as:

- Media and Solution Prep Systems.
- Bioreactor Systems for Fermentation.
- Harvest and Clarification Systems.

In addition to the above, other peripheral sanitary equipment essential for the entire bioproduction process (upstream, downstream, and fill-finish) includes Clean-in-Place (CIP) systems, sterilization systems, decontamination, biowaste systems, and various disposable/single-use systems.

10.9 MEDIA AND SOLUTION PREPARATION SYSTEMS

Vessels and tanks are primarily used for blending, holding bulk liquid volumes, and transport. At the end of the bioreaction, these vessels are used to introduce materials (media, feed, and other solutions) into the bioreactor and transfer either parts or the entire reactor volume to the next unit operation. Stainless steel alloys (particularly 304 and 316) are the most commonly used construction materials for large tanks, but single-use systems are now widely adopted across a broad volume range. These single-use systems are discussed in more detail in Chapter 9.

These vessels can range from simple storage containers to vessels equipped with overhead mixers. Features like temperature control, load cells, pH control, liquid/solid additions, withdrawal, and gassing can determine the specific use of these tanks or vessels. Jacketed vessels are commonly used for temperature control, especially in large-scale preparations, where a temperature control fluid circulates inside the jacket to maintain the required temperature in the process fluid. Other temperature control components that may be used include an immersion heat exchanger and a heating blanket.

For vessels with built-in load cells, all additions are based on weight, eliminating the need to move large tanks for weighing. In large-scale preparations, weight-based solution preparation is more beneficial than volume-based. For filling and transfer, the process length can be established by setting the overall filling time or defining a filling rate (e.g., kg/min) for a vessel with a known volume. pH measurements in bioprocess liquid preparations are typically done offline through manual sampling from the preparation tank. However, in high-end systems, such as bioreactor vessels, continuous online monitoring with a pH probe may be used for pH measurements and adjustments.

10.10   BIOREACTOR SYSTEMS

A bioreactor is a sealed vessel used to support biological systems (e.g., bacterial cells, yeast, mammalian cells) for the production of biopharmaceuticals (such as vaccines and antibodies), primary and secondary metabolites (including ethanol and biofuel), and even in tissue engineering. The first bioreactor was developed in 1857 by Louis Pasteur to study the fundamental principles of fermentation. This milestone in bioprocessing, along with advancements in cell biology and recombinant DNA technology, paved the way for further developments in bioreactor design and their industrial applications beyond food products.

Bioreactor design relies on several factors, including cell type, product throughput, quality control, and mass transfer. The duration required for processes is critical to bioreactor design and establishing operational parameters. The material used for the bioreactor vessel should endure repeated sterilization cycles without affecting long-term performance or durability. The preferred materials are glass (for small-scale benchtop bioreactors) or stainless steel, with 316 SS for wetted parts and 316L SS for animal cell cultures. Non-product contact surfaces can be made of 304-type stainless steel. For microbial cultures, a height-to-diameter ratio of 2:1 or 3:1 is preferred for high gas transfer, while a ratio of 1:1 is common for animal cell cultures. Bioinstrumentation and process control features to ensure sterility are essential design characteristics for bioreactors. Key functionalities include maintaining sterility, providing aeration (oxygen), removing gaseous products (carbon dioxide), controlling and optimizing the environment for cell growth (e.g., temperature control, pH, agitation), minimizing evaporation losses, and enhancing process efficiency.

10.11   BIOREACTOR TYPES

10.11.1   Stirred Tank Bioreactor

In bioprocesses, the stirred tank reactor (STR) is the most common and widely used bioreactor type. They vary in complexity from simple stirred tanks for enzymatic reactions to more advanced aerated fermenters for metabolic bioconversions. A compressor introduces air from the bottom through sub-surface spargers to provide necessary aeration. Agitation via an impeller shaft (equipped with baffles) facilitates mixing and dispersing air bubbles within the vessel's contents, which are crucial for bioreactor performance. Stirred tank reactors are highly adaptable, with high kLa (volumetric mass transfer coefficient) values for gas transfer. Jacketing is often used for heating and cooling. The height-to-diameter ratio depends on the intended use, ranging from 1 for basic vessels with limited surface area per unit volume to 3 for large-scale reactors. This type of reactor operates in one of these modes: batch, fed-batch, or continuous. Various operation modes are explained below (Figures 10.11 and 10.12).

10.11.2   Airlift Bioreactor

An airlift or gas-lift bioreactor is a gas-liquid bioreactor that achieves agitation without mechanical devices, relying on sparged air's convection. A glass grid aerator aids in humidified air dispersion, promoting mixing and oxygenation while using less energy than a stirred tank reactor. Only a specific area of the vessel, called the riser, is sparged with gas. Gas holdup and volumetric mass transfer coefficient (kLa) are influenced by operating conditions. The medium moves upward in the riser due to gas holdup and reduced fluid density. At the top of the reactor, bubbles disengage, and the denser medium flows downward into the downcomer, a non-sparged section of the pipe. Oxygen transfer is often lower than in stirred tank bioreactors due to low shear levels. Airlift bioreactors find extensive use in plant and animal cell growth, as well as immobilized biocatalysts.

However, they tend to form dead zones due to non-uniform nutrient distribution and inadequate mixing (Figure 10.13).

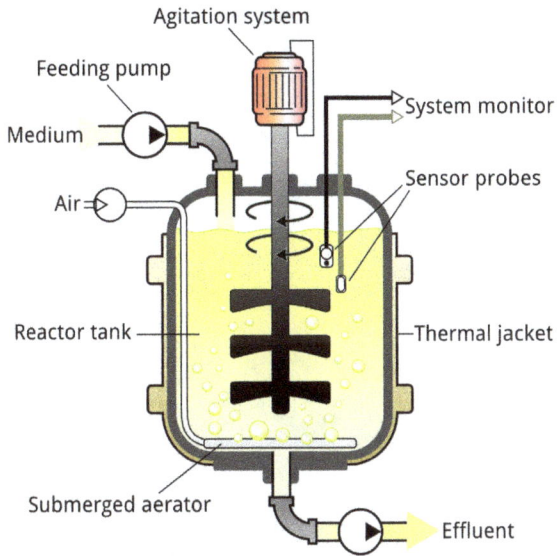

FIGURE 10.11 Stirred bioreactor

Source: Yassine Mrabet–Own work, CC BY-SA 3.0, https://commons.wikimedia.org/w/index.php?curid=8301774

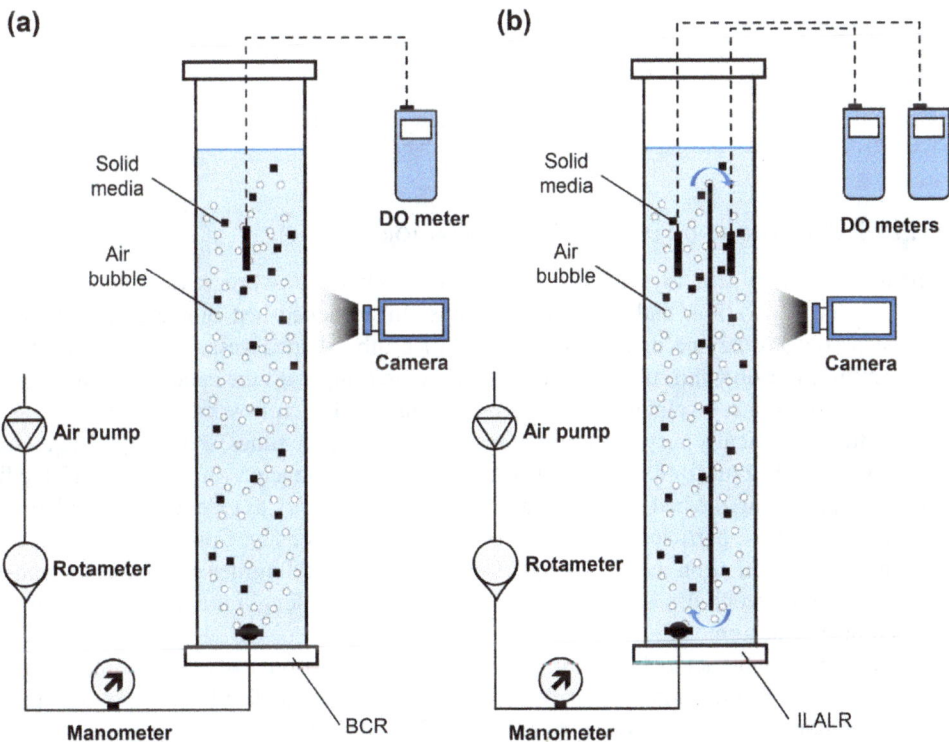

FIGURE 10.12 Schematic of an airlift bioreactor. (a) bubble column reactor (BCR), and (b) internal-loop airlift reactor (ALR)

Source: https://www.mdpi.com/2227-9717/8/6/713/htm; http://creativecommons.org/licenses/by/4.0/

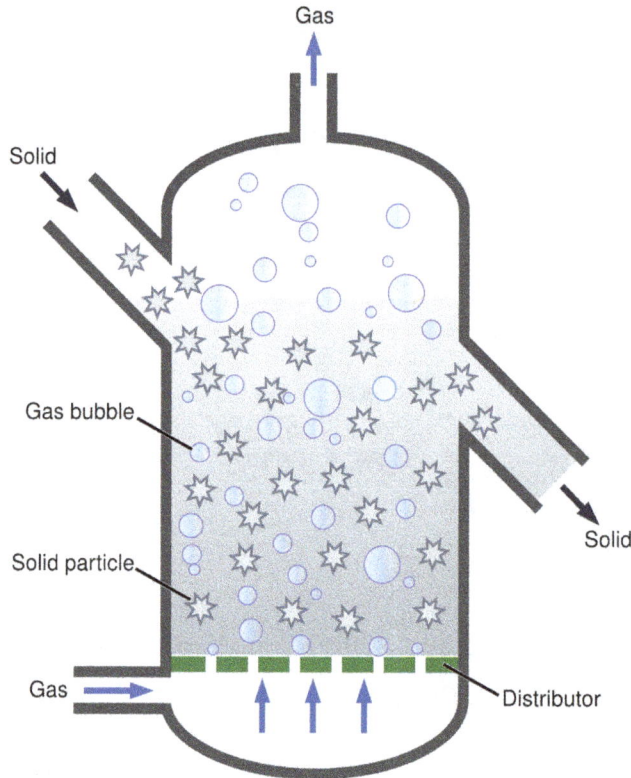

FIGURE 10.13   Fluidized bed bioreactor

Source: YassineMrabet–Own work based on Fluidized Bed Reactor Graphic. JPG (user: Hughesy127), Public Domain, https://commons.wikimedia.org/w/index.php?curid=8278465

10.11.3   PACKED BED AND FLUIDIZED BED BIOREACTOR

The chemical industry employs packed bed reactors for various processes, such as distillation, absorption, separation, and catalytic reactions. In a packed-bed bioreactor, immobilized biocatalyst particles (enzyme or microbial cells) fill a tube-shaped vessel. The liquid medium flows either uphill or downhill through the column, interacting with the catalyst spread along its length. Rapid liquid phase velocity enhances mass transfer. To improve catalyst conversion, the process medium is typically recycled through the column multiple times, often requiring an intermediate storage tank. Fluidized beds are a type of packed bed reactor where the liquid medium flows upwards, allowing the bed to expand at high flow rates, known as extended–or fluidized-bed bioreactors. Biocatalyst particles must have suitable size and density. Continuous movement of particles prevents channeling and clogging. However, understanding mass and energy transfers and accounting for potential pressure drops along the reactor's length are critical challenges in packed bed reactor design.

Different types of bioreactors include the loop reactor, immobilized cell reactor, solid-phase tray reactor, rotary drum reactor, agitated tank reactor with a movable impeller, hollow fiber reactor, and the widely popular disposable WAVE™ bioreactor (Figure 10.14).

Several iterations of the Wave bioreactors have been reported in recent patents by Niazi (author of this book), including a baffled bioreactor (Figures 10.15 and 10.16).

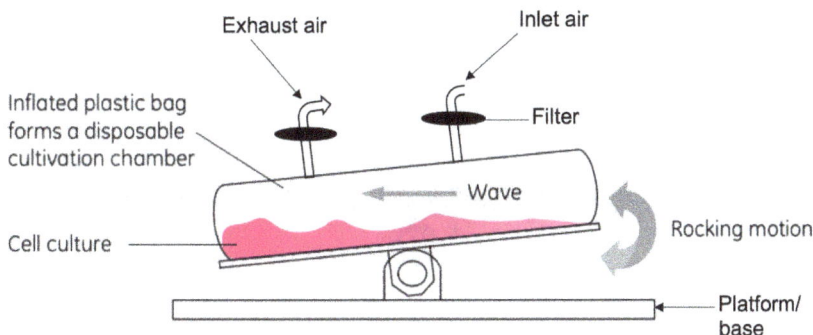

FIGURE 10.14   Schematic of a rocking bioreactor

10.12   MODES OF OPERATION

There are four modes of operation available for bioreactors: batch, fed-batch, perfusion, and continuous fermentation.

In the early days of biopharma manufacturing, the batch mode was predominantly used due to its simplicity. However, over time, fed-batch has become more prominent for microbial and animal cell culture, offering increased productivity compared to the traditional batch mode. Perfusion, originally considered precise, has also gained renewed interest, especially for animal culture, as an alternative to fed-batch mode when culture productivity is exceptionally low.

The choice of operation mode by manufacturers is driven by factors such as the type of expression system used, productivity, manufacturing capacity, facility layout, and output.

10.12.1   BATCH CULTURE

At the start of the process, a batch operation involves a closed vessel system containing all necessary medium components, including the required inoculum for fermentation (cell development). No subsequent feeding or addition of supplement components is performed, maintaining a constant volume throughout the process. Apart from gases, antifoam, and pH adjusting solutions added at the beginning, the medium composition must meet all nutritional requirements to support cell growth and enhance productivity. The substrate concentration remains at its maximum within the reactor, while the cell and product concentration start at their lowest. The entire batch is harvested, and the fermentation end time is typically determined by product kinetics (Figure 10.17).

The simplicity of setup and execution led to the widespread application of the batch process, especially during the initial biotechnology phase involving cell mass production or primary product production (e.g., vaccine production using microcarriers). A batch process typically includes phases that define cell growth: a lag phase, an exponential growth phase, and a stationary phase indicative of harvesting, followed by preparation for a new batch involving cleaning, sterilizing, and filling; Figure 10.17).

The total amount of cell mass-produced in each batch process is calculated per the following equation:

r_b = rate of cell mass production per batch cycle and tc = batch cycle time

$$r_b = \frac{Xm - X}{tc} = \frac{YX/S\ M - So}{tc} \qquad \text{Equation 10.1}$$

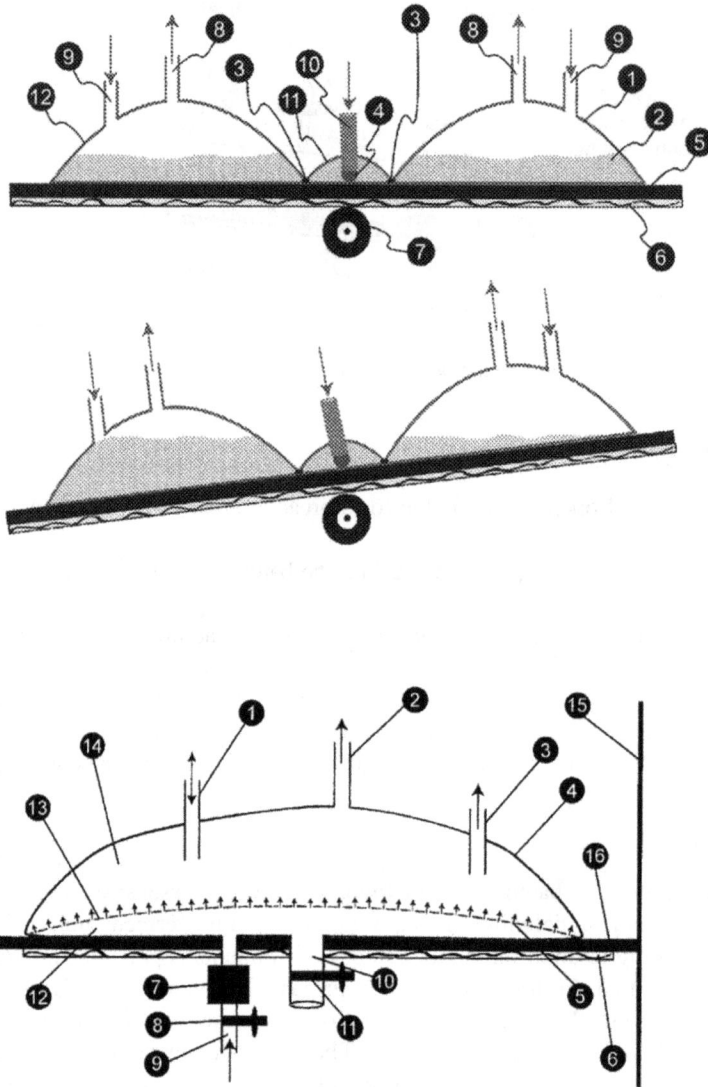

FIGURE 10.15 Baffled pivot bioreactors

Source: Niazi patent US 9238789

$$t_c = \frac{1}{\mu max} \ln \frac{Xm}{Xo} + t_l \qquad\qquad \text{Equation 10.2}$$

where X_m is the maximal attainable cell concentration, and X_0 is the cell concentration at inoculation, t_l is the lag time, and μ_{max} is the exponential growth time.

10.12.2 FED-BATCH

In a fed-batch process, both the substrate (necessary medium components) and inoculum are applied at the start, similar to a batch process. However, it also incorporates periodic feeding of a concentrated solution of the growth-limiting supplement to the cells, allowing for controlled

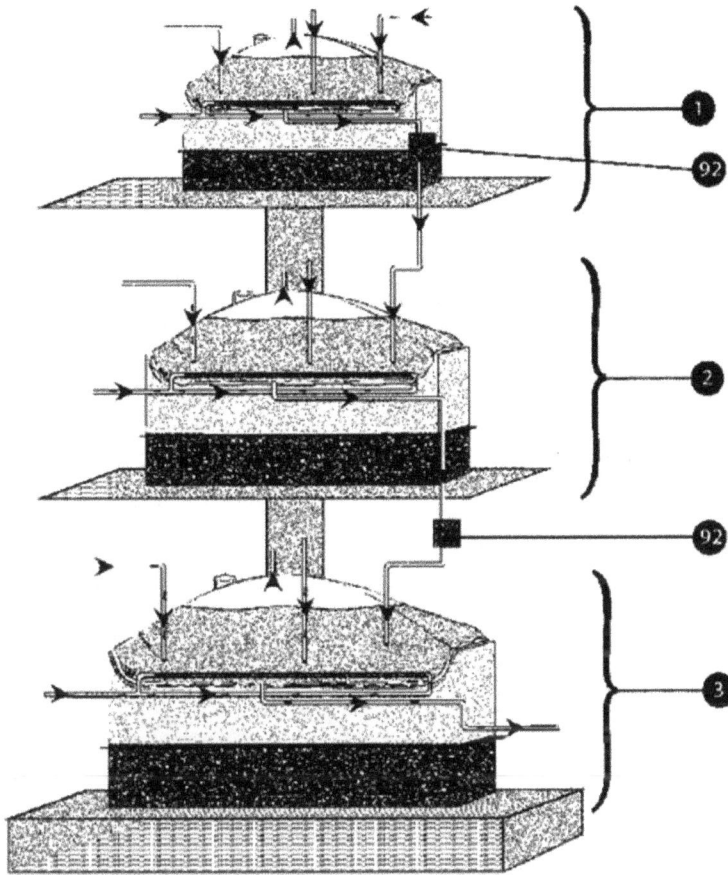

FIGURE 10.16   Exhaust-free bioreactor

Source: Niazi patent US 9469671

cell growth and possibly increased productivity. This process is commonly used in bio-industrial applications requiring high cell density (Figure 10.17 and 10.18).

The feed added to the culture is typically a highly concentrated solution of critical nutrients to extend the growth phase and enhance productivity while avoiding dilution of the fermentation volume. Depending on the culture and components, the feed solution can be a concentrated glucose solution with a single nutrient or a mixture of multiple components depending on the culture, the nature of the components, such as precipitation, in which case it may be better to add various parallels feeds to reduce the risk of precipitation. The feeding is generally intended to resolve any substrate limitation via a sporadic introduction during fermentation. The feeding can either be a bolus feed added intermittently to the culture or a continuous feed that is set up to be continuous, which may be constant, linearly increasing with time, or cascade mode based on sensor measurements (e.g., glucose measurement in the culture). Implementing continuous feeds for large-scale processes can be challenging and requires careful fine-tuning (Figure 10.12).

Fed-batch processes have been successfully employed for microbial (e.g., *E. coli*, Pichia pastoris) and mammalian (CHO cells) cultures. In *E. coli* fermentation, cells are grown to a relatively high density, and a bolus glucose feed is added to achieve a faster growth rate. However, the timing and type of feed addition must be carefully balanced to prevent the accumulation of unwanted by-products or metabolites(e.g., acetic acid in *E. coli* fermentation, ethanol for *Saccharomyces cerevisiae,* and

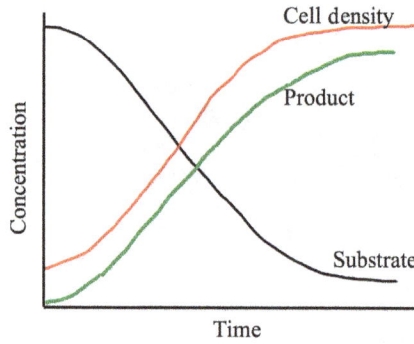

FIGURE 10.17   Cell growth kinetics for a batch process

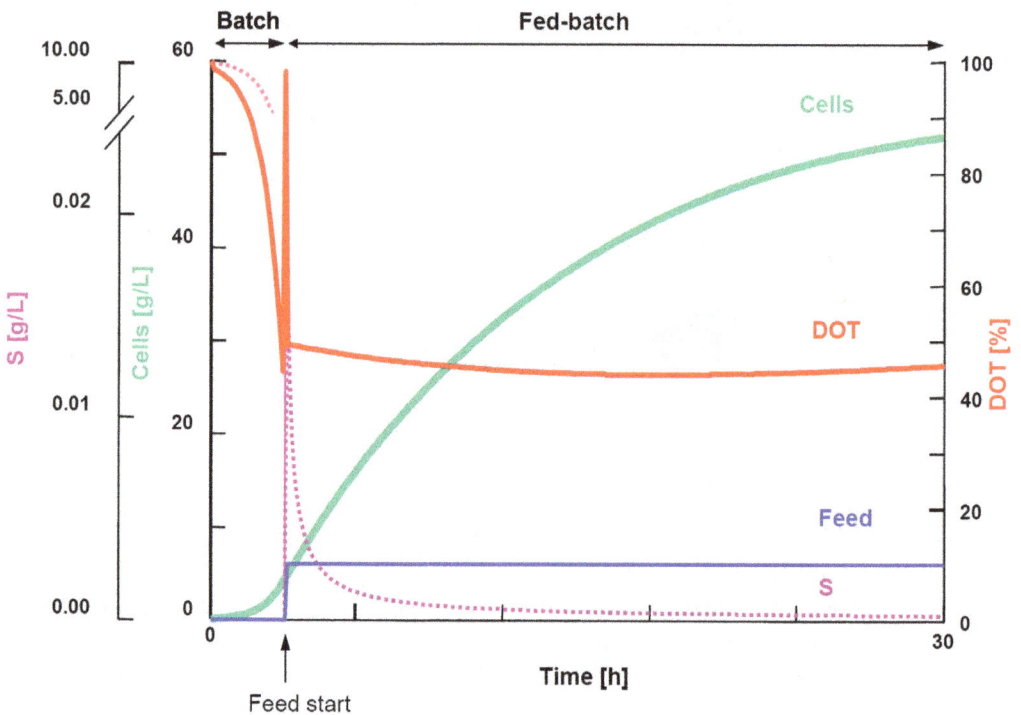

FIGURE 10.18   Fed-batch bioreactor profile

Source: https://upload.wikimedia.org/wikipedia/commons/c/cc/Fed_batch_principle.png

lactic acid in cell culture), which can inhibit growth or affect product impurity profiles. For CHO cell cultures, feeding may increase the medium and culture's osmolality, impacting cellular functions.

In a fed-batch process, the maximal cell density and product production vary depending on factors like the host cell, clone, culture medium, feeding schedule, and bioreactor control regime. Microbial fed-batch operations are considerably faster, with *E. coli* taking 10–48 hours and Pichia pastoris taking 4–7 days, depending on the product. CHO cell fed-batch methods typically take 10–14 days but can extend to 20 days for increased output.

Fed-batch processes have become the preferred choice for bioproduction due to their operational simplicity and ability to address some of the limitations of batch culture. With the application of single-use technology and advanced process control systems, fed-batch processes have become more robust. However, the relatively long process times for mammalian cell culture or yeast cells, required to achieve higher productivity, may be viewed as a disadvantage in terms of operational efficiency. Additionally, non-productive phases, including cleaning, verification, sterilization, and batch preparation, are unavoidable for any type of bioreactor.

10.12.3 CONTINUOUS REACTOR PROCESS

A continuous reactor process includes a steady feeding of the substrate while simultaneously removing an equal volume of culture out from the reactor. The concentration of the substrate can be regulated to a fixed value (Figure 10.19).

The primary form of a continuous process is the steady-state CSTR, also known as a chemostat. In this system, the growth rate is determined by the availability of the limiting substrate or nutrition. The dilution rate, estimated by the chemostat's flow rate, matches the net-specific growth rate, giving users the ability to adjust the growth rate as needed. This control over cell growth allows for precise control over product formation rates. By maintaining a constant dilution rate, specific growth rate remains constant. The lag phase, commonly observed in a batch system, is not present in a continuous operation (Figure 10.21).

Productivity increases with the dilution rate until it reaches a maximum near the specific growth rate (at a steady state). However, when the dilution rate becomes too high, cells can't grow fast enough to reach a steady state, resulting in a washout period without a steady state, leading to decreased productivity (Figure 10.19).

$$\mathrm{Pr\,oductivity} = \frac{Biomass}{(reactor\ volume)(time)} = xD \qquad \text{Equation 10.3}$$

Using a CSTR for cell recycling can significantly enhance volumetric productivity, especially in processes with low-value products and large volumes, such as waste treatment and fuel-grade ethanol production.

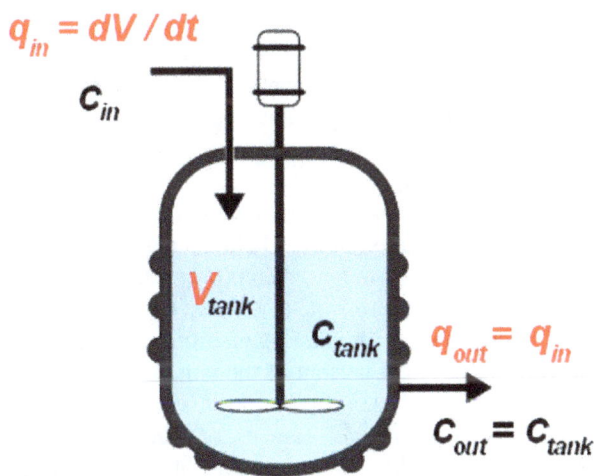

FIGURE 10.19   Schematic of a CSTR

Source: Brijesh Pratap Singh, under Creative Commons Attribution Share-Alike 4.0 International License

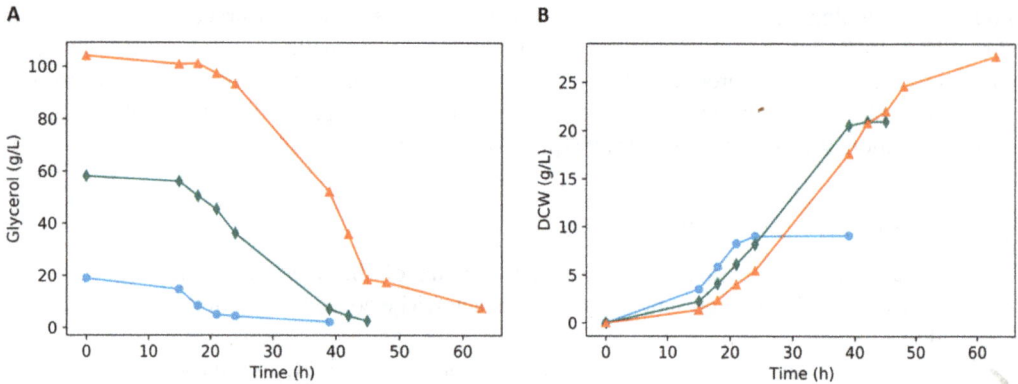

FIGURE 10.20 Genetically modified *Komagataella phaffii* aerobic culture showing the consumption of glycerol (A), biomass (B) in different initial glycerol concentrations: 2% (blue circle), 6% (green diamond), and 10% (orange triangle). Time profile for substrate and cells in a chemostat

Source: Microorganisms 2020, 8(5),781; https://doi.org/10.3390/microorganisms8050781; http://creative commons.org/licenses/by/4.0/

The industrial application of continuous fermentation processes has been limited. While chemostats offer productivity advantages for primary products, concerns related to process flexibility, genetic stability of cells, and contamination risks have restricted their usage (Figure 10.20).

10.12.4 PERFUSION

The perfusion procedure begins as a batch process, initially maintaining a constant volume in the bioreactor. Fresh culture media is continuously supplied while spent medium is withdrawn at the same rate when cells are in the exponential growth phase (typically 2–4 days after inoculation). A cell retention device, such as an ATF or TFF filter, retains reactor cells, allowing the removal of low-molecular components along with spent media. This facilitates continuous harvesting and product preparation for further purification. Although perfusion has been used in cell culture since the 1980s, it has faced challenges related to equipment complexity and scaling up.

Perfusion processes typically run for extended periods, ranging from 20 to as long as 90 days. This approach is less suitable for microbial fermentation due to their faster growth rates, which result in shorter biomass production times. Mammalian cultures, such as CHO cells, are better suited for perfusion processes, as their slower growth requires 15–20 days in a fed-batch process to achieve the desired product yield (Figure 10.21).

During perfusion, the continuous flow of culture medium ensures a steady supply of nutrients to cells. Constant removal and recirculation of cells help maintain low levels of toxic by-products, resulting in higher productivity compared to fed-batch processes. Cell densities ranging from 40 to 80 million cells/mL are achievable with perfusion, in contrast to the 5–20 million cells/mL typically observed in fed-batch processes. However, monitoring viabilities is crucial to prevent cell debris and dead cell accumulation. Bleeding a small portion of the culture helps maintain high cell viability and product quality.

Cell retention is achieved using membranes, screens, or selective cell removal centrifuges. The most common methods are TFF and ATF systems with hollow fiber filters. In TFF, medium is pumped through a membrane filter, while a peristaltic pump recirculates cell culture supernatant over the membrane surface. Smaller molecules pass through the membrane filter as permeate, while larger molecules are retained as retentate. ATF, similar to TFF, uses a diaphragm pump to alternate flow directions over the membrane, minimizing fouling and cell shear. This maintains cells in

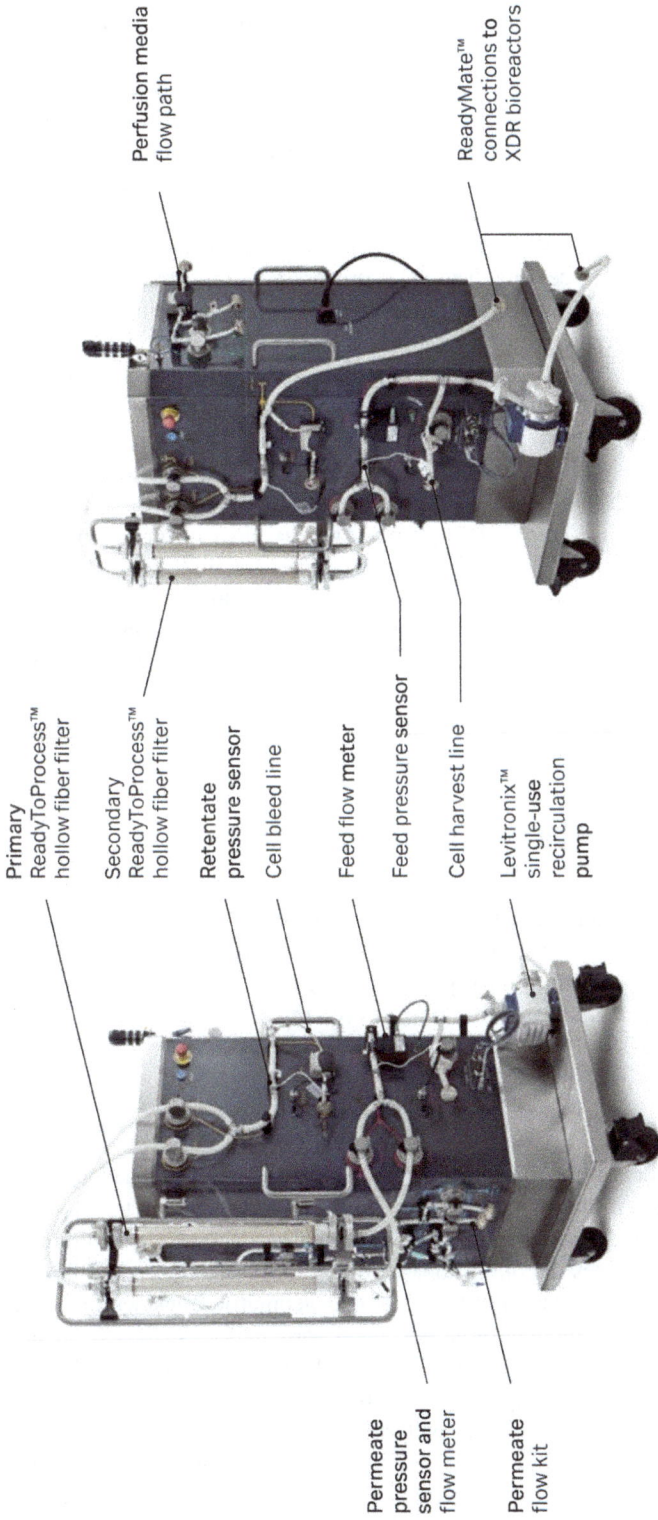

Perfusion media flow path

ReadyMate™ connections to XDR bioreactors

Primary ReadyToProcess™ hollow fiber filter

Secondary ReadyToProcess™ hollow fiber filter

Retentate pressure sensor

Cell bleed line

Feed flow meter

Feed pressure sensor

Cell harvest line

Levitronix™ single-use recirculation pump

Permeate pressure sensor and flow meter

Permeate flow kit

FIGURE 10.21 Bioreactor set up operating in perfusion mode using an ATF system

Source: Copyright Cytiva LifeSciences

constant equilibrium, promoting faster cell growth and higher productivity. Filters come in pore sizes ranging from 10 kDa to 750 kDa with various surface area options, usually made of polysulfone or polyethersulfone. ATF and TFF systems are available as reusable or single-use devices.

The recirculation flow rate is determined by the vessel volume exchanges per day (VVD) or the cell-specific perfusion rate (CSPR) in pL/cell/day. The perfusion rate depends on both the cell density as well as the culture medium. The perfusion rate is increased either manually or automatically, and this increase is decided either based on cell density or nutrient consumption, such as glucose levels in the media. It's advisable to keep the vessel volume exchanges per day to a minimum (typically 0.5–2 VVD) to avoid diluting the desired product and manage medium usage and cost. Higher perfusion rates (> 5 VVD) may require more complex liquid handling and can be more demanding for subsequent processing. The ideal process condition maintains a steady state with manageable high cell densities while controlling the bioreactor environment (foaming, osmolality, pCO_2, and O_2) to sustain productivity.

The primary advantages of the perfusion process over the fed-batch process include improved and controlled nutrient utilization, enabling steady-state conditions crucial for specific cell productivity. This increased cell concentration enhances productivity. When coupled with a microfiltration device for harvesting, the ATF system eliminates the need for laborious clarification processes, such as centrifuge or depth filter systems. Furthermore, perfusion processes contribute to efficient facility utilization and extended production phases. The flexibility to set up perfusion systems with almost any type of bioreactor and scalability are key features preferred for bioproduction processes. However, a drawback is the requirement for large media volumes, which may not fully utilize nutrients compared to fed-batch processes. Media costs are generally prohibitive, especially for chemically defined or custom-made media for specific cell types. Additionally, the preparation time, labor, and media sterilization are challenging and require close supervision. The properties of the media and the chosen cell line significantly impact process efficiency. The complex setups and validation of the systems and processes are areas that would require additional evaluation (Table 10.6).

10.13   KEY SYSTEM COMPONENTS OF A BIOREACTOR

The bioreactor plays a vital role in converting raw materials into the desired product. Running a successful bioreactor operation requires an understanding of its key features, which enable control of critical process parameters determining the bioreactor culture's success. Factors determining the bioreactor environment's suitability for supporting cell growth and the production of interest (biomass or secreted protein) include agitation rate, oxygen transfer, temperature, and pH (as shown in Figure 10.22 and Table 10.7).

10.13.1   AGITATION

The impeller or agitator within the bioreactor vessel maintains homogeneity of the bioreactor contents, suspends solids in the liquid medium, facilitates efficient heat transfer, ensures uniform mass and gas transfer between different phases, and disperses air for aerated culture conditions. Two commonly used impeller types in conventional stirred-tank reactors are axial flow and radial flow impellers, sometimes in combination. Other essential geometric considerations include impeller size, vessel geometry, baffles, number of baffles, width, orientation, sparger form, and location. It's important to note that shear stress due to agitation can be highly damaging to sensitive and fragile cells, so choosing the appropriate impeller type must be done carefully.

Axial flow impellers create an axial flow pattern where the liquid flows parallel to the axis around the impeller shaft. Angled blades pump the liquid downward or upward, evenly mixing contents from the top to the bottom of the bioreactor. The impeller's orientation (clockwise or counterclockwise) determines the flow direction. Axial flow impellers are suitable for heat transfer and

TABLE 10.6
Comparison of Batch, Fed Batch, and Continuous Modes of Operation

Operation Mode	Key Features	Advantages	Disadvantages
Batch	Highest substrate concentration that decreases with residence time, suitable for small-scale production	Easy operation, high biomass accumulation, assurance of quality/sterility for each batch	Extended downtime between runs, high possibility of by-product accumulation
Fed-batch	A medium level of substrate control, process conditions can help prevent by-product accumulation, the residence time of cells can be controlled, distinctive batches, most preferred for microbial and mammalian cell culture processes	High biomass yield, limited by-product accumulation, cost-effective, economically viable	Complex handling, fine-tuning required for feed start times to avoid substrate depletion; demands tight process control
Continuous	Cell growth kinetics is controlled through substrate control, limited by-product accumulation, consistent quality	High-throughput downtime is significantly reduced highest product concentration	Highly complex, time-consuming, increased burden on downstream operations, steady-state is challenging to achieve for fast-growing organisms, scale-up may be a concern, requires a high level of process control, challenging to change operations

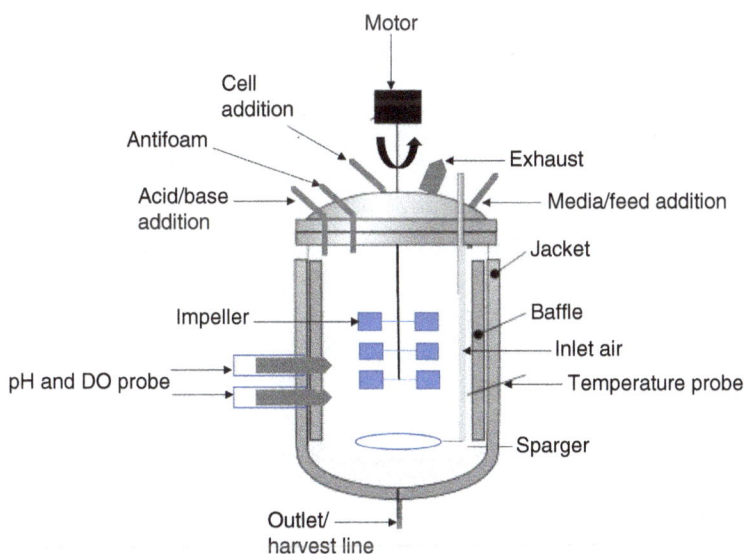

FIGURE 10.22 Schematic of a bioreactor and system components

TABLE 10.7
Parts and Their Function in a Bioreactor

Components	Function
Impeller	Mixing, air dispersion
Sparger	Introduce air, oxygen into the liquid medium to support an aerobic culture
Baffles	Prevent vortex and enable better mixing
Inlet air filter	Filter air before introduction into the bioreactor
Outlet air filter/exhaust	To filter out the released gas
Sensor/probes	Measure and monitor temperature, pH, and DO in the medium
Cooling jacket	Maintain temperature at its set point for the duration of fermentation
Ports (multiple)	Enable sampling, the addition of inoculum, media, feed, and supplements, the addition of acid/base for pH control, the addition of antifoam to control foaming

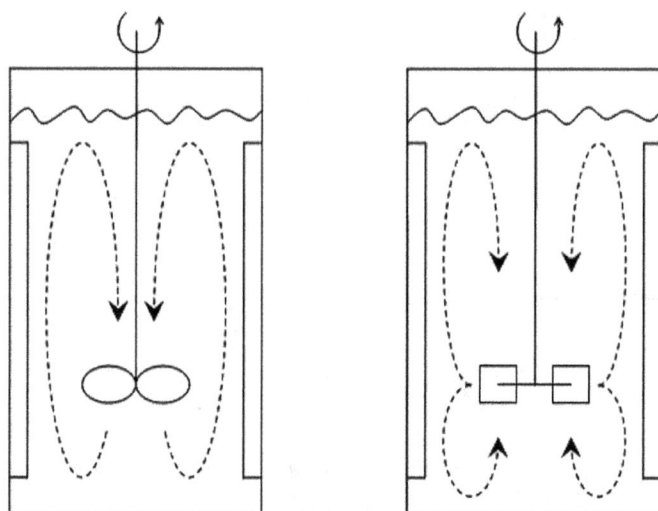

FIGURE 10.23   Impeller types; radial left and axial right

Source: Daniele Pugliesi–Own work, CC BY-SA 3.0, https://commons.wikimedia.org/w/index.php?curid= 4996798

liquid-liquid mixing and are known for their low shear. Examples include marine blade impellers and pitched blade impellers.

Radial flow impellers push liquid away from the impeller along its radius, creating four sections or quadrants within the bioreactor. They are primarily used for gas-liquid and liquid-liquid mixing and have a higher shear (Figure 10.23).

Pitch blade impellers are used for shear-sensitive cells like mammalian and plant cells. They have flat blades positioned at a 45-degree angle to the shaft, promoting both axial and radial flow. This combination enhances mixing and oxygen transfer rates compared to traditional maritime blade impellers.

Pitch blade impellers are used for shear-sensitive cells like mammalian and plant cells. They have flat blades positioned at a 45-degree angle to the shaft, promoting both axial and radial flow. This combination enhances mixing and oxygen transfer rates compared to traditional maritime blade impellers.

TABLE 10.8
Impeller Types and Suitability for Cell Lines

	Suitable Cell Line			
Impeller Type	Bacteria	Yeast	Mammalian (Human and Non-Human Cells)	Insect
Rushton impeller	*Escherichia coli, Bacillus, Streptomyces*	*Sacchromyces cerevisiae*, Baker's yeast, *Pichia pastoris, Candida albicans*		
Pitched blade impeller	*Streptomyces*	*Candida albicans*	HEK 293, HeLa, HL60, CHO, BHK	SF9, Hi-5, Sf21
Marine blade impeller			3T3, MC3T3, NS0	
Spin-filter impeller				SF9, Hi-5, Sf21

Flat-bladed or disk turbines, also known as Rrushton impellers, are commonly used in microbial cultures where shear stress is not a major concern. They feature flat blades set vertically along the shaft, creating unidirectional radial flow (Table 10.8).

The impeller's primary role is to disperse gas, while the sparger introduces air into the liquid medium inside the fermenter. Three basic sparger types used in bioreactors are:

- Porous spargers are used in small-scale applications but limit gas throughput due to high resistance. They are typically made from sintered metal, glass, or ceramics.
- Orifice spargers, also known as perforated pipes, have been utilized in specific applications and involve drilling small holes in piping, which is then shaped into a ring or cross and placed at the reactor's base.
- Nozzle spargers are employed in various bioreactors, providing a low-resistance gas flow and minimal risk of blockage, making them superior to other designs.

Other sparger designs, such as hybrid sparger-agitator designs, have also been developed for smaller fermenters, for example, gas and liquid are injected simultaneously through a nozzle to generate tiny bubbles, while air is delivered through a hollow stirrer-shaft.

The impeller needs to be powerful enough to distribute the gas bubbles in the vessel while also extending the duration it spends there. When adding gas into a liquid media, an important issue is to enhance the surface area to allow for faster gas absorption. Reducing the bubble size by using microspargers to create tiny bubbles will increase the surface area of absorption and enable a higher kLa. A consistent pore structure of the sparger device is key to generating even bubbles. The influence of gas dispersion on cells, on the other hand, must be balanced. Eukaryotic cells can be damaged by air bubbles. In microbial systems, where rapid dispersion and mass transfer across the vessel are required to sustain cell growth and gas transfer rates, high shear impellers are commonly used. For human cells, plant cells, and other cells, an oxygenation device capable of decreasing shear due to bubbles is preferable. A gas basket and bubble-free aeration can be used to accomplish this. A ring sparger, which creates bubbles, is used to introduce gases into the bioreactor tank. Between the exterior surface of the inner tube and an outside membrane, these bubbles travel with the impeller. The gas exchange occurs at the membrane-media interface, resulting in a bubble-free atmosphere for the cells and negating shear induced by bubble breakage.

Baffles are used to increase mixing, prevent vortex formation, and improve gas dispersion and aeration efficiency. Typically, four baffles, accounting for 8–10% of the vessel diameter, are attached radially to the wall. Baffles also help reduce microbial growth on the bioreactor walls.

The bioreactor vessel's size is crucial in determining the impeller diameter, with a common guideline being that the impeller should be approximately one-third of the vessel's diameter.

The combination of the sparger, impeller, and baffles plays a significant role in determining mixing and oxygen transfer efficiency in stirred-tank bioreactors.

10.13.2 AERATION

Aeration provides the necessary oxygen for cells' aerobic requirements as oxygen is an essential substrate for cell development and maintenance in bioreactors. Dissolved oxygen, often referred to as DO, is the primary oxygen source that cells receive in both free and noncompound forms. Hence, one of the critical functions of bioreactor systems is to continuously supply dissolved oxygen to cells through aeration. In industrial bioprocesses, the most common methods for this are using air, air-enhanced oxygen, or pure oxygen.

Aeration occurs in the bioreactor when oxygen diffuses into the cell culture medium at the interface created by the overlay.

The oxygen from the spargers dissolves in the cell culture with the help of agitation.

The total gas flow rate through the sparger varies depending on the type of sparger. For instance, a ring sparger typically has a volume of air per volume of liquid per minute ranging from 0.1 to 0.3 vvm, while a microsparger recommends a maximum gas flow rate of 0.03 vvm for mammalian cell culture processes. Microbial processes can utilize an aeration rate between 0.5 vvm and 2.0 vvm. This aeration rate can also vary significantly during fermentation to accommodate the increase in cell density.

The physicochemical features of the cell culture medium, the geometrical parameters of the bioreactor, and the presence of cells all have an impact on the rate of oxygen transfer (OTR) from gas to liquid interface. The OTR is critical to bioreactor design and scale-up. The DO in the culture medium depends on the OTR and its consumption by the cells (oxygen uptake rate). Agitation disperses the oxygen bubbles and promotes the gas bubbles' mass transfer through the gas-liquid (cell culture medium) interface. The movement of the bubble through the gas-liquid interface and its diffusion through the liquid membrane surrounding the cells into the cytoplasm enable oxygen to be transferred from a gas bubble to the cell. The oxygen uptake (or utilization) rate (OUR) is most often cell dependent. Therefore, monitoring the OUR is essential to assess the viability of the culture.

The rate of oxygen uptake can be expressed as follows:

$$\text{OUR} = Xq_{O2} = \frac{\mu X}{Y_{X/O_2}} \qquad \text{Equation 10.4}$$

Where q_{O2} is the specific uptake rate of oxygen, X is the biomass concentration and, Y_{X/O_2} is the oxygen yield coefficient.

The oxygen uptake rates of cell lines typically used in biomanufacturing are summarized in Table 10.9.

The oxygen transfer rate (OTR) is given by

$$\text{OTR} = k_L a \ (C^* - C_L) \qquad \text{Equation 10.5}$$

where C^* is saturated DO concentration, C_L is the actual dissolved oxygen (DO) in the culture medium, and $k_L a$ is the volumetric mass transfer coefficient.

When oxygen transfer is the rate-limiting step, OUR is balanced by OTR

$$\text{OUR} = \text{OTR} \qquad \text{Equation 10.6}$$

TABLE 10.9
Oxygen Uptake Rates of Cell Lines

Cell Line	OUR [10^{-3} mol/cell/h]
CHO DG44	2
CHO	5.0–8.04
NS0 myeloma	2.19–4.06
MAK hybridoma	4.16
FS-4 (Human diploid cells)	0.5
HFN7.1 Hybridoma	2.0

Source: What do cells need from a bioreactor? (GElifesciences.com)
Cytiva LifeSciences, Ruffieux, P. A. et al. and Xiu, Z. L. et al.

$$\frac{\mu X}{Y_{X/O_2}} = k_{La}\left(C*-C_L\right)$$

Equation 10.7

$$Y_{X/O2} \times OTR = \text{Cell Growth Rate}$$

Equation 10.8

The mass balance for dissolved oxygen in a well-mixed liquid phase is given by

$$\frac{dC}{dt} = OTR - OUR$$

Equation 10.9

Where dC/dt is the accumulation of oxygen rate in the liquid phase.

The mass transfer coefficient, represented by kLa, correlates the oxygen transfer rate with the oxygen uptake rate. kLa depends on various factors, including bioreactor size, media composition, cell type, presence of salts and surfactants, pressure, temperature, agitation speed, aeration rate, and other geometric and operational features. Achieving a high kLa is crucial for bioreactor design and scale-up success. Various physical and chemical methods can measure kLa, such as the unsteady state, steady-state, dynamic, dynamic gassing-out and pressure step, sodium sulfite oxidation, carbon dioxide absorption, and catechol bio-oxidation methods. Changes in specific process parameters can impact kLa, and these must be considered when evaluating different bioreactor systems or scaling up operations. Typically, kLa should be maintained constant during scale-up, as other physicochemical parameters like pH, DO, temperature, and bioreactor geometry are adjusted to achieve the required oxygen transfer rate. If bioreactor designs vary, kLa serves as a metric to guide adjustments to gas flow rates, sparger designs, and more to maintain the desired cell density. The optimal conditions for cell growth are typically met when OTR exceeds OUR.

The key variables that can affect k_La include:

- Gas Flow rate: A higher oxygen supply increases the k_La, powered by increasing the bioreactor's oxygen supply. The oxygen supply may be regulated by changing the concentration, i.e., air versus oxygen and volumetric flow. However, careful evaluation and balance are required to ensure that these changes do not impact the cell culture negatively. For example, a high flow rate could lead to excessive foaming and may also cause cell damage.

- Mixing: Mixing is key to ensuring homogeneity and eliminating concentration gradients within the bioreactor. The impeller type, location, and speed can impact the mixing dynamics and gas dispersion. $k_L a$ increases with tip speed in general; however, tip speed is also proportional to shear forces which can cause cell damage. Therefore, different impeller types and their placements are considered in bioreactor design to ensure these shear forces are not generated while achieving the target $k_L a$.
- Gas bubble size: The gas bubbles that are smaller in size can remain in the culture medium for a more extended period. This increase in residence time increases the $k_L a$.
- Temperature: The $k_L a$ and oxygen solubility in the culture media is inversely influenced by temperature. The oxygen solubility in pure water diminishes.
- Sparger: The number of spargers, the pore size, and surface area are factors that influence the bubble size, flow rate, which in turn impacts the $k_L a$.

The $k_L a$ measurement helps determine the optimum oxygen supply that can support cell growth.

10.13.3 TEMPERATURE CONTROL

Bioreactors commonly use 316 stainless steel for their wetted components. Heat transfer is necessary to regulate and maintain a consistent temperature during fermentation, which is vital for both mechanical agitation and exothermic metabolic activity that generates heat. Most bioreactor designs incorporate a jacketed vessel that circulates a temperature-controlling liquid (e.g., glycol or water) externally connected to the bioreactor to facilitate heating and cooling. In some cases, internal heat transfer coils are used, but microbial growth within the coils often hampers heat transfer efficiency.

The heat is transferred from a heat-transfer fluid to the reactor material through the heat-transfer surface or from the fermenter material to the cooling fluid if cooled. Therefore, the rate of healing depends on the bioreactor volume.

The heat required to heat up or cool down the contents of the bioreactor is represented by the following equation:

$$Q = m \times c_p \times (T0 - T1) = m \times c_p \times \Delta T \qquad \text{Equation 10.10}$$

Where Q is the heat (J), m (kg) = mass of the substance, $c_{p,}$ (J/kg K) = specific heat capacity of the substance, T0 and T1 (K) = start temperature and end temperature, respectively, and

$$\Delta T \text{ (K)} = \text{temperature change}$$

If the substance's specific heat capacity is unknown, then the heat capacity of water is used.

In a fermentation process, cells (irrespective of the microorganism or cell type) have an optimal temperature range that supports their growth. If the temperature is below this range, then the slow growth can reduce the rate of cell production or product synthesis. On the contrary, if the temperature is too high, it can lead to cell death and impact product quality.

The net cell growth rate is expressed as follows:

$$\frac{dX}{dt} = \left(\mu - k_d\right)X, \qquad \text{Equation 10.11}$$

where X and t are cell concentration and time, μ and k_d are cell growth and cell death rate, respectively.

Here, the cell growth, cell death rates are both temperature-dependent and expressed as functions of temperature following the Arrhenius equation:

$$\mu = A \times e^{(-E_a / RT)}$$
Equation 10.12

$$k_d = A' \times e^{(-E_d / RT)}$$
Equation 10.13

The heat generated during a microbial fermentation process is given by the following equation:

$$\frac{\Delta H_{c,S}}{YF_{X/S}} = \Delta H_{c,X} + YF_{H/X}$$
Equation 10.14

Where $\Delta H_{c,S}$ is the heat of combustion of the substrate, $YF_{X/S}$ is the substrate yield factor. $\Delta H_{c,X}$ is the heat of the cells' combustion, and $YF_{H/X}$ is the metabolic heat evolved per gram of cells produced (Figure 10.24).

For mammalian cell culture processes, particularly CHO cell lines, the optimal temperature for cell growth and culture maintenance is typically around 37°C. However, lower temperatures have been shown to extend cell culture viability, although cell growth may not be as robust at 37°C. Lower temperatures can effectively slow down the decrease in cell viability while allowing the cells

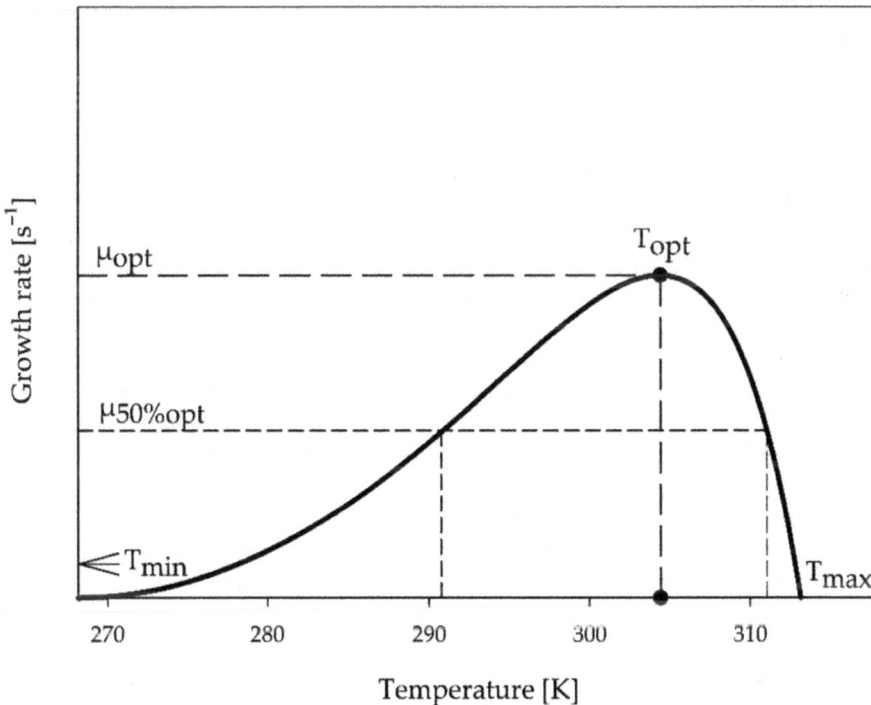

FIGURE 10.24 Effect of temperature on the cell growth rate for *E. coli*

Source: *Processes* 2020, *8*(1), 121; https://doi.org/10.3390/pr801012; http://creativecommons.org/licenses/by/10.0/

to remain in the production phase for protein synthesis for a longer duration. Several studies have demonstrated the impact of temperature on protein synthesis or improving the specific productivity of cells. A successful cell culture process, depending on the specific protein and cell line, may initially begin with temperature control at 37°C to primarily support cell growth and achieve higher densities. Later, the temperature can be adjusted to a lower range to enhance specific productivity. However, the ideal temperature should be evaluated for each cell culture process to ensure it doesn't affect product quality.

10.13.4   pH Control

Similarly to temperature, different biological systems have an optimal pH range. pH levels continually fluctuate during the fermentation process, with many processes requiring constant pH maintenance. Metabolite or by-product accumulation and substrate consumption often lead to shifts in pH in the culture medium. For instance, in microbial fermentation, acetic acid/carbon dioxide accumulation can decrease pH, and ammonia consumption can also lower pH. Consequently, continuous monitoring and pH adjustment are necessary. In mammalian cell culture, glucose consumption leads to lactate accumulation, resulting in pH reduction. pH control is achieved by adding a base or an acid to the bioreactor. Most modern bioreactors utilize a control strategy that automatically adjusts pH using a feedback control loop. In mammalian cell culture processes, sodium bicarbonate is commonly employed to counteract the acidic effects of lactate accumulation and CO_2.

Additionally, CO_2 may be added for pH control, but caution is needed to avoid oxygen depletion, which can impact dissolved oxygen (DO) levels and the culture medium balance, requiring significant amounts of sodium bicarbonate for buffering. Maintaining the pH of the media is critical for the success of the cell culture process, as even minor pH changes can affect cell growth, protein production, and product quality.

10.13.5   Foam Control

Foaming is a common issue in the fermentation process. The combination of agitation and aeration, along with foam-producing and foam-stabilizing chemicals (such as proteins, polysaccharides, and fatty acids), can lead to substantial foam formation in the bioreactor. Excessive foaming can block outlet gas lines and filters, resulting in the loss of fermenter contents, increased equipment pressure that can be detrimental, and potentially providing a route for contamination. Antifoam agents are widely used and added either at the start or during the manufacturing cycle, depending on the level of foaming. Adjusting the agitation rate can also help control foaming to some extent.

In certain cases, cell culture media may be supplemented with antifoam agents (e.g., pluronic acid) before use to minimize foaming. However, antifoam agents can also negatively affect oxygen transport rates and downstream processing due to membrane fouling. Mechanical systems, such as high-speed spinning disks at the top of the reactor, are suitable for addressing mild foam accumulation but consume significant energy in large-scale bioreactors.

Uncontrolled foaming can rise and potentially wet the exhaust filters, causing clogs and increased pressure in the bioreactor or, worse, contamination. Ensuring adequate headspace in a bioreactor allows gas to disengage from the liquid, helping to minimize foaming, especially in large-scale bioreactors.

10.13.6   Controller System

Monitoring bioreactor process parameters is crucial to maintaining optimal conditions that support cell growth and product synthesis. The most common instruments required for bioreactors are related to the physical factors discussed earlier: temperature, agitation, gas flow, and pressure. The fundamental parameters that should be monitored include pH, temperature, and dissolved oxygen (DO). Modern bioreactor designs incorporate new probes and techniques for measuring these parameters and additional metabolites effectively. This involves a combination of online and offline measurements using sensors and probes that provide feedback to the control system. A controller integrated with the bioreactor vessel is responsible for monitoring and controlling these parameters, adjusting them to match the user-defined set point. The sensor and control components of the bioreactor platform, connected to the controller, provide the necessary input and output, forming the control loop. This control loop serves as the medium for process control to ensure system stability and consistent performance. Control loops offer opportunities to enhance process operations. For stable operation, basic control loops for temperature, pH, dissolved oxygen, and agitation are integrated into bioreactor systems. Analysis of this monitoring provides valuable feedback to operators, leading to a deeper understanding of the process and improved stepwise operation. There are two types of control mechanisms: open-loop and closed-loop. In an open loop, the controller's actions are unaffected by the process variable. In a closed-loop system, the controller's actions depend on the setpoint (desired value) and the process variable. Feedback or feedforward loops can be used in a closed-loop system.

In bioreactor systems, the feedback closed control loop is the most common control technique. In this approach, the measured output is continuously examined in a time-dependent manner (typically every second) using a feedback element (i.e., sensor). The value is then compared to the setpoint, and the difference between the measured and setpoint values is fed back into the controller. The controller adjusts the control element to produce the corrected response, which is then fed back into the process. PID controllers (proportional-integral-derivative) are commonly employed in this context.

The other type of control system is feedforward, in which the input is measured by a sensor before being introduced into the process. If necessary, the value is adjusted by the controller and control element to input the control signal into the process. Unlike the feedback loop, there is no measurement of the output in this system (Figure 10.25).

These sensors and probes must be either pre-sterilized (gamma irradiated) or sterilized before use in the process. The insertion of these components should not compromise the sterility of the bioreactor vessel. This may require the use of aseptic connectors or steam sterilization of the bioreactor with the probes/sensors installed. The components must be able to withstand high temperatures (121°C) and humidity. Autoclavable and sterilized-in-place bioreactors, as well as vessel sterilization and decontamination, make sterilization before use in the production process and decontamination after operations convenient. Insertable probes may not always be reliable, especially for long-term mammalian cell culture processes, where probe performance may be a concern. Some other issues with these probes include their positioning in the bioreactor vessel, probe drift affecting their response, lack of in situ recalibration, and, most importantly, a potential route for

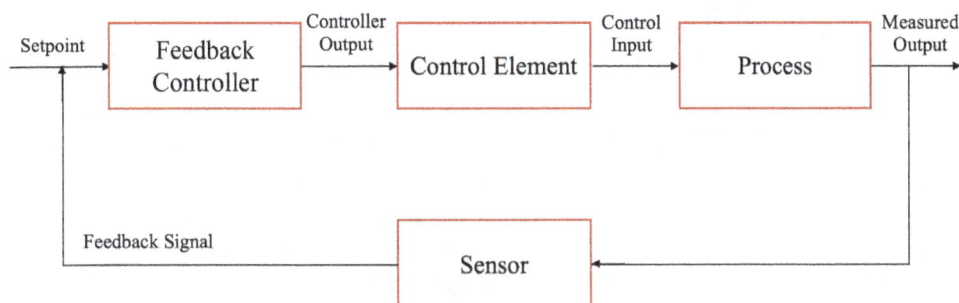

FIGURE 10.25 Illustration of a feedback control loop

TABLE 10.10
Summary of Process Parameters and Associated Measurement Components

Process Parameters	Sensor	Control Element
Temperature	RTD	Heating/cooling jacket/water reservoir
pH	pH probe (optic and conventional)	Pump for base addition and CO_2 from the mass flow controller
DO	Polarographic oxygen sensor, DO electrode	Oxygen mass flow controller
Glucose	Spectroscopic sensor	Pump for glucose solution
Gas flow rate	Rotameters or mass flowmeters	Mass flow controllers
Weight	Load cell	Amount of liquid in the bioreactor vessel
Liquid flow rate	Magnetic-inductive flow meter	Flow valve
Pressure	Pressure gauge	Backpressure regulator in the exit gas line

contamination. SUBs are single-use bioreactors with pre-installed sensors (typically for pH, DO, and cell density), as well as gamma-sterilized and ready-to-use assemblies. Setup and operation are simplified with these single-use sensors. The Celligen BLU (Eppendorf), Cultibag and AMBR (Sartorius), and Applikon Biosep (Applikon) have all successfully utilized pH and DO sensor spot technology (Applikon Biotechnology) (Table 10.10).

The desired features of a control system and its components include precision and accuracy, ease of installation and operation, scalability, compatibility with multiple platforms/sensors/probes (e.g., accommodating single-use or reusable sterilizable probes), and compliance with GMP standards.

In addition to online measurements, offline measurements for cell density, glucose, lactate, and other parameters are also conducted during bioreactor operations. These offline measurements can be used to validate online measurements and for sensor calibration. Several standalone off-line instruments are used for these measurements. Examples include a cell density counter and spectrophotometer for cell density measurements, NOVA, and YSI Biochemistry Analyzer for pH, metabolites, and substrate analysis.

Over the past decade, significant advancements have been made in this field, and with the emergence of single-use technology, online measurements for pH, DO, gas flow rate, agitation rate, temperature, pressure, and glucose concentration in the medium, as well as liquid flow rate, have become possible. Incorporating these controls and data acquisition capabilities has been facilitated by improved analytics. Suppliers and vendors (e.g., Sartorius, Cytiva, Thermo Scientific) have successfully integrated these controls and capabilities into their product offerings. In addition to these advancements, ongoing progress is being made with instrumentation and control systems to fully utilize these systems and move towards a more automated system that requires less intervention.

10.14   HARVEST AND CLARIFICATION SYSTEMS

The primary objective of the harvest process is to separate the cells from the media. In bacterial cells, the product of interest is contained within the cells, whereas in mammalian cultures, the protein is secreted into the medium. The timing of the harvest process is determined based on culture conditions, including cell density, cell viability, productivity, and protein quality. Several harvest methods, such as centrifugation, sedimentation/flocculation, or newer alternatives like crossflow filtration or ultrafiltration (e.g., depth filtration systems, hollow fiber filtration systems), are commonly used, depending on factors such as cell type, product of interest, processing time, and scalability. While the primary recovery steps involve separating cells from the culture medium, a secondary recovery step involves filtration of the harvest using a smaller pore size membrane in mammalian cell culture processes. In microbial cells, biomass/cells are subjected to cell lysis (chemical or a combination of mechanical and chemical) to recover inclusion bodies containing the protein of interest. Chapter 5 provides a detailed description of various clarification/harvest options and considerations for choosing a suitable harvest method for microbial and mammalian culture.

10.15 ANCILLARY AND PERIPHERAL EQUIPMENT

10.15.1 STERILIZATION

In the context of industrial fermenters, associated fittings, and piping, in situ steam sterilization under pressure, commonly known as SIP, is employed. When it comes to large-scale sterilization of equipment and liquids, thermal inactivation is the preferred method, especially for media. This involves introducing saturated hot steam into the vessel/pipe to ensure even distribution throughout the device, eliminating cold spots or dead ends. Successful sterilization requires steam to displace the air in the vessel and pipes. In cases where heat-sensitive devices need sterilization, chemical agents or radiation may be employed. However, it's crucial to ensure that chemical agents don't leave any residue, which could be toxic to the culture or lead to product adulteration. Some of the commonly used compounds for sterilization include ethylene oxide, 70 percent ethanol-water acidified at pH 2 with HCl, formaldehyde, and 3 percent sodium hypochlorite. Radiation sterilization can take the form of gamma rays, electron beams, or UV light. It is an effective method for single-use parts and filter devices, but it is not suitable for larger equipment due to operational challenges. Additionally, radiation can penetrate materials more deeply.

Sterile filtration is a widely used method for both liquids and gases. When it comes to gases, depth filters, surface filters, and membrane cartridge filters are commonly employed. Membrane filters, designed with uniformly small pores, sieve out particles effectively. Pressure drop can affect both depth and surface filters. It is essential to inspect all sterile filters for structural integrity before and after each use. Common methods for assessing the integrity of sterile filters include bubble point diffusion testing, forward flow tests, and pressure hold tests. Filtration with a 0.2–0.45 μm membrane filter can be utilized to remove microbiological components. Inlet and exhaust gases for bioreactors are filtered using sterilizing grade filters. For bioreactor liquid feeds, such as bulk media and heat-labile growth supplements, sterilizing grade filters are also employed. These filters can be directly connected to a sterile line on the bioreactor using a tubing welder in disposable/single-use bioreactor systems.

When it comes to heat sterilization, the key parameters are sterilization temperature and exposure duration. Higher temperatures result in shorter sterilization times for the same degree of effectiveness. There are two methods for heat sterilization: batch and continuous. In the batch method, steam is directly sparged into the vessel, heating its contents to 121°C for a predetermined period (usually 10–20 minutes), followed by cooling with water to return to optimal operating conditions. The use of steam allows for rapid attainment of sterilization temperature. In the continuous method, a heat exchanger is used for both heating and cooling in a continuous operation. Caution must be exercised during heat sterilization, particularly with heat-sensitive materials. Continuous heat sterilization offers energy savings and is a safer option for such materials.

10.15.2 CLEANING-IN-PLACE

Cleaning is a routine procedure for equipment that comes into contact with the product to prepare it for the next batch. CIP is performed without disassembling or disconnecting any parts from the processing system. After completing batch operations, equipment used in upstream production processes, including fermentation production vessels, seed train bioreactors, centrifuges, homogenizers, and tanks, are rinsed with dedicated cleaning agents suitable for the equipment. The specific cleaning agent, required quantity, and incubation period must be specified and validated for successful cleaning. All equipment cleaning for future production runs should adhere to this validated procedure. Commonly used cleaning agents include caustic soda (5 M NaOH) and phosphoric acid (20% w/v). Equipment cleaning involves multiple steps performed under different conditions, including peristaltic pump flow rates for circulating the cleaning agent, circulation times, and, if applicable, temperature. The entire cleaning process can take from a few minutes to several hours or even a day, depending on the contact time required for effective cleaning. A standard cleaning process in the industry starts with circulating water through the system, followed by an acid solution, purified water, and finally a caustic solution. pH and conductivity of the water are checked periodically to ensure no traces of the cleaning solution remain. Chromatography columns, media, and TFF systems also undergo similar cleaning using caustic solutions or a combination of cleaning agents. Packed chromatography columns are often stored in a 0.1–1.0 N NaOH solution.

10.15.3 PUMPS, VALVES, TUBES, AND PIPES

Pumps are routinely used in nearly all unit operations for liquid transfer and circulation. The choice of pump depends on factors such as the nature of the fluid, flow rate, and scale of the process. Commonly used pumps include peristaltic pumps, diaphragm pumps, and rotary lobe pumps. Peristaltic pumps, which do not come into contact with the product, use tubing and molded flow elements for liquid transfer. However, they have limitations, especially with high viscosity fluids, and can generate shearing and tubing shedding due to pulsing, potentially exposing the liquid. It's important to select the right pump head configuration and tubing. Disposable/single-use peristaltic pumps with single-use flow channels are available. Diaphragm pumps are positive displacement pumps that use the reciprocating motion of the diaphragm and valves to pump fluids, making them suitable for high viscosity liquids. Centrifugal pumps, on the other hand, rely on rotational energy from impellers and are best suited for high flow rates and low viscosity liquids. Further details on pumps are discussed in Chapter 6.

Sanitary fittings, primarily constructed from stainless steel alloy, are commonly used in bioreactor frameworks, tri-clamp connections, and skids. These fittings typically include elbows, T-shapes, Y-connectors, and reducers. The choice of piping and fitting depends on the specific unit operation requirements. Fittings used in contact with the product must be sterilized before reuse. Tubing and hoses are employed for liquid transfer. Tubing is typically considered a single-use item and is made from various materials, such as elastomer and silicone, depending on process requirements. In contrast, hoses can be single-use or reusable and are often used for air/gas transfer due to their ability to withstand high pressure and steam. Tubing and hoses are commonly used in various bioreactor operations, including media and feed transfer, inoculum transfer between seed and production bioreactors, air supply to bioreactors, and harvest. Valves are another crucial component, especially in bioreactors for process and flow control. These include sampling valves, drain valves, and pinch valves. Valves can be potential sources of contamination, so it's important to use sterilizable materials, especially for valves reused in the process. The inner surfaces of bioreactor vessels should be smooth and are often electropolished. O-rings are frequently used for small gaps, such as in process control probes, while gaskets are employed for larger openings, such as pipe connections to tanks and agitators.

10.16 SUMMARY

Bioreactor design has evolved over the years, incorporating in-line measurements, spectroscopy, and the constant emergence of advanced sensors and probes to enhance process control. Efforts are ongoing to integrate spectroscopy and advanced sensors to improve process control further. New bioreactor designs and models aim to handle higher cell densities resulting from perfusion by offering improved mixing and volumetric mass transfer coefficients (KLa) for oxygen transfer. Sparger and impeller designs are areas of interest in bioreactor development. Single-use systems have gained acceptance in the late development landscape due to their potential to increase manufacturing capacity. Evaluation of cGMP compliance should be part of bioreactor design considerations.

Single-use bioreactors have gained greater acceptance in the industry, particularly in the past decade. These systems have undergone significant design enhancements, including improved mixing, efficient gassing, and leak-free performance to sustain long-term high-density cultures. Many of these changes are driven by the need to expedite processes due to advancements in cell lines, product compositions, and increased use of perfusion. Computational fluid dynamic modeling and other advanced techniques have been instrumental in optimizing bioreactor design. Another focus area has been optimizing shear while improving cell retention, especially in perfusion systems. Recent trends include using a fixed-bed bioreactor coupled with an automated tangential flow filtration concentrator to improve retention without increasing shear, resulting in enhanced process efficiency, reduced operating costs, and a smaller process footprint.

In general, the industry is moving towards intensified, connected, and continuous bioprocessing, with a focus on enhancing process intensification. Concepts such as automatic perfusion systems integrated directly into bioreactor platforms are becoming more common. The near future is expected to witness the broader adoption of continuous bioprocessing, where unit operations and processes are performed continuously, enhancing bioreactor capabilities and ancillary components. These modifications are likely to increase facility usage, reduce downtime, and maximize overall productivity. Collaboration between biopharmaceutical manufacturers and single-use suppliers is crucial to achieving these improvements, which are essential for a more robust process.

Understanding the capital costs associated with installing new equipment in an existing manufacturing facility and the costs of consumables for solutions or process additives is essential when selecting unit operations. Therefore, process design must take a holistic approach to consider all these factors.

11 Downstream Processes Involved in Protein Production

11.1 OVERVIEW

The crude protein originates in the upstream process, where conditions influence protein type, but the downstream process defines the final product. The therapeutic product, such as secretion in the media (mammalian cell culture) or microbial cell biomass or components, is obtained post-fermentation. Downstream processing involves separation, recovery, and purification of the product from the host system. Typically, the transition from upstream to downstream occurs during the recovery step, i.e., harvest (clarified supernatant or cell pellet). Regardless of the expression system, cell removal is achieved through centrifugation or filtration. The chapter discusses the harvest of culture broth, essential for recovery and purification of biological products, including insights into future trends.

The chapter primarily focuses on the two most utilized production systems, *Escherichia coli* and CHO, outlining purification and product concentration strategies for these systems before final formulation and fill-finish of drug substance (DS)/drug product (DP; Figure 11.1).

The initial step in selecting downstream processing methods involves understanding the protein's features, stability profile, and factors potentially affecting its structure. Downstream processing schemes typically comprise capture, intermediate purification, and polishing stages (Figure 11.2), each serving specific purposes. The capture step, the first chromatographic unit operation, aims to isolate and stabilize the target protein while removing key host cell components. The second-phase of purification eliminates most contaminants such as nucleic acids and host cell proteins; its inclusion depends on succeeding chromatography processes and the purity profile of the target protein. The final stage, polishing, aims for maximum product purity while eliminating product-related impurities such as oxidized or deamidated species. The selection or combination of techniques considers the target protein, product quality, and specific requirements.

The overarching workflow and objective of a downstream process remain constant: ensuring the product meets specified quality attributes and purity profiles, establishing the product profile, and determining critical product quality attributes during the initial phases of process development and design. Purification and efficient recovery are pivotal factors contributing to the success of both the upstream and overall bioproduction processes. The selected purification process needs to be robust, scalable, and capable of effectively removing or reducing both product-related and process-related contaminants to achieve high purity and ensure safety. Maintaining stringent quality standards for recombinant proteins is paramount due to concerns about potential immunogenic effects or other hazards arising from the product's deviation from human-like characteristics or potential contamination by the host cell system (e.g., mammalian cells).

Selection of appropriate chromatography separation methods relies on differences in the properties of the target protein and other substances present in the sample. Chromatography, a fundamental technique in protein purification, continually evolves as a high-resolution method. Both traditional

DOI: 10.1201/9781003392026-11

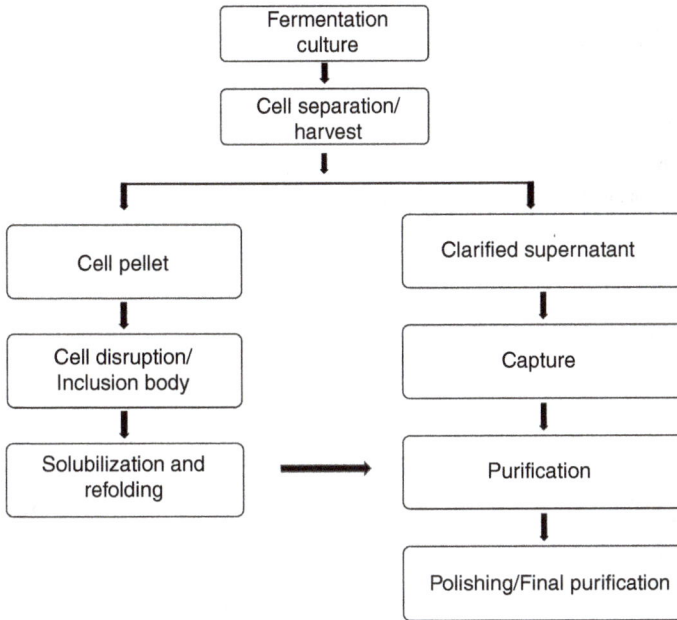

FIGURE 11.1   Overview of downstream unit operations for recombinant protein purification

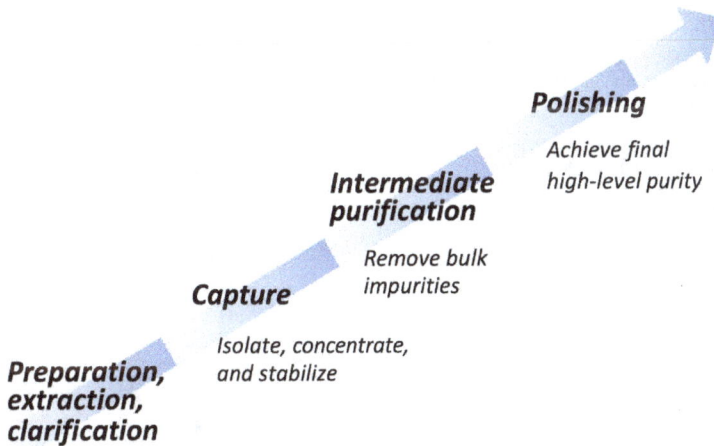

FIGURE 11.2   A three-stage purification strategy

and advanced techniques leverage the physical and chemical properties of the protein, its interactive nature, and the characteristics of product variants. Examples of protein characteristics used in various chromatography methods are illustrated in Table 11.1 and Figure 11.3.

When choosing a resin, consider qualities such as dynamic binding capacity (DBC), yield, quality, HCP removal, and purity.

Maximizing productivity and cost efficiency involves minimizing the number of processes without compromising overall yield. Conversely, downstream processing steps are critical for product protection and therefore require close monitoring. The primary aim of purification is to reduce or eliminate impurities and contaminants to levels that are safe for patient use. Impurities

TABLE 11.1
Protein Property and Applicable Chromatography Methods

Target Protein	Applicable Chromatography Purification Method
Specific ligand recognition	Affinity chromatography (AC)
Metal ion binding	Immobilized metal-affinity chromatography (IMAC)
Charge	Ion exchange chromatography (IEX)
Hydrophobicity	Hydrophobic interaction chromatography (HIC)
Size	Gel filtration (size exclusion chromatography)
Isoelectric point	Chromatofocusing

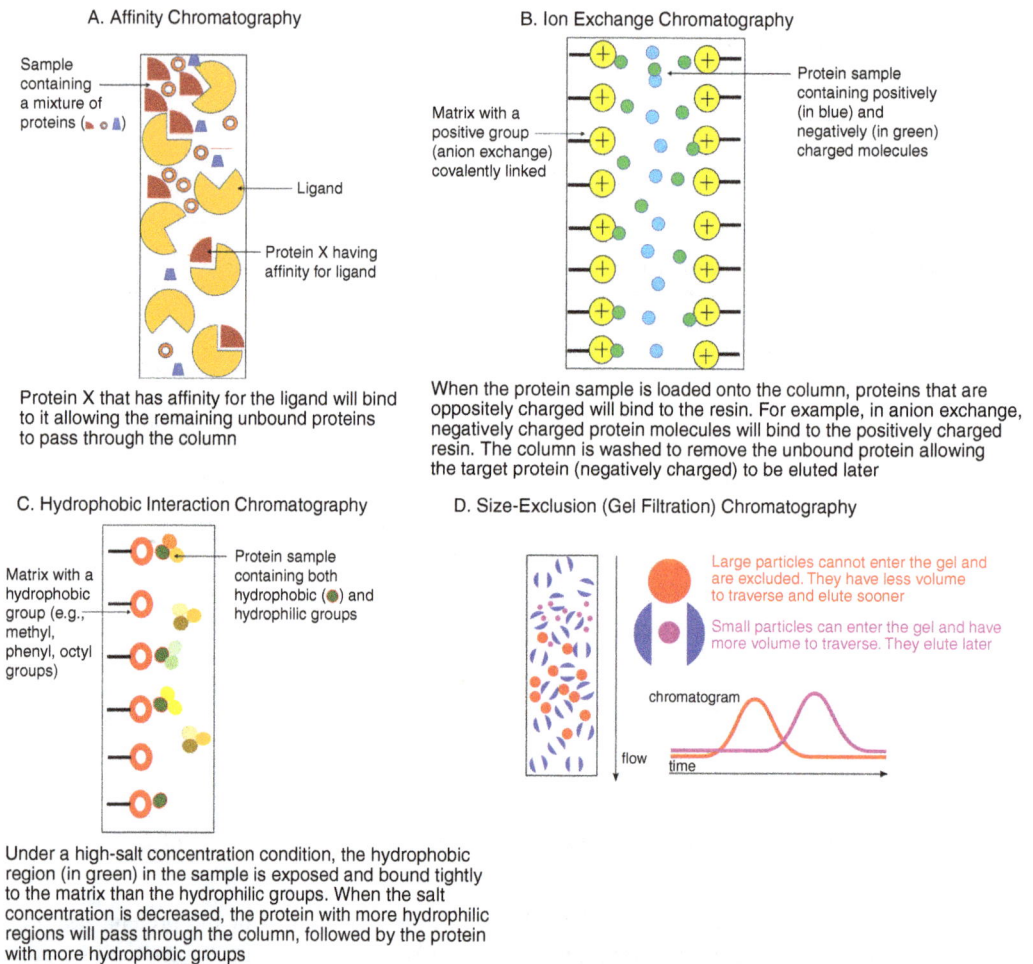

A. Affinity Chromatography

Sample containing a mixture of proteins (▲ ○ ▲)

Ligand

Protein X having affinity for ligand

Protein X that has affinity for the ligand will bind to it allowing the remaining unbound proteins to pass through the column

B. Ion Exchange Chromatography

Protein sample containing positively (in blue) and negatively (in green) charged molecules

Matrix with a positive group (anion exchange) covalently linked

When the protein sample is loaded onto the column, proteins that are oppositely charged will bind to the resin. For example, in anion exchange, negatively charged protein molecules will bind to the positively charged resin. The column is washed to remove the unbound protein allowing the target protein (negatively charged) to be eluted later

C. Hydrophobic Interaction Chromatography

Matrix with a hydrophobic group (e.g., methyl, phenyl, octyl groups)

Protein sample containing both hydrophobic (●) and hydrophilic groups

Under a high-salt concentration condition, the hydrophobic region (in green) in the sample is exposed and bound tightly to the matrix than the hydrophilic groups. When the salt concentration is decreased, the protein with more hydrophilic regions will pass through the column, followed by the protein with more hydrophobic groups

D. Size-Exclusion (Gel Filtration) Chromatography

Large particles cannot enter the gel and are excluded. They have less volume to traverse and elute sooner

Small particles can enter the gel and have more volume to traverse. They elute later

chromatogram

flow   time

FIGURE 11.3   Schematic presentation of the various chromatography methods

influencing downstream purification strategy fall into two categories: process-related and product-related impurities in biological manufacturing.

Product-related impurities in the drug substance are molecular variations that occur during manufacturing or storage, differing from the intended products in terms of function, protection, or efficacy. Structural differences in proteins can arise from the cellular mechanisms of the host organism in protein synthesis or from specific processing activities. These deviations may or may not be acceptable from a patient safety perspective. Product variants are substances with attributes (activity, safety, efficacy) comparable to the target product. Detailed characterization of the product and its variants is necessary to differentiate between contaminants and product-related chemicals.

Process-related impurities are contaminants associated with the manufacturing process, including proteins from the host cell, DNA, and raw materials (e.g., cell culture media, antibiotics, chromatographic media used for purification, and specific buffer components). Upstream process impurities may originate from the cell substrate or the cell culture, influenced respectively by the expression system and upstream process parameters that dictate whether the product is secreted into the medium or remains intracellular. Downstream process conditions and source materials also affect impurities, including chromatographic media, buffer components, and leachable components.

The primary objective of the downstream process is to diminish contaminants through a series of purification procedures to ensure the final product meets purity criteria.

Monitoring downstream unit operations involves screening the product at each stage for its purity profile, stability, and biological activity. Emphasis on characterization, stability, and overall product profile intensifies as the target molecule progresses through developmental stages, from toxicology to clinical and safety and efficacy testing. Testing commences only after finalizing the upstream and downstream processes, underscoring their pivotal role in the biopharmaceutical development timeline.

11.2   *E. COLI* SYSTEM: RECOVERY AND PURIFICATION

Recombinant protein production in *E. coli* occurs in three spaces: intracellular, periplasmic, or extracellular. However, the primary site for production is intracellular, resulting in insoluble aggregates known as inclusion bodies (IBs).

Inclusion bodies, dense protein clumps found in both the cytoplasm and periplasm, possess a higher density than cellular debris, aiding their separation during the process. Proteins within IBs remain generally stable and serve as a suitable stage for halting manufacturing operations. These bodies often contain more than 90%–95% of the protein, lessening the burden of downstream purification. Yet, the protein remains inactive and insoluble, necessitating conversion into its active, native conformation. Once achieved, the functional protein undergoes purification and concentration for final product formulation.

Steps preceding purification involve converting the insoluble protein form to its soluble, active form

- The cells must be broken to release the inclusion body.
- The inclusion body is separated from the cell detritus.
- Co-precipitated pollutants are removed by washing the inclusion body.
- The inclusion body is solubilized to denature it in preparation for refolding.
- The process of restoring a protein to its active state is known as refolding.

Recovering the inclusion body and renaturing the protein into its native state pose additional challenges in the processing stage.

Figure 11.4 depicts a typical downstream process for a recombinant protein generated as inclusion bodies in *E. coli*.

For the expression of soluble proteins in the *E. coli* cytoplasm, inclusion bodies do not form, simplifying the process to recover the desired protein. Certain cytoplasmic proteins can spontaneously fold under optimal conditions.

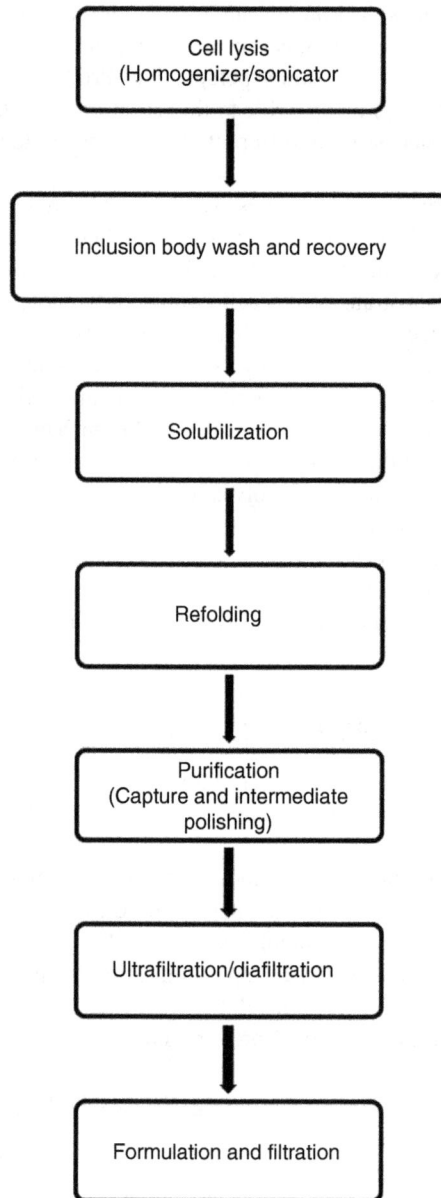

FIGURE 11.4 Flow chart for downstream processing of recombinant protein expressed in *E. coli*

Modifying the expression mechanism and appropriate vector design at the cellular level redirect intracellular protein expression from inclusion bodies to soluble cytoplasmic proteins. While soluble protein expression is an attractive option, its suitability varies among protein types. The success of this strategy relies on expressing the protein abundantly, at least exceeding 5% of the total protein, enabling maximized recoveries without additional steps (IB recovery, solubilization, and refolding).

11.2.1 CELL DISRUPTION

Cell disruption to extract inclusion bodies (recombinant protein) occurs after cell harvest during intracellular protein synthesis in *E. coli*. *E. coli*'s double cell wall consists of an outer lipopolysaccharide

(LPS) membrane, an aqueous periplasmic gap, and an inner thin peptidoglycan cell wall. The breaking of these cellular membranes for accessing the intracellular area is known as cell lysis (involving the outer LPS-rich membrane and the cytoplasmic inner membrane). Cell disruption methods include chemical, enzymatic, mechanical, or a combination thereof.

The appropriate method is determined based on the protein of interest, the technique's impact on product quality, downstream processing, and overall yield. Additionally, considering the product's characteristics (solubility, cellular location, and physical properties), batch size, operational scale, processing time, efficiency, and the protein's stability is crucial for evaluating and determining the optimal method.

11.2.1.1 Physical Methods

Various methods, such as mechanical disruption (e.g., grinding, high-pressure homogenization, and ultrasound), and non-mechanical disruption (e.g., freeze/thaw, heat treatment, and osmotic shock), are utilized to physically lyse cells.

11.2.1.1.1 Mechanical Methods

Mechanical disruption methods are preferred in industries due to their high disruption efficiency and scalability. These methods involve handheld grinders or motorized devices with rotating blades that break down cells. Common devices include the Waring blender, Polytron, hand-held grinders such as Dounce and Potter-Elvehjem homogenizers, and high-pressure homogenizers like the French press.

The Waring blender resembles a typical household blender and is primarily used for grinding. The polytron operates by drawing tissue into a long shaft with rotating blades. Both these devices excel at grinding soft, solid tissues. The Dounce homogenizer functions by pushing the sample between the tube's sides and the pestle, generating shearing forces. The Dounce homogenizer is an effective for lysing tissue culture cells, fine tissue pieces, or applications requiring only mild lysis. Conversely, the Potter-Elvehjem homogenizers grind tissues and also lyse cells. The sample is placed in the sample tube, and the pestle is rotated at a certain speed. This repeated movement of the pestle on the tube causes a shearing force that breaks the cells.

However, the most prevalent industrial device is the high-pressure homogenizer. Samples pass through a narrow space while experiencing high pressure due to piston action (e.g., 20,000 psi), causing cells to expand and rupture as they transition from high to low pressure zones. Typically, samples undergo multiple passes through this homogenizer for enhanced lysis efficiency. To reduce protein denaturation, it's advisable to cool the sample (2–8°C) during homogenization. High-pressure homogenizers offer scalability and accommodate various sample volumes (Figure 11.5).

A bead mill homogenizer is a commonly used mechanical method for disrupting *E. coli*. This method involves beads that are vigorously agitated at high speeds to break and lyse the cells. The cell suspension passes through a grinding chamber (which contains a rotating shaft) filled with beads (approximately 80%). When exposed to high speeds, the sheer force and impact from the beads cause the cells to break. The device does not use any external probes and is relatively self-contained, minimizing contamination risks.

Sonication is another mechanical disruption method used for cell lysis. This technique employs an acoustic transducer to generate pulsed high-frequency sound waves, creating microscopic bubbles that radiate through, leading to agitation and eventual cell lysis. It is useful for homogenizing small sample volumes and effectively targets bacteria and spores. However, excessive heat is typically generated from the ultrasonic treatment, so samples immersed in an ice bath are usually subjected to short bursts.

Despite being commonly used, mechanical disruption methods have challenges. These include heat generation, potential denaturation of proteins, limited selectivity, shear stress that might damage sensitive components (such as specific proteins), and the disintegration of cell debris, making the recovery process more prone to contamination.

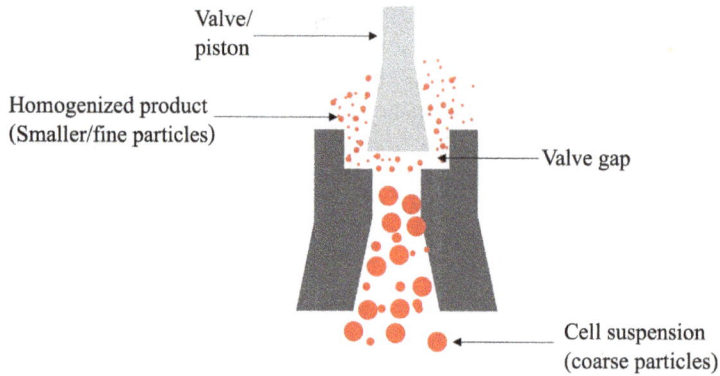

FIGURE 11.5 Schematic of the working principle of a high-pressure homogenizer

11.2.1.1.2 Nonmechanical Physical Methods

Freeze/Thaw   The freeze/thaw method involves freezing a cell suspension (using dry ice, ethanol, or a freezer) and then thawing the cells at ambient temperature or at 37°C. Ice crystals form during freezing, causing cells to expand and lyse during thawing. As a result, multiple freeze/thaw cycles are necessary for effective lysis.

Heat Shock   Thermolysis uses heat to denature membrane proteins and lyse cells at temperatures approximately 50°C for outer membranes or 90°C for cytoplasmic components.

Osmotic Shock   Cell lysis using this method involves a significant alteration in the osmolality of the cells. Initially, cells are immersed in a high osmotic pressure solution (e.g., 1 M sucrose or a high-salt solution; 1M). This is swiftly transitioned to a low concentration solution, inducing osmotic shock within the cells. Consequently, water molecules move from the low-salt concentration to the high salt concentration (into the cells), causing increased pressure within the cells and resulting in an explosion. Conversely, exposing cells first to a low concentration solution and then to a high concentration solution leads to the outflow of water from the cells, causing rupture.

11.2.1.2 Chemical Methods

In addition to mechanical and non-mechanical approaches, chemical disruption methods involving enzymes or chemical additives such as detergents are also utilized to lyse cells. These agents work by enzymatically destroying the cell wall or membrane, increasing osmotic pressure, or precipitating cell wall proteins.

Detergents function by forming micelles, binding to the lipid membrane protein, and causing the rupture of the cell membrane, enabling internal proteins and inclusion bodies to escape. Detergents vary based on physical properties and action type:

- Anionic: Sodium dodecyl sulfate (SDS) reorganizes the cell membrane by disrupting protein-protein interactions.
- Cationic: Ethyl trimethyl ammonium bromide may disrupt LPS and phospholipids in cell membranes.
- Triton X100 is a non-ionic detergent that solubilizes membrane proteins.

Solvent addition, chaotropes, and metal chelators are other chemical additives used for cell disruption. Solvent addition works by extracting the lipid components of the cell wall, increasing cell membrane permeability, and releasing intracellular proteins. Commonly used solvents include toluene, dimethyl sulfoxide, and certain alcohols. Chaotropes such as urea can solubilize membrane proteins. EDTA, a chelator, binds to metal ions Mg^{2+} and Ca^{2+} on the cells' outer membrane, increasing permeability and causing the release of intracellular components.

The use of digestive enzymes that disintegrate the cell wall is another chemical technique for lysing cells. Enzyme selection depends on the variability of cell walls and membranes among different cell types and strains. For instance, lysozyme is commonly used to break down the cell walls of gram-positive bacteria.

The chemical method is easy to implement and scalable compared to mechanical methods but requires substantial capital expenditure. However, limitations include prolonged reaction times for efficient lysis, downstream operations' burden to ensure effective chemical removal, and potential hazards posed to operators by these chemicals.

Typically, a combination of disruption methods is employed in biomanufacturing to overcome efficiency limitations. For example, using chemical detergents (Triton X-100) as a pretreatment followed by mechanical disruption (high-pressure homogenization) enhances lysis efficiency and reduces passes through the homogenizer. Similarly, chelating agents and detergents are included in buffers to suspend the cell pellet before liquid homogenization, improving efficiency compared to using a single method.

In the preparation of soluble proteins expressed in *E. coli*, cells undergo lysis, and the supernatant is cleared to eliminate cell debris, lipids, ribosomes, and other particulate materials. The cleared protein is then introduced to the appropriate chromatographic column for capture.

11.3 INCLUSION BODY RECOVERY AND SEPARATION

After cell rupture and the release of their contents, including inclusion bodies and other cellular components, recovery and separation processes are carried out. These processes are essential for separating insoluble inclusion bodies from soluble components and insoluble cell debris.

Various separation procedures based on inclusion bodies' density and solubility variations have been applied to increase yield and purity. Clarifying, purifying, and concentrating inclusion bodies before solubilization and renaturation require inclusion body recovery and separation. Methods such as centrifugation, filtration, or alternatives such as precipitation and two-phase aqueous extraction may achieve relatively pure inclusion bodies.

Centrifugation is a commonly employed technique for inclusion body recovery. Benchtop/floor and continuous centrifuges may be used depending on the operation's scale and liquid volumes. Adjusting speed and gravitational force (usually between 5,000–20,000 g) allows collection of inclusion bodies as pellets, while the less dense cell debris is removed in the supernatant, reducing the processing volume.

Microfiltration or ultrafiltration is an alternative approach for the recovery of insoluble inclusion bodies. Inclusion bodies are between 50 and 1500 nm in size, and choosing an appropriate large pore size filter (microfiltration: 0.05 μm to 5 μm, ultrafiltration: 0.001 μm to 0.1 μm) achieves a high yield of inclusion bodies. Additionally, filtration aids in enhanced purification by removing soluble impurities, DNA, and toxins released during cell disruption through the large pore size.

Microfiltration is used to remove cells and cell detritus from the cell lysate, targeting a size range of 0.2 μm to 10 μm. Ultrafiltration membranes, with pore sizes spanning from 0.001 μm to 0.1 μm, effectively eliminate larger molecules like proteins, polysaccharides, and IBs. To address impurities potentially co-precipitating with inclusion bodies, a diafiltration step employing an inclusion body wash buffer can aid in their removal. However, its practicality for large-scale operations is limited due to the substantial wash solution consumption required for efficient processing. Moreover, it's advisable to maintain a low transmembrane pressure (TMP) during cell lysate processing, with consideration for factors such as processing time, impact on product quality, membrane fouling, and performance. Essential parameters for filtration operations include membrane pore size, membrane type (hollow fiber, flat sheet), permeate flux/fouling, TMP, and cleaning.

In addition to standard centrifugation or membrane filtration, other methods like expanded bed adsorption, aqueous two-phase liquid extraction, solvent extraction, precipitation, and size exclusion chromatography offer alternative approaches for isolating and purifying inclusion bodies from cell lysate, integrating cell disruption and solubilization.

The selection of the most suitable method—centrifugation separation, membrane filtration, or a combination of cell disruption and solubilization approaches—depends on various factors, such as the protein of interest, operational scale, facility design, buffer consumption, overall production process, and desired purity levels. It is equally crucial to assess the challenges and limitations of each method to ensure reliable, robust, and economically feasible recovery and separation of inclusion bodies.

Depending on the chosen approach, integrating wash solutions might be necessary due to the highly insoluble nature of inclusion bodies, particularly to eliminate cellular impurities that co-precipitate with them. Despite the generally high purity of most inclusion bodies, optimizing wash solutions significantly enhances overall purity and streamlines operations. Enhancing purity before solubilization and refolding of inclusion bodies can lead to increased overall process yield and potentially reduce subsequent processing volumes.

For instance, recovered inclusion bodies may undergo washing with solutions containing specific components (e.g., low levels of chaotropes, detergents, salts, and pH adjustments) to effectively remove cell debris and other co-precipitated impurities. Striking a delicate balance between purity and recovery is vital when selecting chaotropes or agents that could potentially impact inclusion body solubilization and overall yield (e.g., using high concentrations of urea or guanidine-hydrochloride). Typically, centrifugation is employed to recover inclusion bodies post-washing. Finally, purified water serves as the last-step wash, removing chemical agents and debris before yielding a highly pure inclusion body pellet.

At this stage, the concentrated and pure inclusion bodies (IB) can be frozen for long-term storage (typically at $-20^{\circ}C$). This allows for flexibility in production schedules, enabling the pooling of IB pellets from multiple upstream batches for further processing and maximizing downstream operations.

11.3.1 INCLUSION BODY SOLUBILIZATION

Once the IB pellet is recovered, a crucial step is to re-solubilize it in preparation for subsequent renaturation. The aim of the solubilization process is to denature the protein and decrease the amount of aggregated protein in the inclusion body. This denaturation of the insoluble protein aggregate aims to transform it into a soluble linear polypeptide, achieved through a combination of chemical agents and specific operating conditions.

Traditionally, substantial amounts of a denaturant have been used for solubilizing inclusion bodies. Common substances include 6 M guanidine-hydrochloride (GuHCl), 8 M urea, detergents, alkaline pH (>9), organic solvents, or N-lauryl sarcosine. Gu-HCl, being a potent chaotrope, is notably more effective than urea at denaturing excessively aggregated inclusion bodies. However, urea solution containing isocyanate can lead to carbamylation of free amino groups of polypeptides, particularly when exposed to prolonged incubation under alkaline pH, impacting product quality. A challenge with high concentrations of chaotropes is the possibility of precipitation, affecting overall process yield and subsequent purification steps.

Before incorporating the chosen denaturant into the solubilization technique, it is crucial to test it with the target protein.

TABLE 11.2
Example of Solubilization DoE

Process Parameters	Start Condition	Optimization
Buffer	50 mM Tris-HCl, pH 8.0	pH (7.0, 7.5), buffer composition (e.g., EDTA)
Denaturant	8 M urea *or* 6 M Gu-HCl	Concentration of the denaturant
Inclusion body concentration (mg/mL, wet weight)	20	Testing higher and lower concentrations (e.g., 10 and 40 mg/mL)
Temperature (°C)	Ambient	4–30
Time	60 min	15 min to 2+ hours

Factors such as the presence and concentration of a reducing agent, as well as time, temperature, ionic strength, and the denaturant-to-protein ratio, significantly influence the success of solubilization for each denaturant. Table 11.2 provides the initial experimental conditions for solubilizing inclusion bodies, often followed by purification compatible with the solubilized proteins.

Numerous solubilization techniques (e.g., REFOLD database: http://pford.info/refolddb/) have been published, including the use of SDS (10%), N-lauryl sarcosine, or other detergents, and extreme pH levels as alternatives to the commonly used solubilization agents. For proteins with disulfide linkages, reducing agents like dithiothreitol (DTT), beta-mercaptoethanol, or Tris 2-carboxyethyl phosphine (TCEP) are commonly employed to decrease disulfide bonds and stabilize free cysteines.

Milder solubilization solutions with lower chaotrope concentrations have been used for some proteins. Employing mild solubilization conditions has shown to retain native-like secondary structures, potentially improving protein renaturation by denaturing the protein to an intermediate state instead of completely linear polypeptides. This approach might enhance refolding yields, but its applicability heavily depends on the protein and the produced inclusion bodies.

Solubilization significantly impacts the subsequent refolding conditions; hence, the solubilization buffer and operating conditions must align with the renaturation process. For proteins containing cysteine, isolated inclusion bodies often possess non-native intramolecular and intermolecular disulfide bonds. Incorporating reducing reagents with chaotropes can aid in reducing these bonds. The non-native disulfide bonds can likely reduce the solubility of the IBs in the absence of dithiothreitol, cysteine, or beta-mercaptoethanol. The inclusion of thiol agents is unnecessary for proteins that may already be in a reduced state. Arginine is commonly used in solubilization and/or refolding buffers to prevent protein aggregation, while EDTA may be employed to prevent oxidation of free cysteine groups exposed during denaturation and reduction.

Apart from the denaturant type and additive components, parameters such as reagent concentration, solubilization buffer-to-IB pellet ratio, reaction time, pH, and temperature must all be evaluated for optimal solubilization conditions.

11.3.2 INCLUSION BODY RENATURATION

Protein refolding begins with the solubilization of inclusion bodies (IBs) to acquire properly folded proteins. Gradual elimination of excess denaturants and reducing agents occurs, and reduced proteins are then transported to an oxidizing environment, initiating the formation of native disulfide bonds. Renaturation of the solubilized IBs is achieved through dilution, dialysis, or on-column processing. Typically, refolding is conducted at very low protein concentrations, usually approximately 10–100 g/mL, to prevent aggregation and gradually convert denatured proteins to their native, properly folded structure.

11.3.2.1   Dilution

Among refolding methods, dilution stands out as the most common due to its operational simplicity. In this method, the solubilized IB is diluted into a suitable refolding buffer. This process reduces protein and denaturant concentrations, creating an appropriate oxidative environment for disulfide bond formation. Maintaining low protein concentrations throughout the refolding process is crucial to minimize aggregation. Controlled dilution, such as pulse or drip dilution, for converting the solubilized IBs into the refolding buffer over a defined time is a preferred method (slow dilution), is preferred over rapid dilution into excessively large volumes, which can lead to increased aggregation or misfolding due to sudden environmental changes. Continuous mixing of the refolding solution and the denatured protein solution is vital to prevent aggregation. Choosing the optimal dilution that suits the processing volume without compromising protein quality is essential.

11.3.2.2   Dialysis

Dialysis serves as another standard method to reduce or eliminate solubilizing agents by allowing components to diffuse through buffer exchange. During dialysis, the solubilizing agent's concentration gradually decreases, facilitating proper protein refolding. However, dialysis is a slow and cumbersome process, especially when conducted on a large scale.

11.3.2.3   On-Column

Employing packed chromatography columns for refolding offers an appealing alternative to traditional methods. This approach encompasses various techniques:

- Denatured protein immobilization: Immobilizing denatured proteins on a matrix followed by denaturant dilution aids in refolding through non-specific or affinity interactions, spatially separating the protein. An example is affinity chromatography employing fusion tags for on-column buffer exchange and renaturation, necessitating careful optimization of refolding conditions based on protein-matrix interactions.
- SEC-based denaturant dilution capitalizes on partition coefficient differences between proteins and denaturants, preventing aggregation by limiting diffusion of different protein forms into the refolding mixture. The material eluted from the column is fractionated by size, with denatured protein adsorbed, washed to remove denaturants, and eluted in the renaturing solution via bind and elute method.
- Creating a refolding reactor involves immobilizing folding catalysts on the stationary phase of a chromatographic column.

On-column refolding boasts advantages like suppressing unspecific intermolecular interactions, achieving maximum protein concentration, and integrating purification with renaturation. However, challenges like potential precipitation, column fouling, and cleaning difficulty exist. Balancing column chromatography operations with renaturation is crucial for successful refolding.

Denaturant removal facilitates the native protein conformation. Components in the refolding buffer aid correct folding and native disulfide bond (i.e., dilution, dialysis, or on-column) formation. The time required for complete refolding varies from a few hours to days depending on the renaturation method (dilution, dialysis, or on-column). Optimizing refolding conditions significantly impacts the overall yield and efficiency of the process. During renaturation, two critical processes occur: first-order refolding and higher-order aggregation, competing for first and higher-order reactions.

There is no one-size-fits-all refolding process; a method suitable for one protein may not work for another due to various factors, including the refolding buffer, use of additives, and denaturant removal rate. The optimal protein concentration reduces aggregation while considering refolding conditions such as pH, temperature, refolding buffer volume, and processing time. Additives play a

TABLE 11.3
Advantages and Disadvantages of Common Protein Folding Methods

Refolding Techniques	Advantages/Disadvantages
Dialysis	Time-consuming (can take several days)
	Demands large buffer volumes
Dilution	Most preferred
	Slow dilution allows for control over protein aggregation; the dilution ratio is broad (ranging from tenfold to a hundred-fold)
	May demand large buffer volumes and handling capacity depending on the dilution ratio
On-column refolding	Quick, effective, and straightforward
	No volume limitations
	Unlike dilution, working with high protein concentration is possible, eliminating cumbersome equipment handling and even volume reduction steps
	The method is highly dependent on the type of proteins
Size-exclusion chromatography	Volume limitations, columns are designed to handle very small volumes
	Aggregates formed on the column may be difficult to remove
	Similar to on-column refolding, high protein concentrations can be used

crucial role in native disulfide bond formation, proper folding, aggregation inhibition, and protein stability. Achieving these goals often requires several additives to achieve these outcomes. pH and temperature significantly impact protein stability, disulfide bond formation rate, and proper folding. Gradual pH reduction or temperature changes can aid correct folding and precipitate misfolded or unnecessary proteins. Disulfide bond formation is a critical step affecting renaturation rate, influencing the overall process yield. Therefore, controlling reaction conditions is crucial to avoid rapid environmental changes that hinder stable intermediate formation before aggregation, especially when aiming for commercial-scale manufacturing.

To track refolding progress and assess the percentage of unfolded and correctly refolded protein over time, representative samples at specific intervals undergo RP-HPLC analysis. This information is particularly crucial in the early stages of process development when optimizing conditions to maximize recovery. Table 11.3 lists a comparative description of various methods of refolding.

11.3.2.4 Depth Filtration for the Clarification of Refolded Protein

After refolding, the protein is typically clarified before chromatography purification. This clarification involves depth filtration using charged depth filters, normal-flow filtration, and sometimes centrifugation to remove protein aggregates. Due to the diverse particle sizes in refolded proteins, multiple separation steps may be necessary. Combining multigrade depth filters and membrane filtration as a single operation can often address the need for multiple separations. Centrifugation, while still utilized, might not be practical, especially with large processing volumes. Minimizing product loss and obtaining a high-quality filtrate are challenges in the filtration process to maximize subsequent purification steps' efficiency and protect the column.

Cellulose depth filters are commonly used in the biopharmaceutical industry for this purpose. Their thickness and depth trap suspended particles, aided by their positive charge attracting negatively charged particles in the feed stream. Graded structures, created by coupling multiple pore size filters in series, maximize surface area and reduce fouling. The final filtrate undergoes sterile filtration before loading for chromatography. Optionally, adding a microporous membrane before the sterile filter can prevent smaller particles from blocking the final sterile filter, maintaining throughput. Monitoring pressure and filtrate turbidity during depth filtration is essential.

11.4   PURIFICATION

After clarifying the refolded protein solution, the subsequent series of unit operations are dedicated to purifying the protein, producing a highly pure product that meets specific purity requirements. Certain proteins pose challenges in purification, necessitating the use of physicochemical-based chromatography methods to optimize their yield. The selection of suitable chromatographic separation methods depends on variations in the characteristics of the target protein and other chemicals present in the sample.

11.5   CAPTURING

The most appropriate chromatographic separation methods are chosen based on the properties of the target protein and other compounds in the sample. The initial capture step is designed to bind the product to the matrix (due to charge, specific interactions, or affinity) while preventing impurities from binding, facilitating their removal during elution. Elution of the product can be achieved through a step gradient or linear elution method, resulting in a high product concentration but offering a moderate degree of purification. For instance, to prevent interactions with proteases, emphasizing high throughput and shorter processing times becomes crucial. Certain product variants may hinder product recovery and contribute to further degradation that is challenging to remove afterward.

The chromatographic process and capture step strategy may vary depending on the target molecule. For non-antibodies, oligonucleotides, and polysaccharides, ion-exchange chromatography (IEX) or hydrophobic interaction chromatography (HIC) are more commonly used. Conversely, Affinity Chromatography, such as Protein-A or Protein G, is employed to capture antibodies.

In purifying refolded proteins, ion-exchange chromatography (IEX) and, to a lesser extent, hydrophobic interaction chromatography (HIC) have proven effective as initial chromatographic stages. These methods demonstrate increased refolded protein recovery by enhancing stability, reducing aggregation, and efficiently addressing purification challenges associated with both process and product-related contaminants. These methods, employing linear gradient elution for separation, are utilized in purifying refolded proteins. Soluble proteins, expressed in the *E. coli* expression system, are directly loaded onto the chromatography column to separate the target protein from other cellular contaminants. This step occurs subsequent to recovering the proteins through cell disruption and clarification, aiming to remove nucleic acids and lipopolysaccharides, as well as host cell proteins.

Affinity chromatography, primarily used for monoclonal antibody (mAb) purification, is also being explored for the large-scale purification of various recombinant proteins (e.g., recombinant insulin, plasminogen, GCSF, IFN-alpha, Follicle Stimulating Hormone). The key requirements for this capture step are a high degree of recovery, product stability, and the ability to process high capacity.

11.6   INTERMEDIATE PURIFICATION

Following the capture step, high-resolution methods such as hydrophobic-interaction chromatography (both anion and cation exchange), size-exclusion chromatography, and reversed-phase chromatography are employed to remove most impurities like host-cell proteins, nucleic acids, and endotoxins. It's uncommon to use an anion exchange (AEX) as a capture stage followed by cation exchange (CEX) chromatography or vice versa. These choices heavily rely on the target proteins and the impurity profile.

Lower flow rates, gradient elution, and matrices with smaller particles are used to enhance resolution. Typically, the purity of the final product after these stages reaches nearly 99%.

Throughout the chromatography process, there's an inevitable loss of some product at each purification step. Hence, there's a constant drive to minimize the number of purification steps in biomanufacturing processes. Reducing steps not only enhances processing speed but also improves the yield of unstable proteins. After the capture step, an evaluation of the product quality, purity, impurity profile, and objectives of intermediate and final purification steps determines the necessity of an intermediate purification step. Some processes might skip an intermediate purification step, favoring a polishing step to economize biomanufacturing operations.

11.6.1 POLISHING

The polishing phase in purification aims to eliminate traces of aggregates (both low and high molecular weight proteins), degradation products, or other product variants. Previous purification processes have significantly reduced product-related contaminants. This phase prepares the purified product for formulation or storage as an intermediate product. Size-exclusion chromatography and reversed-phase chromatography serve as two polishing procedures for achieving the ultimate product purity.

Occasionally, desalting and buffer exchange are necessary to modify the purified protein composition. Size exclusion chromatography effectively accomplishes this by allowing the removal of low and high molecular weight contaminants while enabling the transfer of the protein into the desired buffer. This facilitates final adjustments to the conditions of the purified protein for storage.

Purification steps may or may not occur sequentially, and sometimes various intermediate processing steps, such as product concentration by tangential flow filtration (TFF), salt precipitation, or desalting, might be integrated between chromatography steps. Desalting is commonly performed when there's a modification in buffer components, either before ion exchange to remove salt and enable the protein sample to bind to the column, after purification to eliminate low molecular weight contaminants, or after purification for the final pure protein.

A generalized downstream process scheme for soluble proteins is depicted in Figure 11.6.

Figure 11.7 illustrates both a three-step and a two-step purification scheme for a protein expressed as inclusion bodies (IBs).

Following the purification process, the concentrated purified protein primarily undergoes TFF to produce the drug substance (either lyophilized or in a sterile solution) before storage for subsequent processing into a drug product.

11.7 MAMMALIAN SYSTEM PURIFICATION

In mammalian cell-based protein production, the product is typically secreted into the culture medium. Consequently, the initial step in product recovery involves separating the cells from the culture medium through depth filtration, centrifugation, or alternative separation methods (Chapter 5). Because the protein is secreted into the media, unlike in *E. coli*, the separation process is less extensive.

The clarified harvest undergoes purification and concentration steps to attain the desired product, meeting specified purity and safety targets. Understanding the protein's properties and its contaminants is crucial in devising the purification strategy. Additionally, proteins produced in a mammalian system may carry a risk of viral contamination. Thus, downstream operations must include steps targeting viral inactivation and removal.

Figure 11.8 outlines a general process for mAb purification. mAbs share a common feature through the Fc region, enabling the development of a platform process. Structurally, mAbs exhibit a symmetrical configuration consisting of identical heavy and light chains linked via disulfide bridges.

A three-phase purification strategy, akin to purifying the refolded protein, can be employed for the clarified harvest (CHO process).

- Capture: Isolate and concentrate the product.
- Intermediate Purification: Remove most bulk impurities (e.g., host cell proteins, nucleic acids, DNA, endotoxin, and viruses).

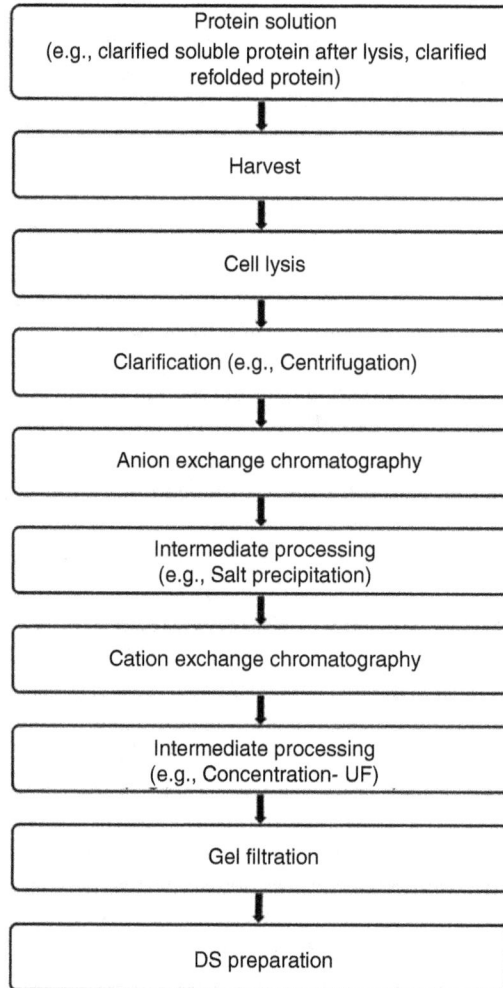

FIGURE 11.6 Scheme for purification of a soluble protein expressed in *E. coli* (three-step purification strategy)

- Polishing: Achieve high purity by eliminating trace impurities and other product-related substances/impurities.

Chromatography methods are chosen and optimized to fit into the purification strategy, aiming to achieve the desired outcomes. The number of steps employed varies depending on protein properties, target purity criteria, yield, impurity identity, and intended use.

Beginning with Protein-A chromatography followed by a series of ion-exchange chromatography steps, most operations are executed in a bind and elute mode, except for anion exchange chromatography, which operates in a flow-through mode for the desired protein.

11.8 CAPTURE–PROTEIN-A CHROMATOGRAPHY

The capture step (e.g., IEX, Affinity Chromatography) designed to isolate and concentrate the product should also effectively remove critical contaminants. Typically, this step substantially increases product concentration and purity, particularly if a highly selective affinity medium is

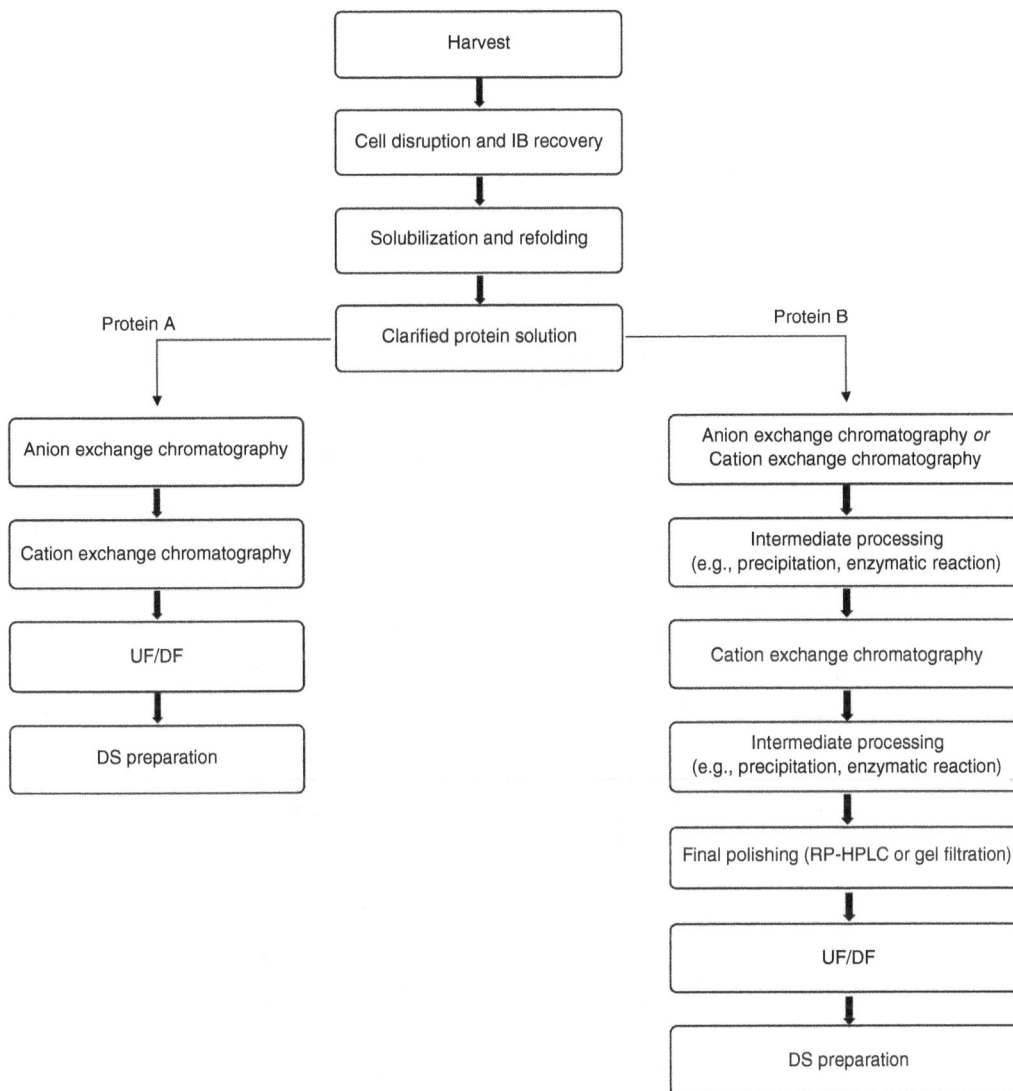

FIGURE 11.7 Multistep purification schemes for expressed proteins

utilized. Other capture methods, such as crystallization and precipitation, are viable but entail additional processing steps (e.g., solid-liquid separation) and are not as successful on an industrial scale.

The primary capture for mAbs from the clarified harvest begins with affinity chromatography, frequently utilizing Protein-A chromatography. The consistent Fc-portion among mAbs, which is the targeted binding region for Protein-A, has made it the predominant choice in downstream purification for capture.

Protein-A chromatography involves antibodies binding to an immobilized protein-A ligand in a specific and reversible manner. Protein-A, a 56-kDa surface protein found in Staphylococcus aureus, possesses five binding domains that can bind to the Fc region of immunoglobulin G (IgG). Both native and recombinant forms of Protein-A are utilized as ligands in Protein-A resins. The ligand, typically coupled to a matrix such as cross-linked agarose (e.g., Sepharose®), exhibits high capacity, capable of binding at least two antibody molecules per single coupled Protein-A molecule.

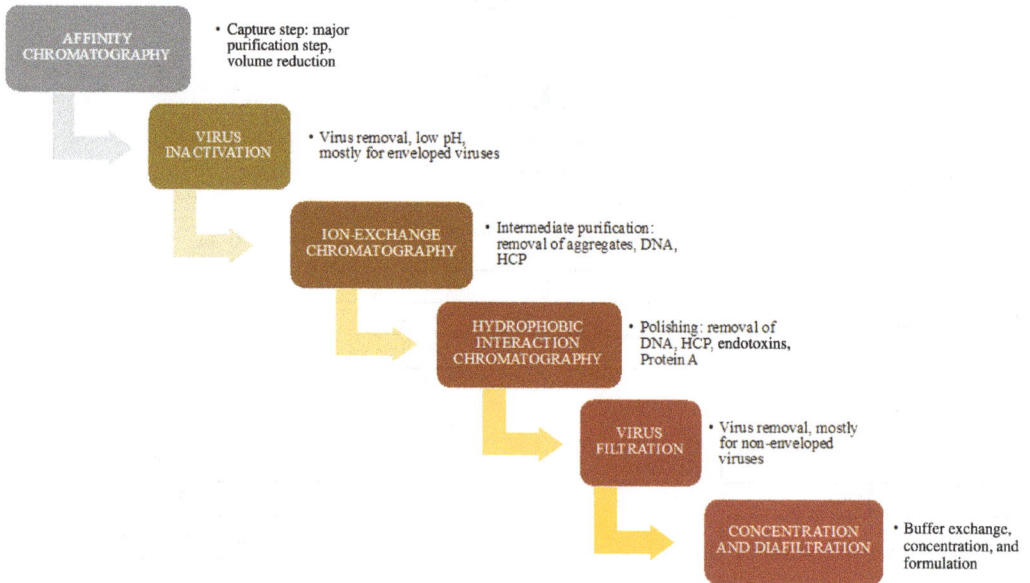

FIGURE 11.8   Overview of a mAb purification process

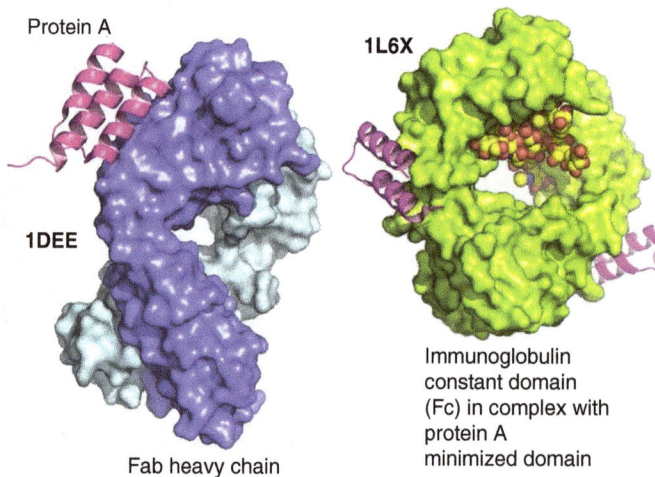

FIGURE 11.9   Protein-A, and it is binding to an immunoglobulin

Source: E A S–Own work, Creative Commons Attribution

Recombinant Protein-A, engineered for enhanced binding capacity, displays robustness and high capacity due to modifications to the ligand, including single domain multimers/single point coupling and multi-point attachment. These alterations offer additional benefits, such as chemical and thermal stability, enabling Protein-A to withstand a wide pH range of 2–11 and resist denaturing and chaotropic agents (e.g., urea, Gu-HCl). Figure 11.9 illustrates the structure of Protein-A and its protein-binding mechanism.

Three major varieties of Protein-A resins are available commercially, based on matrix composition.

- Agarose Based: e.g., Protein-A-Sepharose® Fast Flow, MabSelect (Cytiva).
- Glass or silica-based: e.g., ProSep vA and ProSep vA Ultra (Millipore).

- Organic Polymer-based: e.g., polystyrene-divinylbenzene POROS A™ and MabCapture™ (Applied Biosystems).

These resins are accessible for both laboratory-scale and commercial-scale processes, ranging from less than 1 cm to 2 m column diameter. They exhibit resistance to high concentrations of Gu-HCl, urea, reducing agents, and low pH.

Protein-A also demonstrates an affinity for specific variants of the Fab region, which proves beneficial for purifying Fab fragments. While Protein-A remains the most widely utilized purification system for human and humanized mAbs, certain antibodies may not strongly bind or bind at all to the Protein-A ligand. This selectivity, however, can be advantageous in specific cases.

An alternative to Protein-A is Protein G, an immunoglobulin binding protein found in group G of streptococcal bacteria. It differs from Protein-A in its binding specificities. Depending on the IgG being purified, either of these alternatives can be effectively employed in the capture step. Some key features of these two ligands include:

Protein-A: It displays broad species reactivity, binding well to IgG from various species including humans, rabbits, mice, and cows.

Protein G: Exhibits stronger binding to IgG from mouse rats. The binding site to albumin, present in the native protein G, has been eliminated in the recombinant form.

Protein-A might serve as a better option for segregating certain IgG subtypes and other classes of antibodies, as well as for eliminating other antibodies, such as cross-species IgG contamination from horse or fetal calf serum. When combined with agarose beads, some binding affinities alter; for instance, rat IgG does not bind to Protein-A but binds to Protein-A-Sepharose (Table 11.4).

TABLE 11.4
Antibody Subtypes and Recommended Purification Media

Species	Antibody Subtype	Protein-A Binding	Protein-G Binding
Human	IgG	Strong	Strong
	IgG1	Strong	Strong
	IgG2	Strong	Strong
	IgG3	Weak	Strong
	IgG4	Strong	Strong
	IgA1	Weak	None
	IgA2	Weak	None
	Fab	Weak	Weak
	scFv	Weak	None
Mouse	IgG	Strong	Strong
	IgG1	Weak	Medium
	IgG2a	Strong	Strong
	IgG2b	Strong	Strong
	IgG3	Strong	Strong
Rat	IgG	Weak	Medium
	IgG1	Weak	Medium
	IgG2a	None	Strong
	IgG2b	None	Weak
	IgG2c	Strong	Strong

Source: Adapted from Abcam

Chromatography commonly employs affinity gravity flow or a low/medium-pressure system. The binding capacity is determined by both binding strength and flow rate. Consideration should be given to ligand leakage, with Protein-A point attachment to Sepharose showing minimal leakage under various elution settings. These ligand contaminants are eliminated during the polishing using SEC. Affinity chromatography, as an initial capture step, offers several performance attributes that streamline the process development for new molecules, such as robustness to solution conditions for loading and washing.

In large-scale mAb manufacturing, Protein-A-Sepharose (Cytiva) stands as the most frequently used capture step. Its binding ability surpasses that of protein G Sepharose. Additionally, Cytiva's high-performance medium yields high resolution along with sharp and concentrated peak elution. Table 11.5 presents an example of commercially available Protein-A chromatography medium. Evaluation of each resin for protein A leachability is essential.

Furthermore, the formation of protein aggregates should be considered as a selection factor. Protein A resins exhibit a dynamic binding capacity of 15–100 g mAb/L resin, which varies depending on the mAb type, adsorbent, and flow velocity (Table 11.5).

The suggested typical binding and elution conditions for this media are outlined in Table 11.6. To optimize the performance of Protein-A chromatography, it is crucial to fine-tune certain process variables. This includes optimizing binding conditions, such as buffer composition and pH, to ensure efficient binding. It also involves considering washing conditions, including the ideal composition of the column wash solution, as excessive washing steps can potentially weaken ligand binding and decrease yield. Equally important are the elution conditions, as any variations in these parameters can impact Protein-A's affinity, purity, and impurity levels (Table 11.6).

Protein-A chromatography is a widely favored method for capturing recombinant mAbs due to its resilience. Depending on the intended function of the target protein, such as for diagnostic

---

TABLE 11.5
Purification Options for mAbs and Fc Fusion Proteins Using Commercial Protein-A Chromatography Media

Protein-A Chromatography Media	Features
MabSelect PrismA	Optimal productivity, cleaning, sanitization, bioburden control, alkaline stability, continuous and batch processes, long resin life, easy cleaning, suitable for small-scale purification and screening, prepacked columns suitable for large-scale commercial manufacturing
MabSelect SuRe LX MabSelect SuRe	Higher ligand density, good performance, long resin life, easy cleaning, prepacked columns suitable for large-scale commercial manufacturing
MabSelect SuRe pcc	Continuous processes, long resin life, easy cleaning, prepacked large scale columns suitable for commercial manufacturing, suitable for small-scale purification and screening
MabSelect	Low-to-medium titers, limited number of cycles, suitable for small-scale purification and screening, prepacked columns suitable for large-scale commercial manufacturing
MabSelect Xtra	High titer, higher ligand density, limited number of cycles, suitable for small-scale purification and screening, prepacked columns suitable for large-scale commercial manufacturing
TOYOPEARL AF-rProtein-A HC-650M	IgG binding ability of >65 g IgG/L resin
ProSep Ultra Plus	Large scale, cost-effective, suitable for high titer, increased capacity, and productivity, process flexibility, prepacked, ready-to-use, and disposable columns, high throughput, not suitable for cleaning with sodium hydroxide
Poros MabCaptureA	Highest dynamic binding capacity, process flexibility (shorter bed height, faster flow rate)

TABLE 11.6
Binding and Elution Conditions Commonly Used With Protein-A Sepharose®
Chromatography Purify IgG From Different Species

Species	Subclass	Protein-A Binding pH	Protein-A Elution pH
Human	IgG_1	6.0–7.0	3.5–4.5
	IgG_2	6.0–7.0	3.5–4.5
	IgG_3	8.0–9.0	≤7.0
	IgG_4	7.0–8.0	3.0–6.0
Mouse	IgG_1	8.0–9.0	4.5–6.0
	IgG_{2a}	7.0–8.0	3.5–5.5
	IgG_{2b}	~7.0	3.0–4.0
	IgG_3	~7.0	3.5–5.5
Rat	IgG_1	≥9.0	7.0–8.0
	IgG_{2a}	≥9.0	≤8.0
	IgG_{2b}	≥9.0	≤8.0
	IgG_3	8.0 to 9.0	3.0–4.0 (using 3 M potassium isothiocyanate)

Source: Adapted from Affinity Chromatography Vol 1: Antibodies, Cytiva LifeSciences (Formerly GE Healthcare)

purposes, purification using only Protein-A chromatography may suffice. During this stage, process-related contaminants such as host DNA, HCP, and viruses are significantly removed.

Despite the widespread use of Protein-A chromatography, it does have certain limitations. The high cost of the resin, the procedures required for its repeated use that could potentially lead to cross-contamination, and the impact of caustic cleaning solutions like 0.1 N NaOH on the resin's performance are notable disadvantages. Another concern is the non-specific binding of impurities, such as host cell proteins, DNA, and other cell culture-derived impurities. Consequently, research is underway to explore alternatives, such as ion exchange and other methods, to overcome these limitations associated with Protein-A chromatography. Expanded-bed chromatography is also being considered as a beneficial method for binding proteins from crude cell culture media.

11.9 INTERMEDIATE PURIFICATION AND FINAL POLISHING

The intermediate purification step aims to separate the target protein from contaminants like other proteins, viruses, endotoxins, and DNA. The specifics of this step, including resolution and specifications, heavily rely on the properties of the Protein-A eluate sample and the final product specifications that need to be met. If the protein purity achieved from the capture step is high, the intermediate step might be unnecessary, and the process can proceed to one or more polishing steps to further enhance the final product's purity. High resolution in separating the sample's protein components is expected during the final polishing. Therefore, the binding capacity, resolution, and selectivity for the intermediate purification step are critical, especially if the capture step product had lower purity, as a significant number of impurities may still be present. Eluting the target protein might involve using a continuous gradient or a multi-step elution method.

11.10 POLISHING

The binding of impurities, such as host cell proteins, DNA, and other cell culture-derived impurities, in chromatography is non-specific. For instance, if the target protein has a neutral to basic pI, the flow-through mode would be suitable to eliminate contaminants. In contrast, the chosen conditions would cause acidic impurities to not bind to the column. The "bind and elute" modes are preferable for a target protein with a pI ranging from acidic to below the neutral range. The target protein is eluted first under high salt concentration conditions, leaving most impurities bound to the column.

In CEX or AEX, optimizing the resin, loading conditions, impurity profile, amount of product loaded, charge variant profile, and chromatography conditions is necessary to maximize efficiency and recovery. The primary variables for this step commonly include column loading, wash, and elution buffer compositions.

The impurity profile and the target protein determine the use of hydrophobic interaction chromatography, mixed-mode chromatography, and occasionally ceramic hydroxyapatite, alongside ion-exchange chromatography.

Hydrophobic interaction chromatography serves as a polishing step post-IEX or as an intermediate step after Protein-A purification. In its flow-through mode, HIC effectively eliminates numerous aggregates, ensuring a high yield. It offers excellent resolution and separation of process and product-related contaminants in both bind and elute modes.

Multimodal chromatography uses a resin combining different interaction types to separate the target protein and impurities, such as ion exchange, hydrophobic, and hydrogen bonding. These resins offer different selectivity from standard single-mode chromatography resins, making them suitable for various conditions such as high and low conductivity or pH. Examples of commercially available multimode resins include Capto MMC and Capto Adhere (Cytiva). The multimode chromatography method effectively removes aggregates, host cell protein, and leached Protein-A.

Ceramic hydroxyapatite (CHT) is utilized for its unique separation capabilities, unprecedented selectivity, and resolution in efficiently removing nucleic acids, viruses, macromolecules, and other proteins. CHT serves as a polishing step in large-scale mAb purification, effectively eliminating dimers, aggregates, and leached Protein-A using a gradient elution method.

Polishing steps are crucial to ensure the removal of adventitious and endogenous viruses. Overall, the purification strategy should streamline process development efforts, ensuring the achievement of product quality attributes, reducing production costs to make the process economically viable, and minimizing downstream processing complexities.

11.11 VIRAL REMOVAL, INACTIVATION, AND FILTRATION

The end product must be completely free from any contamination, including bacteria, mycoplasma, and viruses. Mammalian cells are known to naturally produce virus-like particles, which present a significant safety risk. Monoclonal antibodies (mAbs) derived from mammalian cell systems must adhere to strict viral safety specifications due to the potential for contamination from both enveloped and non-enveloped viruses. This process includes characterizing the host cell line, scrutinizing all raw materials for potential adventitious agents—especially those sourced from animals—and conducting tests at various production stages as well as on the finished product. A crucial aspect involves demonstrating through viral clearance that the manufacturing process can effectively handle and eliminate viruses.

According to current regulations, therapeutic products derived from mammalian cells must contain fewer than one virus particle per million doses for safety. This requirement translates to approximately 12–18 log10 clearance for endogenous retroviruses and six log10 clearance for adventitious viruses. Consequently, strategies to remove viruses are integrated into the production process, especially during purification steps. Moreover, multiple virus clearance measures are employed in mAb processes to ensure that viruses are eliminated by at least one mechanism if not by others.

Virus removal or inactivation is achieved by subjecting the solution containing the target protein to conditions that denature virus proteins without affecting the active ingredient. Common methods employed include low pH inactivation, detergents, viral filters, heat treatment, irradiation, and chromatography.

11.11.1 pH Treatment

Treating Protein-A eluate at low pH effectively targets enveloped viruses. Typically, incubating the protein solution at a low pH (approximately 3.0–3.5) for at least an hour has been a common practice in mAb processes. Additionally, high pH treatments, such as using sodium hydroxide for cleaning chromatography columns, have proven effective against both enveloped and non-enveloped viruses. Exposure to extreme pH conditions can significantly reduce the virus count (approximately > 4.0 log10).

11.11.2 Virus Filtration

Virus filtration relies on a size-based approach for viral clearance, often used in conjunction with pH treatment in mAb processes. Virus filters, available as ultrafilters or microfilters with very small pores, are primarily composed of polyethersulfone (PES), polyvinylidene (PVDF), and cellulose. They are categorized as retrovirus and parvovirus filters based on size distribution. Table 11.7

TABLE 11.7
Commercially Available Virus Filters

Company	Product	Material	Virus	Log Reduction Value Claimed by the Manufacturer	Virus Size (nm)
Asahi-Kasei	Planova 15N	Cuprammonium regenerated cellulose	Hepatitis A virus (HAV)	>6.7	27–32
			Parvovirus B19	>6.1	18–26
			Plum pox virus (PPV)	>4.6	18–24
	Planova 20N	Cuprammonium regenerated cellulose	Parvovirus B19	>4.9	18–26
			Plum pox virus (PPV)	>4.0	18–24
			Xenotropic murine leukemia virus (XMuLV)	>3.1	80–110
	Planova 35N	Cuprammonium regenerated cellulose	HIV	>7.3	80–120
			Plum pox virus (PPV)	< 1.0	18–24
			SV40	>7.8	40–50
	Planova BioEX	Hydrophilized PVDF	Mouse minute virus (MVM)	>4.8	18–24
			Amphotropic murine leukemia virus (A-MuLV)	>5.2	80–130
			Plum pox virus (PPV)	>5.3	18–24
Millipore	Viresolve NFR with retropore membrane	PES	Retrovirus	>6	80–130
	Viresolve Pro (Viresolve Pro device, Viresolve Pro Shield prefilters)	PES	Minute virus of mice (MVM)	≥4.0 log	18–24
			Parvovirus	≥4.0	18–26
			Xenotropic murine leukemia virus (XMuLV)	≥5.0	80–110
Pall	Pegasus Prime	PES	Parvovirus	>4	18–26
Sartorius	Virosart® CPV	PES	PPV, MVM	>4	18–24
			MuLV	>6 log	80–130
	Virosart® HF	PES	Small non-enveloped virus (e.g., MVM, vesivirus, parvoviruses)	>4	18–30
			Large enveloped viruses such as MuLV	>6	80–130

summarizes some commercially available viral filters, outlining the most prevalent viruses, though it is not exhaustive, and other potential contaminants may exist.

Filter fouling, caused by aggregates, debris, and DNA, is a common issue impacting the performance of virus filters. Prefilters, such as the negatively charged Pall Mustang S used before the Viresolve Pro virus filter, help prevent this. Controlling the membrane permeability of viral filters within a specific range is crucial for the filtration process. However, throughput can vary between lots due to variability in the protein solution's viral filter burden. Thus, evaluating filters for large-scale manufacturing requires testing their performance using a worst-case protein feed sample.

Ensuring the integrity of virus filters is crucial pre and post-use. These integrity tests confirm the filter's performance, check for defects or damage, verify compliance with manufacturer specifications, validate correct installation, and importantly, conduct end-user virus retention studies. Non-destructive tests such as bubble point, forward flow, water intrusion, and binary gas tests are commonly used. If the post-use filter integrity test fails, the filtration process is repeated. Filter suppliers usually collaborate with drug manufacturers to meet these requirements.

11.11.3 OTHER METHODS

11.11.3.1 Chromatography

Chromatography methods used in mAb purification can efficiently separate enveloped and non-enveloped viruses from the target protein. For instance, affinity chromatography is an example. However, its effectiveness as a complementary method depends on purification conditions and virus properties. Evaluations are necessary to assess chromatography's capability in consistently clearing viruses.

11.11.3.2 Detergent

This method is mainly used in manufacturing blood products. Sodium cholate and Tri (n-butyl) phosphate (TNBP) effectively treat plasma-derived products to deactivate enveloped viruses. Detergent treatment deactivates the virus by dissolving its lipid membrane, preventing it from binding to or infecting cells. However, detergents cannot be used against non-enveloped viruses.

11.11.3.3 Heat Treatment

This method is employed for virus removal in both human plasma-derived and animal-derived products. Wet and dry heat treatments alter the viral protein structure, rendering the virus inactive. Heat treatment is effective against both enveloped and non-enveloped viruses. Yet, non-enveloped viruses require extremely high temperatures for effective inactivation. This could potentially impact the target protein's functionality or denature it, raising concerns.

11.11.3.4 Ultraviolet Irradiation

Gamma irradiation is utilized for animal-derived raw materials. Viruses such as reovirus and CVV have been made non-functional using this method. Precise control of operational parameters is crucial for consistency, effectiveness, and reproducibility. Low-dose UV-C radiation (254 nm) can destroy viral nucleic acid for ultraviolet-based treatment, without affecting the target protein. Some resistant strains of parvovirus have shown increased vulnerability to inactivation using UV-C.

11.12 VIRUS REMOVAL VALIDATION

Regardless of the virus removal method chosen, focus on robustness, reliability, and consistent effectiveness in eliminating the virus is crucial. A risk-based approach might require multiple inactivation or removal methods in the manufacturing process to effectively eliminate both enveloped and non-enveloped viruses. Routine virus validation studies, utilizing model viruses reflecting actual process conditions, are necessary to meet regulatory expectations.

The FDA Guidance "Viral safety evaluation of biotechnology products derived from cell lines of human or animal origin," from 1997, states the following: "Confidence that the infectious virus is absent from the final product will result in many instances are not derived solely from direct testing for their presence, but also from the demonstration that the purification regimen is capable of removing and inactivating the viruses."

The virus protection evaluation procedure includes selecting virus-free cell lines, examining unprocessed bulk, assessing the downstream process's ability to eliminate viruses, and ultimately testing the product to confirm the absence of contaminating viruses.

Validating virus removal throughout downstream processing involves examining cell substrates, raw materials, virus inactivation/removal, and final product testing. Concerns arise with retrovirus or adventitious viral contamination, despite no virus infectivity or reverse transcriptase activity in the master cell bank (MCB) or working cell bank (WCB). Electron microscopy can detect virus-like particles (VLPs). Microscopic examination does not determine the biological relevance of suspicious particles, particularly their infectivity, such as the presence of vast numbers of A-type particles in hybridoma cells, where infectivity is extremely low or non-existent. Despite the discrepancy between the number of virus-like particles and their infectivity, the total reduction factor is often used to calculate the particle number.

It is challenging to dismiss the possibility of an unknown virus with unknown and potentially hazardous physiological implications. Viral contamination complicates the development of specific assays. Without an accurate and responsive assay, monitoring the virus's presence, removal, or inactivation in the protein drug's downstream phase is difficult. Preventive measures include extensive testing of producer cells for specific viruses and testing for adventitious viruses at various fermentation stages.

Therefore, there is a significant emphasis on validating viral clearance steps, often facilitated by a virus challenge or spiking study. This study involves adding viruses to the product at known titers and monitoring them throughout each step of the process using an infectivity assay.

Viral clearance/titer decrease (expressed as log10) is typically calculated at various stages, if not all, of the process. The study of viral clearance or inactivation necessitates the use of identical viruses from the same genus or family as the known or suspected virus, or non-specific viruses closely related to them. The procedure assesses the overall level of viral reduction achieved during operations involving known viruses. Assuming intentional virus insertion into the unit operation application sample shows adequate clearance at specific steps, any downstream unit operation should not be tested under such circumstances. Due to the complexities involved in viral clearance research, focus is placed on a few efficient unit procedures for virus elimination. One-log reduction factors generally do not significantly impact the overall clearance factor, typically 2–3 in a downstream process. While determining excess clearance (clearance minus risk) can be challenging, it should be a critical aspect of any effort to mitigate viral infection risk.

Experiments involving virus spiking should be avoided in cGMP facilities, except in large-scale production, where it's an exception. To prevent potential virus burden at the polishing stage, virus validation experiments should be conducted in small-scale trials using scalable equipment, especially during capture and intermediate phases. Steps likely to clear the virus should be individually considered when there is enough virus for informed conclusions. Confirmation of cleaning in place and the efficiency of frequently used chromatographic columns and filter systems is essential. Fractional factorial designs are ideal for investigations, as downscale factors of 100–1000 can be achieved.

Virus clearance tests are typically conducted twice during the process and product lifecycle. The first is linked to the production of clinical phase I material, demonstrating the eradication of at least two separate viruses. The second involves the eradication of four different viruses during the manufacturing of phase III material. Xenotropic murine leukemia virus (XMuLV), minute virus of mice (MVM), Simian virus 40 (SV40), and pseudorabies virus (PRV) are commonly used as the four virus models due to their representation of various traits reflective of potential adventitious agents.

Validation model viruses must be comparable or identical to suspected viruses in the cell line or closely related to viruses that could infect the cell, such as retroviruses for recombinant or hybridoma cells. To achieve the ideal reduction factor for viruses, the model virus should be produced at high titers and easily detectable with a responsive test. Caution is advised when concentrating a virus solution to improve volumetric titer, as viral particle aggregation can lead to increased but negligible mechanical removal via filtration or decreased inactivation due to viral particle defense at the aggregate's center. Model viruses used as sources of infection include SV40, human poliovirus 1, animal parvovirus, parainfluenza virus or influenza virus, Sindbis virus, RNA viruses, and murine retroviruses.

In cases involving mammalian cell culture or biological materials, virus clearance is achieved through downstream processing, validated similarly to sterility testing for bacterial contamination. Spiking experiments for appropriate unit processes are used to assess the impact of viral clearance. To ensure balanced virus distribution for individual intermediates, the virus titer of the load is compared to the (residual) virus titer of the product-containing fraction after processing, such as the flow-through or eluate of a chromatographic process or the permeate of a filtration process.

In most cases, virus inactivation occurs in a two-step procedure (fast phase 1 and slow phase 2). Samples taken at various time intervals, with at least one time point less than the minimum exposure time, are used to construct an inactivation curve. Quantitative infectivity assays should be sensitive, reproducible, and conducted with enough repetitions to ensure statistical validity. Assays detecting viral contamination often yield highly variable findings due to the biological nature of the test techniques, necessitating extensive validation of assay accuracy, reproducibility, repeatability, linearity, limit of quantitation, and detection limit. Objective statistical assessment is essential, as emphasized in FDA's "Points to Consider," EMEA's "Notes for Guidance," ICH Guidelines, and other sources. Plaque formation and cytopathic assays are the two most common in vitro assay methodologies in quantitative virus clearance research, both validated and routinely used for determining viral titers. Q5A, the fourth phase of the ICH Harmonised Tripartite Guideline, provides deeper insights into tests.

Before titrating process samples, it's crucial to explore how buffer solutions might interact with detector cells or diminish the infectivity of the model virus. Various detector cells for virus titration, such as SC-1 cells (Retrovirus), CV-1 cells (SV 40), L 929 cells (Reovirus), and Vero cells (PI3), are employed. The XC plaque assay is capable of detecting retroviruses over an extended period. The procedure involves inoculating SC-1 cells with the sample, UV-irradiating the cell layer, and overlaying it with XC cells after a specific cultivation period. Once plaques form on the cell layer, they are counted. Retrovirus-infected cell monolayer structure determines the titer in plaque or concentrates forming units (pfu/FFU). For viruses causing cytopathic effects (CPE) without plaques or foci, the titer is expressed as TCID50 (tissue culture infectious dose for 50 percent of the total cell number). Maintaining virus distribution across the process cycle, including washing and regeneration phases of chromatography or filtration retentate, is improbable due to virus denaturation by commonly used caustic solutions or capture within the filter membrane matrix. Approved virus titers typically range of 10^7 to 10^9 mL^{-1} but are reduced by 1 log due to a required 1:10–20 spike for validation experiments. Titration of all process fluids is technically challenging due to limitations set by detection cell volumes, commonly using 0.1–1.0 mL for titration.

Unit activity reduction factor computation involves process fluid volumes and viral titers before and after processing. The reduction factor, expressed in log 10 units, consists of "individual reduction factors" (Ri) for each operation. The combined specific reduction factors during purification generate the overall virus reduction factor. Virus clearance accumulation is only valid for steps with diverse physicochemical measures. A logarithmic reduction factor in the order of 1, indicating a

90% titer reduction, is considered insignificant in virus clearance due to assay variability. Electron microscopy quantifies viral particles in cell culture fluid, yet represents a challenge regarding sample representativeness in various fermentation sizes.

Cells in culture, at densities of 10^6 to 10^7 cells per milliliter, reduce EM-analyzed cells to approximately 10^3/mL after several logarithmic reductions. Identifying virus particles amid particulate matter from the preparation process requires expertise. Sample preparation methods, like high-speed centrifugation, often yield complex aggregates, obscuring virus identification.

Risk assessment for validating a purification process involves evaluating multiple factors on a case-by-case basis, including cell substrate, virus nature, culture methods, target protein, process design, intended product use, patient population, and administration dosage/frequency.

Although outsourcing viral clearance validation to specialized labs is common, replicating certain viral setups in a manufacturing facility might pose challenges due to time, cost, or resource constraints.

11.13   PRODUCT CONCENTRATION

Tangential flow filtration (TFF) is a standard procedure utilized for products derived from *E. coli* and CHO systems. Its primary functions involve clarifying, concentrating, and purifying proteins. In a TFF system, fluid is injected tangentially along the membrane's surface, where some feed components are pressured across the membrane onto the filtrate side. Larger particles and molecules unable to pass through the membrane pores are retained and swept away by a crossflow, preventing membrane clogging and improving throughput (Figure 11.10).

TFF is categorized further based on the size of isolated molecules in the feed. Ultrafiltration (UF) is the most prevalent form, separating proteins from buffer components (e.g., buffer exchange, desalting, and concentration). Membrane pore sizes, ranging from 1 to 20 nm, effectively separate proteins within the 1kD to 1000 kD range (known as the nominal molecular weight limit, NMWL). The pressure-driven ultrafiltration process retains larger molecules (protein products), enabling smaller molecules to pass through. This separation occurs primarily due to variations in filtration rates of components through the membrane under applied pressure.

Ultrafiltration membranes often employ polymers like polysulfone, polyethersulfone, polyvinylidene fluoride, and regenerated cellulose. Their microporous structure controls selectivity, molecule retention, and filtration flux (e.g., polyethylene). These membranes can be reused without significant performance decline or contamination risks, thanks to their resistance to robust cleaning agents, acids, and high temperatures. Cellulose membranes, superior in permeability and retention, are widely used for protein applications, prioritizing high retention crucial for successful processes. When selecting the right membrane, considerations include NMWL rating, chemical compatibility, and fouling limit (Table 11.8).

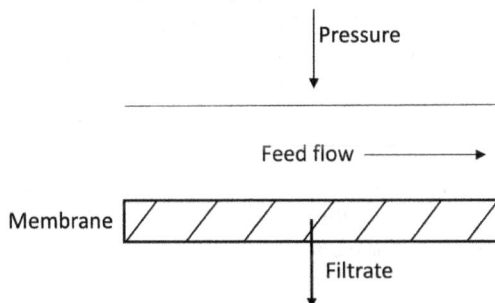

FIGURE 11.10   Tangential flow filtration

TABLE 11.8
Commercial Membranes and Properties

Commercially Available Membranes	Properties
Ultracel®	Regenerated cellulose
Ultracel PL	Regenerated cellulose, NMWL–1 to 300 kD
Ultracel PLC	Composite regenerated cellulose, NMWL: 5–1000 kD
Biomax®	Polyethersulfone-based, NMWL–5 to 1000 kD

In manufacturing processes, two common UF systems include virus filtration and high-performance tangential flow filtration (HPTFF). HPTFF achieves separation by leveraging differences in size and charges. Efficiency is maximized by altering buffer pH and ionic strength to increase disparities between the product and impurities. Particularly in mAb purification techniques, HPTFF effectively removes host cell proteins (HCP) and host cell DNA contaminants.

Diafiltration (DF) is a TFF technique that converts a protein buffer into a preservable and stabilizable form. It collaborates with ultrafiltration or other separation methods to enhance product yield or purity. During diafiltration, the buffer enters the recycle tank while the filtrate exits the device service. Typically, the target protein product resides in the retentate, and diafiltration flushes components out of the retentate into the filtrate, combining buffer exchange and undesired impurity removal/reduction into one technique. Diafiltration can be performed in batch or continuous volume modes. Batch mode involves adding a large buffer volume to the recycling tank, concentrating the retentate, and repeating the process until achieving the desired number of diavolumes. Continuous volume mode maintains the retentate volume by adding buffer at the same rate as filtrate removal, offering more regulated product concentration than batch mode. The primary aim of the DF step is to remove undesirable buffer or contaminant species from the retentate product, affecting yield based on the number of dia-volumes utilized.

The UF/DF formulation step stands as an indispensable and widely adopted stage that handles the highest product concentration, primarily in its final formulation—an integral part of downstream processing. Evolution persists within UF/DF operations, emphasizing robustness, high yield, and cost-effectiveness. Moreover, UF/DF holds a standard position for buffer exchange and product concentration processes before or between chromatography steps.

Within this process, a retentate tank contains the target protein product, while a membrane assembly retains the feed. A feed pump propels the feed through the membrane via tangential flow and pressure. The traditional batch mode operation involves recirculating the feed and retentate through the filter assembly multiple times until achieving the desired protein concentration. Additionally, process monitoring tools, equipment for testing product recovery, and cleaning methods ensure operational consistency and desired yields. TFF systems encompass both traditional stainless steel and more recent single-use methods, constructed using hollow fibers or cassettes. The advent of automated single-use systems with disposable flow routes and lower volume hold-up enhances flexibility, reduces cross-contamination risks, and accelerates turnaround due to minimized cleaning tasks (Figure 11.11).

In recent years, single-pass TFF (SPTFF) has gained prominence—an advanced version of batch mode operation. Here, after a single pass through the filter assembly, the retentate achieves sufficient concentration, eliminating the need for recirculation. This high-throughput and recovery owe credit to increased residence time in the feed channel, brought about by reduced flow rates or longer path lengths. SPTFF proves particularly beneficial for volume reduction steps between chromatography or other intermediate steps with large processing volumes.

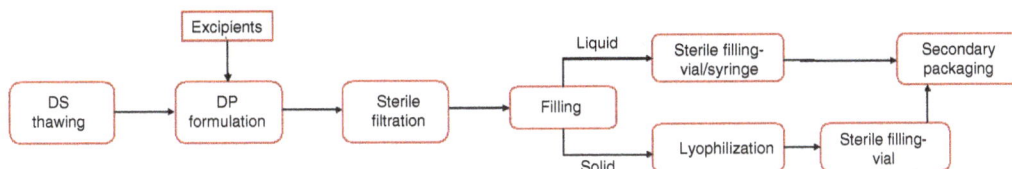

FIGURE 11.11 Schematic of a UF/DF system

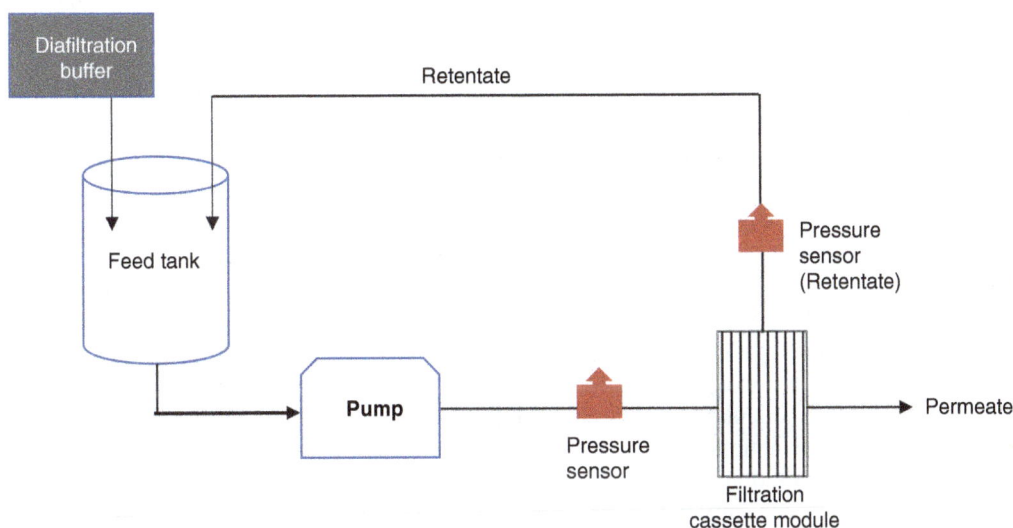

FIGURE 11.12 Schematic for DP preparation activities

Regardless of the operational mode, delineating the process objectives—final product concentration, impurity removal, volume reduction, and buffer exchange—is crucial. Such clarity maximizes process efficiency, enabling precise planning for robust and consistent scale-up operations at the commercial level. Crucially, optimizing process parameters for TFF (UF/DF) minimizes product loss. Several critical process parameters merit consideration for the TFF (UF/DF) process:

- Transmembrane pressure (TMP) refers to the pressure difference across a membrane. It dictates the force needed to drive the feed through the membrane. Filtrate flow increases until it reaches a plateau at a specific TMP level. When protein concentration rises or feed flow rate decreases, TMP decreases until flux hits a plateau (Figure 11.12). Optimal activity occurs at a TMP that sustains high flux without excessive pressure or high protein concentration at the membrane.
- Crossflow rate is determined by the feed channel type and is when the solution moves across the membrane in the feed channel. Higher crossflow rates at the same TMP result in increased flux, potentially causing more product to pass through, leading to product degradation. To counter this, balancing increased flux with more pump passes and holdup volume is crucial for the appropriate crossflow rate.
- Membrane area is determined based on total processing volume and process flux. While opting for a longer process time might reduce membrane area and holdup volume requirements, excessively low values might compromise product quality (causing degradation or contamination). It's advisable to include a safety margin to account for fouling and variations in the feed stream.

- Filtrate control, used in most applications where the target product remains in the retentate, does not have a set point for control and might operate without restrictions.

For diafiltration operations combined with ultrafiltration, determining the starting point for the diafiltration process is essential.

High concentration formulations are generally preferred, especially when the injection volume is low (common in subcutaneous administration of most monoclonal antibodies). However, different drug modalities like antibody-drug conjugates, bispecific antibodies, cell, and gene therapies have prompted adaptations to existing TFF systems (e.g., single-use systems, SPTFF, enhanced monitoring, and pre-sterilized plug-and-play options).

11.14 ANALYTICAL METHODS

Downstream processing primarily aims to reduce or eliminate process and product-related contaminants to yield a pure product. In-process testing during manufacturing adjusts process parameters, ensuring overall process control. These analytical procedures are the foundation of phase analytical technology (PAT). Monitoring product-related impurities such as high-molecular-weight and low-molecular-weight species, glycan variations, and charge variants is critical for overall protection of the products (for mAb products). Currently available methodologies have evolved greatly, making in-process testing a critical tool. Improvements include high-throughput technologies that enable rapid sample processing, a faster turnaround that can support downstream operations effectively and efficiently, particularly for operations that are dependent on a specific analytical testing, example, loading and optimal operation of the downstream unit operation requires knowledge of the product concentration (i.e., titer) in the cell culture media, and subsequent product pools, similarly for product concentration steps. While determining the suitability of testing for large-scale operations, the nature of the product at that stage, e.g., susceptibility to degradation, must be considered for evaluating process hold conditions and minimizing the testing time in such instances.

For recombinant proteins produced by *E. coli*, scanning electron microscopy (SEM) assesses inclusion body morphology and size using Cell Disruption and Recovery Analysis (CDRA). SEM helps evaluate the impact of cell disruption methods and culture conditions on inclusion body development. Traditional plating methods involve plating lysate samples before homogenization on selective and non-selective media, followed by incubation for 12–24 hours. Counting the cells on agar plates determines homogenization efficiency post each pass. Turbidity measurements, as in harvest and clarification procedures, monitor centrifugation processes for inclusion body recovery.

SDS-PAGE serves as a valuable tool in assessing the purity of inclusion bodies during recovery operations. It proves especially useful in devising wash solution strategies and evaluating the reduction of host cell-related protein contaminants. Additionally, this method aids in examining protein solubilization and refolding. Detection of intermolecular (and occasionally intramolecular) disulfide bonds can be achieved analytically through SDS-PAGE under nonreducing conditions. This involves sequentially treating proteins with iodoacetamide (to prevent false disulfide exchange) followed by SDS in the absence of reductant. Techniques such as RP-HPLC, SDS-PAGE, and analytical SEC are clear options for promptly assessing denaturation or refolding degrees. However, even Surface Plasmon Resonance (SPR) and light scattering can be utilized. Both qualitative and quantitative methods prove useful in identifying conditions conducive to solubilization and refolding.

Various standard analytical tests aim to determine protein titer while monitoring process-related and product-related removal across unit operations. Methods for estimating protein titer include UV280nm, RP-HPLC, Bradford Assay, Lowry Assay, Octet, and ProA HPLC. For aggregate analysis, SDS-PAGE, CE-SDS, and analytical size-exclusion methods are commonly used for estimating low and high molecular weight species. Charge variant analysis typically involves CEX-HPLC and iCE.

Several commercial HCP kits are available to monitor process-related impurities, offering options to customize anti-HPC-antibodies. These kits are primarily ELISA-based, and automated immunoassay systems also provide their HCP kits.

11.15 DOWNSTREAM PROCESSING EQUIPMENT AND SYSTEM COMPONENTS

Downstream processing encompasses diverse equipment and supporting components, often referred to as skids, varying in complexity. Equipment specific to downstream operations typically include

- Buffer Preparation and Storage Systems.
- Cell Disruption and Centrifugation (Microbial Processes).
- Purification Systems/Chromatography Separation.
- Filtration Systems (membrane filtration, depth filtration, etc.).

The equipment used in these processes must offer flexibility across various scales (lab, pilot, and commercial-scale production) while ensuring no degradation or damage to the product due to equipment selection. Collaboration between drug manufacturers and equipment manufacturers is crucial to meet user requirement specifications (URS) tailored for the specific process needs. Significant advancements in bioprocessing have led to the development of fully automated skids for purification and membrane filtration operations. Disposable chromatography skids are gaining popularity due to their rapid turnaround and elimination of cleaning and cleaning validation requirements. Skids enable efficient setup and streamlined processing, each unit or system component designed considering the process requirements and functional operation.

Key design features include

- Process control unit/functional system in which the product is processed (e.g., chromatography columns, membrane filter, etc.).
- The automation system enables the sensors' connection/communication with the detection units in the process control system to allow operation and monitoring. Various hardware/software platforms with optional customizable configurations are provided.
- Inlet and outlet systems (e.g., a buffer tank, holding tank, etc.) are connected to the process control unit and other secondary accessories, including piping, valves, pumps, etc.
- Measurement devices/probes/sensors are used to control and monitor the process (e.g., pH, conductivity, UV, pressure sensors).

Manufacturers typically conduct factory tests before delivering manufacturing skids to user facilities. Subsequently, on-site installation and qualification exercises (IQ, OQ) are performed to verify specifications before using the equipment in manufacturing operations.

11.16 SENSORS, PROBES, AND METERS

For upstream bioreactor operations, online or inline monitoring and controlling of process parameters are common. Downstream processes monitor parameters

- flow rate, pH, conductivity, and UV for chromatography unit operations,
- pressure, flow rate/speed for clarification, filtration, and
- flow rate, concentration factor, pressure, conductivity, protein concentration, temperature.

TABLE 11.9
Recommended Online Monitoring for Critical Downstream Processing Steps

Process Stage	Process Parameters Monitored	Process Attributes
Harvest and clarification	Flow rate	Efficiency
	Pressure	Filter membrane clogging
	Turbidity	Clarity of the supernatant
		Protein concentration (product)
Homogenization and IB recovery	Pressure	Homogenization efficiency
	Number of cycles	Protein concentration (product)
	Temperature	Amount of IBs
Purification	pH	Protein concentration (product)
	Flow rate	Purity and impurity profile (e.g., aggregates, residual
	A280 (UV)	DNA, HCP, etc.)
	Conductivity	Column performance/resin lifecycle
	Binding conditions	
	Elution conditions	
Concentration	Diafiltration volumes	Protein concentration (Product)
	Concentration factor	Purity profile
	Flow rate	Impurity profile
	Turbidity	

Monitoring various parameters serves as feedback for control loops, optimizing processes. Data from monitoring is stored in automation systems, allowing trend analysis and inclusion in batch documentation (e.g., UV analysis, chromatogram from purification processes, pressure monitoring in TFF systems (TMP)). pH, conductivity, temperature, and pressure are commonly monitored using in-line or offline probes or sensors (Table 11.9).

Timely monitoring of critical process parameters significantly contributes to product quality, understanding the process impact, and an efficient process. Sensor design depends on unit operations and product/protein type. For instance, in chromatography, in-line sensors should detect proteins, nucleic acids, carbohydrates, salts, flow rates, and perform pressure safety checks. Off-line instruments typically determine product quality resulting from processing conditions.

11.16.1 ULTRAVIOLET MONITORING

UV spectroscopy is crucial for downstream unit operations, measuring absorption from aromatic acids (phenylalanine, tyrosine, tryptophan) around 280nm (sometimes up to 340nm) to scan different proteins eluting from a column. UV monitoring aids chromatographic separation, with systems sometimes featuring an auto-zero function to normalize baseline UV absorption. In certain TFF applications, UV cells monitor the protein breakthrough through the membrane. This is useful for high concentration protein. Alternatively, the UV sensors may also be installed in the retentate line to determine the retentate recovery to minimize the final product's dilution and maximize the overall yield.

FTIR spectroscopy characterizes proteins based on amide bond vibrations in the polypeptide (secondary structure), assessing structural changes.

11.16.2 PH MONITORING

pH measurements serve as in-process controls, buffer criteria, and a suitable reaction environment. pH probes (glass or plastic) are calibrated before each operation but shouldn't be exposed to extreme conductivity values.

11.16.3 CONDUCTIVITY MONITORING

Conductivity measurements play a crucial role in monitoring chromatography and filtration operations. They are utilized to oversee or regulate gradient operations, such as ion-exchange chromatography or hydrophobic interaction chromatography, where increasing salt concentration aids elution. During diafiltration operations, measuring conductivity helps track progress and determine when the target process conductivity is achieved. Additionally, conductivity measurement offers insights into filter equilibration for filtration operations and serves as an endpoint for Cleaning in Place (CIP). Probes are strategically placed in the retentate and permeate lines to monitor buffer exchange and measure conductivity during rinsing operations.

11.16.4 PRESSURE SENSORS

Pressure sensors are widely employed across bioprocessing operations, primarily serving as safety measures for both equipment and operators. For instance, in TFF, pressure sensors monitor trans-membrane pressure (TMP), detecting pressure differentials across cassettes and high system pressure. If pressure spikes, it is critical to halt the feed pump. Similarly, in chromatography columns and depth filtration systems, monitoring pressure drop over time serves as an indicative performance parameter. In product wetted applications, in-line diaphragm sensors are typically used, while other sensors or gauges cover non-product contact areas.

11.16.5 TEMPERATURE

Temperature control is not universally required in downstream processing, but specific operations occasionally demand controlled temperatures. These operations are conducted either in temperature-controlled manufacturing areas . For refolding operations that may require a controlled temperature, tanks (jacketed vessels) are connected to a recirculation chiller to help keep the desired temperature.

The influence of temperature on pH and conductivity measurements is significant. Calibration and measurement should occur at the same temperature, or manual temperature compensation using the meter's control option becomes necessary. Some pH meters feature automatic temperature compensation functions. Given that buffers exhibit varying pH values at different temperatures, it is crucial to use the buffer's value at the calibration temperature. Most new meters include NIST calibration. Monitoring the temperature, pH, and conductivity of samples can be advantageous.

11.16.6 FLOW METERS

Flow meters are pivotal in controlling operational flow rates by providing real-time monitoring. They are commonly integrated into chromatography and filtration systems. High-accuracy inline and non-invasive flow sensors are frequently used as built-in components, capable of bidirectional measurements within pipes. In tangential flow filtration (TFF) systems, mass flow or magnetic inductive flow meters gauge flow on the retentate and permeate sides. Flow rates hold significant importance, especially during operational scale-ups, ensuring consistent system performance across various scales. Magnetic flowmeters, while less expensive than mass flowmeters, require a minimum liquid conductivity for accurate flow rate measurement.

11.16.7 AIR SENSORS

Air sensors play a crucial role in chromatography systems by detecting the end of a sample or buffer solution, thus preventing air from entering the system. This protective function safeguards the column from potential damage caused by air and allows for automatic loading. Notably, the air sensor operates as a non-invasive device.

11.17   FLOW PATH

In chromatography and filtration systems, the flow path stands as a vital component, which can be constructed from either plastic or stainless steel. In bioprocessing operations, a disposable flow path is preferred due to its ease of plug-in/plug-out options. These pre-assembled and pre-sterilized flow paths facilitate quick plug-and-play functionality. Moreover, disposable flow path kits come with documentation on extractables and leachables to meet regulatory requirements (e.g., Cytiva flow path kits, QuantaSep 300 SU system with disposable flow path Sepragen, PROCONNOX by Repligen). Therefore, the flow path should accommodate low-volume processes effectively.

11.18   PUMPS

Pumps hold significant importance in both upstream and downstream operations, serving a wide array of applications from pumping mediums and cultures to buffer solutions and delicate protein solutions. The selection of an appropriate pump for a specific process involves careful consideration of numerous factors, including flow rate requirements, liquid's physical properties, shear sensitivity, and pressure needs.

In a peristaltic pump, as fluid enters the head, it gets trapped between two rollers. This movement creates a void, leading the tubing to be occluded by the rollers. This alternation between fluid and void causes the flow to pulse rather than operate smoothly. Pulsations exist in all pumps but having a pulse-free flow ensures better control of flow rates and more precise timed operations. Methods to reduce pulsation include using a pump head with adjustable occlusion, employing a multiple roller design, utilizing pulse-dampening mechanisms, or modifying the discharge tubing layout.

Suction lines, often overlooked in pump systems, transport the source fluid material through piping or tubing. Priming the suction lines is necessary, and this feature may be part of the pump itself – either self-priming or non-self-priming. Self-priming pumps can draw feed liquid even from an empty pipe, while non-self-priming pumps require liquid in their lines before operation.

A shorter suction line can enhance operational efficiency by reducing energy consumption and extending the pump's lifespan. Additionally, it helps minimize cavitation, a phenomenon that significantly compromises the pump's performance and durability. Cavitation arises from the formation of air pockets within the fluid due to fluctuating pressure, causing the liquid stream's pressure to drop below the vapor pressure of the pumped liquid. These minute bubbles collapse, leading to damage to nearby components. Different pump types have specific suction line requirements for optimal functioning. For instance, centrifugal pumps necessitate a direct and concise suction line. The highest point on the suction line is the pump inlet, which must maintain a tight, air-leak-free connection for proper pump operation. In magnetic drive pumps, keeping the suction line length to a minimum and mounting it gradually to the pump prevents air pocket formation. The diameter of the suction pipe should match or exceed the pump's suction size. Diaphragm pumps, on the other hand, require a non-collapsible, reinforced suction line.

Regarding the most commonly used pumps in bioprocesses

- Peristaltic pumps are commonly used for single-use or disposable applications due to their compatibility with flexible tubing (e.g., silicone). However, these pumps have limitations, such as susceptibility to tubing breakage due to constant movement and friction from the pump head. Therefore, caution is advised against using them for highly viscous liquids or high flow rates, which may risk product loss or contamination.
- Rotary Lobe Pumps: Suitable for high-viscosity liquids and large volumes, but susceptible to damage from hard particles in the fluid. Speed control via a variable frequency drive using a flow meter is common.

- Diaphragm Pumps: Predominantly used in downstream operations such as chromatography, available in various pressure ratings suitable for high-pressure chromatography applications requiring pressures more than 100 bar.

11.19 VALVES

Valves regulate product and buffer flow within the system, affecting pressure-flow characteristics. Materials like stainless steel, polypropylene (PP), polyvinylidene difluoride (PVDF), and polyether ether ketone (PEEK) are commonly used in valve construction. Various types of valves cater to different biopharmaceutical manufacturing operations: pinch valves for soft, flexible tubing in single-use systems, diaphragm valves for low-pressure operations, and ball valves widely used in HPLC systems.

11.20 IN-LINE FILTRATION (STERILE FILTRATION AND PARTICLE FILTRATION)

Filtration is a vital operation in downstream processes, applied in stages such as harvest clarification, buffer and solution preparation, chromatography, and final filtration for the finished product. Operations like microfiltration, ultrafiltration, nanofiltration, and direct flow filtration through sterilizing-grade filters are commonly employed.

Standard flow filtration involves passing the feed directly through the membrane without cross-flow, known as direct flow or dead-end filtering. This method, often employed in chromatography unit operations and sterile filtration like virus filtration, effectively protects the chromatographic column by removing particles from the buffer and feeds, reducing bioburden. To optimize filtration parameters, it's essential to assess the filtration area, porosity, and cartridge configuration. Pressure sensors placed upstream and downstream of the filter unit monitor and control the filtration operation by estimating pressure differentials, signaling when the filter requires replacement. For particle and microbiological removal, membrane pore diameters range from 0.1 μm to 10.0 μm. Pre- and post-use filter integrity testing is performed on all filters used in upstream and downstream operations. Tests like the bubble point test, forward flow test, water intrusion test, and binary gas test are conducted. These tests gauge a wet membrane's ability to prevent gas from flowing freely is measured using the bubble point and forward flow tests. A dry hydrophobic membrane is utilized as a barrier to the free flow of water, and a non-wetting fluid is used in the water intrusion test (HydroCorr test). A mixture of two gases with large permeability variances is used in the binary gas test. The test entails determining the composition of the gas mixture upstream and downstream of a wetted membrane. If the post-use integrity test fails, refiltration is conducted.

When considering a bioproduction process, selecting and specifying equipment should primarily align with operational needs. With the emergence of process intensification in bioprocessing, smaller-scale equipment holds potential advantages, especially in meeting product quantity requirements for toxicology and clinical studies. Additionally, smaller skids offer compatibility benefits and facilitate the implementation of single-use technologies.

Most downstream processing equipment is constructed from stainless steel, posing limitations for operations requiring extreme conditions due to corrosion risks. Plastics like polypropylene, EPDM, PTFE, and PEEK are commonly used in tubing, measuring cells, valves, and gaskets. pH and UV sensors typically utilize glass components. Many elements, including stainless steel, are considered extractable, necessitating collaboration between drug manufacturers and suppliers for testing and documentation purposes. As the target product moves towards increased purity in the final drug substance or drug product preparation, the demand for sterile or aseptic conditions intensifies, mandating hygienic design for process flow paths and product contact surfaces. Conventional cleaning methods involve using caustic solutions of varying concentrations for tasks such as column and filter membrane cleaning, equipment maintenance, and other consumables. If needed, steam sterilization may also be applied. Single-use systems replace several components, significantly reducing cleaning procedures and expediting turnover times.

11.21 SUMMARY

The success of developing a robust downstream process and meeting product quality requirements hinges on the efficiency and recovery of each unit operation. Product losses can substantially impact the economic feasibility of the product, emphasizing the need for a systematic approach in identifying the objectives and expectations of each unit operation. For instance, a three-stage purification plan does not necessarily require three chromatography phases in all manufacturing processes. Decisions should be guided by purity standards and the intended usage of the protein. While a platform process streamlines operations in a multi-product facility dealing with similar products, adaptations to this approach warrant evaluation.

Downstream operations often have inherent limitations. Chromatography resins, for instance, present challenges concerning their lifespan, lot-to-lot variability, cleaning, regeneration processes, and viral clearance capacity in chromatographic procedures.

Optimization efforts targeting reduced processing times and process simplification through process intensification should be explored. Strategies like adjusting media volume based on impurity levels can minimize resin and buffer consumption while enhancing economic viability. Prioritizing process efficiency, robustness, and scalability is crucial. Innovative approaches such as integrating chromatographic steps into multimodal processes, continuous processing, and embracing single-use systems that eliminate complexities associated with packaging, cleaning, and maintenance have gained traction. Although their implementation remains limited, these technologies offer opportunities for enhanced productivity and flexibility.

12 Formulation of Biopharmaceuticals

12.1 OVERVIEW

The development requirements for biopharmaceuticals differ significantly from small chemical molecule drugs due to their larger molecular size and the variability of molecular structure. These properties impact the body's immune systems in unique ways.

Firstly, as most protein drugs are administered via parenteral routes, the science of protein drug formulation primarily focuses on injectable formulations. The choice of delivery route is limited due to the instability of protein structures in many administration environments. Factors such as acidity in the gastrointestinal tract, the large molecular size, high hydrophilicity hindering absorption across biological membranes, and high dose-response sensitivity restrict significant variations in bioavailability.

Secondly, proteins possess structural features like functional groups susceptible to oxidation, including methionine, cysteine, histidine, tryptophan, and tyrosine. These require common approaches for stabilization. Additionally, conformational changes and aggregation, unique to large molecules, necessitate specific formulation components.

Thirdly, proteins are sensitive to temperature, light, and agitation during storage, shipping, and handling. The formulation challenges are compounded due to various factors not commonly considered in small molecule drugs, potentially affecting the quality and efficacy of biopharmaceuticals.

The formulations of biopharmaceuticals vary significantly based on the delivery route, predominantly parenteral, but advancements are diversifying to noninvasive routes. The choice of administration route considers practicality and probability factors, requiring a detailed understanding of biopharmaceutical interactions with the administration route's environment. Computational tools over the past two decades aid in rapidly creating decision matrices for optimizing formulations.

Different biological barriers confront each route of administration due to anatomical and physiological characteristics. To surmount these barriers, various formulation approaches have been developed, incorporating advancements in information technology, biotechnology, nanotechnology, and sophisticated medical devices, including electric or magnetic forces and sonic waves, to maximize noninvasive drug delivery effectiveness.

A formulation aims to deliver a biopharmaceutical active to the administration site, crossing biological barriers into the bloodstream and ultimately reaching the site of action. Given the high likelihood of product degradation during shelf-life, proprietary technology, including numerous patents, has been developed to enable a dosage form to deliver the drug effectively to the site of action.

An appendix in this chapter details the physicochemical properties of proteins and peptides, crucial for designing formulations.

Due to the high cost of biopharmaceutical development, scientists engage in evaluating intellectual property related to biopharmaceutical manufacturing and delivery systems. Chapter 8 provides details on intellectual property management, essential reading for scientists involved in the formulation of biopharmaceuticals.

Managing biopharmaceutical stability involves either chemically modifying the molecule or selecting proper excipients. These combinations ensure stability without compromising product safety or efficacy. Structure modifications, such as creating protein scaffolds and PEGylation of molecules, among other technologies, are elaborated in Chapter 1.

12.2 PROTEIN STRUCTURE

12.2.1 BASIS

A comprehensive understanding of protein structure and the associated risks in formulating these products is necessary to comprehend the complexities of formulating biopharmaceutical products. Proteins consist of amino acid chains with reactive groups forming multidimensional structures, defining their chemical and physical properties are based on this reactivity.

Protein instability arises from both chemical and physical reactions. Chemical instability involves the formation or dissolution of covalent bonds within a polypeptide or protein structure, leading to oxidation, deamidation, reduction, and hydrolysis. Physical or conformational instabilities encompass dissociation, denaturation, accumulation, and precipitation. When a chemical event, like oxidation, triggers a physical reaction like aggregation, the protein degradation pathways synergize. Unlike small molecule drugs, physical changes in biopharmaceuticals, apart from the PK profile, can significantly impact safety.

Table 12.1 lists several formulation variables triggering uncertainty, grounded in the chemistry of chemical and biopharmaceutical molecules. However, biopharmaceuticals have a distinct effect on protection and efficacy.

Understanding the intricate degradation mechanisms causing chemical and physical instability in biopharmaceutical formulations has historically posed challenges. However, advancements in analytical chemistry have significantly facilitated this comprehension. The FDA-approved Appendix Physicochemical Properties of Proteins and Peptides, as of March 2020, serves as a comprehensive compilation of critical product properties. This database enables formulators to adopt a focused scientific approach in developing formulations by comparing and selecting stable formulations based on similar molecular properties.

Compared to small molecule drugs, biopharmaceuticals are less tolerant of minor variations in solution chemistry. Their stability in terms of composition and conformation is confined within a narrow pH and osmolarity range. To maintain solubility throughout the product's shelf life,

TABLE 12.1
Impact of Formulation and Environmental Factors on the Degradation of Proteins

Factor	Impact
Buffer species	Deamidation
Light	Photo decomposition
Metal ions	Hydrolysis, oxidation
Other excipients	Maillard reaction
Oxygen	Oxidation
pH	Hydrolysis, deamidation
Temperature	Most routes

TABLE 12.2
Protein Biopharmaceuticals Stability Issues

Problems	Potential Causes	Possible Solutions
Cleavages	Protease impurity, other unknown mechanisms	pH, product purity, inhibitors
Covalent aggregation	Disulfide scrambling, other unknown mechanisms	pH, inhibit non-covalent aggregation
Cyclic imide	pH around 5	pH optimization
Deamidation	pH < 5.0 or pH >6.0	pH optimization
Non-covalent aggregation	Solubility, structural changes, heat, shear, surface, denaturants, impurities	pH, ionic additives, amino acids, surfactants, protein concentration, raw material purity
Oxidation	Active oxygen species, free radicals, metals, light, impurity	Excipient purity, a free-radical scavenger, active oxygen scavengers, methionine
Surface denaturation, adsorption	Low protein concentration, specific affinity, protein hydrophobicity	Surfactants, protein concentration, pH

supportive formulation components are often necessary for multiple molecules. Even lyophilized protein products are susceptible to substantial degradation, unlike small-molecule drugs, which tend to be highly stable in most lyophilized formulations.

Table 12.2 succinctly outlines prevalent stability issues encountered in protein formulation development along with potential solutions. However, given the unique nature of each molecule, this list should serve as a guideline rather than an exhaustive directive.

12.2.2 PHYSICAL DEGRADATION

Protein degradation stems from various factors including hydrophobic surfaces, boiling, lyophilization, reconstitution, interaction with organic solvents, shaking, and other physical and chemical influences. Physical stressors can lead to denaturation, adsorption, accumulation, or deposition on container walls.

12.2.2.1 Structural Changes

Biological macromolecules like antibodies possess a three-dimensional tertiary structure crucial for their folded state, involving complex intramolecular and intermolecular interactions with functional amino acid groups and external environments. Non-covalent interactions (electrostatic, van der Waals, hydrogen bonding, hydrophobic) play a pivotal role in maintaining the native structure's stability. Disruption of this interaction balance by external sources leads to structural changes, rendering large molecules unstable. For instance, in an aqueous solution, more soluble amino acid residues interact with solvent molecules while non-polar residues are shielded, creating a hydrophobic core.

The amino acid sequence determines protein folding into its biologically active form. However, proteins can also unfold, transitioning to an intermediate or denatured state from their native structure. Such variants tend to assemble into more stable complexes, such as aggregates, due to higher free energy. Aggregates consist of multiple monomers held together by covalent or non-covalent bonds. Dilution, for example, can dissociate native monomer cluster aggregates due to monomer association. Precipitation or irreversible aggregates can occur as a result of the nucleation of different monomers. Aggregation is caused by a variety of stressors, the most common of which are temperature, mechanical agitation, and freeze/thaw stress during manufacturing. Aggregation can be caused by a pH change, and high temperatures can cause conformational destabilization or partial/complete unfolding. IgG4 forms more soluble aggregates than IgG1 at lower pH and higher temperatures, for example, due to lower conformational stability caused by lower unfolding temperature and changes in tertiary structures.

Because protein tertiary structures are vulnerable to environmental physical stress, structural changes in mAbs can occur at any stage during the manufacturing process, starting from protein expression to processing and storage. Structural transformation is attributed to non-physiological conditions during manufacturing processes contribute to structural variants in the final product. Stressors such as buffer selection, fabrication techniques, and container type may exacerbate these issues.

12.2.2.2 Aggregation

Aggregated proteins pose significant concerns in biopharmaceuticals, diminishing bioactivity and increasing immunogenicity. Macromolecular protein complexes can trigger an immune response, recognizing the protein as foreign and prompting an antigenic reaction.

Buffer selection significantly impacts product stability. For example, acetate buffer causes precipitation in IgG3 formulations, unlike when arginine and histidine are used. Adjusting buffer salt concentrations can mitigate phase changes. The lyophilizate's pH is crucial in preventing recombinant vaccine antigen aggregation, often necessitating additional stabilizers such as trehalose.

Non-native proteins should be avoided in finished mAb-based biopharmaceutical products. When protein solutions are drawn from vials, aggregation might occur, leading to inconsistent dosing. For instance, aggregating IFN– promotes the development of neutralizing anti-drug Abs (NAb), hindering the IFN receptor from binding and thus reducing clinical efficacy. Induced NAbs can disrupt the normal function of endogenous proteins, especially hormones and cytokines. NAb interference with endogenous erythropoietin led to Eprex®-related severe anemia and pure-red cell aplasia (PRCA) in patients receiving recombinant human erythropoietin. The NAb formation was due to aggregation, often facilitated by prefilled syringes containing ingredients like polysorbate 80 and silicone oil. Therefore, any progress in the formulation or manufacturing process of biopharmaceuticals requires further research following the ICH Q5E guidelines (https://database.ich.org/sites/default/files/Q5E%20Guideline.pdf). The creator of Eprex did not conduct essential studies and believed that minor formulation changes would not impact erythropoietin's protection or efficacy.

Aggregation is a prevalent issue in protein production and storage. Exposure to liquid–air, liquid–solid, or liquid–liquid interfaces enhances a protein's aggregation tendency. Mechanical agitation, including shaking, stirring, pipetting, or pumping through tubes, and freezing and thawing also contribute to aggregation. Solvent conditions such as temperature, protein concentration, pH, and ionic force can affect the nature and amount of aggregates formed.

Several mechanisms lead to protein aggregate formation, including domain swapping (ds), strand association (sa), edge-edge-association (ee), and beta-strand stacking. Aggregators include protein multimers such as dimers, trimers, tetramers, and large polymers. These aggregates can be non-covalent or covalent (disulfide-linked). Non-covalent aggregates are completely soluble in a clear solution, partially soluble in a turbid solution, and mostly insoluble as sediment at the container's bottom. Interactions between exposed hydrophobic groups in proteins trigger non-specific protein-to-protein interactions, leading to aggregation. While covalent aggregation is irreversible, weakly associated non-covalent aggregates might be reversible but progress to multimers in most cases. Strongly associated non-covalent aggregates are not reversible through dilution and can precipitate.

Aggregates are categorized based on their size range: (1) submicron particles (<1 μm), also known as soluble particles; (2) sub-visible particles (1–100 μm), and (3) visible particles (>100 μm size).

Aggregation models exist in various forms and sizes. In the "Native to Unfolded to Aggregate" model, hydrophobic interactions lead denatured or unfolded molecules to aggregate. These interactions occur due to the release of submerged hydrophobic regions, inducing aggregate formation. As temperature increases, unfolding intensifies, and since reactions typically follow first-order kinetics, the reaction rate rises in this model.

The "Native to Intermediate to Unfolded" model involves the intermediate stage producing the aggregate. These misfolded intermediates are thermodynamically stable and are part of the native state ensemble. Therefore, protein aggregation isn't necessarily an abnormal state and can occur even under conditions favoring the native state.

Protein aggregation comprises two stages: nucleation expanding to a critical mass after the nucleation process. Although turbidity measurements track aggregation extent, they aren't always reliable predictors. When native and folded proteins interact, irreversible non-native structures with elevated non-native intermolecular-sheet formations may develop. Solution conditions such as pH, salt species, concentration, co-solutes, excipients, and surfactants significantly influence the aggregate's onset, rate, and final morphology. The precise existence of an aggregate is determined by the relative intrinsic thermodynamic stability of the native state.

Biopharmaceuticals can aggregate at various process stages, including hold points, shipping, and long-term storage due to necessary physical and chemical manipulations in production, downstream processing, formulation, and filling. Agitation of protein solutions (shaking, stirring, or shearing) at air-liquid interfaces aids protein molecules in joining and unfolding, exposing hydrophobic regions, fostering aggregation.

Agitation-induced aggregation is observed in proteins like recombinant factor XIII, human growth hormone, hemoglobin, erythropoietin, and insulin. Preventing significant protein activity loss or visible particulate matter formation requires minimizing foaming caused by agitation in manufacturing and product use. Antimicrobial preservatives used in multidose formulations, such as benzyl alcohol, accelerate protein aggregation by producing partially unfolded protein conformations. Increasing preservatives' amounts can increase hydrophobicity, decreasing aqueous solubility. Phenol and m-cresol significantly destabilize proteins, with m-cresol causing protein precipitation and phenol promoting both soluble and insoluble aggregates.

Freezing and thawing can occur several times during growth, which may reduce the shelf-life of the product and have a significant effect on protein aggregation. When water-ice crystals form at the container's rim, the effect is known as "salting out" (where heat transfer is greatest). Protein and excipients become increasingly concentrated in the eventually freezing center of a container.

Precipitation and accumulation occur during freezing owing to high salt and protein concentrations, which will not be completely reversed upon thawing. Thyroid-stimulating hormone, for example, retains its potency for up to 90 days when stored at −80°C, 4°C, or 24°C but loses more than 40% of its potency when frozen at −20°C due to subunit dissociation.

Repeated freezing and thawing cycles have a cumulative effect on subvisible and visible particulate generation. Buffer component crystallization during freezing can induce pH changes, with potassium phosphate buffers exhibiting smaller pH transitions than sodium phosphate buffers. Oxidation can accelerate pH-dependent reactions, leading to precipitate appearance within minutes.

The causes of aggregation related to the manufacturing process are listed in Table 12.3.

TABLE 12.3
Process-Related Causes of Protein Aggregation

Process	Factor
Administration	Diluents, component materials and surfaces, leachable
Fermentation/Expression	Inclusion bodies
Fill/Finish	Surface interaction, shear, contamination (e.g., silicone oil)
Filtration	Surface interaction, shear
Freeze/Thaw	Cryo-concentration, pH changes, Ice-solution interfaces
Lyophilization	Cryo-concentration, pH changes, ice-solution interfaces, dehydration
Purification	Shear, pH, ionic strength
Shipping	Agitation, temperature cycling

Note that the liquid is frozen in cryo-concentration, and the water is removed as ice as it thaws.

Dispensing proteins in prefilled syringes with silicone oil lubrication poses challenges. Variations in protein absorbance at 350 nm among syringe brands are common based on silicone type and quantity. Contact with silicone in syringes can cause properly folded monoclonal antibodies to form an intermediate, leading to partial unfolding, soluble aggregate formation, and visible precipitation depending on silicone concentration. Insoluble particles result from combining subvisible and visible particles, with sub-visible particles having a diameter of 0.1–1 micron.

Sucrose-based formulations can cause protein aggregation over time due to protein glycation during sucrose hydrolysis. Aggregate formation can be facilitated by ligands such as ions. Interactions with metal surfaces can cause epitaxic denaturation (the formation of an aggregate by growing a crystal layer of one mineral on the crystal base of another mineral with the same crystalline orientation as the substrate), while foreign particles from the atmosphere, manufacturing processes, or container systems can also trigger aggregation, such as silicone oil. Protein handling at compounding pharmacies often leads to multiple-fold aggregation.

Developing formulations preventing protein aggregation or precipitation requires comprehensive evaluations of optimum pH and osmotic conditions. Surfactants, polyols, or sugars can be added to prevent irreversible denaturation aggregation.

Nonionic detergents (surfactants) are used to improve product stability and prevent aggregation. Because hydrophobic interactions occur between proteins and surfactants, these compounds stabilize proteins by lowering the surface tension of the solution and binding to hydrophobic sites on their surfaces, thereby reducing the potential for protein-protein interactions that can lead to aggregate formation. Tween 20 and Tween 80 are nonionic detergents that can prevent the formation of soluble protein aggregates at surfactant concentrations below the critical micelle concentration (CMC); chelating agents can prevent the aggregation of metal-induced proteins.

12.2.3   Chemical Degradation

Chemical instability involves the formation or destruction of covalent bonds within a protein structure. Oxidation, deamidation, reduction, and hydrolysis are the most common chemical modifications of proteins. Although a protein molecule has thousands of active functional groups, the identity of these groups is limited because they are made up of a fixed number of amino acids. Table 12.4 highlights hotspots for protein degradation.

Figure 12.1 depicts the most common chemical degradation routes for antibodies used to make most biopharmaceuticals.

Diketopiperazine is an amino acid degradation intermediate of dipeptide esters and amides. A nucleophilic attack of N-terminal nitrogen on the amide carbonyl occurs between the second and

---

TABLE 12.4
Protein Sequence Hotspots for Degradation

Pathway	Site
Beta-Elimination	Ser, Thr
Deamidation	Asn, Gln, –Asn-X-, –Asn-Gly-, Asn-His-, –Asn-Ser-, –Asn-Ala-,–Asn–Asp-,–Asn-Thr-
Diketopiperazine	X-X-Gly, X-Pro-
Glycation	Lys
Hydrolysis	Asp,–Asp-Pro-,–Asp-Gln-,–Pro-Asp,–Asp-Tyr-,–X-Ser-,–X-Thr-
Isomerization	Asn, Asp, –Asn-Gly-,–Asp-Ser-,–Asn-Ser-,–Asp-Ser-
Oxidation	Met, Cys, His, Trp, Tyr
Pyroglutamic acid	H2N-Gln-, H2N-Gln-Gly-, H2N-Glu-

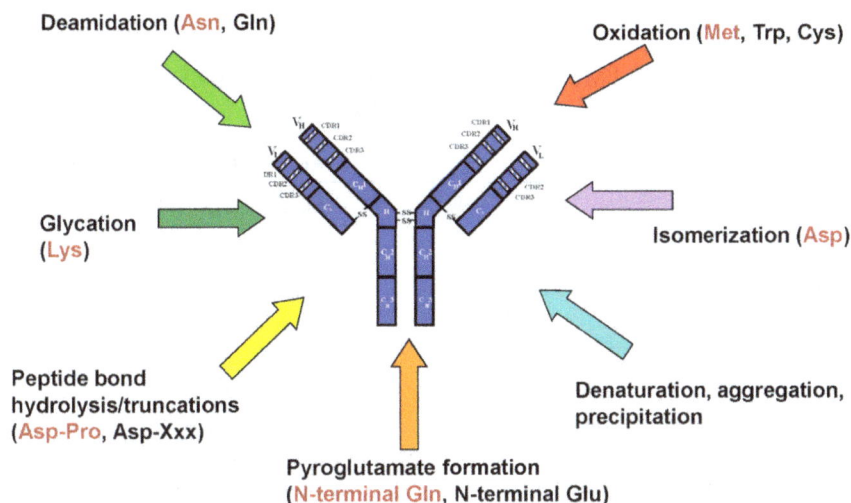

FIGURE 12.1 Common routes of protein degradation

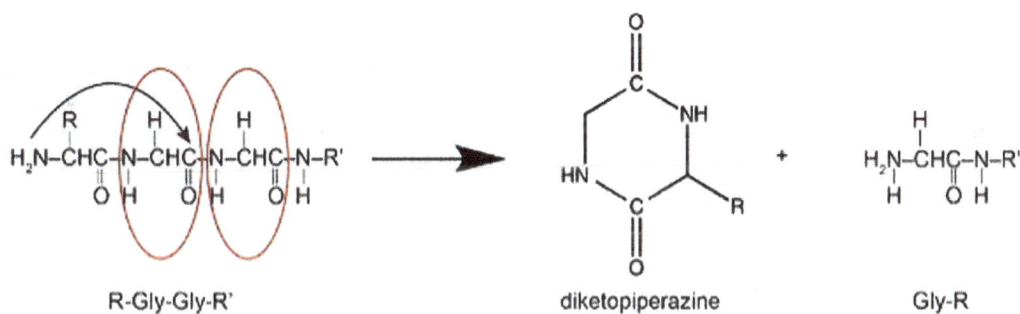

FIGURE 12.2 Diketopiperazine formation in the degradation of recombinant growth hormone

third residues. Therefore, peptides containing Gly as the third residue or Pro as the second residue from the N-terminus are particularly vulnerable; this reaction occurs best in a neutral or alkaline medium. The diketopiperazine from X-Pro [(X = Gly, Ala, Val, Phe, beta-cyclohexylamine, and Arg] is influenced by the cis-trans equilibrium of Pro and the charge distribution around the peptide bond. The Cis type facilitates ring closure. Figure 12.2 shows an example of a diketopiperazine formulation. Switching the amino acid preceding the proline residue has a significant effect on the rate of diketopiperazine formation at pH 7.0.

Another chemical modification intermediate is pyrogalacmic acid. Because the terminal Gln will spontaneously cyclize to form PyroE, Gln-Glyn responds much faster than Gln-Glyn. The N-terminal Glu cyclization results in a −17 Da mass change and a −1 or loss of critical residues; the N-terminal Glu cyclization results in no charge change but an 18 Da mass shift.

Although predicting specific chemical reaction effects is challenging, their consistent impact on acidity, as shown in Table 12.5.

12.2.3.1 Deamidation

Deamidation, a chemical reaction extracting the amide functional group from an amino acid, is the most common chemical degradation in biopharmaceutical products based on mAbs. It can lead to isomerization, racemization, and protein truncation as potential outcomes.

TABLE 12.5
Effect of Chemical Modifications of Proteins on Acidity Function and Charge Heterogeneity (See also Appendix)

Chemical Modification	Acidity/Charge Heterogeneity
Deamidation	More acidic ($z = -1$)
Succinimide formation	More basic or neutral
Glycation	More acidic
Pyroglutamate formation	More acidic ($z = -1$)
Peptide Bond Hydrolysis	Either acidic or basic

The rate of protein deamidation is significantly influenced by side-chain branching in the (n+1) th residue. The charge of the residue is generally unimportant, except in the case of His, Ser, and Thr. Conversely, the (n−1)th residue has only a minor effect on the deamination rate. The half-life of deamidation ranges from one day to over a thousand days, contingent upon the identity of the carboxyl side residue. The rate of deamidation is also influenced by the protein's secondary structure. Changes in the helical structure of certain proteins can slow down the deamidation rate. The resulting structural alterations from deamidation can have various effects on the physicochemical and functional stability of proteins.

Steric hindrance can also influence the deamidation rate. Bulky asparagine residues may impede the formation of the intermediate succinimide during the deamidation reaction. By substituting a glycine residue with bulkier leucine or proline residues, the rate is reduced by 30 to 50 times. Deamidation rates are typically lower in lyophilized formulations due to the limited availability of free water required for the reaction.

The key features of the deamidation reaction include:

- Non-enzymatic reaction that takes place at Asn and Gln.
- Water is needed for the hydrolysis reaction.
- pH affects the pathways.
- Under slightly acidic to essential conditions, the cyclic imide pathway is activated.
- Under acidic conditions, direct hydrolysis occurs.
- In the pH range of 3–4, the minimum rate is optimized.
- In the pH range of 7–12, the buffer has a catalytic effect.
- For Asn, the rate is 5–10 times higher than for Gln.
- Both normal and beta-peptide bonds are formed.
- The N+1 residue affects the rate.
- isoAsp-Y to Asp-Y interconvertibility.

Table 12.6 presents examples demonstrating the diverse effects of deamidation observed.

12.2.3.2 pH

The pH, buffer, and ionic strength significantly impact deamidation. Using formulations within a pH range of 3–5 reduces peptide deamidation. Insulin isoaspartate or aspartate forms of AsnA-21 and AsnB-3 are utilized based on the pH of the solution.

Deamidation can occur at lower pH, primarily through a succinimide-independent mechanism. For instance, deamidation of Asn in the A insulin chain is favored at pH 5, mediated by the appearance of an intermediate cyclic anhydride; although there are examples of deamidation occurring at lower pH, this occurs primarily through a mechanism independent of succinimide formation. Factors such

TABLE 12.6
Examples of the Effects of Deamidation of Various Biopharmaceutical Molecules

Biological Molecules	Effect of Deamidation
Growth hormone-releasing factor analogs	Methanol raises the degree of helicity, thus decreasing the rate of deamidation
RNAase	The relatively rigid backbone in the loop, which is stabilized by a disulfide between Cys-8 and Cys-12 and by the–turn at residues 66–68, helps prevent the cyclic formation imide. However, when the enzyme is reduced and denatured before being refolded, aspartic and isoaspartic forms are formed, demonstrating different enzymatic activities. As Asp-67 is replaced with Iso-Asp-67, the isoaspartic form refolds at half the rate of the completely amidated form
Human growth hormone	Alters proteolytic cleavage decreasing biological activity
IFN-beta	Increase in biological activity
Peptide growth-hormone-releasing factor	As compared to the native peptide, converting to aspartyl and iso-aspartyl types decreases bioactivity by 25 and 500 times, respectively
Hemoglobin	Hemoglobin's propensity for oxygen improves when an Asn-Gly site is deamidated
Class II major histocompatibility complex molecules	Asparagine deamidation perturbs antigen presentation
Human epidermal growth factor	Isomerization of Asp 11 decreases its mitogenic activity by fivefold
Triose-phosphate isomerase	Subunit dissociation occurs when two Asn-Gly sequences are deamidated

as sequence and local structure, including steric effects, influence the deamidation rate. The presence of amino acids at Asn's carboxyl end significantly impacts the deamidation rate, which decreases as side-chain size and branching increase.

As pH increases, deamidation rates rise, and phosphate and carbonate buffers act as deamidation catalysts. At low pH, deprotonation of the amide group on the asparagine side chain of peptides and protein deprotonates. The nitrogen atom of the asparagine residue undergoes nucleophilic attack by the nitrogen atom of the amide anion peptide carbonyl carbon. In this series of reactions, the peptide chain is cleaved, yielding a fragment of succinimide peptides. Asparaginyl and asparaginyl peptides are formed after the succinamide ring is hydrolyzed.

Deamidation via unstable cyclic imide formation occurs at pH > 5.0, spontaneously hydrolyzing thereafter. Under highly acidic conditions (pH 1–2), direct hydrolysis of the amide side chain predominates over cyclic imide formation. Indirect hydrolysis of the amide is primarily responsible for peptide bond cleavage.

12.2.3.3 Racemization and Isomerization

Isomerization, a common chemical degradation pathway, results in outcomes similar to deamidation. It frequently occurs directly from the Asp residue or indirectly through the succinimide intermediate. Isomerization, like deamidation, is more prevalent at neutral and basic pH levels and is affected by steric effects.

One of the most common non-enzymatic degradation outcomes is structural isomerization and racemization, especially isomerization of aspartate to isoaspartate residues caused by neutral pH deamidation. Isomerization often involves Asn, Asp, and Gln, all containing an intermediate succinimide. Asp degrades much slower than Asn due to this mechanism. Deamidation produces iso-Asp and Asp in a 3:1 ratio, influenced by location and mobility. Mechanisms for aspartate–isoaspartate deamidation and isomerization are alike, involving a cyclic intramolecular imide intermediate.

Isomerization can induce racemization as part of the deamidation reaction. Succinimide intermediates formed during asparagine deamidation are prone to racemization, producing d-asparagine residues. Except for glycine, other amino acids racemize at alkaline pH. The deamidation rates of individual amide residues are determined by their primary sequence, three-dimensional structure, and solution properties such as pH, temperature, ionic strength, and buffer ions. Typically, the deamidation rate of glutamine residues is lower than that of asparagine residues.

12.2.3.4   Temperature

Storage temperatures affect deamidation rates, varying with the buffers used. Amines with high temperature coefficients, like tris and histidine, alter pH when stored at temperatures differing from preparation temperatures. Formulation pH changes can affect deamidation rates since both deamidation and isomerization are pH-dependent reactions. Indirectly, the water dissociation constant, influenced by temperature, affects deamidation rates via variations in hydroxyl ion concentration.

12.2.3.5   Excipients

Organic solvents reduce deamidation rates by lowering solution dielectric constants. Addition of co-solutes like glycerol, sucrose, and ethanol decreases the dielectric strength, resulting in notably lower rates of isomerization and deamidation. Decreasing the medium's dielectric strength from 80 (water) to 35 (PVP/glycerol/water formulations) leads to a six-fold reduction in peptide deamidation concentrations due to less stabilized ionic intermediates. Insulin prepared in neutral solutions containing phenol eliminates deamidation by stabilizing tertiary structure (-helix formation) around the deamidizing residue, reducing intermediate imide formation.

12.2.3.6   Hydrolysis

Hydrolysis, akin to deamidation, leads to succinimide formation, racemization, and isomerization. In the hydrolysis cycle,–x-Asp-y is termed labile, reacting 100 times faster in dilute acids than other bonds. Asp-Pro bonds are 8–20 times more prone to hydrolysis than other Asp-x or x-Asp bonds. Asp-Gly is vulnerable in highly acidic conditions (pH 0.3 to 3). Other peptide bonds cleave faster at the N-terminus than–x-Ser or–x-Ther.

Hydrolysis of peptide bonds such as Asp-Gly and Asp-Pro causes protein fragmentation. Asp-Y is 100 times more susceptible to hydrolysis than any other peptide bond. Hydrolysis typically occurs post-deamidation of Asn residues, as observed in insulin formulations.

Asp–Gly and Asp–Pro peptide bonds are most susceptible to cleavage in hydrolytic proteins. The hinge area, an antibody's most flexible domain, is also prone to hydrolysis. Altering pH from 9 to 5 can change the hydrolysis sites in a recombinant monoclonal antibody (mAb) peptide, causing increased cleavage beyond that area.

Multimeric proteins can degrade into peptide fragments after dissociating into monomers (or single peptide chain proteins) with two or more subunits. Non-enzymatic fragmentation of peptide bonds yields lower molecular weight polypeptides than the intact parent protein.

To minimize hydrolytic fragmentation, formulations must be adequately buffered to maintain an appropriate pH for each protein type. For instance, calcitonin undergoes hydrolysis at a simple pH but not at pH seven, even at room temperature. Buffer composition also influences hydrolysis. Recombinant human macrophage colony-stimulating factor fragments in phosphate-buffered solutions but not in histidine-buffered solutions at the same pH and ionic strength.

Limiting the role of proteases in protein purification, whether from the manufacturing process (e.g., host-cell proteins) or external contamination (e.g., adventitious microbes), is critical.

12.2.3.7   Disulfide Bond

The disulfide bond plays a crucial role in the three-dimensional structure, influencing the activity and antigenicity of biopharmaceutical products. Various chemical stresses can break these bonds, leading to a significant loss of activity.

Cross-linking, whether mediated by disulfide bond formation or not, can cause chemical degradation. In cases where disulfide bonds are involved in cross-linking, the reaction occurs through the formation of new disulfide bonds or exchanging existing ones. Intramolecular disulfide bonding can alter the tertiary structure, while intermolecular or inter-domain disulfide bonding can affect the quaternary structure or result in covalent aggregate formation. At higher pH levels, the formation of reactive thiolate ions (S) from the Cys residue thiol group (–SH) is favored, potentially increasing the likelihood of disulfide bond formation.

12.2.3.8 Glycation

The presence and positioning of oligosaccharides impact the rate of peptide hydrolysis under low pH conditions. The location does not affect hinge-region cleavage but reduces fragmentation in the CH2 domain. (For more information, see Figure 12.1.) Acidic and simple hydrolytic cleavage of peptide bonds may yield different results. Recombinant human macrophage-stimulating factor generates diverse peptide fragments under acidic and simple pH solutions. Enzymatic protein fragmentation can result from residual or contaminating proteases or, in some instances, autoproteolysis of an enzymatic protein.

Most proteins undergo glycosylation and some experience post-translational modifications like phosphorylation, altering their degradation pathways and kinetics. Conversely, reducing sugars interact with highly susceptible amino groups such as Lys–amino and N-terminal–amino groups through the Maillard reaction. Glycation affects acidification (loss of positive charge), insolubility, cross-linking, and chromophore formation. A change in solution color might signal unexpected glycation reactions sensitive to pH, temperature, amino acid group pKa, adjacent amino acids, sugar reduction concentration, and protein concentration. The concentration dependence of glycation is a significant concern, with several mAbs now formulated at high concentrations to minimize dose-volume for subcutaneous injection or infusion rather than intravenous administration.

12.2.3.9 Oxidation

Reactive oxygen intermediates or oxidants like hydrogen peroxide, found in formulations as contaminants of polysorbates or leached from disposable tubing, along with oxygen, metal ions, and other excipients, cause protein oxidation. Residues Met, Cys, Trp, His, and Tyr are susceptible to oxidation, altering a protein's physicochemical properties, leading to aggregation or fragmentation. The location of oxidized amino acids concerning a protein's functional or epitope-like domain can impact its potency and immunogenicity.

Amino acids in the system interact with oxygen radicals, rendering proteins and peptides vulnerable to oxidative damage. Methionine (Met), cysteine (Cys), histidine (His), tryptophan (Trp), and tyrosine (Tyr) are highly prone to oxidation (Tyr). Met and Cys contain sulfur atoms, while His, Trp, and Tyr contain aromatic atoms.

The key products of oxidation are listed in Table 12.7.

Table 12.8 lists some of the key catalysts for the oxidation of proteins.

External factors causing oxidation include light exposure, interaction with trace amounts of transition metal ions, and the presence of excipient degradation products (e.g., hydrogen peroxide from polysorbate degradation). Oxidation can lead to increased aggregation. Methionine residue is the most commonly oxidized, resulting in sulfoxide and sulfone as the main by-products. The oxidation rate is influenced by the local structure around the oxidation-prone group (e.g., surface exposure and steric hindrance) and solution pH. While increasing the solution's pH can accelerate oxidation in some cases, this is not a frequent occurrence.

Oxidation can diminish potency and induce conformational changes, leading to aggregation depending on the oxidation site. Clinical protection cannot usually be extrapolated from knowledge of degradation pathways. For instance, the biological activity of parathyroid hormone differs based on whether it undergoes single or double oxidation of Met-8 or Met-18 (Met-8 with Met–18).

TABLE 12.7
Key Degradation Products of Oxidation

Residues	Oxidation Products
Met	Met-Sulfoxide
Cys	-S-S-disulfide cross-links, sulfenic acid/sulfinic acid/sulfonic acid
His	2-oxoimidasoline, aspartate/asparagine
Trp	N-formylkynurinine, kynurenine
Tyr	Try-Try cross-link, 3,4-dihydroxy phenylalanine

TABLE 12.8
Oxidation Source and Process

Source	Element that Contributes
Reagents for chemical analysis	Oxidative burst operation (H_2O_2, Fe^{2+}, Cu^{1+}, Glutathione, HOCl, HOBr,
Irradiation of activated phagocytes in the presence of oxygen UV light, Ozone	$1O_2$, ONOO)
	Potential for oxidation
Peroxides of lipids	Radicals with a lot of capacity
Mitochondria are the cells that make up the mitochondria (electron transport chain leakage)	HNE, MDA, and acrolein are all terms for the same thing.
	Xanthine oxidase, Myeloperoxidase, and P-450 enzymes are examples of oxidoreductase enzymes
Medications and their metabolites	Oxidative products, free radicals

Similarly, oxidation of Met-36 and Met-48 in human stem cell factor (SCF) by *Escherichia coli* reduces potency by 40% and 60%, respectively, increasing the constant dissociation rate SCF dimer by 2–3 times, implying improved binding and tertiary structure of the subunit. These examples stress the need to thoroughly assess any molecule's behavior changes due to degradation.

Met, Tyr, Trp, His, and Cys are oxidation-sensitive residues commonly found in mAbs.

While less common than deamidation and isomerization, oxidation is a major degradation mode for some proteins, such as OKT3 (IgG2), exhibiting oxidation at several Met residues and free Cys when stored at 5°C.

Species that act as buffers: Buffer species primarily impact contaminants, possess metal chelating abilities, and exhibit potential interactions with reactive oxygen species. Tris functions as an iron and copper chelator and a hydroxyl radical scavenger. Citrate also acts as a chelator, while phosphoric acid (weak) and tartaric acid serve as buffers. In Fenton chemistry, a bicarbonate ion is necessary, but generalizations regarding this requirement are not straightforward.

Chelators: Metal-ion concentrations in the atmosphere influence metal-ion–catalyzed oxidation. The presence of Fe^{3+}, Ca^{2+}, Cu^{2+}, Mg^{2+}, or Zn^{2+} at 0.15-ppm chloride salts has no effect on the oxidation rate of human insulin-like growth factor-1. However, a significant increase in oxidation occurs when the metal concentration is raised to 1 ppm.

Cys, Met, and His are particularly prone to oxidation in the presence of metals. Potent 1:1 chelators (e.g., EDTA, desferrioxamine, nitrilotriacetic acid) can affect oxidation rates based on stoichiometry (chelator/Fe ratio). Oxidation rates increase until all Fe is sequestered, reaching a maximum ratio of 1. At ratios of 1.1 to 1.2, almost complete protein inhibition is observed. A significant excess (5–20) is required to counteract the effects of poor chelators (e.g., o-phenanthroline). Chelate-Fe (III) complexes inhibit site-specific oxidation while increasing non-site-specific oxidation. These complexes prevent iron from binding to potential sites and promote the formation of ROS species unlike metal-binding sites. Peptide bond hydrolysis, pyroglutamate (more acidic; $z=-1$), deamidation (more acidic; $z=-1$), succinimide (more simple or neutral), and glycation (more acidic; acidic or essential).

Cysteine: Cysteine oxidation is more common at alkaline pH, which deprotonates thiol groups. This oxidation leads to the formation of intermolecular or intramolecular disulfide bonds, further oxidizing to form sulfenic acid. Transition metals strongly catalyze cysteine oxidation at higher pH (optimum approximately 6). However, this reaction is less susceptible to mild oxidants such as hydrogen peroxide compared to Met or Cys. In the absence of a nearby thiol for disulfide formation, oxidation can produce sulfenic, sulfinic, and sulfonic acids. In a reducing environment, cysteine oxidation results in a nucleophilic attack on disulfide bonds by thiolate ions, forming new disulfide bonds and separate thiolate ions. The newly formed thiolate can further react with another disulfide bond to regenerate cysteine.

Protein degradation generates intermolecular disulfide connections, accumulating mispaired disulfide bonds and scrambled disulfide bridges, altering the protein's conformation and subunit associations. By-products of cysteine residues that spontaneously oxidize in the presence of metal ions or adjacent thiol groups include sulfinic acid and cysteic acid. Human fibroblast growth factor (FGF-1) can undergo copper-catalyzed oxidation, leading to homodimers.

Cysteine oxidation impacts the spatial orientation of thiol groups in proteins, with the rate of oxidation inversely proportional to the distance between such groups. This can result in the formation of large oligomers or non-functional monomers, as seen in basic fibroblast growth factor (bFGF) containing easily oxidized cysteines that form intermolecular or intramolecular disulfide bonds, inducing conformational protein modifications. Cysteine oxidation has a significant impact on the spatial orientation of thiol groups in proteins. The rate of oxidation is inversely proportional to the distance between such thiol groups, possibly resulting in the development of large oligomers or non-functional monomers in the long term, as in the case of basic fibroblast growth factor (bFGF), which contains three easily oxidized cysteines and forms intermolecular or intramolecular disulfide bonds that trigger conformational protein modifications. The volume of the protein's side chains is increased by cysteine disulfide bonds, resulting in unfavorable van der Waals interactions.

Excipients: Peroxides (e.g., in polysorbates) and trace metals, particularly Fe and Cu, significantly affect common excipient organisms. High concentrations of sugars and polyols inhibit peroxide contamination caused by polysorbates and polyethylene glycols (PEGs), possibly through a metal complexation mechanism. Peroxide contamination from polysorbates and polyethylene glycols (PEGs), commonly used as pharmaceutical excipients, can lead to oxidation. The degree of oxidation in rhG-CSF correlates with the amount of peroxide in Tween-80, with peroxide-induced oxidation being more pronounced than that caused by atmospheric oxygen. Plastic or elastomeric materials in primary packaging container closure systems, such as prefilled syringes, may also leach peroxide. The degree of oxidation in rhG-CSF was related to the amount of peroxide in Tween-80, with peroxide-induced oxidation appearing to be more extreme than atmospheric oxygen. Peroxide is leached from plastics and elastomers used in packaging.

Exogenous variables: pH, Temperature, and Excipients Buffer.

Histidine: Histidine residues are highly susceptible to oxidation when reacting with their imidazole rings (metal or photocatalyzed catalyzed oxidation), resulting in additional hydroxyl species. During light and metal oxidation, oxidized histidine can produce asparagine/aspartate and 2-oxo-histidine (2-O-His), acting as a transient moiety causing protein aggregation and precipitation, complicating the isolation of 2-O-His as individual degradants. Photooxidation through singlet oxygen occurs commonly with photosensitizers. The inclination and rate of oxidation are influenced by surrounding residues and amino acid conformation, resulting in colored solutions.

Light: Photooxidation levels are in the following order: non-site-specific processes (e.g., hydrogen peroxide, light) oxidize buried residues at a higher rate. Photo-induced oxidation primarily targets Trp and His. Ultraviolet light is essential for protecting proteins from light-induced damage. Photooxidation can alter primary, secondary, and tertiary protein structures, impacting their long-term stability, bioactivity, and immunogenicity. Even after turning off the light source, biochemical cascades affecting a protein can persist. The effects depend on the energy provided to a protein and the available oxygen from the atmosphere. When a compound absorbs enough light at a specific wavelength, it gains sufficient energy to enter an excited state known as photooxidation. The excited molecule transfers its energy to molecular oxygen, splitting it into reactive singlet oxygen atoms. Tryptophan, histidine, and tyrosine are light-modified in the presence of oxygen. Various hydroxy tyrosine byproducts arise from tyrosine photooxidation. The cross-linking of oxidized tyrosine residues causes protein aggregation. In human growth hormone exposed to intense light, oxidation occurs mainly at histidine-21. Photodegradation of the peptide backbone is also possible. Alternatively, energetic proteins can directly photosensitize other proteins, commonly through low pH methionine and tryptophan residues. Excipients and leachants can collaboratively promote protein oxidation and degradation. Some formulating components influence the rate of photooxidation, such as phosphate buffer that accelerates methionine degradation more than other buffer systems. Stabilizing excipients such as polyols and sugars that help stabilize protein structure can reduce oxidation rates, while denaturing/unfolding reagents increase protein oxidation. Ascorbic acid enhances the oxidation of human ciliary neurotrophic factor, whereas using a reducing agent such as ascorbate can boost oxidation.

Photooxidation has the potential to alter the primary, secondary, and tertiary structures of proteins, impacting their long-term stability, bioactivity, and immunogenicity. Even when the light source is switched off, the impact of light exposure can set off a series of biochemical events that affect proteins. These effects hinge on the energy and oxygen levels the protein receives from its environment. When a compound absorbs sufficient light at a specific wavelength, it gains enough energy to enter an excited state, a phenomenon known as photooxidation. In this excited state, the molecule transfers its energy to molecular oxygen, leading to the creation of reactive singlet oxygen atoms. Tryptophan, histidine, and tyrosine are particularly affected by light in the presence of oxygen. Tyrosine photooxidation generates mono-, di-, tri-, and tetrahydroxy byproducts. Furthermore, oxidized tyrosine residues can cause aggregation in certain proteins. The concentration of metal ions in the atmosphere can catalyze oxidation reactions. For instance, the presence of 0.15 ppm Fe^{3+}, Ca^{2+}, Cu^{2+}, Mg^{2+}, or Zn^{2+} chloride salts does not significantly impact the oxidation rate of human insulin-like growth factor-1, but there's a marked increase in oxidation when the metal concentration is raised to 1 ppm. The hierarchy of photooxidation levels follows this order: its > Trp > Met > Tyr; with Trp and His being the primary targets of photo-induced oxidation. Non-site-specific pathways (e.g., H_2O_2, light) encounter difficulty in oxidizing buried residues. Ultraviolet light plays a crucial role in safeguarding proteins. Notably, primary, secondary, and tertiary amines can undergo structural alterations due to photooxidation.

12.3   FORMULATION COMPOSITION

The route of administration and the physicochemical properties of a product, such as those of other drugs, determine the composition of biopharmaceutical formulations. The large molecular size and high molecular mass of drug molecules lead to low membrane permeability, thereby limiting available delivery routes. Passive diffusion facilitates the passage of drugs with a molecular mass below 500 Da through membranes in the gastrointestinal tract and the skin. However, the inner and outer plexiform layers of the human retina restrict the diffusion of macromolecules larger than 76 kDa, with those larger than 150 kDa unable to enter the inner retina. Nasal mucosa exhibits low membrane permeability for molecules larger than one kDa. The hydrophilicity of biopharmaceuticals restricts most administration routes because proteins larger than 3–5 kDa are considered peptidyl molecules, and antibodies larger than 150 kDa are categorized as such.

Given that most protein drugs have a log P value less than zero, their permeation through biological membranes is challenging, complicating protein drug delivery to intracellular targets. [See the Appendix at the end of the chapter.] The lipophilic nature of biological membranes and the 3–10 paracellular space impede the diffusion of proteins, necessitating active transport or endocytosis for cellular uptake. However, endosome entrapment remains a major drawback of the endocytic pathway for proteins, leading to lysosomal enzyme degradation.

Another physicochemical property influencing absorption is the surface charge of a biopharmaceutical, determined by the protein's amino acid sequence and the surrounding pH. Deamination, isomerization, or post-translational alterations often lead to changes in the protein's net charge and the formation of acidic and basic variants. Due to their surface charge, protein drugs can interact with molecules on cell surfaces or tissue components, impacting protein absorption, distribution, and elimination in the body.

12.3.1 EXCIPIENTS AND PROPERTIES

Preformulation involves assessing the biochemical and biophysical characteristics of a biopharmaceutical product based on its amino acid sequence, influenced by factors such as pH, ionic strength, and excipients. A systematic approach such as the design of experiment (DoE) or the empirical phase diagram helps establish stability-indicating assays and define lead excipients (EPD) in the presence of stress, resulting in structural and functional changes.

Excipients in biopharmaceutical formulations aren't licensed as finished products but range from well-known organic or inorganic molecules to complex and challenging-to-classify structures. The choice of excipient is influenced by statutory requirements across different jurisdictions. The US Food and Drug Administration (FDA) maintains a searchable database (IID) of approved concentrations, dosage forms, and administration routes (www.accessdata.fda.gov/scripts/cder/iig/index.cfm), while the Japanese Pharmaceutical Excipients Dictionary (JPED) compiles excipients used in approved medications in Japan (www.yakuji.co.jp/wpyj-002/wp-content/uploads/2020/05/jpe2018 order form.pdf).

Health Canada publishes a list of permitted non-medicinal agents, but the European Medicines Agency lacks a comparable list or database for European products.

Table 12.10 lists the different types of pharmaceutical excipients that are commonly used in biopharmaceutical products and some examples.

While formulations vary widely in their composition, Table 12.11 lists the most common ranges of quantities used.

TABLE 12.10
Common Pharmaceutical Excipients

Category	Example
Amino acids	Arginine, aspartic acid, glutamic acid, lysine, proline, glycine, histidine, methionine
Buffer	Phosphate, acetate, histidine, glutamate
Buffers	Acetate, succinate, citrate, histidine, phosphate, tris
Cyclodextrins	Hydroxypropyl beta-cyclodextrin
pH	Buffers
Preservatives	Benzyl alcohol, m-cresol, phenol, 2-phenoxyethanol
Solubilizer	Salts, amino acids, surfactants
Stabilizer	Surfactants, sugars, salts, antioxidants
Stabilizers/bulking agents	Lactose, trehalose, dextrose, sucrose, sorbitol, glycerol, albumin, gelatin, mannitol, dextran
Surfactants	Tween 20, Tween 80, Pluronic F68
Tonicity, bulk modifier	Sodium chloride, sorbitol, mannitol, glycine, polyanions, salts

TABLE 12.11
General Ranges of Formulation Components

Component	General Range
Buffer	5–100 mM
Component	General range
pH	4–8
Salts	0–300 mM
Stabilizers	1%–10%
Surfactants	0.01%–0.1% (w/v)

Dosing criteria determine the quantity of the active ingredient in a formulation, with concentration linked to the product's solubility. Protein solubility refers to the average amount of protein soluble in co-solvents, yielding a visibly transparent solution without precipitated proteins, crystals, or gels. Factors such as ionic strength, salt form, pH, temperature, and specific excipients influence protein solubility, impacting bulk water surface tension and protein binding to water and ions or self-association. Protein binding to certain excipients or salts alters the protein's conformation or masks specific amino acids involved in self-interaction, influencing solubility. Some salts, amino acids, and sugars preferentially hydrate proteins, leading to altered solubility by stabilizing more compact conformations.

A variety of excipients are used to stabilize protein formulations. To improve the product's safety and efficacy, excipients, and buffers for formulation (Table 12.8) are used.

The most common ingredients in biopharmaceutical drug formulations, according to an analysis, are:

- Buffering agents such as phosphates, citrates, and acetates ensure that the pH remains as stable as possible.
- Stabilizers such as surfactants and sugars include polysorbates, albumin, mannitol, sucrose, and sorbitol.
- Sugars and electrolytes like sodium chloride are examples of ingredients that change tonicity and conductivity.

Figure 12.3 shows the percentage of the most common components used in the approximately 200 biopharmaceutical injectable drugs.

12.3.1.1 pH

pH stands out as the most critical among the mentioned formulation variables. Other formulation methods pose significant challenges in resolving physical property issues, such as precipitation due to solubility and stability. pH optimization emerges as a simple yet effective solution to combat these problems. pH triggers various chemical reactions including deamidation, cyclic imide formation, disulfide scrambling, peptide bond cleavage, and oxidation. Careful evaluation of the properties of other functional excipients is necessary. For instance, sucrose, used to stabilize proteins during lyophilization and in solid-state storage, warrants thorough examination.

Adjusting the pH and ionic strength of a protein solution, incorporating sugars, amino acids, polyols, and utilizing surfactants are effective strategies to prevent oxidation and precipitation. An in-depth assessment of optimal pH and osmotic conditions stands as a critical element in formulation production to circumvent protein aggregation or precipitation, which is irreversible and is prevented by surfactants, polyols, or sugars.

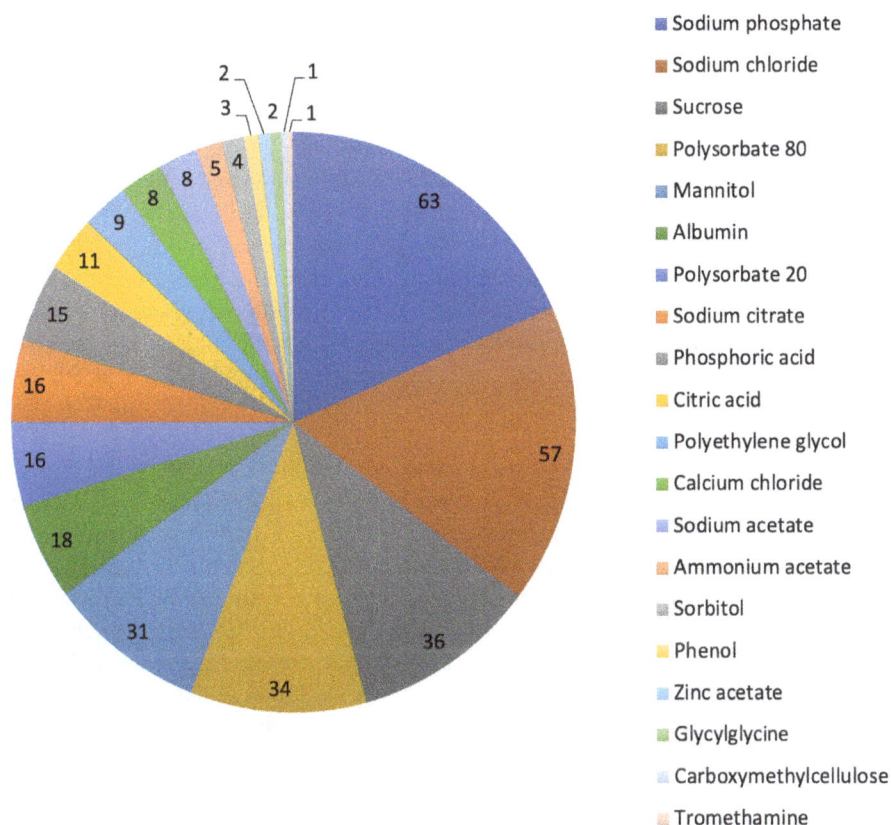

FIGURE 12.3 Percentage occurrence of common formulation components in biopharmaceutical drugs

12.3.1.2 Surface Tension

Surfactants, like sodium polyacrylate, possess both hydrophobic and hydrophilic portions (e.g., an alkyl chain carboxyl and carboxylate groups).

Nonionic detergents, known as surfactants, are utilized to enhance stability and prevent aggregation. These compounds establish stability by lowering the surface tension of the solution and binding to hydrophobic sites on the proteins, thereby reducing the likelihood of protein-protein interactions leading to aggregate formation. Notably, nonionic detergents such as Tween 20 and Tween 80 prevent the formation of soluble protein aggregates below the critical micelle concentrations (CMC). When introduced into IgG solutions, polysorbate (Tween) 80 stabilizes small aggregates and prevents their enlargement into larger particles.

12.3.1.3 Tonicity

The osmotic pressure of an "isotonic" solution mirrors that of human blood, typically ranging between 250 to 350 mOsmol/kg. Buffering agents, including phosphate, glycinate, carbonate, and citrate buffers utilizing sodium, potassium, or ammonium ions as counterions, maintain aqueous solutions against pH changes resulting from the addition of acid, alkali, or solvent dilution.

12.3.1.4 Protectants

Novel excipients play a crucial role in enhancing protein/peptide stability, as commonly used excipients provide only limited stabilization. Examples like resveratrol, a natural phenol, hydroxybutyrate, polyamines, octanoic acid, and quinone-tryptophan derivatives illustrate this trend. Additionally, hydrophobic salts such as pentane-1,5-diamine salts and camphor-10-sulfonic acid salts reduce the viscosity of mAb solutions by tenfold. However, using uncommon excipients might necessitate extensive safety testing, potentially including in vivo studies.

Lyoprotectants, when employed alongside a protein of interest, aid in preventing or minimizing the chemical and physical instability of proteins during lyophilization and subsequent storage.

Preservatives serve to inhibit bacterial activity and can be optional in formulations. For instance, developing a multi-use formulation becomes easier by incorporating a preservative. Various preservatives like octadecyldimethylbenzyl ammonium chloride, hexamethonium chloride, benzalkonium chloride (a mixture of alkyl benzyl dimethylammonium chlorides with long-chain alkyl groups), benzethonium chloride, and aromatic alcohols such as phenol, butyl, and benzyl alcohol, alkyl parabens such as methyl or propylparaben, catechol, resorcinol, cyclohexanol, 3-pentanol, and m-cresol, as well as alkyl parabens such as methyl or propylparaben.

One common method of preventing aggregation is to limit protein mobility is a common method to prevent aggregation by reducing molecular collisions. Excipients such as surfactants (e.g., polysorbate 20 and 80), carbohydrates (e.g., cyclodextrin derivatives), and amino acids (e.g., arginine and histidine) help prevent aggregation by adsorbing to the air-liquid interface and safeguarding the protein. However, certain excipients such as polysorbate 80 can lead to micelle formation, heightening the risk of immunogenicity. Cyclodextrin stabilizes commercially available antibody-based drugs in a hydrogel formulation. Pluronic F68, trehalose, glycine, and amino acids such as arginine, glycine, glutamate, and histidine, which are found in many commercial protein therapy products, are all considered safe excipients (GRAS). Avastin® (bevacizumab, 25 mg/mL) contains ingredients such as trehalose dehydrates, sodium phosphate, and polysorbate 20. Histidine hydrochloride, histidine, trehalose dehydrate, polysorbate 20, methionine, and water for injection are all excipients in subcutaneous Herceptin® (trastuzumab, 600 mg). Chelating agents are used to prevent metal-induced protein aggregation.

12.3.1.5 Stabilizers

Utilizing large polymeric excipients allows for protein stabilization, where neutral polymers function as crowding agents to stabilize proteins by eliminating steric repulsion. Examples include PVP, Ficoll70, hydroxyethyl (heta) starch, or PEG 4000. Recent compositions involving functionalized trehalose-containing dextrans and glycopolymers aim to enhance process and storage stability. Additionally, polyanions/polycations like heparin, dextran sulfate, pentosan polysulfate, polyphosphoric acid, poly-L-glutamic acid, and poly(acrylic acid) or poly(acrylamide) are potential stabilizers due to their role in protein-polyion interactions (methacrylic acid). Activity between polycationic chitosan and negatively charged lactate dehydrogenase (LDH) results in significant stabilization during air-jet nebulization. When agitated, however, negative heparin and keratinocyte growth factor 2 (KGF-2) activity promotes protein aggregation.

Strong interactions can lead to protein destabilization, exemplified by the preferential interaction mechanism. The fibrillation process, responsible for the formation of amyloid fibrils linked to various human diseases, involves interactions between crystalline and non-native protein species. (Under certain conditions and over time, proteins lose their native folded state and form amyloid fibrils, a mechanism linked to a variety of human diseases. Foreign surfaces, such as nanoparticles with different surface properties, can disrupt this fibrillation process.)

Utilizing recombinant hyaluronidase enzyme in protein formulation facilitates rapid tissue distribution, allowing for larger-than-normal injection volumes. However, incorporating polymers or proteins in protein formulations increases complexity, posing challenges in formulation characterization and stability studies.

12.3.2 Liquid Formulations

When designing liquid formulations, various interactions like electrostatic, Van der Waals, hydrogen bonding, and hydrophobicity are taken into account. High concentrations of saccharides such as sucrose, trehalose, and lactose, along with polyhydrated alcohols like sorbitol, mannitol, and polyethylene glycol, aid in maintaining the native conformation of biologics. This prevents their interaction with the protein surface. Saccharose isn't used due to increased surface tension. The process of "salting in" enhances protein solubility by adding small salt amounts. While salts serve as tonicity regulators, they can sometimes negatively impact conformational stability. Consequently, counterions and their concentrations, as per the Hofmeister series, are employed to alter the stability profile—a critical consideration in pre-formulation screening. For instance, different buffer species at varying concentrations affecting ionic strength can achieve identical pH states, thereby influencing protein stability. The binding of Zn2+ to human growth hormone illustrates how ligand binding preserves the native protein state.

Surface-active agents prevent protein adsorption, denaturation, and aggregation at interfaces (air-water and solid-water). They affect protein stability by binding differently to native and denatured protein states. Surface denaturation can also result from agitation, freeze-thaw stress tests, or low surfactant concentrations like Polysorbate 20, Polysorbate 80, Pluronic F68, or others adept at reducing both soluble and insoluble aggregates. Addressing issues like metal ions, barium from glass vials, vulcanizing agents from stoppers, tungsten oxide from prefilled syringes, and silicone oil penetration is crucial. EDTA removes metal leachates from stoppers. Similar to pre-formulation, counterions and their concentrations based on the Hofmeister series critically impact the stability profile. Varying buffer species at different concentrations affecting ionic strengths can yield the same pH state, thereby impacting protein stability. Binding ligands such as Zn^{2+} to human growth hormone also aid in maintaining native protein structure.

Antimicrobial preservatives are commonly used in multi-dose biopharmaceuticals, constituting a third of all such products. They can induce protein aggregation, complicating biopharmaceutical stabilization. Commonly used preservatives include m-cresol, benzyl alcohol or phenol, phenoxyethanol, and chlorobutanol. Screening various preservatives before their standalone or combined usage is advisable.

12.3.3 Lyophilized Formulations

Lyophilization with suitable excipients enhances protein stability by reducing protein mobility and limiting conformational flexibility. This process minimizes hydrolytic reactions due to water removal. Proper excipients, like lyoprotectants, prevent aggregate formation during lyophilization and final product storage. Achieving adequate stability depends on the lyoprotectant-to-protein molar ratio. Ratios of 300:1 or higher are necessary, especially for room temperature storage. However, such ratios can cause undesirable viscosity increases.

Lyophilization may be necessary due to protein instability in an aqueous solution without preservatives. When stability, storage, and shipping requirements align with the target product profile, lyophilization becomes an important alternative to liquid formulation, especially for highly thermolabile products and live virus vaccine items. Freezing is a prerequisite for lyophilization, followed by vacuum-assisted primary and secondary drying. The drying process, however, presents its unique challenges. Denaturation can occur during freezing, caused by freeze-concentrate conditions, frozen surface interfaces, or cold-denaturation. Formulations during the freeze-concentrate phase should consider local salt and buffer concentrations' effects, along with increasing trapped oxygen concentrations.

Similarly, in lyophilized products, changes in pH due to buffer crystallization must be factored into the formulation design space. Buffering at physiological pH with a low concentration of potassium phosphate buffer (including ten mM) is preferable to sodium phosphate buffer due to the significant pH shift during freezing for sodium phosphate. Citrate, Tris, and Histidine are good buffer choices if the pH range is appropriate. To minimize oxidation, antioxidants (e.g., ascorbic acid) and scavengers (e.g., thiourea) can be utilized.

Lyoprotectants, external stabilizers, might be necessary in addition to cryoprotectants. For instance, sorbitol may appear as a good stabilizer during liquid pre-formulation screening, but it's not favored in dried formulations due to its low glass transition temperature. Lyoprotectants, such as sucrose and trehalose, with high glass transition temperatures, act as solid water substitutes, preserving the native state in the dry state. However, the use of reduced sugars (e.g., lactose) requires careful assessment in risk evaluation. Excipient combinations, especially in a multi-stabilizer system, can be limited due to the possibility of phase separation (e.g., PEG-Dextran). Trehalose is preferred over sucrose due to its acid hydrolysis ability at a lower pH.

To prevent "blowout" of low-concentration products, bulking agents (1 percent solid) are added to lyophilized products. Examples include amorphous bulking agents like sucrose, trehalose, lactose, raffinose, dextran, hydroxyethyl starch (HES), or crystalline ones like glycine and mannitol, for amorphous or high eutectic temperature (Teu) crystalline excipients. Mannitol's selection is limited due to mannitol hydrate presence, posing risks of glass breakage during manufacturing (due to high fill volume, incorrect freezing procedure, and high concentration).

Isotonicity plays a role in pain relief. Achieving isotonicity in a lyophilized product is challenging due to the concentration of both protein and excipients during reconstitution. A 500:1 protein molar ratio may result in hypertonic preparations if the protein concentration exceeds 100 mg/mL.

While freeze-drying is extensively used for protein drugs, it has drawbacks, leading to the development of alternative drying methods (e.g., spray-drying, spray-freezing, supercritical fluid drying, foam drying) for proteins like insulin, trypsin, human growth hormones, and monoclonal antibodies.

12.3.4 Higher-Concentration Formulations

Higher concentrations are often needed for subcutaneous administration's lower volume. Yet, as protein concentrations increase, their physical properties can drastically change, affecting opalescence, viscosity, and protein aggregation/immunogenicity. Manufacturing, administration, and marketability of biotherapeutic products are at risk due to these altered properties.

Subcutaneous routes have a limited volume of 1.5 mL. Formulations requiring large doses, over 1 mg/kg or 100 mg per dose, are formulated at concentrations exceeding 100 mg/mL. Developing high concentration formulations for proteins prone to aggregation is challenging. At higher concentrations, protein interactions can induce reversible self-association, leading to the formation of insoluble aggregates. Increased concentration heightens the probability of reversible oligomers, such as dimers and tetramers, due to enhanced molecular collisions. Aggregates can form through mechanisms like covalent linkages, for instance, disulfide exchange, even with minor native structure conformational changes, particularly at higher concentrations.

A high-concentration solution entails solutes occupying a substantial space. Another definition is when molecular size aligns with the distance between Van der Waals' surfaces, termed "high concentration" due to molecular proximity. The primary hurdle in achieving high concentration formulations is the solubility of the target protein, influenced by molecular properties (sequence, charge distribution) and solution conditions (pH, ionic strength, etc.). Solubility defines the maximum protein amount in a solution without visible particles, precipitates, or clumps after 30 minutes of centrifugation at 30,000 g with a co-solute. Besides solubility, factors like opacity, viscosity, and aggregation are vital in mAb formulation. Opacity, expressed in turbidity units in nephelometry, results from reversible protein-protein and liquid-liquid phase separations. Protein-protein interaction significantly impacts opalescence and viscosity at high concentrations, potentially leading to reversible self-association, increased viscosity, opalescence, and aggregation in closely packed molecules.

Viscosity escalation directly impacts manufacturability and injectability in high concentrations. Tangential flow filtration (TFF) is a common technique for buffer exchange and protein concentration in large-scale manufacturing (clinical and commercial). Elevated viscosity induces back pressure surpassing the pump's capacity due to cavitation and shear stress from rapid pumping through narrow tubing. This high pressure stresses the mAb, elevating manufacturing costs by prolonging production time at the very least.

Elevated viscosity significantly affects subcutaneous dosage administration. Glide force, determining the ease of subcutaneous injection by measuring the force to propel liquid through the syringe, is predominantly influenced by viscosity. As viscosity increases, injection site pain rises, potentially reducing patient compliance.

An emerging concept to tackle protein stability and high viscosity involves "nanoclusters" – densely packed protein molecules developed in the presence of a crowder like trehalose. At extremely high concentrations (up to 320 mg/mL), these form colloidally stable dispersions of nanoclusters (35–80 nm). Nanoclusters have protein molecules packed more closely than in bulk solution. While shorter distances between proteins may enhance interactions, they could compromise protein stability. The nanocluster concept requires further development.

12.3.5 EXAMPLES OF FORMULATIONS

The following is a list of a few commercial product compositions.

- Oprelvekin injection (interleukin [IL]-11).

Bill of Materials (Batch Size 1 L):

Scale/mL		Item	Material	Quantity	UOM
1.00	mg	1	Oprelvekin (interleukin [IL]-11)	1.00	g
4.60	mg	2	Glycine	4.60	g
0.32	mg	3	Dibasic sodium phosphate heptahydrate	0.32	g
0.11	mg	4	Monobasic sodium phosphate monohydrate	0.11	g
qs	mL	5	Water for injection, qs to	1.00	L

- Interleukin injection (IL-2).

Bill of Materials (Batch Size 1 L):

Scale/mL		Item	Material	Quantity	UOM
0.25	mg	1	IL-2	0.25	g
0.70	mg	2	Sodium laurate	0.70	g
10.00	mM	3	Disodium hydrogen phosphate	10.00	M
50.00	mg	4	Mannitol	50.00	g
Qs	mL	5	Hydrochloric acid for pH adjustment 1 M	qs	
qs	mL	6	Water for injection, qs to	1.00	L

- Interferon Alfa-2a injection.

Bill of Materials (Batch Size 1 L):

Scale/mL		Item	Material	Quantity	UOM
3MM	IU	1	Interferon alfa-2a	3B	IU
7.21	mg	2	Sodium chloride	7.21	g
0.20	mg	3	Polysorbate 80	0.20	g
10.00	mg	4	Benzyl alcohol	10.00	g
0.77	mg	5	Ammonium acetate	0.77	g
qs	mL	6	Water for injection, qs to	1.00	L

- Interferon Beta-1b.

Bill of Materials (Batch Size 1 L):

Scale/mL		Item	Material	Quantity	UOM
0.30	mg	1	Interferon beta-1b	0.30	g
15.00	mg	2	Albumin human	15.00	g
15.00	mg	3	Dextrose	15.00	g
5.40	mg	4*	Sodium chloride	5.40	g
qs	mL	5	Water for injection, qs to	1.00	L

This item is packaged separately as 0.54% solution (2 mL diluent for lyophilized product).

- Interferon Beta-1a injection.

Bill of Materials (Batch Size 1 L):

Scale/mL		Item	Material	Quantity	UOM
*33.00	mcg	1	Interferon beta-1a	33.00	mg
15.00	mg	2	Albumin (human)	15.00	g
5.80	mg	3	Sodium chloride	5.80	g
5.70	mg	4	Dibasic sodium phosphate	5.70	g
1.20	mg	5	Monobasic sodium phosphate	1.20	g
qs	mL	6	Water for injection, qs to	1.00	L

- Interferon Alfa-n3 injection.

Bill of Materials (Batch Size 1 L):

Scale/mL		Item	Material	Quantity	UOM
5 MM	U	1	Interferon alpha-n3	5B	U
3.30	mg	2	Liquefied phenol	3.30	g
1.00	mg	3	Albumin (human)	1.00	g
8.00	mg	4	Sodium chloride	8.00	g
1.74	mg	5	Sodium phosphate dibasic	1.74	g
0.20	mg	6	Potassium phosphate monobasic	0.20	g
0.20	mg	7	Potassium chloride	0.20	g
qs	mL	8	Water for injection, qs to	1.00	L

- Interferon Alfacon-1 injection.

Bill of Materials (Batch Size 1 L):

Scale/mL		Item	Material	Quantity	UOM
0.03	mg	1	Interferon Alfacon-1	0.03	g
5.90	mg	2	Sodium Chloride	5.90	g
3.80	mg	3	Sodium Phosphate	3.80	g
qs	mL	4	Water for Injection, qs to	1.00	L

- Interferon Gamma-1b injection.

Bill of Materials (Batch Size 1 L):

Scale/mL		Item	Material	Quantity	UOM
200.00	mcg	1	Interferon Gamma-1b*	200.00	mg
40.00	mg	2	Mannitol	40.00	g
0.72	mg	3	Sodium Succinate	0.72	g
0.10	mg	4	Polysorbate 20	0.10	g
qs	mL	5	Water for Injection, qs to	1.00	L

- Infliximab for injection.

Bill of Materials (Batch Size 1 L):

Scale/mL		Item	Material	Quantity	UOM
10.00	mg	1	Infliximab	10.00	g
50.00	mg	2	Sucrose	50.00	g
0.05	mg	3	Polysorbate 80	0.05	g
0.22	mg	4	Monobasic Sodium Phosphate Monohydrate	0.22	g
0.61	mg	5	Dibasic Sodium Phosphate Dihydrate		
qs	mL	6	Water for injection, qs to	1.00	L

- Daclizumab for injection.

Bill of Materials (Batch Size 1 L):

Scale/mL		Item	Material	Quantity	UOM
5.00	mg	1	Daclizumab	5.00	g
3.60	mg	2	Sodium Phosphate Monobasic Monohydrate	3.60	g
11.00	mg	3	Sodium Phosphate Dibasic Heptahydrate	11.00	g
4.60	mg	4	Sodium Chloride	4.60	g
0.20	mg	5	Polysorbate 80 (Tween®)	0.20	G
qs	mL	6	Water for injection, qs to	1.00	L
Qs	mL	7	Sodium Hydroxide for pH adjustment	qs	
Qs	mL	8	Hydrochloric acid for pH adjustment	qs	
Qs	Cu ft	9	Nitrogen gas	qs	

- Coagulation factor VIIa (recombinant) injection.

Bill of Materials (Batch Size 1000 vials):

Scale/vial		Item	Material	Quantity	UOM
*1.20	mg	1	rFVIIa	1.20	g
5.84	mg	2	Sodium chloride	5.84	g
2.94	mg	3	Calcium chloride dihydrate	2.94	g
2.64	mg	4	Glycylglycine	2.64	g
0.14	mg	5	Polysorbate 80	0.14	g
60.00	mg	6	Mannitol	60.00	g

- Reteplase recombinant for injection.

Bill of Materials (Batch Size 1000 vials):

Scale/vial		Item	Material	Quantity	UOM
18.10	mg	1	Reteplase	18.10	g
8.32	mg	2	Tranexamic acid	8.32	g
136.24	mg	3	Dipotassium hydrogen phosphate	136.24	g
51.27	mg	4	Phosphoric acid	51.27	g
364.00	mg	5	Sucrose	364.00	g
5.20	mg	6	Polysorbate 80	5.20	g

- Alteplase recombinant injection.

Bill of Materials (Batch Size 1000 vials):

Scale/vial		Item	Material	Quantity	UOM
58MM	IU	1	Alteplase	100.00	g
3.50	g	2	L-arginine	3.50	kg
1.00	g	3	Phosphoric acid	1.00	kg
11.00	mg	4	Polysorbate 80	11.00	g
qs	mL	5	Water for injection, qs to	1.00	L

12.4 ROUTES OF ADMINISTRATION

Each administration route has its own set of limitations based on anatomical size and location, microclimate, complex physiological conditions, and formulations. The volume and viscosity of the fluid in the rectum affect drug absorption.

pH conditions in various biological environments affect the ionization, chemical stability, and absorption of protein-based drugs and their delivery mechanisms. For instance, protein drugs become unstable at physiological pH. The highly acidic gastric environment (pH 1–3) causes protein drug destabilization in the stomach, while higher pH reduces chemical degradation in the ileum and colon. Therefore, the buffering agent in an ocular delivery system plays a critical role, as hyperosmotic solutions cause transient dehydration of anterior chamber tissues, and hypotonic solutions can cause edema.

Oral protein delivery and bioavailability face challenges due to enzyme degradation in the gastrointestinal tract. Protease activity is higher in the small intestine but much lower in the colon. Hence, colon-targeted delivery systems have garnered attention as a viable mechanism for protein drug delivery. This approach can enhance drug absorption and duration of action. Colon-targeted drug delivery systems also prove useful in treating local bowel disorders like colon cancer, ulcerative colitis, Crohn's disease, and amoebiasis. Despite non-oral routes bypassing the hepatic first-pass effect, enzymatic barriers create a "pseudo-first-pass effect." For example, low metabolic enzyme activity can impede protein drug delivery through nasal and pulmonary routes.

Mucus and epithelial cell membranes act as major absorption barriers for non-injectable drugs. Mucus, coating all mucosal epithelia, acts as the first line of defense against mechanical damage and the entry of harmful substances into the eye, respiratory tract, and gastrointestinal tract. It physically shields large molecules and, due to its hydrophilic nature and negative charge, interacts with the drug, slowing drug diffusion and limiting absorption in the intestine (Figure 12.4).

Mucus comprises mucin-type glycoproteins and varies greatly in thickness throughout the body. For example, airway mucus ranges from 5 to 55 microns thick, while nasal tract mucus is very thin, creating a porous surface. In the eye, the precorneal mucin gel covering the conjunctiva measures 30–40 um thick. The thickness of the gastrointestinal mucus layer varies significantly by location and digestive system activity, being thickest in the stomach and colon, ranging from 10 to over 170 μm. Despite the colon's lack of proteolytic activity, drugs must penetrate this thicker mucus layer, making it an advantageous site for protein absorption.

Parenteral routes, excluding the mouth and alimentary canal (e.g., rectal), commonly deliver biopharmaceuticals via intravenous bolus, intravenous infusion, subcutaneous injection, and intramuscular injection. Despite its precision, parenteral injection faces challenges due to invasiveness, discomfort, infection risks, high cost, and low patient compliance.

Developing noninvasive drug delivery routes like oral, nasal, pulmonary, ophthalmic, rectal, or transdermal proves challenging due to biopharmaceuticals' large molecular size, hydrophilicity, low permeability, and chemical/enzymatic instability. Alternative drug delivery approaches have two major drawbacks. First, the drug's route of administration is hostile to polypeptides; for example, orally administered proteins are subjected to harsh conditions before absorption through

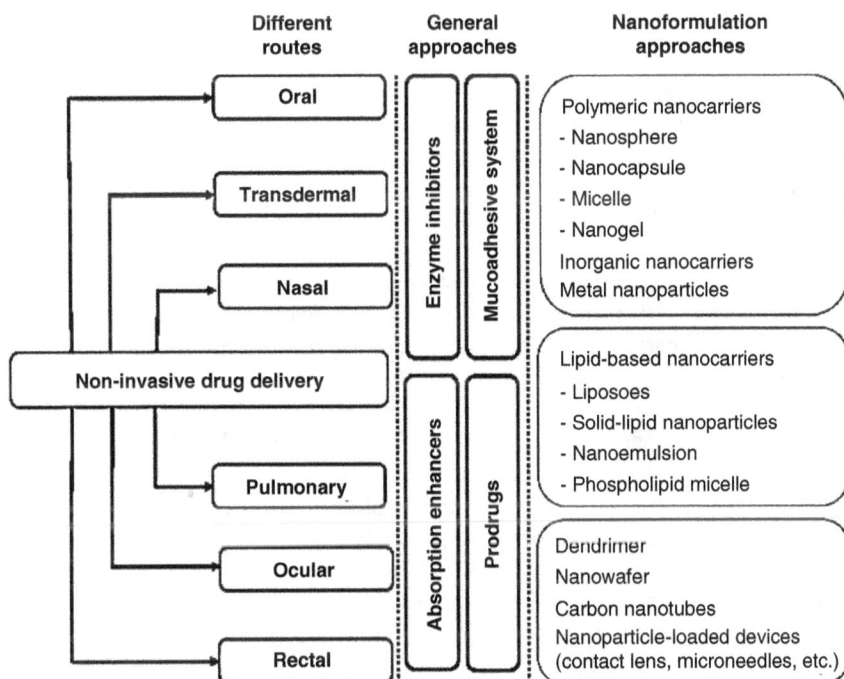

FIGURE 12.4   Barriers to absorption in various routes of administration

the gastrointestinal tract or absorption through the nasal mucosa, which can cause significant metabolism. After administration, adequate drug absorption through the respective barrier layers may be a significant factor in achieving a pharmacological response. Encapsulation in hydrophobic carriers, penetration enhancers, electrical transport, or chemical modification to increase hydrophobicity are all strategies for improving absorption of hydrophilic (thus poorly absorbed) compounds. Given the advances in nanotechnologies, new nano-formulations with regulated particle size and surface modification are being developed, which improve target selectivity, systemic half-life, and bioavailability of protein drugs.

However, newer approaches, like devices administering drugs orally into the gastrointestinal tract, face approval challenges due to dosing variability, akin to the withdrawal of inhalation insulin. Additionally, risks of gastrointestinal bleeding and dose limitations deter their approval.

12.4.1 Intravenous Administration

Intravenous bolus, intravenous infusion, and subcutaneous delivery stand as the most commonly utilized methods for administering biopharmaceuticals. Typically, medications exhibiting poor or highly variable bioavailability, like oncology drugs, are administered intravenously to ensure precise dosing. Drugs that might provoke irritation in subcutaneous tissue are better suited for intravenous injection. However, this approach isn't recommended for self-administration due to the significant costs associated with drug therapy. Formulation challenges are minimal, except for the requirement that the drug be in a solution or a very fine emulsion to prevent vein blockage. Some biopharmaceuticals initially designed for intravenous injection or infusion have recently been reformulated for subcutaneous administration, enabling patients to self-administer them.

12.4.2 Subcutaneous Administration

Insulin holds the distinction of being the first biopharmaceutical accepted for subcutaneous use. Intravenous bolus or infusion remains the most common route for medications necessitating precise dosing calculations, particularly oncology drugs, and is typically administered by healthcare professionals. However, there has been a recent shift from intravenous to subcutaneous administration due to economic reasons. After the introduction of subcutaneous formulations of trastuzumab and rituximab in Europe between 2013 and 2014, numerous medications are now reformulated as subcutaneous dosage forms, moving away from intravenous administration. This shift enables self-injection of therapies for rheumatoid arthritis, multiple sclerosis, or primary immunodeficiency, where mixed dosing (not based on body weight) is recommended.

Biopharmaceutical products given subcutaneously have a different pharmacokinetic profile than those given intravenously. The pharmacokinetic profile of biopharmaceutical products injected subcutaneously is typically marked by a slow rate of absorption from the subcutaneous extracellular matrix, resulting in lower C_{max} levels lower than those obtained with intravenous dosing.

The absorption of molecules into the bloodstream follows a particular pattern, attributed to the reduced permeability of macromolecules through the vascular endothelial layer. Consequently, lymphatics serve as an alternative route for absorption into the circulatory system. Despite this function, lymphatic absorption poses a barrier to complete penetration for molecules injected subcutaneously. Interactions with interstitial glycosaminoglycans, proteins, and enzymatic degradation collectively contribute to the incomplete bioavailability of molecules injected subcutaneously.

In contrast to small molecules, biopharmaceutical products with molecular weights exceeding 20 kDa exhibit limited transportation through blood capillaries, predominantly entering the circulatory system via lymphatics. Subcutaneous administration of biotherapeutics is more immunogenic compared to intravenous dosing due to heightened exposure to the lymphatic system. Presently, regulatory agencies mandate immunogenicity testing for subcutaneous dosages over intravenous

TABLE 12.12
Examples of Biopharmaceuticals Delivered in Subcutaneous Dosage Forms

Molecule	Brand Name (Originator)	Dosing Frequency	Injection Volume	Device
Abatacept	Orencia (Bristol-Myers Squibb)	q1w	1 mL	Prefilled syringe, prefilled pen/ autoinjector
Adalimumab	Humira (AbbVie)	q2w	0.4–0.8 mL	Prefilled syringe, vial, prefilled pen
Anakinra	Kineret (Swedish Orphan Biovitrum GmbH)[a]	q1d or q2d	0.67 mL	Prefilled syringe
Certolizumab pegol	Cimzia (UCB-Euronext and BEL20)[a]	q2w and q4w	1 mL	Prefilled syringe, vial, prefilled pen
Etanercept	Enbrel (Amgen)	q1w or twice weekly	0.5–1 mL	Prefilled syringe, vial, prefilled pen/ autoinjector, prefilled cartridge for reusable autoinjector
Glatiramer acetate	Copaxone (Teva)	q1d or three times per week	1 mL	Prefilled syringe, pen/autoinjector
Golimumab	Simponi (Janssen)	q1m	0.5–1 mL	Prefilled syringe, prefilled pen/ autoinjector
Insulin	Several	PRN	variable	Vials, prefilled pen, syringes
Interferon-beta-1a	Rebif (EMD Serono/Pfizer)	Three times per week	0.2–0.5 mL	Prefilled syringe, prefilled pen/ autoinjector, electronic injection system
Interferon beta-1b	Betaseron/Betaferon (Bayer)	q2d	0.25–1 mL	Prefilled syringe. vial, autoinjector
Interferon beta-1b	Extavia (Novartis)	q2d	0.25–1 mL	Prefilled syringe, vial, autoinjector
Peg-interferon beta-1a	Plegridy (Biogen)	q2w	0.5 mL	Prefilled syringe, prefilled pen/ autoinjector
Rituximab	MabThera/Rituxan Hycela (Roche)	q3w–q3mc	11.7–13.4 mL	Vial and syringe
Sarilumab	Kevzara (Sanofi-Aventis)	q2w	1.14 mL	Prefilled syringe, prefilled pen
Tocilizumab	Actemra (Roche)	q1w and q2w	0.9 mL	Prefilled syringe, prefilled pen
Trastuzumab	Herceptin (Roche)	q3w	5 mL	Vial and syringe

ones. Instances requiring administration of a biological drug via both subcutaneous and intravenous routes necessitate the demonstration of the safety of subcutaneous administration over intravenous administration.

Subcutaneous administration of biopharmaceutical products suffers from incomplete bioavailability of the injected molecule, typically ranging from 50% to 80% for monoclonal antibodies (mAbs). Understanding the enzymes involved and their translation across species in the pre-systemic catabolism at the subcutaneous administration site or the lymphatic system remains limited. For mAbs, subcutaneous bioavailability correlates inversely with clearance after intravenous dosing; mAbs exhibiting lower intravenous clearance demonstrate higher subcutaneous bioavailability. Hematopoietic cells, such as macrophages or dendritic cells, play a role in both subcutaneous first-pass clearance and systemic clearance after intravenous dosing. Due to poor bioavailability, subcutaneous infusions generally necessitate higher dosages compared to intravenous infusions, resulting in higher costs for subcutaneous formulations.

To enhance the subcutaneous bioavailability of a biotherapeutic, subcutaneous infusions employing the dispersion-enhancer hyaluronidase can be administered or developed as co-formulations. This enzyme aids in the spread of injected fluid within subcutaneous tissue, potentially increasing the bioavailability of co-injected molecules due to enhanced dispersion in the interstitial tissue.

Subcutaneous injections, typically administered in a buffered aqueous solution, may induce pain, especially with solutions containing citrate buffer. For instance, Humira, a top-selling biopharmaceutical drug, initially contained a citrate buffer causing discomfort upon injection. After the gene sequence patent expired, AbbVie reformulated the medication without the buffer, asserting that the large proteins themselves function as a buffer, a fact known to the developer. The reformulated version, being more concentrated, reduces injection volume and inflammation, as stated in AbbVie's new patent that now protects the company.

Subcutaneous administration offers sustained activity, as seen with insulin glargine, which precipitates upon subcutaneous injection, allowing for prolonged release. Recent advances in polymer science have led to the development of hydrogels for sustained drug release, high tissue compatibility, and patient self-administration. Hydrogels produce a deformable drug depot that steadily elutes a high drug concentration to surrounding tissue over time. However, most hydrogels chemically bind to drugs rather than covalently, resulting in rapid drug release over hours to days, limiting their suitability for long-term drug delivery.

12.4.3 ORAL ADMINISTRATION

While oral administration is the most common route, it's nearly impossible for protein drugs due to permeability issues and chemical instability. Oral formulations often exhibit inconsistent bioavailability, particularly problematic for biological drugs with a narrow therapeutic range. Investigations into lipophilic insulin and thyrotropin-releasing hormone derivatives, created by fatty acylation with palmitic or lauric acid for oral administration, are ongoing. These transformed drug molecules form vesicle-like structures (Prosome®, Pharmacosome®), significantly enhancing drug bioavailability and circulation time in patients.

Microspheres, liposomes, or nanoparticles encapsulate polypeptide drugs within polymeric, phospholipid, or carbohydrate particulate delivery systems.

12.4.4 NASAL/PULMONARY ADMINISTRATION

The lung provides rapid and high drug absorption due to its expansive surface area (around 80–140 m²), thin alveolar epithelium (0.1–0.5 mm), and ample blood supply. Pulmonary drug delivery avoids hepatic first-pass effects, is noninvasive, effective at lower doses, and can be used locally or systemically, pulmonary drug delivery is advantageous. Although lung tissue exhibits lower enzymatic activity compared to the gastrointestinal tract, the pulmonary epithelium possesses several immunological properties. However, pulmonary delivery has certain drawbacks, including a short

---

TABLE 12.13
Orally Administered Biopharmaceuticals

Product	Drug	Route	Indications
Minirin	Desmopressin	Oral, Nasal	Cranial diabetes insipidus or nocturia associated with multiple sclerosis
Sandimmune	Cyclosporine A	Oral	Immunosuppressants
Colomycin	Colistin	Oral	Intestinal infection (caused by sensitive gram-negative organisms)
Cytorest	Cytochrome C	Oral	Leukopenia
Cachexon®	Glutathione	Oral	AIDS-related cachexia
Ceredist OD	Taltirelin	Oral	Spinocerebellar ataxia
Anginovag	Tyrothricin	Oral	Pharyngitis
Vancocin	Vancomycin	Oral	Infection, *Clostridium difficile*-associated diarrhea
Oral-Lyn	Insulin	Buccal	Diabetes mellitus

duration of action due to the rapid removal of the drug. Inhaled drugs deposited in the lungs are swept towards the mouth, where they are phagocytosed by alveolar macrophages and eliminated. Therefore, achieving a sustained drug release requires a method to circumvent or suspend the normal clearance mechanisms of the lungs before administering encapsulated drugs effectively. Generally, proteins within the molecular weight range of 6000 to 50,000 D exhibit high bioavailability after inhalation. Consequently, pulmonary administration has gained significant attention as a promising method for delivering protein drugs.

Only a handful of drugs currently in development for pulmonary delivery encompass interleukin-1 receptor (asthma therapy), heparin (blood clotting), human insulin (diabetes), alpha-1 antitrypsin (emphysema and cystic fibrosis), interferons (multiple sclerosis and hepatitis B and C), and calcitonin and other peptides (osteoporosis). Inhalation delivery targeting specific tissues or organs can also be employed for gene therapy. Innovative dry powder formulations, packaging, and filling technologies like those by Inhale enable patients previously receiving injections to inhale medication into the deep lung independently and painlessly, facilitating natural and effective bloodstream absorption.

Given its critical role in the efficacy of pulmonary drug administration, selecting an appropriate delivery system is vital in the formulation design for pulmonary drug delivery. Nebulizers (e.g., jet nebulizers, ultrasonic nebulizers, and vibrating mesh nebulizers), metered-dose inhalers, and dry powder inhalers are commonly used instruments to administer therapeutics as aerosols.

Various nanotechnology-based approaches have been extensively studied for successful protein delivery via the pulmonary route. Nanoparticles, in general, are promising as a protein delivery carrier in the lungs due to their ability to target and release drugs in a controlled manner. Nanoparticles smaller than 200 nm can also avoid detection by alveolar macrophages, resulting in better absorption and drug action. In addition to polymeric nanoparticles, other nanocarriers such as liposomes, and solid lipid nanoparticles have all been utilized as nanocarriers for delivering protein drugs through pulmonary administration. Subsequent sections will explore these nanocarriers in more detail.

Inhalable insulin, a powdered form of insulin, is inhaled and absorbed through the lungs. Inhaled insulins work faster than subcutaneously injected ones, resulting in a higher peak blood concentration and faster metabolism. Pfizer introduced Exubera, the first inhaled insulin medication, in 2006, initially developed by Inhale Therapeutics (later renamed Nektar Therapeutics). However, due to poor sales, it was withdrawn in 2007. The FDA approved Mannkind's monomeric inhaled insulin, Afrezza, in 2014. Dypreza inhaled insulin by Highlands Pharmaceuticals received approval for sale in Europe in 2013 and in the United States in 2016. Achieving precise dosing with inhalable insulin can be challenging, particularly when administered through a specific system.

While the nasal route offers advantages such as increased bioavailability and ease of administration, it can also result in delivery to the brain. Macromolecules pass through the lungs easily, making pulmonary delivery a feasible noninvasive option for protein delivery. Inhaled insulin is absorbed faster than subcutaneously injected insulin, leading to an improved physiological response to a meal. However, an inhalation insulin device was recalled due to dose inconsistency. The nasally administered items are listed in Table 12.14.

The blood-brain barrier poses a significant challenge in treating many neuronal degenerative disorders as it regulates the passage of most therapeutics, including proteins, into the central nervous system. In this context, the nasal route might be more effective than oral or parenteral routes. Strategies involving absorption enhancers to promote permeation through the membrane, mucoadhesive formulations to enhance nasal residential time, and prodrug approaches aim to optimize absorption. Various absorption enhancers, such as bile salts, surfactants, fluidic acid derivatives, phosphatidylcholines, fatty acids (Tauro dihydro fusidate), cyclodextrins (CDs), cationized polymers, chelators, and cell penetration peptides, aid in facilitating drug passage through the nasal membrane. Mucoadhesive systems extend nasal retention time, enhancing protein bioavailability. For instance, the use of Carbopol 941 and carboxymethyl cellulose led to increased calcitonin and insulin nasal

TABLE 12.14
Nasally Administered Biopharmaceuticals

Product	Drug	Route	Indications
Antepan	Protirelin	Nasal	Hypothyroidism and acromegaly
Desmospray	Desmopressin	Nasal	Cranial diabetes insipidus or nocturia associated with multiple sclerosis
FluMist® Quadrivalent	Vaccine	Nasal	Influenza
Fortical®	Salmon calcitonin	Nasal	Hypercalcemia or osteoporosis
Kryptocur	LHRH	Nasal	Cryptorchism
Miacalcin	Salmon calcitonin	Nasal	Hypercalcemia or osteoporosis
Minirin	Desmopressin	Oral, Nasal	Cranial diabetes insipidus or nocturia associated with multiple sclerosis
Suprecur	Buserelin	Nasal	Prostate cancer, endometriosis
Suprifact	Buserelin	Nasal	Prostate cancer, endometriosis
Synarel	Nafarelin	Nasal	Endometriosis
Syntocinin	Oxytocin	Nasal	This medication is used to start or strengthen uterine contractions

bioavailability. Mucoadhesive polymers also enhance permeation by loosening the tight junctions in the nasal epithelium. Consequently, mucoadhesive micro-/nanoparticles, providing longer residence time and better permeation through the membrane, serve as useful carriers for protein drug delivery via the nasal route.

12.4.5 TRANSDERMAL ADMINISTRATION

Numerous cytokines are topically applied, yet using liposomes to deliver human epidermal growth factor significantly improves its effectiveness. Peptide drugs could utilize the skin's pilosebaceous pathway through niosomes (liposomes made of nonionic surfactants). For instance, vesicles made of glyceryl dilaurate cholesterol and polyoxyethylene-10-stearyl ether enhance the absorption of interferon-alpha and cyclosporine. Transfersomes (a phosphatidylcholine/sodium cholate mixture) have also been employed to deliver insulin through topical application in vivo.

Penetration enhancers, such as N-alkylazacycloheptanones (Azone) for desglycinamide arginine vasopressin, temporarily compromise the skin's integrity or physicochemical characteristics to facilitate peptide transmission through the skin. In vitro studies demonstrate that the nonionic surfactant n-decyl methyl sulfoxide enhances Leu-enkephalin penetration through hairless mouse skin, while a urea/ethanol/menthol/camphor/methyl salicylate hydroxypropyl cellulose gel improves the absorption of the nonapeptide leuprolide (a luteinizing-hormone-releasing-hormone analog) by increasing hydration and exhibiting a keratolytic effect.

Recently, researchers have explored iontophoresis, employing electrical stimulation of skin permeability to enhance the delivery of short peptides (model tripeptides, vasopressin), growth hormone-releasing factor (amino acids 1–44), insulin, and luteinizing hormone-releasing hormone. Ultrasonic vibration has shown some success in delivering insulin in vivo.

Microneedles enhance patient compliance and provide a versatile platform for hydrophilic and high molecular weight drugs, including protein drugs, to overcome the skin barrier without causing pain. Comprised of silicon, plastics, biodegradable polymers, and carbohydrates, microneedles represent a painless instrument. The initial generation of microneedles utilized sturdy needles to perforate the skin membrane and enhance drug permeability. While solid microneedles seemed effective in delivering insulin, their usage is limited due to poor delivery performance, complicated administration, imprecise dosing, and the risk of infection. Recent advancements involve directly coating the drug payload onto the microneedle surface, resulting in more robust microneedles. Various methods like dip-coating, casting, and deposition are used to coat microneedles. Biodegradable microneedles ensure continuous drug release upon the hydrolysis of the biodegradable polymer matrix. Polymers with high molecular weights and crosslinking density are preferred in the construction of these microneedles.

Sonophoresis utilizes ultrasonic waves to enhance drug permeability in the skin. Ultrasound waves cause expansion and oscillation of air pockets in the stratum corneum, disrupting the lipid bilayer and creating cavities that boost drug permeability. The degree of drug delivery via sonophoresis depends on the physicochemical properties of the drug, the duration of ultrasound exposure, and the pulse "on" length. While sonophoresis aids in biopharmaceutical transdermal delivery, caution is necessary due to the risk of protein instability from ultrasound exposure. Combining sonophoresis with methods such as chemical enhancers, electroporation, and iontophoresis significantly improves drug delivery through the skin compared to using sonophoresis alone.

Electroporation, a recent approach in transdermal delivery of proteins and peptides, uses ultra-short pulses and electrical strength to alter the skin, enabling hydrophilic compounds to penetrate. Unlike iontophoresis, which propels a drug directly into the skin, electroporation primarily changes membrane permeability to enhance drug penetration.

12.4.6 Ocular Administration

Ocular protein delivery faces challenges due to the blood-retinal barrier and efflux transporters. Formulation viscosity affects ocular drug delivery, where higher viscosity increases corneal contact time but induces reflex weeping and blinking.

Two products, an anti-vascular endothelial growth factor (anti-VEGF) aptamer and a monoclonal antibody (Lucentis; Ranibizumab), have gained approval for ocular delivery. Traditional topically applied dosage forms, such as eye drops, suffer from low bioavailability and therapeutic efficacy. Hence, new strategies have emerged to overcome ocular delivery barriers and enhance protein bioavailability through the ocular route. For instance, coadministration of chemical chaperones and recombinant human hyaluronidase facilitates protein delivery via the ocular path. To address protein aggregation concerns in ocular disease treatment, a novel strategy involving chemical chaperones, which act as protein aggregation inhibitors, has been devised to prevent misfolding and self-assembly of aggregation-prone protein sequences. Additionally, combining recombinant hyaluronidases with biopharmaceutical drugs has long been practiced to enhance drug penetration through ocular tissue barriers by breaking down hyaluronic acid, a vital tissue component. Research into nanocarriers like polymeric micelles, liposomes, nanospheres, nano wafers, and dendrimers focuses on controlled and targeted protein delivery through the ocular route, aiming to overcome ocular delivery barriers. Table 12.15 lists drugs administered through the eyes.

TABLE 12.15
Ocular Biopharmaceutical Products

Product	Drug	Route	Indications
Cenegermin	Oxervate	Eye drop	Neurotrophic keratitis
Eylea	Aflibercept	Ocular	Wet age-related macular degeneration (WAMD), diabetic macular
Lucentis	Ranibizumab	Ocular	edema (DME) or diabetic retinopathy (DR) in DME, macular edema following retinal vein occlusion (MEtRVO) WAMD, DME or DR in DME, MEtRVO, myopic choroidal neovascularization (mCNV)

Nano wafers are small, transparent circular or rectangular membranes containing arrays of drug-loaded nano reservoirs that release drugs in a more controlled and long-lasting manner compared to eye drops (lasting from a few hours to several days). Among the polymers used are polyvinyl alcohol, polyvinyl pyrrolidone, hydroxypropyl methylcellulose, and carboxymethyl cellulose. Placed on the patient's fingertip, nano wafers can endure continuous blinking without being dislodged. They slowly release the drug, extending drug residence time, enhancing absorption into ocular tissues, and improving therapeutic efficacy. Moreover, as the drug is released, the nano wafer gradually dissolves, leaving the ocular surfaces free of polymers.

For ocular drug administration, drug-loaded contact lenses can be utilized. These lenses prolong drug residence in the eye, thereby enhancing drug permeation into the cornea. Sustained drug release is achievable as drug molecules diffuse slowly from the lens matrix. Encapsulating the drug in nanocarriers and dispersing these loaded nanocarriers in the lens matrix further increases residence time and drug release rate. However, using contact lenses has downsides such as drug leaching during storage and delivery, along with safety concerns related to surface roughness that need addressing.

12.4.7   RECTAL ADMINISTRATION

Protein drugs, highly susceptible to physicochemical and enzymatic destabilization, benefit from absorption enhancers, protease inhibitors, prodrugs, and nano formulations. Insulin, heparin, calcitonin, recombinant human granulocyte colony-stimulating factor (rhGCSF), and human chorionic gonadotrophin require absorption enhancers. However, certain enhancers used in rectal drug delivery may cause irritation and damage to the mucous membrane. Protease inhibitors enhance rectal bioavailability by minimizing protein degradation. Using prodrugs shields proteins from peptidases and mucosal enzyme degradation, boosting protein and peptide absorption. Nanotechnology-based formulation methods further aid in enhancing protein drug delivery via rectal administration.

12.5   FORMULATION TECHNOLOGIES

12.5.1   HYDROGELS AND IN SITU FORMING GELS

Hydrogels, three-dimensional polymeric networks composed of crosslinked hydrophilic and biocompatible polymers that swell in aqueous media due to their thermodynamic compatibility with water, have diverse clinical applications. These applications include contact lenses, biosensors, tissue engineering components, and drug delivery carriers. Hydrogels aid in safer and more comfortable delivery of protein drugs. Notable polymers employed in protein delivery hydrogels encompass 2-hydroxyethyl methacrylate, ethylene glycol dimethyl acrylate, N-isopropyl acrylamide, acrylic acid, methacrylic acid (MAA), poly (ethylene glycol) (PEG), and poly (vinyl alcohol) (PVA).

A hydrogel-based particulate formulation releases the protein in its active state and maintains therapeutic concentration for at least three months. Hydrogels, polymeric materials that do not dissolve in water and expand significantly in an aqueous medium under physiological conditions, are formed through crosslinking. Crosslinking involves covalently linking polymer main chains, sometimes including strong non-covalent interactions, preventing complete dissolution of the polymer. Hydrophilic polymer-based hydrogels absorb water, causing their network to swell due to the high water content, making them biocompatible and suitable for tissue regeneration. However, despite the potential advantages in drug delivery, designing extended formulations for drug release becomes challenging due to the high water content of hydrogels.

The mechanical properties of hydrogels are crucial in pharmaceutical applications. Adjusting the degree of hydrogel crosslinking is essential, as higher crosslinking yields a stronger but more brittle structure. Copolymerization produces hydrogels that are both solid and elastic.

Physiological stimuli such as pH, ionic strength, and temperature are often employed in designing hydrogels. Responsive hydrogels change their swelling behavior, network structure, permeability, and mechanical strength in response to environmental stimuli. pH-triggered drug release systems protect proteins in harsh gastric environments, facilitating more efficient oral delivery. Ionic hydrogels with groups that ionize in response to pH changes cause the hydrogel network to swell, known as pH-responsive hydrogels.

Nanogels, crosslinked polymer nanoparticles with hydrodynamic sizes ranging from 10 to 100 nanometers distributed in an aqueous medium while retaining their fixed conformation, offer tailored properties. They can control their scale, surface charge, network density, and chemical functional groups for specific structural and functional needs.

Insulin molecules bound covalently to highly hydrophilic and multifunctional nanogels for nasal delivery have shown promising results. Poly (N-vinyl pyrrolidone)-based nanogels covalently bound to insulin cross the blood-brain barrier, displaying neuroprotection against amyloid ß-induced dysfunction post intranasal administration, compared to free insulin.

12.5.2 Nanoparticles

Nanoparticles increase protein physicochemical stability in the gastrointestinal tract by encapsulating them in a polymeric matrix within a size range of 10–1000 nm. Non-toxic, non-immunogenic nanoparticles are crucial as oral protein carriers. They play pivotal roles in absorption, distribution, removal, and in-vivo action in the gastrointestinal tract. Nanoparticles smaller than 100 nm are more readily absorbed through the intestinal mucosa, while those larger than 500 nm have significantly lower absorption rates. Custom ligands on nanoparticle surfaces can target receptor-mediated transport pathways.

Nanoparticles can be delivered topically, periocularly, suprachoroidally, or intravitreally. However, intravitreal injection of nanoparticles can cause vitreous clouding due to the light scattering properties of polymeric particles. Challenges in delivering nano-formulations of proteins include loss of bioactivity, low protein stability due to interactions with the nanoparticle matrix, and comprehensive nanoencapsulation methods, limiting the development of ocular delivery systems employing nanoparticles.

Nanoparticles utilize both natural and synthetic polymers for preparation. Common materials include polylactic acid, polylactic-co-glycolic acid, chitosan, gelatin, polymethylmethacrylate, and poly-alkyl-cyanoacrylate. Chitosan is a deacetylated chitin copolymer made up of glucosamine and N-acetyl-glucosamine., due to its biocompatibility, muco-adhesion, and low toxicity, stands out as an excellent choice for protein delivery carriers, improving cellular uptake by opening close junctions.

Alginate, a natural anionic polymer, serves as a commonly used drug carrier in the pharmaceutical industry. Its anionic surface charge facilitates gel formation when interacting electrostatically with cationic materials. However, high porosity in alginate beads often leads to drug leakage. Combining alginate with substances like chitosan or dextran sulfate mitigates this issue.

Various synthetic polymers, alongside natural polymer-based nanoparticles, serve as oral delivery carriers for protein drugs. One representative polymer is polylactic-co-glycolic acid (PLGA), formed from lactic acid and glycolic acid, creating a ring-opening copolymer known as PLGA. Its excellent biodegradability and biocompatibility make PLGA an exceptional drug delivery vehicle for oral protein delivery.

Redox-activated nanocarriers, sensitive to glutathione as a cellular redox regulator, have been proposed as effective mechanisms for drug and gene delivery.

In recent years, the use of nanoparticles for delivering protein drugs through the nose has garnered significant interest. Mucoadhesive nanoparticles, particularly, tend to spend more time in the nasal cavity. Chitosan nanoparticles have been extensively studied for insulin delivery through the nose. Their positive charge enables prolonged contact with the nasal mucosal membrane, thereby enhancing insulin bioavailability. Intranasal administration of chitosan-N-acetyl-L-cysteine nanoparticles and PEG-g-chitosan nanoparticles has shown improvements in insulin bioavailability. In intranasal vaccination, chitosan, PLGA, and polystyrene polymeric nanoparticles have proven effective in terms of antigen absorption. Trimethyl chitosan nanoparticles extend the antigen's residence time, enhancing IgA and IgG efficiency. Similarly, nasal administration of mucoadhesive chitosan nanoparticles significantly improves nerve growth factor uptake in the brain.

Polymeric nanoparticles, due to their biocompatibility and ease of surface modification and copolymerization, are commonly employed as carriers for pulmonary drug delivery. Among natural polymeric carriers, chitosan, alginate, and gelatin are prevalent. In the realm of synthetic nanocarriers for pulmonary drug delivery, Poloxamer, poly(lactic-co-glycolic) acid, and polyethylene glycol stand out as the most frequently used.

Polymeric nanoparticles and a polymer-based thermo-gelling method prove beneficial in ocular drug delivery.

Carbon nanotubes, cylindrically shaped carbon structures with unique physicochemical properties, are easily manipulated on the surface and belong to the fullerene family. These nanotubes are ideal for targeted or controlled drug delivery, biosensing, and bioimaging due to their exceptional mechanical properties, high thermal conductivities, and capacity to penetrate cell membranes.

Nanoparticles exhibit lipid-fluidizing properties, which influence skin permeability by altering the extracellular lipids in the stratum corneum.

Lipid-based nanocarriers, such as liposomes, solid lipid nanoparticles, and nanostructured lipid carriers, have been studied extensively for ocular protein delivery. Prolonged drug release may help reduce the risk of ocular complications associated with multiple intravitreal injections, such as vitreous hemorrhage, endophthalmitis, retinal detachment, and cataracts.

Solid-lipid nanoparticles offer several advantages, including physical stability, targetability, controlled release, fast scale-up, and non-toxicity, owing to their composition of physiological lipids. They enhance drug absorption through the cornea, thereby increasing the ocular bioavailability of both hydrophilic and lipophilic drugs.

Niosomes, self-assembling nanovesicles composed of nonionic surfactants resembling liposomes, are preferred for topical ocular drug delivery due to their chemical stability, biodegradability, biocompatibility, lack of immunogenicity, and low toxicity. They exhibit structural flexibility, encapsulating both lipophilic and hydrophilic drugs. Discomes, a type of niosome with wide structures (12–16 mm) as a result of the addition of Solulan C24 (nonionic surfactant), are advantageous for ocular administration, preventing drainage into the systemic pool due to their size and shape, fitting comfortably into the eye's cul-de-sac. However, their development is still in the early stages.

While polymeric nanoparticles have demonstrated benefits across various delivery routes, there has been limited progress in developing them for rectal administration. Commonly used materials for polymeric nanoparticles in rectal drug delivery include chitosan and its derivatives such as PLGA, PLA, and methacrylic acid copolymers. Surface modifications of these nanoparticles offer additional benefits such as site-specificity or prolonged circulation periods.

Nano-sized liposomes are employed for rectal administration of macromolecules, with some studies investigating liposomal formulations. For mucosal immunization, updated nanoliposomes containing hepatitis B surface antigen are suggested consisting of a 1,2-dipalmitoyl-sn-glycerol-3-phosphocholine bilayer engulfing a solid fat center (mainly glyceryl tripalmitate) and using monophosphoryl lipid A as an adjuvant and containing hepatitis B surface antigen for mucosal immunization, showing higher stability and significant humoral and cellular immune responses in rats following intracolonic administration. Solid lipid nanoparticles are also utilized for rectal drug delivery, but evidence of their superiority over traditional formulations is yet to be provided.

Considering the hydrophobic nature of the stratum corneum, nanocarriers in lipophilic vehicles should effectively penetrate it. Nano-emulsions, low viscosity isotropic dispersed systems composed of two immiscible liquid phases, are generated through high-pressure homogenization, phase-inversion temperature, and micro-fluidization. Their major disadvantage lies in physical instability during long-term storage due to their thermodynamically unstable nature. Nano-emulsions achieve a metastable state by optimizing particle size and surfactant composition. While less common in transdermal antigen delivery due to their instability, nano-emulsions have shown promise in trans-cutaneous immunization when used as nano-dispersions.

Polymeric micelles, sized between 10 and 100 nm, consist of amphiphilic block copolymers forming a shell of hydrophilic chains and a core of hydrophobic chains. They self-assemble in aqueous media, forming an organized supramolecular structure at concentrations surpassing their critical micellar concentrations. Poloxamer 407, poloxamer 188, methoxy poly (ethylene glycol)-poly(e-caprolactone), poly (butylene oxide)-poly (ethylene oxide)-poly (butylene oxide), polyhydroxyethylaspartamide, and isopropylacrylamide are some polymers used to create poly-meric micelles for ocular distribution.

Dendrimers, small polymeric carriers capable of capturing and conjugating high-molecular-weight molecules, exhibit treelike structures with well-defined, homogeneous, and monodisperse radial symmetry. Commonly utilized dendrimers include polyamidoamines, polyamines, polyamides (polypeptides), poly (aryl ethers), polyesters, and carbohydrates.

12.5.3 LIPOSOMES

Liposomes serve as carriers to encapsulate proteins within the aqueous core, enhancing membrane permeability for protein drugs. The structural similarity of liposomes to cellular membranes aids in intestinal absorption. However, they do have drawbacks as oral protein carriers due to chemical and enzymatic instability in the gastrointestinal tract. To address stability issues, surface coating becomes essential for oral drug delivery in liposomes. Various approaches, such as altering the liposomal surface using ligands interacting with specific receptors on cellular membranes, present promising possibilities. Lectins, a type of plant-derived glycoprotein, are a potential ligand for spe-cific binding to mucosal carbohydrate receptors.

Liposomes, bilayer vesicles comprising phospholipids, encapsulate hydrophilic and hydrophobic compounds within their aqueous core or bilayer structure. These phospholipid molecules arrange molecularly in water, exposing hydrophilic phosphate head groups to the aqueous environment due to their amphiphilic nature. Upon linking of hydrocarbon chains, a lipid film forms. Upon addition of water and stirring, this lipid layer transforms into covered vesicles. Liposomes may exist as single bilayer (unilamellar) or multiple bilayers (multilamellar), with sizes ranging from 20–100 nm for small unilamellar vesicles to 100–1000 nm for large unilamellar vesicles (large unilamellar vesicles). Various methods such as dry lipid hydration, freeze-thawing extrusion, reverse evapor-ation, and double emulsification are employed to produce liposomes. The main steps involve lipid film hydration, mechanical dispersion for liposome formation, and solvent removal. While vigorous shaking is commonly used, it results in polydispersed multilamellar vesicles. Extrusion through a narrow orifice manipulates liposome size to produce monodispersed small unilamellar vesicle liposomes. Several physical stresses during liposome preparation, including heat, organic solvents, and agitation, can impact protein stability.

Proteins in liposome polymeric particles exhibit prolonged release when encapsulated. Bilayer destabilization causes liposome breakdown, releasing encapsulated agents. Processes like proton-ation of phospholipid head groups and acid-catalyzed bilayer hydrolysis contribute to biolayer breakdown in vivo, consequently altering the drug's kinetic profile. Surface PEGylation reduces protein interactions with biological fluids, preventing liposome aggregation and enhancing stability.

Archaeosomes, a lipid-based oral delivery system derived from polar lipids of various Archaeobacteria, possess unique structural features enabling stability under extreme conditions, including high temperatures, varying pH levels, and in the presence of phospholipases and bile salts. This potential for improved gastrointestinal stability has led to considerable interest in their use as protein carriers, including in vaccines. Nasal administration of drug-loaded liposomes has proven effective in intranasal distribution of biopharmaceuticals and peptides, facilitating direct nose-to-brain drug delivery via nanoparticles.

Liposomes are efficient carriers for delivering therapeutics into the skin due to their identical components to skin lipids. They are rapidly absorbed by the epidermis, reaching deep skin layers. Additionally, hydration layers enhance absorption by molecular mixing of the liposome bilayer with intracellular lipids in the stratum corneum.

A non-invasive macromolecule transdermal delivery system has been developed by encapsulating proteins in liposomes. Advanced liposomes have increased macromolecule permeation through the stratum corneum, overcoming limitations in drug delivery through the skin. To enhance macro-molecule delivery into the skin, liposomal formulations are integrated into dissolving microneedle arrays.

Liposomes stand out as highly effective pulmonary carriers for protein drugs due to their enhanced and sustained drug release, biocompatibility, biodegradability, and non-immunogenicity. Altering a drug's physicochemical properties (increasing hydrophobicity) and reducing mucociliary clearance with liposomes may enhance drug permeation through the alveolar epithelium due to increased surface viscosity. This has led to the development of liposomal formulations for protein drug delivery to the lungs.

Apart from liposomes, solid lipid nanoparticles (SLN) have been investigated as carriers for delivering biopharmaceuticals through the lung epithelium. For instance, spray-dried powders containing SLNs have addressed the issue of low inertia, preventing nanoparticles from settling in the lungs.

12.6 SUMMARY

Drug delivery necessitates a dosage form delivering the active molecule at a predetermined rate and concentration to the site of action. Biopharmaceutical products, being large and inherently unstable molecules in various administration environments, often rely on the parenteral route. The safety and efficacy of biopharmaceuticals significantly depend on the applied formulation and manufacturing technology, unlike chemical products. Research exploring novel administration routes aims to expand biopharmaceutical applications. This chapter outlines model formulations for various classes of biopharmaceuticals.

APPENDIX: PHYSICOCHEMICAL PROPERTIES OF PROTEINS AND PEPTIDES APPROVED BY THE FOOD AND DRUG ADMINISTRATION

Name	MOA	MW	Formula	IEP	Hydrophobicity	MP	Half-Life
Abarelix	IIIc	1416	C72H95ClN14O14	NA	NA	NA	13.2 ± 3.2 d
Abatacept	IIa	92300	C3498H5458N922O1090S32	NA	NA	NA	12–23 d
Abciximab	IIa	145651	C6462H9964N1690O2049S48	6.16	−0.424	71	0.5 hrs
Adalimumab	Ic	144190	C6428H9912N1694O1987S46	8.25	−0.441	NA	240–480 hrs
Aflibercept	Ib	115000	C4318H6788N1164O1304S32	NA	NA	NA	7.13 d
Agalsidase beta	Ia	45352	C2029H3080N544O587S27	5.17	−0.307	NA	45–102 min
Albiglutide	Ib	72970	C3232H5032N864O979S41	NA	NA	NA	4–7 d
Aldesleukin	Ib	15315	C690H1115N177O202S6	7.31	−0.192	NA	0.22–1.42 hrs
Alefacept	IIa	51801	C2306H3594N610O694S26	7.86	−0.432	NA	270 hrs
Alemtuzumab	IIa	145454	C6468H10066N1732O2005S40	8.76	−0.431	NA	288 hrs
Alglucerase	Ia	55597	C2532H3854N672O711S16	7.41	−0.168	NA	3.6–10.4 min
Alglucosidase alfa	Ic	105271	C4435H6739N1175O1279S32	NA	NA	NA	2.3 ± 0.4 hrs
Alirocumab	Ic	146000	C6472H9996N1736O2032S42	NA	NA	NA	17–20 d
Aliskiren	IIa	552	C30H53N3O6	NA	NA	NA	24 hrs
Alpha-1-proteinase inhibitor	IIa	44325	C2001H3130N514O601S10	5.37	−0.302	59	NA
Alteplase	Ib	59042	C2569H3928N746O781S40	7.61	−0.516	60	NA
Anakinra	IIa	17258	C759H1186N208O232S10	5.46	−0.412	NA	4–6 hrs
Ancestim	Ib	18500	NA	NA	NA	NA	NA
Anistreplase	Ic	59042	C2569H3928N746O781S40	7.61	−0.516	60	NA
Anthrax immune globulin human	IIa	NA	NA	NA	NA	NA	24.3 d
Anti-inhibitor coagulant complex	Ia	NA	NA	NA	NA	NA	4–7 hrs
Anti-thymocyte Globulin (Equine)	IIIb	NA	NA	NA	NA	NA	1.5–13 d
Anti-thymocyte Globulin (Rabbit)	IIIb	NA	NA	NA	NA	61	2–3 d
Antihemophilic Factor	Ia	264726	C11794H18314N3220O3553S83	6.97	−0.533	NA	8.4–19.3 hrs
Antithrombin Alfa	Ia	57215	C2191H3457N583O656S18	NA	NA	NA	11.6–17.7 hrs
Antithrombin III human	Ia	58000	NA	NA	NA	NA	2.5–4.8 d
Antithymocyte globulin	IIa	NA	NA	NA	NA	61	2–3 d
Aprotinin	IIa	6511	C284H432N84O79S7	NA	NA	>100	10 hrs
Arcitumomab	IIb	144483	C6398H9900N1714O1995S54	8.26	−0.423	61	1 hr
Asfotase Alfa	Ia	180000	C7108H11008N1968O2206S56	NA	NA	NA	5 d

(continued)

Name	MOA	MW	Formula	IEP	Hydrophobicity	MP	Half-Life
Asparaginase	Ic	31732	C1377H2208N382O442S17	4.67	0.059	NA	8–30 hrs
Asparaginase erwinia chrysanthemi	Ic	140000	C1546H2510N432O476S9	NA	NA	NA	16 hrs
Atezolizumab	IIa	145000	NA	NA	NA	NA	27 d
Autologous cultured chondrocytes	Ia	NA	NA	NA	NA	NA	NA
Basiliximab	IIa	143801	C6378H9844N1698O1997S48	8.68	−0.473	61	7.2 ± 3.2
Becaplermin	Ib	12294	C532H892N162O153S9	9.38	−0.16	NA	NA
Belatacept	IIa	92300	C3508H5440N922O1096S32	NA	NA	NA	9.8 d
Belimumab	IIa	147000	C 6358 H 9904 N 1728 O 2010 S 44	NA	NA	NA	19.4 d
Beractant	Ia	NA	NA	NA	NA	NA	20–30 hrs
Bevacizumab	IIa	149000	C6538H10034N1716O2033S44	NA	NA	61	NA
Bivalirudin	Ia	2180	C98H138N24O33	3.91	−0.985	NA	0.42 hrs
Blinatumomab	IIIc	54100	C2367H3577N649O772S19	NA	NA	NA	2.11 hrs
Botulinum Toxin Type A	Ic	149323	C6760H10447N1743O2010S32	6.06	−0.368	NA	NA
Botulinum Toxin Type B	Ic	150804	C690H1115N177O202S6	NA	NA	NA	NA
Brentuximab vedotin	IIb	149200–151800	C6476H9930N1690O2030S40	NA	NA	NA	4–6 d
Brodalumab	IIa	144000	C6372H9840N1712O1988S52	NA	NA	NA	NA
Buserelin	IIIc	NA	C62H90N16O15	NA	NA	NA	50–80 min
C1 Esterase Inhibitor (Human)	Ia	105000	NA	NA	NA	NA	56 hrs
C1 Esterase Inhibitor (Recombinant)	IIa	67000	NA	NA	NA	NA	2.4–2.7 hrs
Canakinumab	IIIb	145200 (deglycosylated)	C6452H9958N1722O2010S42	NA	NA	NA	26 d
Canakinumab	IIa	145200	C6452H9958N1722O2010S42	NA	NA	NA	26 d
Capromab	IV	NA	NA	NA	NA	NA	NA
Certolizumab pegol	IIb	91000	C2115H3252N556O673S16	NA	NA	NA	14 d
Cetuximab	IIIc	145782	C6484H10042N1732O2023S36	8.48	−0.413	71	114 hrs
Choriogonadotropin alfa	Ib	25720	C1105H1770N318O336S26	8.61	−0.258	55	29 ± 6 hrs
Chorionic Gonadotropin (Human)	Ia	25719	C1105H1770N318O336S26	NA	NA	NA	NA
Chorionic Gonadotropin (Recombinant)	Ia	25720	C1105H1770N318O336S26	8.61	−0.258	55°C	4.5 ± hrs
Coagulation factor ix	Ia	46548	C2041H3136N558O641S25	5.2	−0.431	54	19.4 4 hrs
Coagulation factor VIIa	Ib	45079	C1972H3076N560O597S28	6.09	−0.311	58	NA
Coagulation factor X human	Ib	NA	NA	NA	NA	NA	NA
Coagulation Factor XIII A-Subunit (Recombinant)	Ia	NA	NA	NA	NA	NA	5.1 d

Collagenase	Ic	112023	C5028H7666N1300O1564S21	5.58	−0.714	NA	NA
Conestat alfa	Ia	NA	NA	NA	NA	NA	2.4–2.7 hrs
Corticotropin	IV	4541	C207H308N56O58S	NA	NA	NA	15 min
Cosyntropin	IV	2933	C136H210N40O31S	NA	NA	NA	15 min
Daclizumab	IIa	142612	C6332H9808N1678O1989S42	8.46	−0.437	61	11–38 d
Daptomycin	IIa	1621	C72H101N17O26	NA	NA	NA	7 d
Daratumumab	IIIc	148000	NA	NA	NA	NA	18 d
Darbepoetin alfa	Ib	18396	C815H1317N233O241S5	8.75	−0.188	53	a few hrs
Defibrotide	NA	NA	NA	NA	NA	NA	1.16–1.3 hrs
Denileukin diftitox	IIb	57647	C2560H4042N678O799S17	5.45	−0.301	NA	25.4 d
Denosumab	IIIc	144700	C6404H9912N1724O2004S50	NA	NA	NA	2–3 hrs
Desirudin	Ib	6964	C287H440N80O110 S6	NA	NA	NA	15–20 hrs
Digoxin Immune Fab (Ovine)	IIa	47302	C2085H3223N553O672S16	8.01	−0.343	NA	10 d
Dinutuximab	IIIc	145000	C6422H9982N1722O2008S48	NA	NA	67	NA
Dornase alfa	Ib	29254	C1321H1999N339O396S9	4.58	−0.083	NA	5.5 hrs
Drotrecogin alfa	Ib	55000	C1786H2779N509O519S29	6.78	−0.291	NA	5 d
Dulaglutide	Ib	59670	C2646H4044N704O836S18	NA	NA	NA	272 hrs
Eculizumab	Ia	148000	NA	NA	NA	NA	5 d
Efalizumab	IIa	150000	NA	NA	NA	NA	NA
Efmoroctocog alfa	Ib	NA	NA	NA	NA	NA	7.52–35.9 min
Elosulfase alfa	Ia	110800	C5020H7588N1364O1418S34	NA	NA	NA	NA
Elotuzumab	IIIc	148100	C6476H9982N1714O2016S42	NA	NA	NA	NA
Enfuvirtide	IIa	4492	C204H301N51O64	4.3	−0.875	NA	3.8 hrs
Epoetin alfa	Ib	18396	C815H1317N233O241S5	8.75	NA	53	7.37 hrs
Epoetin zeta	Ib	18200	C809H1301N229O240S5	NA	NA	NA	7.37 hrs
Eptifibatide	NA	832	C35H49N11O9S2	NA	−2.3	NA	29 ± 6 hrs
Etanercept	IIa	51235	C2224H3475N621O698S36	7.89	−0.529	71	102 ± 30 hrs
Evolocumab	IIa	141800	C6242H9648N1668O1996S56	NA	NA	NA	2.4 hrs
Exenatide	Ib	4187	C184H282N50O60S	NA	NA	NA	11–28
Factor IX complex (human)	Ib	NA	NA	NA	NA	NA	78.7 ± 18.13 hrs
Fibrinogen concentrate (human)	Ia	340000	NA	NA	NA	NA	24 hrs
Fibrinolysin aka plasmin	Ic	88400	C3848H5912N1096O1185S60	5.65	0.209	60	3.5 hrs
Filgrastim	Ib	18800	C845H1343N223O243S9	NA	NA	NA	3.5 hrs
Filgrastim-sndz	IIIc	NA	NA	NA	NA	NA	3.5 hrs

(continued)

Name	MOA	MW	Formula	IEP	Hydrophobicity	MP	Half-Life
Follitropin alpha	Ib	NA	NA	NA	NA	NA	24–53 hrs in females
Follitropin beta	Ib	22673	C975H1513N267O304S26	7.5	−0.33	55	35–40 hrs
Galsulfase	Ia	56013	C2534H3851N691O719S16	NA	NA	NA	6–40 min
Gastric intrinsic factor	Ib	NA	NA	NA	NA	NA	NA
Gemtuzumab ozogamicin	IIb	151000–153000	NA	NA	NA	61	NA
Glatiramer acetate	IIa	5000–9000	C254H422N70O72	NA	NA	NA	NA
Glucagon recombinant	IV	3767	C165H249N49O51S1	9.52	−1.197	NA	NA
Glucarpidase	Ic	44017	C1950H3157N543O599S7	NA	NA	NA	5.6 hrs
Golimumab	IIb	146943	C6530H10068N1752O2026S44	NA	NA	NA	2 weeks
Gramicidin D	IIa	1882	C99H140N20O17	NA	NA	229	NA
Hepatitis A vaccine	IIIa	NA	NA	NA	NA	NA	NA
Hepatitis B immune globulin	IIIa	NA	NA	NA	NA	NA	22–25 d
Human calcitonin	Ib	NA	NA	NA	NA	NA	NA
Human clostridium tetani toxoid immune globulin	IIIb	NA	NA	NA	NA	NA	NA
Human rabies virus immune globulin	IIIa	NA	NA	NA	NA	NA	NA
Human Rho(D) immune globulin	IIIb	NA	NA	NA	NA	NA	24–30.9 d
Human serum albumin	Ia	66472	C2936H4624N786O889S41	5.67	−0.395	62	NA
Human Varicella-Zoster Immune Globulin	IIIa	NA	NA	NA	NA	NA	26.2 d
Hyaluronidase	Ic	53871	C2455H3775N617O704S21	5.73	−0.117	NA	NA
Hyaluronidase (Human Recombinant)	Ib	61000	NA	NA	NA	NA	NA
Ibritumomab	IIb	143376	C6382H9830N1672O1979S54	7.91	−0.359	NA	0.8 hrs
Ibritumomab tiuxetan	IIIc	143376	C6382H9830N1672O1979S54	7.91	−0.359	61°C	0.8 hrs
Idarucizumab	Ib	47766	C2131H3299N555O671S11	NA	NA	NA	4.5–10.8 hrs
Idursulfase	Ia	76000	C2654H4000N688O774S14	NA	NA	NA	44 ± 19 min
Imiglucerase	Ia	55597	C2532H3854N672O711S16	7.41	−0.168	NA	0.06–0.173 hrs
Immune globulin human	IIIb	142682	C6332H9826N1692O1980S42	NA	NA	NA	>20 hrs
Infliximab	IIa	144190	C6428H9912N1694O1987S46	8.25	−0.441	NA	9.5 d
Insulin aspart	Ia	582580	C256H381N65O79S6	NA	NA	NA	81 mins
Insulin beef	Ia	5734	C254H377N65O75S6	NA	NA	NA	NA
Insulin Degludec	Ia	6104	C274H411N65O81S6	NA	NA	NA	25 hrs
Insulin detemir	Ia	5917	C267H402N64O76S6	NA	NA	NA	425 ± 78 min

Insulin Glargine	Ia	6063	C267H404N72O78S6	6.88	0.098	81	30 hrs
Insulin glulisine	Ib	5823	C258H384N64O78S6	NA	NA	NA	42 min
Insulin Lispro	Ia	5808	C257H387N65O76S6	5.39	0.218	81	1 hr
Insulin Pork	Ia	5796	C257H387N65O76S6	5.39	0.218	NA	NA
Insulin regular	Ia	5808	C257H383N65O77S6	5.39	0.218	81	NA
Insulin, porcine	Ia	5796	C257H387N65O76S6	5.39	0.298	NA	NA
Insulin,isophane	Ia	5808	C257H383N65O77S6	9	NA	NA	NA
Interferon alfa-2a, recombinant	Ib	19241	C860H1353N227O255S9	5.99	−0.336	NA	6–8 hrs
Interferon alfa-2b	Ib	19271	C860H1353N229O255S9	5.99	−0.339	61	2–3 hrs
Interferon alfa-n1	Ib	19241	C860H1353N227O255S9	5.99	−0.336	61	1.2 hrs
Interferon alfa-n3	Ib	NA	NA	5.99	NA	61	NA
Interferon alfacon-1	Ib	19271	C860H1353N229O255S9	5.99	0.339	61	2–3 hrs
Interferon beta-1a	Ib	20027	C908H1408N246O252S7	8.93	−0.427	NA	10 hrs
Interferon beta-1b	Ib	20011	C908H1408N246O253S6	9.02	−0.447	NA	10–20 min
Interferon gamma-1b	Ib	17146	C761H1206N214O225S6	9.54	−0.823	61	NA
Intravenous Immunoglobulin	Ia	142682	C6332H9826N1692O1980S42	8.13	−0.331	61	20 hrs
Ipilimumab	IIIc	148000	C6572H10126N1734O2080S40	NA	NA	NA	14.7–15.4 d
Ixekizumab	Ic	146158	NA	NA	NA	NA	13 d
Laronidase	Ia	69899	C3160H4848N898O881S12	9.09	−0.3	NA	1.5–3.6 hrs
Lenograstim	Ib	18668	C840-H1330-N222-O242-S8	NA	NA	NA	2.3–3.3 hrs
Lepirudin	Ia	6963	C287H440N80O110S6	4.04	−0.777	65	1.3 hrs
Leuprolide	IIa	1209	C59H84N16O12	NA	0.1	NA	3 hrs
Liraglutide	Ib	3751	C172H265N43O51	NA	NA	NA	13 hrs
Lucinactant	Ib	2470	C126H238N26O22	NA	NA	NA	NA
Lutropin alfa	Ib	30000	C1014H1609N287O294S27	8.44	−0.063	55	4.4 hrs
Mecasermin	Ib	7649	C331H518N94O101S7	NA	NA	NA	2 hrs
Menotropins	Ib	23390	C1014H1609N287O294S27	8.44	−0.063	55	NA
Mepolizumab	Ib	149000	NA	NA	NA	NA	16–22 d
Methoxy polyethylene glycol-epoetin beta	Ib	60000	NA	NA	NA	NA	134 ± 65 hrs
Metreleptin	Ib	16155	C714H1167N191O221S6	NA	NA	NA	3.8–4.7 hrs
Muromonab	IIa	146190	C6460H9946N1720O2043S56	8.31	−0.513	61	0.8 hrs
Natalizumab	IIa	NA	NA	NA	NA	61	11 ± 4 d

(continued)

Name	MOA	MW	Formula	IEP	Hydrophobicity	MP	Half-Life
Natural alpha interferon OR multiferon	IIa	19300–22100	NA	NA	NA	NA	NA
Necitumumab	IIIc	144800	NA	NA	NA	NA	14 d
Nesiritide	Ib	3464	NA	NA	NA	NA	18 mins
Nivolumab	IIIc	143597	C6362H9862N1712O1995S42	NA	NA	NA	26.7 d
Obiltoxaximab	IIIa	148000	NA	NA	NA	NA	NA
Obinutuzumab	IIb	146100	C6512H10060N1712O2020S44	NA	NA	NA	28.4 d
Ocriplasmin	Ic	272500	C1214H1890N338O348S14	NA	NA	NA	NA
Ofatumumab	IIIc	146100	C6480H10022N1742O2020S44	NA	NA	NA	2.3–61.5 d
Omalizumab	IIa	145058	C6450H9916N1714O2023S38	7.03	−0.432	61	624 hrs
Oprelvekin	Ib	19047	C854H1411N253O235S2	11.16	−0.07	NA	6.9 hrs
OspA lipoprotein	IIIa	27743	C1198H2012N322O422S2	6.72	−0.652	NA	1.2 Hrs
Oxytocin	Ib	1007	C43H66N12O12S2	5.51	−2.7	NA	1–6 min
Palifermin	Ib	16193	C721H1142N202O204S9	9.47	−0.65	NA	NA
Palivizumab	IIIa	NA	NA	NA	NA	61	18–20 d
Pancrelipase	Ia	131126	C5850H8902N1606O1739S49	6.44	NA	48–50	NA
Panitumumab	IIa	NA	NA	NA	NA	NA	7.5 d
Pegademase bovine	Ia	40788	C1821H2834N484O552S14	5.33	−0.428	NA	NA
Pegaptanib	IIa	NA	NA	NA	NA	NA	10 ± 4 d
Pegaspargase	Ic	31732	C1377H2208N382O442S17	4.67	0.059	NA	NA
Pegfilgrastim	Ib	18803	C845H1343N223O243S9	5.65	0.209	60	15–80 hrs
Peginterferon alfa-2a	Ib	60000	NA	5.99	NA	61	80 hrs
Peginterferon alfa-2b	Ib	31000	C130H219N43O42	5.99	NA	61	40 hrs
Peginterferon beta-1a	Ia	20000	NA	NA	NA	NA	78 hrs
Pegloticase	Ib	34193	C1549H2430N408O448S8	NA	NA	NA	14 d
Pegvisomant	IIa	22129	C990H1532N262O300S7	5.27	−0.411	76	6 d
Pembrolizumab	IIIc	146286	C6504H10004N1716O2036S46	NA	NA	NA	28 d
Pertuzumab	IIIc	148000	NA	NA	NA	NA	18 d
Poractant alfa	Ia	NA	NA	NA	NA	NA	NA
Pramlintide	Ia	3949	C171H267N51O53S2	NA	NA	NA	48 min
Preotact	Ib	9420	C408H674N126O126S2	NA	NA	NA	1.5 hrs
Protamine sulfate	Ib	NA	NA	NA	NA	NA	4.5 min
Protein S human	Ib	69000	NA	NA	NA	NA	NA
Prothrombin complex concentrate	Ia	NA	NA	5.05.5	NA	NA	48–60 hrs
Ragweed Pollen Extract	IIIa	NA	NA	NA	NA	NA	NA

Name							
Ramucirumab	IIIc	143600	C6374H9864N1692O1996S46	NA	NA	NA	15 d
Ranibizumab	IIa	48350	C2158H3282N562O681S12	NA	NA	NA	9 d
Rasburicase	Ic	34110	C1521H2381N417O461S7	7.16	-0.465	NA	18 hrs
Raxibacumab	IIa	142845	C6320H9794N1702O1998S42	NA	-0.435	NA	16–19 d
Reteplase	Ib	39590	C1736H2671N499O522S22	6.86	NA	60	NA
Rilonacept	IIa	251000	C9030H13932N2400O2670S74	NA	NA	NA	8.6 d
Rituximab	IIa	143860	C6416H9874N1688O1987S44	8.68	-0.414	61	0.8 hrs
Romiplostim	Ib	59000	C2634H4086N7220790S18	NA	NA	NA	3.5 d
Sacrosidase	Ia	100000	NA	NA	NA	NA	NA
Salmon Calcitonin	Ib	3432	C145H240N44O48S2	8.86	-0.537	NA	0.83–1.33 hrs
Sargramostim	Ib	14435	C639H1006N168O196S8	5.05	NA	NA	NA
Satumomab Pendetide	IV	141479	C6268H9708N1666O1971S48	7.02	-0.427	61	0.80 hrs
Sebelipase alfa	Ia	55000	C1968H2945N507O551S15	NA	NA	NA	5.4–6.6 min
Secretin	IV	3056	C130H219N43O42	9.45	-0.463	NA	NA
Secukinumab	IIa	147940	C6584H10134N1754O2042S44	NA	NA	NA	NA
Sermorelin	Ia	3358	C149H246N44O42S	9.99	-0.33	NA	11–12 min
Serum albumin	IV	66472	C2936H4624N786O889S41	5.67	-0.395	62	NA
Serum albumin iodonated	IV	66472	C2936H4624N786O889S41	5.67	-0.395	62	NA
Siltuximab	IIa	145000	C6450H9932N1688O2016S50	NA	NA	NA	20.6 d
Simoctocog Alfa	Ia	170000	NA	NA	NA	NA	14.7 hrs
Sipuleucel-T	IIIc	NA	NA	NA	NA	NA	NA
Somatotropin Recombinant	Ib	22129	C990H1532N262O300S7	5.27	-0.411	76 at pH 3.5	NA
Somatropin recombinant	Ib	22129	C990H1532N262O300S7	5.27	-0.411	76	NA
Streptokinase	Ic	47287	C2100H3278N566O669S4	5.12	-0.728	NA	NA
Sulodexide	IIIc	5000–8000	NA	NA	NA	NA	11.7 ± 2.0 hrs
Susoctocog alfa	Ib	NA	NA	NA	NA	NA	~17 h
Taliglucerase alfa	Ia	56638	C2580H3918N680O727S17	10.54	NA	NA	NA
Teduglutide	Ia	3752	C164H252N44O55S	NA	NA	NA	2 hrs
Teicoplanin	IIa	1880	C88H97Cl2N9O33	NA	NA	NA	70–100 hrs
Tenecteplase	Ib	58951	C2561H3919N747O781S40	7.61	-0.528	60	1.9 hrs
Teriparatide	Ib	4118	C181H291N55O51S2	NA	NA	NA	NA
Tesamorelin	Ib	5136	C221H366N72O67S	NA	NA	NA	38 min
Thrombomodulin Alfa	Ib	52124	C2230-H3357-N633-O718-S50	NA	NA	NA	2–3 d
Thymalfasin	Ib	3108	C129H215N33O55	NA	NA	NA	2 hrs

(continued)

Name	MOA	MW	Formula	IEP	Hydrophobicity	MP	Half-Life
Thyroglobulin	Ib	660	NA	7.5	-0.33	55	65 hrs
Thyrotropin Alfa	IV	22673	C975H1513N267O304S26	NA	NA	NA	5 ± 10 hrs
Tocilizumab	IIa	148000	C6428H9976N1720O2018S42	8.68	-0.4144	NA	11 d
Tositumomab	IIb	143860	C6416H9874N1688O1987S44	8.45	-0.415	61	0.8 hrs
Trastuzumab	IIa	145532	C6470H10012N1726O2013S42	NA	NA	NA	28.5 d
Tuberculin Purified Protein Derivative	IV	NA	NA	NA	NA	NA	NA
Turoctocog alfa	Ia	NA	NA	NA	NA	NA	NA
Urofollitropin	Ib	980	C42H65N11O12S2	7.5	-0.33	55	35–40 hrs
Urokinase	Ib	31127	C1376H2145N383O406S18	8.66	-0.466	76	12 min
Ustekinumab	IIIb	14690	NA	NA	NA	NA	NA
Vasopressin	Ib	1050	C43H67N15O12S2	NA	-4.9	NA	10–20 min
Vedolizumab	IIa	146837	C6528H10072N1732O2042S42	7.6	NA	NA	336–362 hrs
Velaglucerase alfa	Ia	63000	C2532H3850N672O711S16	NA	NA	NA	11–12 min

Notes: MOA (Mode of Action) Group Ia–Replacing a protein that is deficient or abnormal; Group Ib–Augmenting an existing pathway; Group Ic–Providing a novel function or activity; Group IIa–Interfering with a molecule or organism; Group IIb–Delivering other compounds or proteins; Group IIIa–Protecting against a deleterious foreign agent; Group IIIb–Treating any harmful disease; Group IIIc–Treating cancer; Group IV–Protein diagnostics.

13 Quality and Compliance Systems

13.1 COMPLIANCE

A detailed survey of common QA missteps found in audits is presented.

The core principles articulated in cGMP regulations forming a contemporary quality system include

- Every product must exhibit distinct identity, strength, purity, and other quality attributes ensuring safety and effectiveness standards.
- Quality-by-design involves creating and developing manufacturing processes during product creation to consistently maintain predefined quality at the manufacturing phase's end.
- A robust quality system facilitates the flow of process information from production to commercial manufacturing and post-development improvements.
- The quality control unit (QCU) responsibilities, according to cGMP regulations, generally encompass quality control (QC) and quality assurance (QA) functions.
- QC involves evaluating in-process materials and finished goods to assess manufacturing process efficiency and compliance with requirements.
- QA primarily encompasses reviewing and authorizing manufacturing, maintenance, associated records and procedures, and conducting audits and trend analysis.

13.1.1 CURRENT GOOD MANUFACTURING PRACTICE COMPLIANCE

For a biopharmaceutical product to enter the market, it must receive approval (authorization in the EU and licensure in the US), necessitating a successful inspection by regulatory authorities. Understanding deficiencies recorded by regulatory authorities is crucial in establishing a contemporary quality system.

13.1.1.1 Food and Drug Administration

A comprehensive analysis of FDA observations over the past two decades reveals the most common issues companies overlook. The top-ten frequently cited observations by FDA inspections from 2006 to 2017 are outlined.

1. QC (quality control): Procedures not available in writing or followed.
2. QC: Controls of identity, strength, quality, and purity lacking due to missing specification, standards, sampling plans, or test procedures.
3. QA (quality assurance): CAPA not in place or practiced.
4. MFG (manufacturing): Written methods inadequate.

DOI: 10.1201/9781003392026-13

5. MFG: Cleaning and maintenance procedures not present or followed.
6. QC: Release not appropriate.
7. QA/QC/MFG: Computer controls and login not appropriate.
8. MFG: Sterile area maintenance not adequate.
9. MFG: Calibration of equipment not appropriate.
10. QC: Written stability program not in place.

The recurrence of these observations signifies that many companies neglect basic requirements. Ensuring these listed observations are addressed can significantly enhance the chances of a successful inspection. Monitoring and controlling these practices fall under the responsibility of the QA team, a focus of this chapter's detailed exploration of the quality system comprising QC, QA, and its integration with manufacturing for cGMP compliance.

Receiving a warning letter from the FDA escalates the stakes for corporations. For instance, Schein Pharmaceuticals received a warning letter in 2000 citing inadequate controls over computerized laboratory systems, leading to data integrity issues. Increased FDA scrutiny on facility compliance with data integrity rules has resulted in heightened inspections. Consequences for non-compliance include facility closures, product recalls, import/export restrictions, delayed or denied pharmaceutical approvals, substantial repair costs, and damage to consumer due to a tarnished reputation are all possible consequences of the FDA's compliance measures for failing to comply with data integrity rules. Manufacturers who are found in breach of data integrity requirements may lose the FDA's trust and face more frequent and in-depth inspections.

For more serious enforcement violations, such as earlier Form 483s that have not been satisfactorily addressed, inspectors from the FDA's Office of Regulatory Affairs (ORA) deliver warning letters. Data integrity issues were prevalent in over half of global medication 483s between 2014 and 2018 and in 79% of global medication warning letters during the same period. The frequency of FDA warning letters citing data integrity issues has notably increased in recent years.

Despite data integrity regulations in part 11 of 21 CFR, these issues are seldom addressed in 483s or warning letters. Most identified flaws relate to failure in meeting cGMP predicate standards, particularly 21 CFR parts 210, 211, and 212. Notably, parts 211.68 and 211.194 are frequently cited:

Part 211.68 outlines requirements for "Automatic, Mechanical, and Electronic Equipment" and commonly cited issues include

- The company failed to establish an effective computer system control to restrict access to authorized individuals only.
- Access permissions were inconsistent with appropriate roles and responsibilities. For instance, laboratory analysts possessed the ability to delete or alter data, modify configuration settings (such as disabling audit trails), and manipulate date and time stamps of electronic data to falsify the date/time acquisition timing.
- Data were inadequately backed up, hindering future data reconstruction efforts.
- Discrepancies existed between audit trail data and the data printed on chromatograms.

Additionally, in reference to Part 211.194, companies may receive citations for not reviewing and including all pertinent data in release decisions. Common citations in this domain include

- Failure to review crucial data and metadata essential for identifying out-of-specification (OOS) events requiring investigation in lot release decisions.
- Falsification of test results, data destruction, or lack of necessary data supporting a test result.
- Laboratory analysts manipulating data by reprocessing or deleting OOS data to meet acceptance criteria.

Miscellaneous issues observed include

- Utilizing 'pre-injections' of product samples outside full sample sets to determine if results meet acceptance criteria, subsequently deleting or disregarding failed results.
- Intermittent disabling of audit trails to obscure results.
- Alterations or deletions of results.
- Use of integration suppression settings to minimize data likely to cause an OOS result.
- Unjustified aborting of test runs with no justification.

13.1.2 European Directorate for the Quality of Medicines and Healthcare

Deficiencies found during European Directorate for the Quality of Medicines and HealthCare (EDQM) inspections are categorized as important, major, or other, based on their potential risk to public health and the extent of deviation from EU GMP, the associated CEP dossier, and the European Pharmacopoeia (Ph. Eur.; Figure 13.1).

The most common deficiencies identified in each GMP area during EDQM inspections include

- Inadequate oversight of quality units in GMP activities, for example:
  - Failure to adequately control documentation (both paper and electronic).
  - Inadequate supervision of production and laboratory activities.
  - Underreporting and insufficient investigation of quality events (complaints, deviations, OOS results, change controls).
- Fraudulent documentation practices (as noted in FDA warning letters):
  - Rewriting documents to demonstrate acceptable, expected, or presentable results, values, or dates.

Top 10 Citations
Fiscal Years: 2009–2022

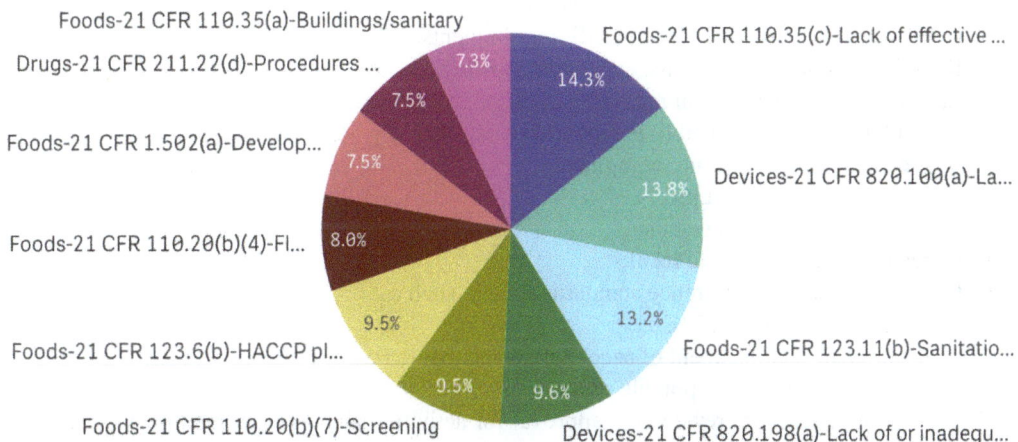

Foods-21 CFR 110.35(a)-Buildings/sanitary
Drugs-21 CFR 211.22(d)-Procedures ...
Foods-21 CFR 1.502(a)-Develop...
Foods-21 CFR 110.20(b)(4)-Fl...
Foods-21 CFR 123.6(b)-HACCP pl...
Foods-21 CFR 110.20(b)(7)-Screening
Foods-21 CFR 110.35(c)-Lack of effective ...
Devices-21 CFR 820.100(a)-La...
Foods-21 CFR 123.11(b)-Sanitatio...
Devices-21 CFR 820.198(a)-Lack of or inadequ...

14.3%
13.8%
13.2%
9.6%
9.5%
9.5%
8.0%
7.5%
7.5%
7.3%

FIGURE 13.1 The overall distribution of deficiencies from EDQM inspections between 2006 and 2018 by GMP area and CEP compliance

Source: Council of Europe 2019 EDQM Inspections and Trends of Deficiencies, Overview 2006–2018 PA/PH/CEP(18) 56

- Delayed recording of operations.
- Unavailability of records.
- Use of loose sheets instead of bound logbooks.
- Lack of application or inadequate implementation of quality risk management principles in production activities, deviations, change control, etc.
- Non-utilization of annual quality review as a quality tool by companies, for instance:
  - Inadequate reflection of all batches (especially "non-CEP" grade, despite being manufactured by the same process).
  - Trends not detected or investigated.
- Failure to detect or investigate trends, and insufficient personnel training, including:
  - Lack of GMP-related training for upper management.
  - Inadequate assessment of training effectiveness or limited value.
- Inadequate validation, such as:
  - Incomplete coverage of processes like the use of recovered solvents, blending, or micronization.
  - Lack of comprehensive knowledge of different approaches to cleaning validation.
- Other deficiencies include: Inadequate approval and management of vendors supplying key starting materials or intermediates (e.g., unreliable on-site audits).
- Risk of traceability loss due to insufficient container identification.
- Improper storage conditions (temperature, humidity, non-controlled storage facilities).
- Risks of contamination and cross-contamination from:
  - Poor facility design.
  - Inadequate equipment cleaning.
  - Insufficient maintenance of equipment.
- Lack of appropriate user requirement specifications for equipment qualification.
- Inadequate scientific approach in managing computerized systems used for material management, production, laboratory controls, etc., including:
  - Lack of suitable user requirement specifications.
  - Limited understanding of validation requirements.
  - Insufficient management of access levels, leading to potential traceability loss.
  - Lack of controls to prevent data manipulation.
  - Inadequate or absent audit trail reviews.
  - IT staff lacking knowledge of GMP requirements.
- Blending batches without prior appropriate testing.
- Lack of control over solvent recovery.
- Fraudulent practices related to testing activities, like:
  - Pretesting or "testing into compliance."
  - Omission of OOS results.
  - Unreliable analytical results.
- Unreliable microbiological results.
- Issues with chemical reference standards (CRS), such as:
  - Absence of Ph. Eur. CRS.
  - Insufficient establishment of secondary standards.
- Inadequate monitoring of potable water.
- Lack of or insufficient review and approval for activities such as equipment/instrument calibration, computerized systems validation, further powder processing.
- Most breaches of data integrity occurred in documentation practices and laboratory controls. Additionally, issues such as the absence of gaps in validation and controls on computerized systems were observed. Notably, between 2015 and 2018, 44% of critical and 25% of significant deficiencies were related to data integrity issues.

13.1.3 WORLD HEALTH ORGANIZATION

The World Health Organization provides extensive guidelines for pharmaceutical products, including guidance on sterile products, that are useful in establishing quality systems. The WHO also certifies companies for GMP compliance, such as the EU certification. However, it is important to note that a WHO or EU certification does not hold value for FDA submissions. The WHO's general guidelines for cGMP compliance are similar to the FDA and EMA guidelines, but not as detailed or demanding.

The WHO's charter mandates collaboration with regulatory agencies, primarily in emerging markets, often waiving inspection requirements based on GMP compliance certification by regional agencies. Regulatory agencies in emerging markets prioritize physical compliance more than the detailed documentation aspects that are focal points for the FDA and the EDQM.

13.1.4 HARMONIZATION

Collaboration among various regulatory bodies including the European Union Member States, the United Kingdom's Medicines and Healthcare products Regulatory Agency (MHRA), the United States Food and Drug Administration (FDA), the Australian Therapeutic Goods Administration (TGA), Health Canada, the Japanese PMDA, and the WHO aims to harmonize the evaluation of cGMP enforcement for sterile products in a pilot program lasting at least two years. Post this period, participating authorities will assess the program's effectiveness and determine future steps.

The EU legislation, specifically Eudralex volume 4 of "The laws regulating medicinal products in the European Union," provides recommendations for interpreting principles and guidelines of good manufacturing practices for medicinal products for human use. Similarly, FDA 21 CFR 210 and 21 CFR 211 contain comprehensive details on GMP regulation. In 2009, the FDA and EMA initiated a joint inspection program under the Good Clinical Practice (GCP) initiative focusing on investigator sites, sponsors, and contract research organizations (CROs) in the United States and the European Union.

Most countries have their regulations for cGMP. However, there are fundamental differences between how EMA (EU) GMP conducts evaluations compared to FDA cGMP:

- *Cleaning validation*: (i) According to EMA—Annex 15, Clause 41, the method "Test until clean" is deemed invalid for cleaning validation. (ii) *FDA* guidelines emphasize testing the product until it's deemed safe. Resampling is discouraged for systems or equipment with an approved cleaning procedure and should only be considered in exceptional circumstances, aligning with EMA's clause 41, but reserved for rare cases.
- *Personal growth and development*: (i) EMA—Clause 2.9, Chapter 2: mandates ongoing training provision, with a requirement to regularly assess its effectiveness. There is no FDA equivalent specifically addressing periodic evaluation.
  (ii) Under EMA—Clause 2.8, Chapter 2: All personnel requiring access to production areas or control laboratories, including technological, maintenance, and cleaning staff, must undergo training. No corresponding FDA directive exists for this criterion.
- *Sample*: (i) While the FDA terms it as a reserve sample, EMA categorizes samples into retention and reference samples, with additional criteria outlined for the retention survey. (ii) EMA lacks an equivalent to 21 CFR 211.176 of the FDA, which pertains to penicillin contamination.
- *Internal quality assurance audits*: (i) Notably, the FDA doesn't stipulate the necessity for internal quality assurance audits or the obligation to maintain records of such audits. (ii) However, the EMA incorporates a section on self-inspection within its instructional documents (Chapter 9: Self inspection).

- *Air room classification*: (i) The FDA classifies air based solely on 0.5 microns, whereas EMA categorizes it into 0.5 and 5 microns, respectively. (ii) FDA's air classification requirements pertain only to "in operation," while EMA covers both "dynamic" and "in operation." (iii) Specifically, ISO 6 classification is exclusively defined in the FDA. (iv) EMA provides details regarding the appropriate clothing for each cleanroom grade. (v) For Blow/fill/seal technology, FDA standards recommend a Class 100,000 (ISO 8) or better environment surrounding BFS machinery should generally meet Class 100,000 (ISO 8), or better, standards, depending on the design of the BFS machinery and the surrounding room. EMA: Blow/fill/seal equipment used for aseptic production fitted with an effective grade A air shower may be installed in at least a grade C environment, if grade A/B clothing is used. (vi) EMA specifies a minimum sample volume of 1 m cubic for classification purposes in grade A zones, lacking a corresponding listing in FDA directives.
- *Outdoor attire*: According to Annex 1, Clause 44 of the European Medicines Agency, wearing outdoor clothing is prohibited in changing rooms leading to grade B and C rooms. There's no corresponding FDA directive for this regulation.
- *Expiry date*: (i) EMA's Annex 13, Clause 26(j) mandates including an expiry date on the packaging of an investigational medicinal product (IMP). (ii) Contrarily, the FDA exempts IMP from the expiry date requirement unless the medication is reconstituted at the time of dispensing, as per the 21st Century Code of Federal Regulations, section 211.137.
- Tamper-Evident Packaging: FDA regulations, under 21 CFR 211.132, oversee tamper-evident packaging for over-the-counter (OTC) human drug items. No equivalent directive exists in the EMA guidelines for this specific regulation.
- *Inspection method*: (i) FDA investigators conduct site checks on specific items such as pharmaceuticals, biologics, and medical devices. Site inspectors closely adhere to FDA requirements, including 21 CFR 312 (Investigational New Drug Application) and 21 CFR 812 (Investigational Device Exemption). While inspecting sponsors, CROs, and monitors, the FDA compares their policies and procedures to the commitments outlined in the FDA application. (ii) In the EU, the GCP Inspection Services Group of the EMA supervises inspections. The EMA conducts inspections either upon request from their division, due to a particular interest in a product, or to ensure adherence to GCP rules. Inspectors utilize the Joint Program to ensure Member State compliance and conduct trials as per international agreements. Regulations for clinical trial conduct in the EU, including GCP, GMP, and inspections, are established in the Clinical Trial Directive (Directive 2001/20/EC) and the Good Manufacturing Practice (GMP) Directive (Directive 2005/28/EC), along with related guidance documents.
- Credentials are essential. When initiating an inspection, the FDA inspector presents credentials along with the original signed FDA-482 form, known as the Notice of Inspection, to the individual most accountable within the company, typically the management representative. Conversely, the EU follows a different procedure, not furnishing standardized documents at the inspection's outset. Instead, an initial meeting takes place where the inspection's goals, objectives, and any necessary documents or individuals for interviews are discussed verbally. Neither FDA nor EU inspectors are mandated to sign any documents requested by the company. While FDA inspectors are not obliged to sign non-FDA paperwork, they are required to note these requests in their written Establishment Inspection Report (EIR). The EMA and the FDA share a similarity in this aspect. Both the FDA and the EU request a site tour and pose inquiries to ensure adequacy of the trial's resources, staff, and overall facilities. During the tour, queries may encompass procedures and documentation, such as temperature controls and records of the product's storage location. However, in contrast to EU inspections, FDA inspections incorporate fewer plant tours, with a stronger emphasis on documentation.
- *Documentation*: (i) EU inspectors maintain a log tracking all requested and obtained papers. This log is provided to the inspected site to confirm that all demands are duly recorded.

(ii) The FDA solely makes formal verbal requests for documents. Additionally, the FDA stipulates that records must be made available expeditiously; failure to do so could lead to severe penalties, including suspension, denial, restriction, or refusal of a drug inspection.

- *The final meeting*: (i) If significant problematic findings related to products, practices, or violations of acts like the FD&C Act are uncovered during an FDA inspection, inspectors issue an FDA-483, a List of Objectionable Conditions, in writing before leaving the site. The FDA-483 outlines important findings relevant to the investigated items or procedures. Recurring or unresolved findings from previous inspections are also noted on the FDA-483.

   (ii) Unlike FDA inspectors, EU inspectors do not provide a written list of unsatisfactory findings at the inspection's conclusion. Instead, they informally discuss results during the closeout conference. The EMA issues an inspection report and an Integrated Inspection Report (IIR) for each inspected location. The reports are prepared in English, with on-site inspection reports copied to the investigator and sponsor, while CRO/sponsor inspection reports are sent only to the auditees.

- *Certification*: "Certification" refers to the process of obtaining a license. The EU allows the issuance of cGMP compliance certifications for product approval but does not grant product approval. Claiming to be "FDA authorized" results in severe penalties by the FDA due to its focus on facility systems capable of mass production. Facilities approved for a specific item in a particular item. Additional submissions in the same dosage form do not require another inspection if a facility has received approval for a sterile material in a vial dosage form. However, if a prefilled syringe is mentioned in the new applications, an inspection will be performed. There is inconsistency in dosage kinds, needing additional examinations. For several commodities, the EU may allow cGMP-certified companies to manufacture them. The EU approvals have a lesser ultimate guarantee in this regard, although their cGMP inspections are more rigorous and extensive than FDA inspections.

The discussion in this chapter encompasses fundamental elements for establishing a globally compliant quality system.

13.2   QUALITY SYSTEM

The definition of a quality unit aligns with modern quality systems, ensuring the correct execution, authorization, and monitoring of numerous operations within production and testing systems. According to cGMP regulations, the quality unit holds explicit authority to establish, monitor, and enforce the quality system. However, it's important to note that the quality unit isn't intended to take on the responsibilities of other components within a manufacturer's organization, such as production employees, engineers, and development scientists.

Other mandated functions of the quality unit, in line with a modern quality system approach, include:

- Ensuring appropriate application and execution of controls during the manufacturing process.
- Validating and implementing developed procedures and standards, including those used by a company contracted to the manufacturer.
- Approval or rejection of in-process materials and medication products. These actions, though critical, don't substitute for or prevent production personnel from ensuring consistent product quality routinely.
- Reviewing output records and investigating any unexplained variations.

The manufacturing and quality units operate separately yet cohesively within the overarching principle of delivering high-quality goods through a robust quality framework. In very small operations, a single person may serve as the quality unit, responsible for establishing controls and verifying manufacturing outcomes to meet product quality requirements.

The quality mechanism forms the foundation for interconnected and interdependent manufacturing processes. In the quality systems model, multiple manufacturing processes aren't viewed as distinct entities but are integrated into an acceptable model. Evaluating the state of control within these processes is a central theme of a systems-based inspection enforcement program (e.g., six sigma). This model aids businesses in achieving the necessary level of control, consisting of four main parts:

- Management responsibilities.
- Resources.
- Manufacturing operations.
- Evaluation activities.

13.2.1 MANAGEMENT RESPONSIBILITIES

Management plays a crucial role in designing, implementing, and overseeing modern and robust quality systems models. Administration, for instance, determines the appropriate quality framework structure for the company. The overall responsibility for providing the necessary leadership for the effective operation of the quality system lies with management.

13.2.2 PROVIDING LEADERSHIP

Senior management must demonstrate commitment to establishing and sustaining a strong, modern quality system that aligns with the manufacturer's goals and strategies. Ensuring alignment of quality system plans with business plans signals leadership. Senior management defines execution goals and formulates action strategies. Managers can support the quality system in various ways:

- Active participation in the design, implementation, and monitoring of the system, along with its analysis.
- Continuous improvement of operations and the quality system.
- Allocating necessary resources.

Managers should unequivocally support the quality framework and ensure its implementation across all levels (e.g., across multiple sites). Additionally, they can facilitate internal communication on quality issues throughout the organization, maintaining continuous contact between research and development, regulatory affairs, manufacturing, quality unit staff, and, where possible, management regarding quality matters.

13.2.3 ORGANIZATIONAL STRUCTURE

To ensure a robust quality system, management is responsible for establishing the organization's structure and ensuring that assigned roles and authority support the manufacturing, quality, and management operations necessary for delivering high-quality products. Senior management holds the responsibility of registering the organization's structure.

Managers are tasked with elucidating staff responsibilities, obligations, and authority within the system while ensuring clear comprehension and communication of interactions.

It is the corporation's duty to delegate authority to the individual overseeing the quality system for identifying issues and implementing solutions. Typically, a senior manager administers the quality system, ensuring timely feedback on quality issues for the organization.

13.2.4 BUILDING A QUALITY SYSTEM

Management is tasked with establishing a comprehensive quality system that defines the organization's structure and ensures alignment of delegated authority and roles to support manufacturing, quality, and management operations for delivering superior goods. Senior management holds the responsibility of ensuring the registration of the organization's structure.

Managers are in charge of explaining staff responsibilities, obligations, and authority within the system, as well as ensuring clear understanding and communication among team members.

By building a complete quality system, the management is tasked with determining the organization's structure and ensuring that delegated authority and roles support the manufacturing, quality, and management operations required to provide excellent goods. Senior management is responsible for ensuring that the organization's structure is registered.

Delegating authority to the individual overseeing the quality system to identify issues and implement solutions is a corporate responsibility. Typically, a senior manager administers the quality system, guaranteeing timely feedback on quality of the organization The quality system should comply with laws concerning protection, identification, strength, quality, and purity, meeting the minimal standards of cGMP regulations and the producer's requirements. Senior managers must guarantee that the established quality system offers consistent operational guidance and facilitates systematic problem assessment, aligning with the quality systems model.

In a modern quality systems approach, a structured mechanism for submitting modification requests to directives is recommended. Manufacturers operating under a quality system must design and document record control procedures for the completion, security, maintenance, and archiving of records, including data, serving as evidence of operational and quality system functions. This approach aligns with cGMP regulations, mandating manufacturers to establish and record controls for requirements, plans, and procedures guiding operational and quality system activities, ensuring correctness, proper checks, approvals, and easy accessibility of directives.

13.2.5 ESTABLISHING POLICIES, OBJECTIVES, AND PLANS

Within a modern quality system, senior managers utilize policies, goals, and strategies to communicate their quality vision across all organizational levels.

Under a quality structure, senior management must deeply embed a commitment to quality into the company's purpose. They should design a compatible quality policy, commit to meeting standards, enhance the quality framework, and establish quality policy objectives. For success, the quality system must be conveyed to and understood by employees and applicable contractors, requiring regular updates as needed.

Managers operating within a quality framework must define the quality policy's priorities. Senior management ensures the determination of the organization's quality priorities through a comprehensive quality planning process at the top level (and at other levels as necessary), aligning with the firm's business plans. The quality framework aims to ensure managers have necessary resources to achieve their goals and regularly track targets.

Managers will be needed to allocate resources and develop strategies to achieve quality goals within the quality framework through quality planning.

Documented quality strategies should be communicated to employees, aligning organizational practices with strategy and quality priorities.

13.2.5.1 Review of the System

System evaluation is crucial in any comprehensive quality system to ensure ongoing suitability, sufficiency, and effectiveness. Under a quality system, senior management are required to review the complete quality chain on a predetermined timetable. In most cases, such a study includes a product review as well as user expectations (in this section, the customer is defined as the recipient of the product, and the product is the goods or services being provided). The review should consider the following aspects in a quality system:

- Quality strategy and priorities.
- Results of audits and other assessments.
- Customer feedback, including complaints.
- The findings of the data trends research.
- Current condition of preventative measures to avoid a potential problem or recurrence.
- Actions taken based on prior management evaluations.
- Reporting any changes in market practices or conditions impacting the quality system (e.g., volume or form of operations). Consumer requirements are met through product qualities.

Reviews may be more frequent during the design and implementation of new quality programs than in mature systems. The quality system is usually a standard agenda item in general management meetings outside scheduled evaluations. The following are common review outcomes:

- The quality system and associated quality processes have been improved.
- Material and production process improvements.
- Reorganization of resources.

13.2.5.2 Change Control

Change management is a fundamental cGMP regulatory guideline designed to address changes and mitigate unforeseen consequences. In the context of cGMP requirements, the primary focus of change control lies within the functions assigned to the quality management unit. Specific alterations in production necessitate regulatory filings and prior approval, particularly those that modify requirements, vital product features, or bioavailability. A comprehensive quality framework encompasses change management activities such as quality planning and control of changes related to requirements, process parameters, and procedures. Manufacturers are encouraged to establish a regulatory framework conducive to continual improvement. This implies that manufacturers can enhance processes over time by leveraging insights gained from the diverse array of items utilized in the production process.

13.2.5.3 Corrective and Preventive Action

Corrective and preventive action (CAPA) is another well-recognized cGMP regulatory concept aimed at identifying, rectifying, and preventing anomalies.

13.2.5.4 Data Management

An effective quality framework mandates the reporting of management assessment outcomes. Planned actions, corrective measures, preventive actions, and change management protocols form integral parts of this framework. The cGMP regulations are specifically applied to certain components within the quality systems model described in this section, as outlined in Table 13.1. Manufacturers are advised to consistently reference relevant guidelines to ensure compliance with all laws.

13.2.5.5 Resources

Proper allocation of resources is crucial in establishing a robust quality framework and adhering to cGMP regulations.

TABLE 13.1
21 CFR cGMP Regulations Related to Management Responsibilities

Quality System Element	Regulatory Citations
1. Leadership	
2. Structure	Establish quality function: § 211.22(a) (see definition§ 210.3(b)(15))
	Notification: § 211.180(f)
3. Build QS	QU procedures: § 211.22(d)
	QU procedures, specifications: § 211.22(c), with reinforcement in §§ 211.100(a), 211.160(a)
	QU control steps: § 211.22(a), with reinforcement in §§: 211.42(c), 211.84(a), 211.87, 211.101(c)(1), 211.110(c), 211.115(b), 211.142, 211.165(d), 211.192
	QU quality assurance; review/investigate: § 211.22(a), 211.100(a–b) 211.180(f), 211.192, 211.198(a)
	Record control: § 211.180(a–d), 211.180(c), 211.180(d), 211.180(e), 211.186, 211.192, 211.194, 211.198(b)
4. Establish policies, objectives, and plans	Procedures: § 211.22(c–d), 211.100(a)
5. System review	Record review: § 211.180(e), 211.192, 211.198(b)(2)

13.2.6 GENERAL ARRANGEMENTS

Sufficient resources should be allocated to quality procedures and organizational activities within a robust quality framework. Senior management, or a designated authority, holds the responsibility of ensuring adequate resources for the following purposes:

- Maintaining necessary facilities and equipment to consistently produce high-quality products.
- Acquiring appropriate items suited for their intended use.
- Converting raw components into finished pharmaceutical products.
- Selecting, storing, and examining in-process, stability, and reserve samples for laboratory analysis of the completed drug product, including in-process, stability, and reserve sample collection, storage, and inspection for laboratory analysis of the final drug product.

13.2.7 DEVELOPING PERSONNEL

Within a quality framework, senior management should foster a problem-solving and communicative corporate culture. Managers are expected to cultivate collaboration by creating an environment that values employee feedback and is receptive to change proposals. Management can also facilitate cross-functional groups to exchange ideas for improving procedures and processes.

Given the nature of operational activities and their potential impact on product quality, the quality framework emphasizes the qualification of personnel assigned to specific tasks. Managers must identify relevant requirements for each function within the quality framework to ensure suitable task assignments for individuals. Personnel should understand the impact of their activities on both the product and the consumer, a quality system parameter also defined in the cGMP standards. This includes considerations such as education, training, experience, or a combination thereof.

Continuous training is imperative within a quality system to ensure employee competence and compliance with cGMP standards. Typical quality systems training should encompass regulations, processes, procedures, and written instructions linked to operational practices, the product/service, the quality system, and the desired work culture (e.g., team building, communication, change, behavior). Under a quality framework, education should emphasize employees' essential job duties and relevant cGMP regulatory criteria.

Managers are tasked with developing training programs within a quality system that encompass the following:

- Assessment of preparation requirements.
- Provision of preparation to meet these requirements.
- Training effectiveness is assessed, and training and retraining are recorded.

Supervisory managers must ensure that skills acquired from training are effectively integrated into day-to-day operations within a comprehensive quality system environment.

13.2.8 FACILITIES AND EQUIPMENT

Within a quality framework, technical specialists (e.g., engineers, production scientists) familiar with biopharmaceutical research, risk factors, and applicable manufacturing processes are responsible for specific facility and equipment specifications.

Per cGMP rules (refer to 211.22(c)), the quality control unit (QCU) holds the responsibility of examining and approving all initial design requirements and procedures for facilities and equipment, along with any future modifications. The FDA conducts pre-operational inspections of manufacturing facilities when resources permit.

cGMP regulations necessitate that equipment be qualified, calibrated, cleaned, and maintained to prevent contamination and mix-ups. In terms of calibration and maintenance, most standard quality device types require standards higher than those outlined in cGMP requirements. While cGMP rules give equal importance to both process and testing equipment, most quality programs primarily focus on testing equipment.

13.2.9 CONTROL OUTSOURCED OPERATIONS

When a producer outsources, they enlist a third party to handle operational processes that are inherently their responsibility. For instance, a manufacturer might outsource packaging and labeling tasks or cGMP compliance training. Quality systems involve contracts (termed quality agreements) that outline materials or services, quality prerequisites, obligations, and communication protocols. The producer ensures that the contracted company is accredited under a quality scheme. Personnel from both the contracting firm and the contracting manufacturer should be appropriately qualified and managed for performance in accordance with the contracting firm's quality framework. The quality standards of the contracting firm and contracting manufacturer should align. It's crucial within a quality scheme that officers of the contracting manufacturer are well-versed in the contract's precise specifications. Concurrently, the QCU holds the responsibility of authorizing or rejecting goods or services provided under the agreement, adhering to cGMP requirements.

Table 13.2 illustrates various aspects of cGMP regulations within this section, aligning with elements of a quality system.

13.2.9.1 Manufacturing Operations

The elements of a quality framework and cGMP regulation standards for manufacturing operations share many similarities. It's important to reiterate that FDA compliance and inspection systems primarily focus on cGMP regulations.

TABLE 13.2
21 CFR cGMP Regulations Related to Resources

Quality System Element	Regulatory Citation
1. General arrangements	
2. Develop personnel	Qualifications: § 211.25(a)
	Staff number: § 211.25(c) Staff training: § 211.25(a–b)
3.	Facilities and equipment
	211.173
	Equipment: § 211.63–211.72, 211.105, 211.160(b)(4), 211.182
	Lab facilities: § 211.22(b)
4.	Control outsourced operations
	Consultants: § 211.34 Outsourcing: § 211.22(a)

13.2.9.2   Design and Develop Product and Processes

Critical characteristics of the product must be specified in a contemporary quality system in manufacturing settings, and overall modifications should be controlled from design to delivery. Processes and procedures for quality assurance and manufacturing, as well as enhancements, must be defined, accepted, and monitored. It is crucial to establish responsibility for creating or modifying goods. Essential variables can be identified if related processes are recorded.

This documentation includes:

• Resources and infrastructure.
• Procedures to follow to complete the procedure.
• Identification of the process owner, who is responsible for maintaining and updating the process as required.
• Identification and regulation of essential variables.
• Quality control measures, required data collection, monitoring, and effective controls for the product and process.
• Validation operations, such as operating ranges and approval conditions.

Managers must ensure that product specifications and process parameters are determined by qualified technical specialists (e.g., engineers, development scientists). Biopharmaceutical experts should be well-versed in biopharmaceutical research, risk factors, manufacturing procedures, and how variations in materials and methods can impact the final product.

13.2.9.3   Monitoring the Packaging and Labeling Processes

Packaging and labeling controls, critical elements in biopharmaceutical production processes, are not directly addressed by quality systems models. As a result, the FDA recommends manufacturers adhere to packaging and labeling control standards outlined in 21 CFR 211 Subpart G.

In today's quality systems environments, when new or re-engineered processes are established, it is assumed they will follow regulated protocols. Design plans must encompass authorities and responsibilities, design and implementation phases, thorough evaluation, verification, and approval. In scenarios where multiple parties are involved in the design and development process, the model suggests reporting the roles of various groups to avoid neglecting crucial responsibilities and ensuring effective interaction among groups. Plans should be revised during the design process as required. A comprehensive quality system ensures that processes (or the shipment of a product) can function as intended before implementation, while change controls should be maintained throughout the design process.

13.2.9.4   Examining Inputs

In modern quality systems models, the term "input" refers to any material used in the finished product, irrespective of whether it is purchased or manufactured for processing by the manufacturer. Materials encompass components (e.g., products, process water, gas), containers, and closures. A robust quality system guarantees accuracy in all inputs to the manufacturing process, as quality controls have been designed for the reception, processing, storage, and utilization of all inputs.

Manufacturers and contractors are mandated to scrutinize the components and services they provide under the quality systems model; however, the testing framework differs from cGMP rules.

Moreover, cGMP standards require testing or the use of a Certificate of Analysis (COA) along with identification analysis. The initial checks should suffice to demonstrate reliability, with a schedule for regular rechecks. Data on commodity acceptance and rejection should be examined as part of purchasing controls to ascertain supplier efficiency.

Under the quality systems plan, suppliers must undergo regular audits. The manufacturer may observe the supplier's tests or inspections during the audit to evaluate the reliability of the supplier's COAs. An audit should comprehensively assess the supplier's quality system to ensure consistent reliability. The FDA suggests a hybrid approach (reviewing suppliers' COAs and conducting supplier audits). Even if comprehensive analytical testing isn't conducted, the audit may cover the supplier's analysis, but a clear identity test remains necessary.

A quality systems approach should include procedures to verify that materials are from approved vendors (specific sources are specified in submissions for application and licensed products). Additionally, procedures for acceptance, use, rejection, and disposal of facility-generated items (e.g., purified water) should be established. Systems creating these in-house materials should be developed, maintained, verified, and validated as needed to ensure they meet approval requirements.

Changes to products (specifications, suppliers, or materials processing) should be managed through a change management system (certain changes require review and approval by the quality control unit). It is crucial to have a system in place to respond to changes in supplier materials to make necessary process adjustments and prevent unforeseen consequences.

13.2.10   PERFORM AND MONITOR OPERATIONS

The primary aim of implementing a quality systems approach is to help manufacturers conduct and monitor operations more efficiently and effectively. Identifying, adhering to, reviewing, and reporting specific specifications and process parameters aims to objectively determine whether an operation meets its design and product performance goals. A comprehensive quality system should encompass production and process controls to verify that the finished goods possess the claimed or assumed identity, strength, quality, and purity.

A design model developed during product development typically transforms into a commercial design following process experimentation and progressive adjustments within a contemporary quality system. It's crucial to pinpoint flaws in the process and thoroughly examine variables that influence critical quality aspects. According to the FDA, scale-up experiments can demonstrate the full realization of a fundamentally sound concept. A reliable manufacturing process should be established before commercial production commences. Validating a manufacturer's manufacturing process involves ensuring good design and efficient transmission of process information from development to commercial production. Method validation within a quality system provides initial evidence that the process design achieves the desired product quality through commercial batch manufacturing. Adequate testing data provides crucial insights into the success of the new process and offers avenues for quality improvement. Incorporating modern equipment with continuous monitoring and control capabilities can enhance this knowledge base. While initial commercial batches may validate the process's validity and accuracy, the quality system should encompass the entire lifecycle by instituting continuous improvement mechanisms. Thanks to the quality systems approach, process validation becomes an ongoing operation rather than a one-time event.

Opportunities for process enhancements can emerge as experience in commercial manufacturing grows. Complying with cGMP requirements involves studying and evaluating documentation to ascertain the need for any adjustments. These documents contain product information and details providing insights into the product's control condition. Change management systems serve as a solid foundation for promptly executing technically sound manufacturing modifications.

In a quality system, written protocols are followed, and any deviations are justified and documented. This enables the manufacturer to monitor the product's history in terms of personnel, goods, facilities, and chronology as necessary. It ensures that the processes for product release are comprehensive and well-documented.

Both cGMP requirements and quality system models mandate monitoring critical process parameters during development.

A validated computer system or a second person might be utilized to verify process stages. Batch production records should be updated upon completion of each manufacturing step. While time limitations may be specified for crucial product quality, in-process criteria such as desired process endpoints determined through real-time testing or monitoring equipment can establish production controls (e.g., blend until mixed versus blend for 10 minutes).

Procedures must be in place to prevent microbial contamination of supposedly sterile finished products and the presence of undesirable microorganisms in non-sterile finished items. Validating sterilizing processes is critical.

Pharmaceuticals must meet stringent specifications, and production operations must adhere to strict criteria. In a quality system, selected data are used to assess the quality of a process or product. Additionally, data collection can facilitate and assess future ideas for change. Manufacturers must develop procedures to track, evaluate, and analyze operations using a quality systems approach that includes analytical methods and statistical techniques. Information continues to accumulate from product production to its commercial end within a well-managed quality system. Significant unforeseen variables should be identified, and necessary changes made. Procedures should be reviewed as needed to improve the functional design based on new information. With experience, identifying the need for change to achieve quality improvement becomes clearer. When implementing data collection procedures, consider:

- Are the methods of selection documented?
- When will the data be obtained during the product lifecycle?
- Measurement and tracking tasks are to be delegated in what way and to whom?
- When should laboratory data be analyzed and evaluated (for example, trending)?
- What documents are required?

A modern quality systems approach emphasizes that change control is crucial when data analysis or other information indicates a need for improvement. Managing and documenting changes to an existing process ensures meeting the required attributes of the finished product.

The cGMP elaborates further on change control for biopharmaceuticals. When making process modifications, it's crucial to consider product design and scientific competence. Significant design issues due to process practices might necessitate rethinking the design of manufacturing facilities, equipment, production and control methods, or laboratory controls within a company. Evaluating the impact of a change should focus on tracking and analyzing specific areas that may be affected, based on a comprehensive understanding of the implemented process. This enables a complete analysis of the steps taken to implement a change and its influence on the approach. Determining the results of a shift might require more tests or examinations of subsequent batches (e.g., additional in-process testing or stability studies).

Identified components within a quality framework significantly aid manufacturers in managing change and executing continuous improvement in their production processes. As an integral part of this framework, it's crucial to establish procedures ensuring the accuracy of test results. Any out-of-specification test results should undergo thorough scrutiny, as they might stem from research or production issues. Utilizing empirical and statistical data is recommended to justify invalidating test results. Upon completing production, it's advisable for manufacturers to align shipping specifications with special handling needs to maintain consistency, such as refrigeration in biopharmaceuticals.

Regular definition and review of trends serve as essential elements within a quality management framework. One effective method to achieve this is through statistical process management. Analyzing trends enables continuous monitoring of quality, early detection of potential deviations before they escalate into problems, supplements the data collected for annual reviews, and aids progress throughout the product lifecycle. Assessing process capabilities helps determine necessary changes, thereby contributing significantly to process performance and development.

13.2.10.1   Address Nonconformities

Every quality system must include procedures to address nonconformities and exceptions. Documentation of investigation, conclusions, and follow-up actions is essential. Ensuring a product meets specific specifications and expectations necessitates assessing both process and product qualities, like defined control parameter strength. Employees should be vigilant for inconsistencies at any stage of the process or during quality control. While not all irregularities lead to product defects, it's crucial to track and manage them appropriately. Promptly initiating a discrepancy inquiry when inconsistencies affecting product quality are identified is essential.

In a quality framework, it's critical to define and document procedures for halting and restarting operations, monitoring nonconformities, reviewing inconsistencies, and taking corrective actions. Re-evaluating the repaired product or technique for compliance and the significance of any nonconformities is important. If a nonconformity significantly impacts process performance, product quality, safety, or availability, strategies to prevent its recurrence are crucial.

Detecting or segregating products or procedures failing to meet standards and haven't been released for use is vital to prevent inadvertent supply to users. Remedial actions might involve rectifying the nonconformity, proceeding with sufficient approval, registering the issue, repurposing the product, or rejecting it. Products released without meeting specifications might necessitate a recall. Customer reports should be treated as anomalies warranting investigation.

Table 13.3 shows how cGMP regulations apply to various quality system components. Manufacturers should consistently refer to relevant regulations (Table 13.4).

TABLE 13.3
21 CFR cGMP Regulations Related to Manufacturing Operations

Quality System Element	Regulatory Citation
Design and develop product and processes	
Production: § 211.100(a)	
Examine inputs	Materials: §§ 210.3(b), 211.80–211.94, 211.101, 211.122, 211.125
Perform and monitor operations	Production: §§ 211.100, 211.103, 211.110, 211.111, 211.113
	QC criteria: §§ 211.22(a-c), 211.115(b), 211.160(a), 211.165(d)
	QC checkpoints: §§ 211.22 (a), 211.84(a), 211.87, 211.110(c)
Address nonconformities	Discrepancy investigation: §§ 211.22(a), 211.115, 211.192, 211.198
	Recalls: 21 CFR Part 7

TABLE 13.4
21 CFR cGMP Regulations Related to Evaluation Activities

Quality System Element	Regulatory Citation
1. Analyze data for trends	Annual review: § 211.180(e)
2. Conduct internal audits	Annual review: § 211.180(e)
3. Risk assessment	
4. Corrective action	Discrepancy investigation: § 211.22(a), 211.192
5. Preventive action	
6. Promote improvement	

13.2.10.2 Evaluation of Activities

The quality system aspects are directly associated with the requirements in the cGMP rules, as stated in the preceding section.

Trend analysis entails continuous tracking of outputs to identify any patterns. It involves monitoring data, problem recognition and resolution, and anticipation and prevention. Gathering data from reports, measurements, complaint handling, and other processes, tracking it over time, are integral to quality control methods. Analyzing data helps identify diminishing controls' performance, crucial for resolution or prevention. The cGMP mandates annual analysis of representative batches, a practice often requested by quality systems. Trend detection is instrumental in early identification of potential issues, enabling swift corrective and preventive measures. It aligns with the approach of annual evaluations and emphasizes internal audits.

An internal audit should be conducted as it is an essential part of a quality system strategy. Audits play a crucial role in determining whether processes and products meet defined criteria and specifications, while also assessing the implementation and maintenance of the quality system. Audit procedures need to be established and published, ensuring the proposed audit schedule takes into account various factors, including the relative risks of different quality system operations, previous audit results and corresponding corrective actions, and the necessity to audit the entire system at least once annually. Quality programs recommend guidelines that detail how auditors should acquire objective data, their duties, and audit methods. Protocols should outline auditing tasks such as audit scope, methodology, auditor assignment, and completion (including audit plans, opening and closing meetings, interviews, and reports). It is crucial to track audit results and assign responsibilities for follow-up to minimize difficulties. Managers overseeing audited areas must promptly address audit findings and ensure that follow-up activities are executed, evaluated, and documented, as per the quality systems model.

13.2.11 Risk Assessment

Effective decision-making within a quality systems environment relies on a comprehensive understanding of quality challenges. In the case of biopharmaceuticals, addressing risk issues related to intended use and patient safety, as well as ensuring the availability of medically appropriate pharmacological products, is crucial. Risk evaluation, involving assigning priorities to actions based on the risks of action or inaction, is a critical practice. Analyzing repercussions requires the involvement of all relevant stakeholders such as customers, pertinent manufacturing personnel, and other stakeholders. The assessment process involves resolving hazards using the manufacturer's risk assessment model, formulating a plan by choosing appropriate options, implementing the strategy, and evaluating the outcomes. Risk management is an iterative process that should be revisited if new insights emerge that alter the need for, or nature of, risk management.

Risk evaluation plays a significant role in establishing product requirements and essential process parameters within manufacturing quality systems. Coupled with process awareness, risk evaluation assists in managing and controlling change effectively.

13.2.11.1 Corrective Action

Corrective action is a proactive approach aimed at system improvement to prevent recurring severe problems. Both quality programs and cGMP requirements endorse corrective measures. According to the quality systems approach, processes must be established and documented to evaluate the necessity for action in terms of potential impacts, investigate the root cause of the issue, identify potential actions, take a chosen action within a specified timeframe, and assess the effectiveness of the action taken. Keeping track of any disciplinary actions taken is critical.

Understanding and using information from sources such as non-compliance records and rejections are necessary to determine actions needed to prevent problem recurrences. Both internal and external audits are conducted as part of this process.

Proactivity is essential in quality systems management, involving tasks such as succession planning, training, recording institutional data, and planning for staff, legislative, and process adjustments.

Establishing potential conditions and root causes, analyzing potential effects, and considering actions are integral to a preventive action procedure. The effectiveness of the chosen preventive intervention should be measured, documented, and monitored. Predicting problems allows the utilization of data reviews and risk assessments in organizational and quality system processes, enabling alignment with shifts in scientific and regulatory requirements.

13.2.11.2 Promote Improvement

The quality activities discussed in this chapter are geared towards enhancing the effectiveness and efficiency of the quality system. Additional enhancement activities can be employed by management as needed, with the involvement of senior management being crucial in assessing this improvement process.

The table below demonstrates how cGMP regulations apply to various aspects of the quality systems model described in this section. Manufacturers must refer to applicable regulations to ensure compliance with all laws (Figure 13.1).

13.3 VALIDATION MASTER PLAN

13.3.1 Overview

Quality control methods are in place to ensure consistency in each batch produced. While good QA practices encompass in-process controls, standard operating procedures, and meticulous documentation control, the unique process demands of recombinant production and the inherent variability of biological systems make QA systems more challenging. Recorded occurrences involving biological product usage emphasize the necessity for tighter controls. Quality assurance procedures aim to prevent out-of-spec products, adverse effects, or lack of efficacy within the process. Regulatory standards from ICH, FDA, EMEA, and Japan specify requirements and tolerances for each test. However, manufacturers often establish stricter internal standards, limits, and quality assurance methods, sometimes including tests that are neither necessary nor disclosed to regulatory agencies.

Current good manufacturing practice (cGMP) requires the validation of biopharmaceutical output for finished biopharmaceuticals, as outlined in 21 CFR 210 and 211. Validation involves manufacturing facility certification and process validation, which comprehensively evaluates all aspects of a new product and its manufacture. This process ensures that items are manufactured safely and efficiently, requiring control not only of the finished product but also of the manufacturing process.

While process validation starts early in the process, it becomes mandatory during cGMP manufacturing phase 3.

The validation master plan (VMP) is a comprehensive document within the quality assurance system. It initiates with process creation and evolves over time, reducing the risk of overlooking crucial components in the CMC section and ensuring batch compliance through effective validation techniques. Process validation, a key part of the VMP, encompasses various aspects such as:

- All in-process components, API, and DP analytics must meet the acceptance criteria.
- The analytical methods employed, as well as plans for certification and validation, must all be identified.
- Cells utilized in cell culture propagation are characterized. Cell line history, substrate, raw material characterization, microbial agents, fungi, mycoplasmas, viruses, and prions are all included in the software. Characterization of cells is usually carried out in accordance with ICH recommendations.
- The essential parameters of each unit function are defined. A statistical factorial architecture is used to establish important parameters.
- Short- and long-term stability tests for intermediate commodities that have been processed for some time. Product consistency under the stipulated storage conditions must be achieved throughout the storage term.
- Parameter intervals and statistical analysis to determine key parameters, recoveries, yields, batch data, column and filter performances, columns, and filter lifetimes are among the output parameters of process robustness testing.
- Flowsheets are used to define any unit activity.
- Impurities must be found and eliminated.
- Every unit operation is described in flowsheets.
- Impurities must be identified and removed.

The protocol for any validation study includes a declaration of experimental purpose, specification of what is to be qualified or validated, experimental plans, sampling plans, test plans with approval requirements, and a summary of statistical tests to be applied.

It is essential to specify parameter intervals for unit operations, covering proven appropriate ranges, regulatory ranges, control ranges, and operating ranges.

Addressing identity, security, process criticality, release processes, and analysis certificates is vital. ISO 9000–9004 standards are frequently applied in the following areas:

- Descriptions, procedure qualification, and validation were used as analytical tools.
- Protocols for pilots and production, as well as batch documentation.
- Related production documents, overview notes, unit process details, procedures, and batch records, whether direct or indirect (development report).
- Short- and long-term stability reports.

Sampling and testing strategies involve end-of-production monitoring, in-process tracking, quality control, target protein characterization, holding times, and stability tests.

Analytical test software for drug substance (DS) and drug product (DP) is specified in the specifications, along with various reports such as product development overview, lot summary report, process output report, in-process monitoring report, and validation protocol completion report.

Identifying essential raw materials and ensuring identity, purity, suitability, and traceability are needed.

Chapter 7 discusses general process validation considerations, process validation phases, and particular practices for each stage of the product lifecycle.

Information about the target protein, the chosen expression strategy, and specific post-translational modification requirements (like glycosylation, acylation, phosphorylation, or pegylation) serve as justifications for the process. The process plan should cover aspects such as product safety, process robustness, scaling up, cGMP production, and cost considerations. This plan should allow for updates in the process, aligning it with evolving stages from phase 1 to the mature phase 3. A visual flow chart detailing all process unit actions, including the entry and exit points of key raw materials or adventitious agents, is provided. The chart encompasses impurities from the host cell, the drug, and procedural elements. A solid foundation in process awareness and comprehension forms the basis for designing an effective process management strategy for each unit activity and the overall process. Management solutions can be devised to reduce input variance, adjust during production to limit its impact on output, or a combination of both.

To ensure in-process materials and finished products consistently meet established quality standards efficiently, manufacturing processes must comply with CGMP regulations.

13.3.2 ANALYTICAL METHODS

Process knowledge relies on precise and accurate measuring procedures for evaluating and analyzing medication components, in-process materials, and completed products. Validated analytical methodologies play a crucial role in product development, device characterization studies, and other phases where validated methods are not readily available. These analytical methods should be scientifically sound, offering specificity, sensitivity, accuracy, and consistent results. Maintaining well-functioning laboratory equipment is crucial, and protocols for analytical techniques, equipment maintenance, documentation, and calibration procedures should be established. The adaptation of existing technology or the integration of new analytical technology is advantageous in defining a process or a product. These methods significantly aid in reducing risks by providing better control over the product's quality. However, analytical procedures used for commercial batch release must comply with CGMP guidelines in sections 210 and 211, while clinical supplies should adhere to suitable CGMPs for the respective trial stages.

Quality Assurance (QA) systems ensure the reliability and suitability of analytical processes for their intended tasks. Evaluating the quality of raw materials, personnel, facilities, and manufacturers is essential, along with thorough validation of the analytical methods in compliance with Good Manufacturing Practice (GMP) criteria. The extent of validation varies based on the development stage; during initial phases, techniques are still evolving, focusing primarily on effectiveness and toxicity testing. However, procedures must be fully validated before creating clinical test batches. Critical validation factors encompass specificity, linearity, range, accuracy, precision, detection limit, quantification limit, robustness, and system suitability testing. These requirements align with other CMC (Chemistry, Manufacturing, and Controls) testing methods. More detailed information can be found in the ICH harmonized tripartite guideline Q2B (www.ich.org/MediaServer.jser?@ ID=418&@ MODE=GLB). Revalidation might be necessary if there are changes in the manufacturing process, drug product structure, or analytical method. The extent of revalidation required depends on the nature of the changes. The empirical validation plan outlines the steps for completing empirical validation, included within the master validation plan. A formal report on analytical technique description encompasses sample preparation instructions, raw material lists, process descriptions, data collection procedures, results, data interpretation, and a systematic validation process with relevant sample and control replication analytical sequences, validation features, data analysis, and reporting methodologies.

A manufacturer must ensure a high level of confidence in the performance of the manufacturing process before commercially distributing any batch for consumer use. This ensures that both active pharmaceutical ingredients (APIs) or active biological drugs, and the resultant drug products, adhere to critical attributes such as identity, strength, quality, purity, and potency. Objective evidence and data from laboratory, pilot, and commercial-scale investigations are utilized to provide this assurance. Statistical information can demonstrate the consistent production of satisfactory quality goods under commercial manufacturing settings.

An effective validation program relies on information and expertise gained during product and process development. This knowledge serves as the basis for developing a manufacturing process control strategy that ensures goods meet specified quality attributes. Manufacturers must acknowledge various sources of variance by:

- Determining whether or not there is a difference and, if so, how much.
- Recognizing how variance affects the process and, as a result, product qualities.
- Controlling variance in proportion to the danger it poses to the process and the final product.

Each producer must assess whether they possess sufficient expertise to ensure high assurance during the manufacturing process before permitting commercial distribution of the product. Focusing solely on certification efforts without considering production processes and variability may not offer adequate quality assurance. Manufacturers must maintain process control throughout the product's lifecycle, adapting to changes in products, equipment, production conditions, personnel, and manufacturing methods.

To evaluate the process, manufacturers can utilize ongoing initiatives to gather and analyze product and process data. These systems can identify process or product issues and highlight opportunities for process improvement, which can be implemented using actions from phases 1 and 2.

Legacy product producers can leverage knowledge acquired during the original process creation and qualification, as well as their manufacturing experience, to continuously enhance their processes.

13.3.3 DOCUMENTATION

In complex and lengthy projects spanning multiple disciplines, documenting each stage of the process validation lifecycle is crucial for effective communication and success. Documentation ensures that information about a product or process is accessible and understandable to all involved in each lifecycle stage. Transparency and accessibility of information are fundamental principles of the scientific method, crucial for informed decision-making by responsible organizational units, ultimately leading to a product's commercial release.

Current Good Manufacturing Practice (cGMP) necessitates varying levels and types of documentation throughout the validation lifecycle. Stages 2 and 3, particularly during process qualification and verification, demand extensive documentation. Compliance with GMPs is imperative, with the quality unit responsible for overseeing studies in accordance with regulations (see 211.22 and 211.100). Even when conducted on a small scale, tests for viral and impurity clearance require supervision by the quality unit.

Stage 1 process design produces cGMP documentation for industrial manufacturing (i.e., the initial commercial masterbatch development and control record (211.186) and supporting procedures). Firms should draw up a process flow diagram for the full-scale process.

Process flow diagrams should outline each unit's function, its placement in the overall process, monitoring and control points, and the inputs such as parts and other processing materials (e.g., processing aids) as well as expected outputs (i.e., in-process materials and finished products). As the process design progresses, creating and preserving process flow diagrams at various scales aids in comparisons and decisions regarding their compatibility.

13.4 GOOD LABORATORY PRACTICES

13.4.1 Overview

Good Laboratory Practice (GLP) constitutes a quality management system for research laboratories and organizations involved in non-clinical experimental research. It ensures uniformity, consistency, reliability, reproducibility, quality, and integrity of products in development for human or animal health (including pharmaceuticals) through non-clinical safety tests. Scientific measures (whether they are used to detect pollutants in pharmaceutical products, make clinical blood glucose determinations, characterize forensic evidence, or test materials for space missions) are widely acknowledged to influence life and death decisions. As a personal acknowledgment of their responsibility, scientists have historically employed sound laboratory procedures to ensure the accuracy of their findings. However, until recently, these policies faced inconsistent acceptance, application, and auditing. Because of well-known historical instances of incorrect data leading to disastrous outcomes, national and international agencies have established GLP guidelines for various industries (food, agricultural, pharmaceutical, medicinal, environmental, etc.) outlined in 22 CFR Part 58.

Federal agencies in the United States, such as the FDA and the EPA, have published documents outlining laboratory standards that must be met for technical results from laboratory studies to be acceptable for legal or contractual purposes. Laboratories engaging with these entities must adhere to GLP regulations. Ensuring compliance has become paramount, with many companies investing considerable effort, ranging from 10% to 50% of their overall resources, in internal quality assurance. On average, companies allocate about 25% of their efforts towards this.

Given the critical role of GLP in modern laboratory operations and its significance for competent scientists, it is highly recommended that all bioprocess engineers thoroughly review these guidelines. The guidelines are accessible on the websites mentioned in the reference section of this chapter.

13.4.2 Elements of Good Laboratory Practice

13.4.2.1 Quality Assurance: Establishing Confidence in Reported Data

The laboratory's analytical data, the primary outcome of chemical analysis, undergoes meticulous quality assurance (QA) procedures. These tasks encompass ensuring accurate chemical and physical measurements, interpreting and recording data with sufficient error estimates and confidence levels. QA activities also involve maintaining comprehensive records of specimen/sample sources, background information (sample tracking), procedures, raw data, and findings associated with each specimen/sample. Although each of these QA components might warrant extensive volumes, I'll briefly touch upon each here. Standard Operating Procedures (SOPs) are validated and certified procedures crucial for specific determinations. Regulatory bodies like the EPA or FDA typically approve and publish these procedures, disallowing the use of alternative procedures for collecting analytical data on specific analytes. It is imperative for any commercial laboratory to have SOPs aligned with appropriate standards. This ensures that analytical data obtained and recorded can be traced back to a documented procedure, allowing for replication of determinations using the SOP for similar specimens.

13.4.2.2 Instrumentation Validation

Instrument validation stands as a critical procedure in every analytical laboratory. Although default instrument data may seem reliable, modern computer-controlled systems, isolating analysts from data collection and instrument control functions, make it challenging to detect inaccuracies. Thus, it's crucial to establish objective protocols for regularly assessing instrumental data validity. These protocols guarantee the continued safe operation of laboratory instruments within defined parameters. Control charts, as time-related graphical records, depict outcomes of instrument validation procedures. Typically, the "control limits," which are assigned as upper and lower ranges around the projected instrumental output, are linked to some agreed-upon estimation of the expected random error for the entire process. Typically, the control limits are set at two standard deviations. When an instrument's performance exceeds these limits, QA procedures mandate its non-use for analytical reports until the issue is identified, rectified, and certified to operate within control limits again before being returned to service for determinations.

13.4.2.3 Reagent and Materials Certification

Reagents and product testing are integral to QA, following GLP guidelines that stress adherence to established protocols and proper documentation. Guidelines necessitate labeling each laboratory reagent/material container with certification details, date, and expiration. This protocol aims to ensure that SOP-specified reagents are used.

QA also requires an Analytical Qualification (COA), demanding evidence of analyst training and experience with suitable laboratory procedures. As the American Chemical Society lacks a 'certification' policy for chemists or analysts, certification standards are usually set by the lab, meeting FDA or EMA requirements.

13.4.2.4 Certification of Laboratory Facilities

Certification of laboratory facilities is usually performed by a third-party entity. Representatives from a government agency with which they have a contract, for example, may be audited at an analytical laboratory. An independent laboratory should submit paperwork to the appropriate state or federal agency. The evaluation considers space (quantity, efficiency, and relevance), ventilation, facilities, storage, hygiene, and other factors.

13.4.2.5 Specimen and Sample Tracking

The emergence of computer-based Laboratory Information Management Systems (LIMSs) highlighted the significance of tracking specimens and samples in quality control. Sample monitoring, whether manual using paper files or modern bar-coding techniques, remains an essential part of quality assurance. Although the terms "specimen" and "sample" are often interchangeable, "specimen" typically refers to a chemically determined substance, while "sample" generally denotes a finite portion of the specimen taken for analysis. In homogenous specimens, the sample mirrors the overall composition, but in heterogeneous ones (e.g., metal alloys, rock, soil, foods, etc.), a sample might not accurately represent the overall composition (e.g., metal alloys, rock, soil, textiles, foods, polymer composites, and vitamin capsules). Maintaining analytical result reports' context is crucial for data interpretation.

Different laboratories may employ varied procedures for proper specimen/sample monitoring, but they all must preserve the unmistakable link between analytical data and the specimens/samples they were derived from. Additionally, the source of the specimen/sample(s) must be documented and unequivocally linked to the analytical data collection. In specific situations, establishing and validating a "chain of custody" becomes necessary. This is particularly crucial for forensic samples in criminal cases but could be relevant in various other circumstances. For instance, a pharmaceutical company might need to demonstrate the authenticity of specimens used in clinical trials to eliminate doubts about data validity. These safeguards might involve ensuring that trial specimens were not tampered with and providing a complete chain of custody to eliminate any doubts about the validity of specimens submitted for chemical analysis.

13.4.2.6 Documentation and Maintenance of Records

Protection of specimen/sample origin records, chain of custody, raw analytical data, processed data, SOPs, instrument validation and reagent certification reports, and analyst certification papers aligns with GLP guidelines. These records allow for post-evaluation of performance, often after several years have passed. In the event of legal disputes, maintaining all specified records offers evidence that may be needed because of the effect of decisions concerning original analytical findings.

GLP's record-keeping function is critical, with many features now incorporated into modern instrument service computer packages. For instance, modern computer-based instruments allow unrestricted storage of raw analytical data for specific samples in a secure, tamper-proof environment. They also ensure the preservation of historical control chart data, crucial for determining an instrument's operational quality during data acquisition.

The duration for retaining laboratory records varies. In supervised laboratories, the general rule is to maintain records for at least five years, with the possibility of extending this period thanks to higher-density storage devices for digitized data. This kind of record-keeping is increasingly crucial, especially with the rise in chemistry-related commercial goods lawsuits. For businesses dealing with potential lawsuits, safeguarding stored data integrity becomes a significant security concern.

All of the record-keeping ingredients described above are captured in the traditional laboratory notebooks serve as repositories for the record-keeping elements described earlier, providing scientists with a detailed guide for laboratory maintenance. Detailed instructions on maintaining a lab notebook will be provided in a subsequent section.

Data collection in laboratories involves meticulous recording in notebooks using indelible ink, strictly avoiding erasable materials. Corrections are not made by overwriting; instead, incorrect entries are minimally crossed out for legibility. A new entry, accompanied by the operator's initials, follows. This practice, mandated by GLP, applies universally, even in simple or preparatory experiments. In instances where data is initially noted on loose paper (such as napkins) and later transcribed, the original writing must remain intact, a requirement extending to the final document.

The value of data hinges on several crucial questions: What is its intrinsic value? How confident are the results? How precise is the measurement, and what's the reproducibility of recorded numbers? Contrary to popular belief, the number of significant figures does not necessarily equate to accuracy. An excessive number of figures often hampers data presentation and might misrepresent its accuracy.

A data value represents a material property with an element of uncertainty. This data may be accurate, inaccurate, or a combination of both. The level of uncertainty associated with a value is reflected in how it is written, typically by the number of figures included, indicating potential uncertainty. Sometimes, there's an excessive number of figures after the decimal point, but even the figures before the decimal point can be tailored to represent the data accurately. A simple way to gauge this necessity is by counting the significant numbers. For instance, the numbers 19,490 and 10.098 both contain five significant figures each. The required number of significant figures depends on two factors. First, the value's significance, i.e., how relevant it is. For instance, if an instrument can only detect a 1% difference, significant figures should not exceed two after the decimal point. Second, the numerical multiplicative value matters. Consider the number π (22/7); while it can be extended to an infinite number of significant figures, a standard calculator rounds it to 3.14285714285714 due to the digits' remainder.

13.4.3 Electronic Data Handling

13.4.3.1 Overview

Entering data directly into electronic devices like computers, tablets, or through handwriting conversion is now common. However, electronic data handling poses new challenges and requirements that must be thoroughly understood by all handling such data. In the past five years, the FDA has issued more citations for non-compliance with electronic data handling than for any other reason, including adherence to GMP. These citations have been given to companies of various sizes, from small regional businesses to large multinational corporations. Consequently, many facilities generating data for regulatory submission continue using manual recording systems until they feel comfortable transitioning to electronic systems.

Electronic data management requires establishing an elaborate validation and security system, often inaccessible to smaller institutions. Stringent FDA requirements mandate validated hardware, secure operator identification, multi-level passwords, and active data monitoring. Although non-regulatory research institutions might bypass these requirements, compliance becomes imperative when planning a regulatory submission.

These regulatory requirements are detailed in CFR 21 Part 11 of the Federal Register. Students should familiarize themselves with at least the basic aspects of this law to grasp the system's requirements.

13.4.3.2 Code of Federal Regulations 21 Part 11: Electronic Records

Part 11 of Title 21 of the Code of Federal Regulations acts as a reference for those keeping or uploading records electronically to comply with FDA regulations. It covers all electronic records produced, updated, maintained, archived, retrieved, or distributed in line with FDA Regulations. Part 11 also encompasses electronic documents submitted to the FDA under the Federal Food, Drug, and Cosmetic Act (the Act) and the Public Health Service Act (the PHS Act), even if these records aren't expressly defined in FDA regulations (11.1). Predicate laws are the foundational criteria outlined in the Act, the PHS Act, and the FDA, other than Part 11.

The FDA enforces the provisions of part 11 including, but not limited to, certain controls for closed systems in § 11.10, for example, the following controls and requirements:

- Limiting device access to only those who are allowed.
- The application of operating framework tests.
- Tests for authority.
- Unit checks are used.
- The determination that people who design, operate, or use electronic systems have the necessary qualifications, training, and experience to do their jobs.
- Individuals are held responsible for acts taken with their electronic signatures if written policies are developed and followed.
- Additionally, there are requirements for system documentation controls, acceptable controls over systems documentation for open systems (11.30), and requirements related to electronic signatures (e.g., 11.50, 11.70, 11.100, 11.200, and 11.300).

For full compliance, individuals must adhere to relevant predicate rules, ensuring the preservation and accuracy of the documents intended for preservation or submission.

Part 11 applies when people opt for electronic documents over paper format. When computers generate paper printouts of electronic records that meet all relevant predicate rule criteria and these printouts are relied upon for controlled activities, the FDA typically doesn't classify this as 'using electronic records in place of paper records' under 11.2(a) and 11.2(b). In such cases, the use of computer systems in creating paper records doesn't trigger part 11.

Part 11 of the FDA's regulations pertains to specific electronic records or signatures (part 11 records or signatures)

- Records must be held following predicate rule provisions and kept in electronic format rather than paper format. Part 11 records, on the other hand, are records (and any related signatures) that are not supposed to be kept under predicate rules but are kept in electronic format.
- Records that are supposed to be kept under predicate rules are kept in both electronic and paper formats and are used to carry out supervised activities.

Real business practices may determine whether electronic records or paper records are used under 11.2(a) in certain cases. For example, if a predicate rule requires record maintenance and a machine generates a paper printout of electronic records, the dependency for supervised operations is on the electronic record. In such cases, the FDA might opt for an electronic record over a paper one. Essentially, when determining the applicability of part 11, the FDA considers your business practices.

Records submitted to the FDA in electronic format under predicate rules (even if not explicitly listed in FDA regulations) (assuming identification in docket number 92S-0251 as acceptable electronic submissions). However, a record used to generate a request is not considered part 11 compliant unless allowed under a predicate rule and maintained in electronic format.

Predicate laws mandate handwritten signatures, initials, and other signings, with electronic signatures intended as substitutes. Part 11 signatures include electronic signatures used to document specific events or activities per the predicate rule (e.g., accepted, checked, verified).

13.4.4 Validation

FDA requires validation of computerized systems (11.10(a)) and corresponding criteria (11.30). Assess the scope of computerized system validation based on their impact on meeting predicate rule requirements and the accuracy, reliability, credibility, availability, and validity of necessary records and signatures. Even without predicate rule requirements for validation, cases may necessitate validation.

Clients should focus their strategy on a documented risk assessment to evaluate system impacts on product quality, protection, and record integrity. Validation may not be necessary for a word processor generating SOPs exclusively.

Computer systems encompass hardware and software; hardware validation protocols are well-defined, but software validation poses significant challenges. Most off-the-shelf software programs do not meet FDA validation requirements.

13.4.5 Audit Trails

Unique part 11 standards govern computer-generated, time-stamped audit trails, requiring compliance with relevant predicate rule provisions for recording date (e.g., 58.130(e)), time, or event sequencing. Any modifications to records must not obscure prior entries.

Even if no predicate rule requirements are available to track, for example, the date, time, or sequence of events in a specific case, audit trails or other physical, logical, or procedural security measures may be necessary to ensure the records' trustworthiness and reliability. We should base our decision on whether to use audit trails or other necessary steps on the need to comply with predicate rule requirements, a justified and recorded risk assessment, and a determination of the possible impact on product quality, protection, and record integrity. Based on such an assessment, the FDA recommends that we implement effective controls. When users are required to build, alter, or remove controlled records during regular operations, audit trails can be particularly useful.

The copies of electronic records are provided to the FDA as follows:

- When records are held in common portable formats, making copies of them is a simple task.
- Where possible, using existing automated conversion or export methods to create copies in a more popular format (examples of such formats include, but are not limited to, PDF, XML, or SGML).

13.4.6 Record Retention

Predicate rule criteria, a justified and recorded risk evaluation, and a calculation of the records' worth over time should all be considered when deciding how to keep records.

The FDA permits archiving necessary records on non-electronic media like microfilm, microfiche, paper, or standard electronic file formats (e.g., PDF, XML, or SGML). Predicate rule provisions must be followed, and both content and purpose of the required documents and their copies must be preserved. The electronic version of records may be discarded if all predicate rule conditions are met, and content and context are maintained and archived. A hybrid situation where paper and electronic recording and signature components coexist is acceptable as long as predicate rule criteria are met, and the records' accuracy and meaning are preserved.

13.4.7 DATA ERRORS

13.4.7.1 Absolute and Relative Errors

The significant digits are also decided frequently on the output of the instrument recording the data; for example, if a balance is capable of giving ±1 g, then there is no sense reporting weight even to a single decimal place. The last number should be rounded off, for example, a weight machine recording 138.7 g (yes the output may be provided to any significant value) then the number should be reported as 139 g. In the example given above, we have introduced another concept of absolute error, meaning that within a range of 1 g on each side, the values are not accurate. When the absolute error is compared with the total value, we obtain a relative error. In the example above, 139 g weight recorded on a machine with ± 1 g uncertainty represents a relative error of $(1/139) \times 100 = 0.72\%$ relative error.

As absolute error is an estimation rather than an actual measurement, reporting it to more than two significant figures is unnecessary. In the example calculation, reporting a relative error of 0.7269% wouldn't provide meaningful information.

Absolute errors and relative errors, as discussed earlier, pertain to individual data sets. When multiple datasets are incorporated into a mathematical formula, the error can become substantial. As a rule of thumb, relative errors are additive when performing multiplication or division. In the previously mentioned example, the relative error for weight measurement was 0.72%. If the volume measurement (for density determination) has a relative error of 2%, then the overall error for density will amount to 2.72%. For addition or subtraction, absolute errors, not relative errors, are combined. However, when subtracting large numbers, the absolute errors may result in smaller values, transforming into considerably large relative errors. For instance, if a value of 2890 is subtracted from 2900, both with an absolute error of 10, the final answer of 10 will possess an absolute error of 10 or a 100% relative error.

13.4.8 SYSTEMATIC AND RANDOM ERRORS

The preceding paragraphs detailed significant figures in numbers and addressed handling data reliability. Errors in measurements can stem from a fixed factor, such as lack of calibration, or unpredictable human errors. The former is termed a systematic error; for instance, if the user overlooks the 42g weight of the sample container, all measurements should be adjusted downward by 42 g. Additionally, calibration errors, resulting in all readings being 10% higher, can be rectified after data collection. Systematic errors produce highly reproducible results, hence precise although not accurate. The latter type, random or accidental error, arises from unknown causes such as human or machine errors leading to varying measurements or a scattered distribution. For accuracy, results should exhibit minimal systematic and random errors.

Finally, some errors fall in the category of blunders—needless to say; it takes a man to err, a computer to blunder.

The goal of obtaining data remains to obtain accurate data recorded to reasonable significant figures, thus obviating systematic and random errors.

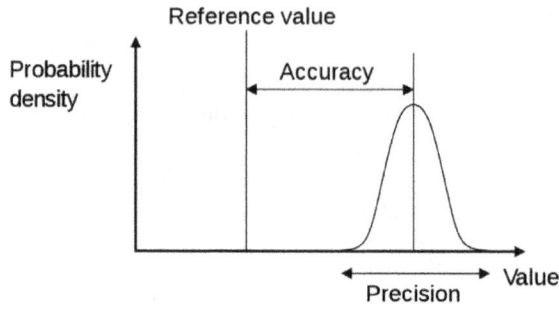

FIGURE 13.2   Precision-accuracy relationship chart.

Source: Copyright Millipore Sigma

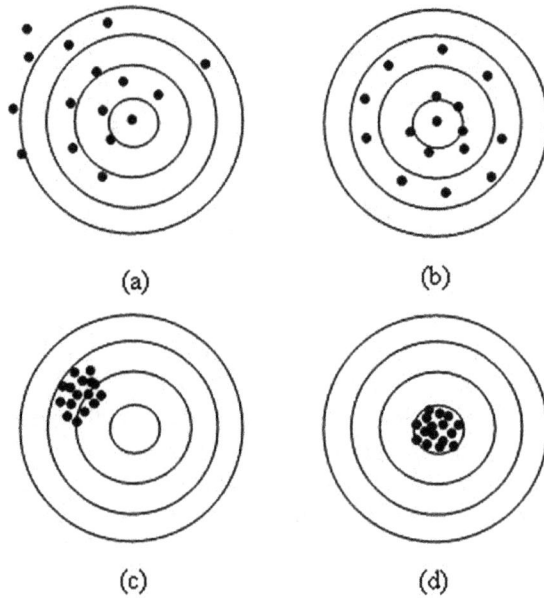

FIGURE 13.3   Darts thrown representing how precision and accuracy are defined: (a) imprecise and inaccurate (b) imprecise and accurate (note: the decision to call this observation accurate depends on the range of precision required; for example, in most circumstances, a 5% lack of precision will be readily accepted, in others a much lower range is desired); (c) precise and inaccurate; and (d) precise and accurate.

Source: Copyright Millipore Sigma

In cases where absolute and correct figures are reported, there's no limit to significant figures, as seen with the value of π or an exact dollar amount. However, in collected data, reporting more than three significant figures often surpasses the sensitivity of the methods used, giving a false impression of higher accuracy and reliability.

To represent the above discussion in a graphical form, Figure 13.2 shows the relative errors.

On a more graphical base, Figure 13.3 shows the description of precision and accuracy on a dartboard.

Interestingly, the next time you look at the advertisement of a high-end manual Swiss watch, notice that they tout their "precision movement", not "accurate movement" because none of the watches, particularly the manual ones, are accurate.

13.4.9   STATISTICAL ANALYSIS

Randomness in data is associated with unpredictable errors; however, another aspect of randomness involves the data measured. While an electronic instrument might produce an electrical signal with a random range of responses to an impulse, universal values encountering randomness are common occurrence.

The age distribution of the American population reflects a bell-shaped curve, termed a Gaussian distribution phenomenon, when plotted against age groups and corresponding population numbers. This bell curve might be ideally symmetrical (representing a truly randomized sample) or skewed due to an overall bias. For instance, the Japanese curve skews rightward, signifying longer life expectancy and slower population growth. Conversely, in many developing countries, the curve skews leftward (lower age), symbolizing a high birth rate and elevated mortality at older ages.

When a coin is flipped numerous times, the outcomes would be represented as a flat bar indicating the two outcomes rather than a bell-shaped curve, owing to the discrete nature of the results. It's crucial not to confuse the randomness in these examples with the randomness observed in the data output that constitutes our dataset. These random measurement errors can be analyzed through statistical procedures to determine the best estimate of the measured variable and assess how random error influences the data.

It is pertinent to note that, similar to the age distribution example, random errors also adhere to a Gaussian (or normal) distribution. Theoretically, an infinite number of readings would yield an error-free arithmetic mean. However, a reasonable number of readings suffice to understand the actual value.

The process begins with calculating the arithmetic mean by adding all values and dividing the sum by the number of readings.

This represents an initial attempt to define the real value. However, this value doesn't account for measurement precision, which is indicated by how each reading deviates from the arithmetic mean—the residual value. This residual provides a statistical parameter known as standard deviation (σ).

$$\sigma = \sqrt{\frac{n}{\Sigma(x-x)^2}} \tag{13.1}$$

$$\frac{\sqrt{(x_1-x)^2+(x_2-x)^2+(x_3-x)^2+}}{(x_n-x)^2}$$

Hence, in reporting the results of repeated measurements, the mean is quoted as the best estimate of the variable, while the standard deviation gauges the confidence in the result. Both mean and standard deviation share units and dimensions with the variable (x), and the variable is reported as mean ± standard deviation. As the number of observations (n) increases, the standard deviation decreases while simultaneously bringing the arithmetic mean closer to the real value. In cases where a high standard deviation is observed, the focus should be on system improvement rather than reducing the deviation through repeated measurements. Typically, a few dozen readings suffice to grasp the extent of deviation. Notably, systematic errors stemming from poor calibration or validation are constant modulators linked to accuracy and aren't subject to statistical analysis.

13.4.10   CONCLUSIONS

Data analysis encompasses techniques for describing evidence, identifying patterns, forming theories, and testing hypotheses. Numerical results of data analysis tend to be straightforward, often revealing the most representative number and comparing them. It unveils averages (e.g., average pH or temperature) and variations (e.g., differences in optical density during fermentation). However, data analysis is not solely about numbers; it utilizes them. The challenge arises not in contemplating "How does it work?" but in the realm where data analysis operates. For instance, in an 8-hour bacterial culture, the optical density increased from an initial 0.1 to 12. Mathematically, the culture averaged an optical density increase of 1.49 h^{-1}. However, without further data collection and analysis, the question "How does it work?" remains unanswered. Additional data analysis in this scenario might reveal that the culture doubled in density every 20 minutes until reaching around 12 and then stabilized, which occurred approximately 4.5 hours in. Consequently, data analysis assists in testing a particular model's applicability to a process, estimating the significance of coefficients in process models, and visualizing a variable's general pattern influencing another.

Experimental data can be categorized into independent variables and dependent variables, with the latter representing the uncontrolled response. Examples of independent variables include time, pH, or temperature, while the dependent variable, such as optical density, is expressed as a function of the independent variable.

Flow diagrams serve as visual representations of processes, effectively summarizing a vast amount of data. They can be complex, outlining pertinent process information and data. Figure 13.2 illustrates a flow diagram depicting the manufacture of a recombinant protein. Experiment conditions and recorded outputs can be integrated into flow diagrams. Some flow diagrams transform into decision trees, determining a specific path based on true or false conditions. Engineering flow diagrams contain extensive details and are routinely used to describe large complex systems.

Data are typically represented through tables, graphs, or equations. Tables offer a way to display data of varying lengths and levels of detail, but longer tables can become difficult to interpret. Graphs, on the other hand, provide a quick visualization of results and trends. Understanding these aspects of data analysis is crucial for grasping the overall process and identifying outliers. It also facilitates the design of additional experiments based on different phases of the experiment. Conventionally, independent variables are plotted on the abscissa (X-axis), while one or more dependent variables are plotted on the ordinate (Y-axis). One simple method for plotting data is by using Microsoft Excel, which provides extensive mathematical and statistical tools. Proficiency in Microsoft Excel is highly recommended for anyone working in a laboratory setting. However, it's important to note that these data manipulations might not comply with CFR 21 Part 11, which may or may not be an issue depending on whether the data are submitted for regulatory approval of products.

The relationship between independent and dependent variables can often be presented in equation form, establishing a mathematical relationship. A regression fit might yield a linear relationship, such as $y = Ax + B$, where B represents the intercept of the straight line on the ordinate and A is the slope; A and B are also known as coefficients or adjustable parameters.

Non-linear regression involves incorporating another mathematical function, such as an exponential growth model like $X = X_0 e - kt$, where k is the rate constant and t is time. This relationship implies a natural log-linear relationship, where plotting the natural log of X against time produces a straight line with a slope equal to $-k$. Fitting data to these equations allows for understanding and predicting outcomes based on a certain equation.

Considering inherent errors in each data point and those that can be analyzed through statistical methods is crucial when drawing conclusions from data analysis. This emphasizes the use of regression analysis to ensure proper understanding of a dataset. While Microsoft Excel simplifies the creation of various regression fits or models, it's essential for students to manually calculate the goodness of fit to appreciate the role of data variability. Understanding statistical principles behind calculations is fundamental, as human errors often contribute significantly to experimental errors. Recognizing the significance of random errors, systematic errors, and blunders is essential for those working in laboratories. Collecting data inaccurately severely limits their meaningfulness, adhering to the principle of "garbage in, garbage out." Therefore, a thorough understanding of basic statistical methods and their limitations is crucial in laboratory work.

When data are plotted, either manually or by computer, and a best-fit line is drawn through them, the question arises regarding the significance of certain points over others. This concern becomes more pronounced when employing manual data smoothing techniques. Computers, however, mitigate this bias by drawing lines that minimize variance between predicted points and actual values at different intervals. Nevertheless, this method tends to give more weight to data points with larger values. To address this, models are available that assign specific weights to data points, thereby preventing such biases in automated computations. The least-squares analysis, a prevalent technique for determining the line or curve that minimizes residuals, involves minimizing the sum of squares of the residuals in this statistical method. Different approaches exist for this operation. For instance, Legendre's approach decreases the number of squares of the residuals for the dependent variable, while Gauss's and Laplace's methods reduce the sum of squares of weighted residuals, with weights determined by the scatter of replicate data points. It's crucial to note that each approach yields distinct results; determining the "correct" fitting curve is essentially subjective. In the least-squares analysis, the generated curve may not closely align with specific data points known to be more accurate, as it minimizes the number of squares of the residuals. Alternatively, characterizing the best fit by raising the number of residuals to the fourth power minimizes the absolute values of the residuals. The selection of the sum of squares is somewhat arbitrary, as several other mathematical methods are equally valid. Outliers, points with large residuals, strongly influence regression. In some cases, these outliers can be excluded, but only after analyzing the data both with and without them. Statistical models specifically designed to handle outliers exist, requiring a deeper understanding of statistical modeling. It is important to note that Good Laboratory Practice (GLP) standards prohibit the exclusion of any outliers.

To summarize, note that the least-squares analysis applies solely to data containing random errors, necessitating independent variables. In essence, y cannot be a function of x and be determined by the process's nature. For instance, if x represents time and y is optical density, regardless of the time readings taken, y should not depend on the clock hour. If readings at 2 pm consistently show a 10% increase, there exists a dependence between x and y. Such instances require more sophisticated models for analysis. Moreover, it assumes uniform data output regardless of the experiment. Consider whether equipment heating up over time might introduce more random error measurements.

That will require necessitating additional corrections and potentially requiring weighted least-square analysis.

In the past, graph paper plotting was commonplace. However, in today's electronic age, it's advisable to refrain from this practice. Not only is it time-consuming, but it also tends to result in significant errors and hinders electronic data storage. Instead, students are encouraged to develop proficiency in tools like Microsoft Excel. Computer plotting offers added benefits such as error bars, standard deviation bars, regression coefficients, and measures of goodness of fit.

13.5 QUALITY CONTROL

13.5.1 OVERVIEW

For biopharmaceuticals and chemically derived drugs, in-process testing, release testing based on DS and DP specifications, and product characterization testing follow similar protocols. Monitoring various parameters and responses is part of a robust quality management program. This encompasses essential parameter descriptions, in-process control of intermediate substances, and testing of both drug substance and product. Quality control standard definitions include process management, substance/product control, and a summary of analytical methods employed to classify intermediate and final products. In-process measurements like pH, conductivity, total protein, and redox potential are common. Testing of drug substances/products adheres to ICH standards, focusing on identity, biological activity, immunoreactivity, purity, and quantity, comparing data against predetermined acceptance criteria. Release monitoring applies to drugs with a compendial monograph (e.g., interferon, erythropoietin, growth hormone, insulin). Methods are checked (and tested if a compendium method exists) and necessary documentation generated.

13.5.2 IN-PROCESS CONTROL

When comparing biological products to chemical ones, safety emerges as a more significant concern. Impurities in biological systems carry greater importance than in chemical systems as they have the potential to modify the three-dimensional structure of proteins, thereby impacting their immunogenicity. Despite impurity levels falling well below unsafe or detectable thresholds, they can still adversely affect the product. Consequently, product quality is intrinsically linked to various factors: process design, robustness, compliance with cGMP, and comprehensive quality management systems. These systems encompass product requirements, process specifications, process control, drug substance and product testing, as well as regulatory policies, all rooted in scientific comprehension. In-process controls, such as raw material control, process variable regulation, and analytical testing at intermediate stages and post-cell culture termination, are critical. Process controls are commonly integrated to ensure quality by monitoring process parameters and responses. This mandates a meticulous characterization of procedures early in process development and scale-up, particularly in the manufacture of phase 1 and phase 2 clinical supplies. The finalization of process validation occurs during the production of phase 3 materials, encompassing both regulatory and operational scopes. While retrospective validation is prevalent in biopharmaceutical manufacturing, it might not be sufficient to optimize all critical parameters for tracking inline, on-line, and at-line processes.

The FDA's Process Analytical Techniques (PAT) aim to comprehend and monitor the production process, aligning with our current drug quality system. Quality cannot be added to products; it must be inherently designed within them. PAT functions as a system for designing, analyzing, and controlling manufacturing processes through timely measurements of critical quality and performance attributes of raw and in-process materials. Notably, the term 'analytical' in PAT encompasses various activities, spanning chemical, physical, microbiological, mathematical, and risk analyses. These tools, existing and novel, enable risk-managed biopharmaceutical production, manufacturing, and quality assurance when integrated within a framework. They facilitate data collection, process awareness, risk mitigation, quality enhancement, and the exchange of information and expertise. Categorically, within the PAT framework, these tools fall into several groups:

- Tools for collecting and analyzing multivariate data.
- Process analyzers, also known as process analytical chemistry instruments, are modern tools for analyzing processes.
- Tools for tracking and controlling processes and endpoints.
- Instruments for continuous development and information management.

Optimal combinations of these methods, whether singly or collectively employed, can enhance a unit operation or an entire manufacturing process. The PAT system's goal is to design and implement processes that consistently ensure predefined quality at the end of the manufacturing phase. These procedures must adhere to the quality-by-design principle, potentially reducing performance risks and regulatory concerns while enhancing reliability. The gains in quality, safety, and efficiency might vary based on the product and are anticipated to arise from the following:

- Using on-, in-, and at-line measurements and controls to shorten output cycle times.
- Rejects, scrap, and reprocessing are avoided.

- The prospect of a real-time release is being considered.
- To increase operator protection and reduce human error, more automation is being implemented.
- Increasing performance and managing variability by facilitating continuous processing.
- Using small-scale equipment and dedicated production facilities (to avoid such scale-up issues).
- Growing capability and improving energy and material use.
- Human error is reduced, continuous processing is facilitated, and processing time parameters are shortened due to a combination of increased automation and real-time analysis.

Biological manufacturing processes are segregated into distinct unit operations, each typically consisting of a single technical procedure. This sequence involves processing a sample according to a protocol, resulting in an output such as a pool, precipitate, supernatant, or filtrate. While managing sample and procedural parameters is feasible, controlling performance proves challenging due to the numerous variables governing upstream and downstream operations. In typical upstream processes, parameters like pH, redox potential, and dissolved oxygen significantly impact cell growth and stability. Likewise, temperature, agitation rate, and flow rates affect cell growth, redox potential, and metabolic activity, regulated further by glucose and glutamine supply. Similarly, downstream processes involve crucial parameters influencing outcomes:

- Protein aggregates and other high-molecular increase pressure are affected by backpressure (should be kept constant).
- Stability, binding to chromatographic media, viscosity, turbidity, and holding times are all affected by conductivity.
- Flux, fouling, and cross-flow velocity are all affected by filtration inlet pressure.
- Flux, fouling, and cross-flow velocity are all affected by filtration outlet pressure.
- The amount of time you hold something affects its stability and solubility.
- Protein binding capacity in chromatographic media is affected by linear flow.
- The ability of chromatographic media is affected by load (adjust accordingly).
- Stability, precipitation reactions, des-amido type composition, elimination, racemization, disulfide bond and cleavage, binding to chromatographic media, solubility, and holding times are all affected by pH.
- Stability, solubility, viscosity, turbidity, and retention times are all affected by protein concentration.
- The stability of intermolecular and intramolecular disulfide bonds, the formation of oxidized forms, and holding times are all affected by redox potential.
- Stability, solubility, the development of protein derivatives, the enzymatic activity of proteolytic enzymes, reaction kinetics, and holding times are all affected by temperature.
- Filtrate flow, flux, and fouling are all affected by transmembrane strain.
- The ability to pass filters and chromatographic media is affected by turbidity.
- The ability to pass filters and chromatographic media is affected by viscosity.

Due to the complex composition of samples, comprehensive characterization remains challenging yet essential for operational control. The procedures applied can yield unexpected results concerning parameters such as cell density, viability, production rates, ammonia concentration, expression levels, amino acid concentration, NADH/NADPH ratio, and lactate dehydrogenase activity.

The parameters are expressed as intervals rather than fixed points to accommodate changes, especially in large-scale operations. Specifying lower and upper limits allows for statistical multivariate data analysis and in-process optimization without needing to redefine the process. Internal action limits, referred to as a proven reasonable range (PAR) based on small-scale experiments and enforced for worst-case scenarios as stipulated by the FDA, are further refined according to regu-latory documents. Factorial designs are used to determine the statistical methods for validating the interval ranges, as detailed in the quality assurance section.

To avoid such tests during manufacturing processes, intermediate products are thoroughly analyzed during development stages. Tests for microbial agents, fungi, mycoplasma, viruses, endotoxins, 1D-SDS, HP-IEC, HPRPC, HP-SEC, and ELISA are common in process control studies. More details about some of these tests and their drawbacks are provided below.

Continuous probe systems are widely used to monitor parameters, notably in automatic controls used in modern fermenters. In biological manufacturing monitoring, an unusual circumstance arises when the properties of the monitored medium change over time. For instance, a pH change might be followed by alterations in temperature, ionic strength, other solute strengths, and redox potential. Validating pH probes to account for all these variables is crucial. This work is typically part of the PAT exercise, but selecting all relevant factors before completing the method creation requires probe revalidation. Furthermore, issues arise from the probes' stability and robustness due to changes induced by chemical or biological reactions in probed solutions. Determining each probe's shelf-life is essential. Factors affecting parameter calculation, such as the ionic strength of the solution and temperature, impact pH measurements and need to match the calibration conditions. Obtaining stable measurements for redox potential calculation is often challenging. In biological systems, the presence of proteins shields the slow exchange of electrons with the platinum electrode in the redox core. To achieve fast measurements, a redox mediator capable of rapid electron exchange with the electrode is utilized. The choice of the mediator's Em7 (midpoint redox potential at pH 7.0) should be similar to the estimated redox potential of the solution at a given pH (Em values adjusted for different pHs considering pH 2–10: approximately −400 mV or −50 mV per pH unit increase). The mediator's volume should be minimal compared to the solution's volume. Using a few drops of a 0.05% solution to 100 mL of the test solution often yields good results. Redox titration is commonly performed in oxidative and reductive series with mediator concentrations ranging from 10^{-6} to 10^{-3}, and mediators within the Em (±60 mV) range of the tested redox couple.

The E region of greatest resistance in the E region closely aligns with the redox E_m value of the mediator, a fact known for pH buffer pKs. Considering temperature variations in all redox potential calculations is necessary. When accounting for the influence of oxygen, additional precautions are required, such as utilizing an oxygen-free safety gas (e.g., nitrogen).

13.5.3   Specifications

To establish the criteria for drug substance, drug product, or intermediary compound conformity, specifications consist of a list of tests, references to analytical procedures, and appropriate criteria such as numerical limits, ranges, or other test criteria. The alignment of batch data with specification acceptance criteria is a vital component of the certificate of analysis (COA).

Specifications are formulated during the early stages of process and product development (process design, scale-up, non-GMP manufacture, and cGMP manufacture for clinical phases 1 and 2), once the active drug's physicochemical properties, biological activity, immunochemical properties, purity, and quantity have been thoroughly characterized. The acceptance criteria are linked to the chosen analysis method and established as early as possible. However, these specifications evolve during the development process, partly due to scale-up and partly due to an improved understanding of parameter relevance, such as detecting product and process impurities. Characterization parameters recommended by the ICH include appearance (color and clarity), identity (amino acid composition, amino acid sequence, CD, DSC, EPR, MS, IE focusing, isoform pattern, native elec-trophoresis, NIR, NMR, peptide map, 2D electrophoresis, X-ray diffraction), biological activity (animal assays, cell assays, receptor assays, as applicable), and immunochemical properties (amino acid composition).

Tests for primary, secondary, and tertiary structure, posttranslational changes, and physico-chemical properties of the therapeutic substance/product are utilized for active product identification. Assays include molecular determination weight, isoform pattern, extinction coefficient, electrophoretic patterns, liquid chromatography patterns, and spectroscopic profiles. Structural characterization commonly includes amino acid sequence, amino acid composition, terminal amino acid sequence, peptide map, sulfhydryl group(s) and disulfide bridges, x-ray diffraction, NMR analysis, and carbohydrate structure. Biological activity determination relies on animal, cell, receptor, ligand, and biochemical assays. Potency, given in units, represents the quantitative measure of biological activity and should ideally be compared to that of the natural product.

Additional testing for biopharmaceuticals involves evaluating their potential to generate immunogenicity, which is challenging to estimate accurately. The true test of immunogenic potential is determined during actual use, with millions of doses provided over an extended period. Early trials can only detect substantial hypersensitivity and allergic responses. However, assays based on antibody binding, capable of detecting antibodies at nanogram levels, are gaining wider acceptance. Changes in molecules, such as pegylation, heighten the relevance of immunogenicity potential due to the possibility of unexpected immunogenic reactions.

In biological products, impurities may arise from accidental agents, processes, or product contaminants. Utilizing a bacterial expression system reduces the risk of virus infection. Even with an in vitro folding process, scrambled versions of the target protein could pose a problem. Therefore, ensuring protein purity should not rely solely on a few analytical methods but also on the expression system used, process design, and target protein derivatives resulting from upstream and downstream processing.

As even minor impurity concentrations can significantly impact protein structure, identifying and quantifying impurities is crucial, even if they aren't hazardous. Host-related impurities originate from the manufacturing of the recombinant organism, cell infections, co-expressed chemicals with the target protein, or cells undergoing apoptosis and lysis. Examples include endotoxins, viruses, prions, nucleic acids, host cell lipids and proteins, and proteolytic enzymes. Process-related impurities encompass those from upstream, downstream, and formulation phases, such as bacteria, yeast, fungus, mycoplasmas, viruses, prions, endotoxins, raw materials, and cell culture substrates. This category also includes unintentional agents like mycoplasma infections in cell cultures that aren't actively utilized in the process. Product-related impurities encompass des-amido, oxidized, scrambled, glycosylated, cleaved, carbamylated forms, and polymeric forms, which might be physically and chemically similar to the target protein and may possess complete or partial biological function. Particularly, polymeric forms might trigger an immune response. In regulatory terms, some derivatives are not considered contaminants if they exhibit similar properties (activity, efficacy, and safety) to the desired product.

The quantity of total protein in a sample of highly purified recombinant products is commonly used to determine its quantity. Quantitative methods, including amino acid analysis, Kjeldahl, and UV absorption, are employed. Immunogenic assays, such as ELISA, may determine the quantity of active medication in less pure goods.

13.5.4 Regulatory Compliance

Regulatory inspections occur at different drug development and registration filing stages; typically, FDA inspections happen post-application submission. Other regulatory agencies, including the EMA, may conduct audits at the manufacturer's request to grant GMP compliant status. Facilities aren't labeled "FDA Approved" since it is only the product approved by the FDA for manufacturing in a specific facility.

Manufacturers can conduct a self-audit of their compliance based on the details provided by the agencies such as the EMA (EU Guidelines EUDRALEX volume 4 https://ec.europa.eu/health/documents/eudralex/vol-4_en) and at the FDA (https:// practice-cgmp-regulations).

13.6 SUMMARY

cGMP compliance is universally observed for all human products, but in biopharmaceuticals, poorly executed quality systems can lead to significant safety concerns. Achieving quality necessitates compliance from everyone within the system, although an independent group within manufacturing personnel monitors compliance. This chapter acts as a primer for all involved in biopharmaceutical development, manufacturing, and regulatory compliance. Quality control at in-process and release stages requires scientific understanding, as outlined in this chapter. Validation ensures flawless system functioning despite inevitable variations. Understanding the limitations of reproducibility is crucial for all personnel involved in biopharmaceutical development and manufacturing.

14 Intellectual Property Issues for Scientists

14.1 OVERVIEW

Intellectual property is crucial for every industry (Figure 14.1), extending beyond mere patents. This book focuses on the patenting process in new drug development.

The term "patent" originates from "letters of patents patent," an open letter granting specific privileges or rights to a subject. Since Filippo Brunelleschi received the earliest recorded patent in 1421 for an agricultural invention in Florence, countries have developed their patent rules, including the duration of patent awards, patent categories, and filing procedures.

Patenting biopharmaceutical discoveries is essential for commercialization. The development of these products involves a lengthy, expensive cycle, often exceeding a billion dollars. Such investment necessitates protecting product exclusivity to recover costs. Two types of exclusivity exist: one from a granted patent and the other, in the US, as regulatory exclusivity lasting 12 years from the launch date, irrespective of patent protection.

Manufacturers strive to avoid patent infringement to prevent lawsuits or market entry barriers. Many scientists and technicians who have not been trained in and are unfamiliar with patenting may not realize that patents differ significantly from scientific publications; patents are legal documents requiring precise detail crucial for new biologics.

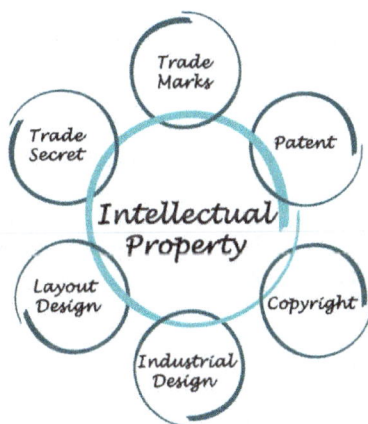

FIGURE 14.1 Types of intellectual properties

DOI: 10.1201/9781003392026-14

New drug entities can be protected by their chemical structure, synthesis method, or new use. While manufacturing methods for chemical entities might not be exclusive for product synthesis, biological drugs can secure multiple patents covering upstream and downstream processes and purification.

Table 14.1 lists 51,566 patents safeguarding biological drugs, ordered by the number of patents protecting each entity. This database aids in deciding which products to develop and assists in creating freedom-to-operate documents for approved biological products.

TABLE 14.1
Patents Protecting Biopharmaceuticals

Parathyroid hormone: (3396); interferon alfa-2b: (3168); peanut: (3139); gonadotropin, chorionic: (3099); somatropin: (2605); urokinase:(2436);botulismantitoxinheptavalent:(1757); bevacizumab: (1712); albumin (human): (1702); hyaluronidase: (1588); rituximab: (1390); rituximab); hyaluronidase: (1330); zoster vaccine live: (1170); histamine: (1151); alemtuzumab: (972); albumin human: (847); panitumumab: (837); trastuzumab: (828); filgrastim: (816); adalimumab: (796); collagenase: (782); trastuzumab; hyaluronidase-oysk: (720); darbepoetin alfa: (700); etanercept: (598); insulin human: (592); asparaginase: (583); cetuximab: (552); epoetin alfa: (518); insulin recombinant human: (504); nivolumab: (399); bacillus anthracis: (369); infliximab: (338); pancrelipase (amylase); lipase; protease: (315); anakinra: (303); immunoglobulin G: (282); peginterferon alfa-2b: (264); aprotinin: (254); tocilizumab: (253); alteplase: (243); interferon beta-1a: (238); palivizumab: (236); sargramostim: (230); basiliximab: (222); insulin aspart: (207); insulin lispro: (195); ocrelizumab: (45); reteplase: (44); insulin detemir: (42); interferon gamma-1b: (39); palifermin: (39); elotuzumab: (38); menotropins (fsh);lh): (37); fibrinogen (human): (33); fibrinogen human: (33); hepatitis b vaccine (recombinant): (33); durvalumab: (32); urofollitropin: (32); insulin lispro recombinant: (31); rabies vaccine: (30); ado-trastuzumab emtansine: (28); daratumumab: (28); obinutuzumab: (28); canakinumab: (27); agalsidase beta: (26); alirocumab: (26); thrombin human: (26); insulin aspart recombinant: (25); insulin detemir recombinant: (25); menotropins: (25); necitumumab: (25); dermatophagoides farinae: (24); siltuximab: (24); thyrotropin alfa: (24); bacillus calmette-guerin substrain tice live antigen: (23); rilonacept: (23); dermatophagoides pteronyssinus: (22); reslizumab: (21); autologous cultured chondrocytes: (20); romiplostim: (20); becaplermin: (19); belatacept: (19); blinatumomab: (19);

onabotulinumtoxina: (190); ipilimumab: (185); denosumab:(184);abciximab:(179);insulinglargine:(178); pertuzumab: (175); golimumab: (173); human immunoglobulin G: (165); natalizumab: (163); ranibizumab: (158); daclizumab: (154); ibritumomab tiuxetan: (137); aldesleukin: (134); belimumab: (129); ustekinumab: (129); chymopapain: (128); hemin: (113); pembrolizumab: (112); ofatumumab: (111); gemtuzumab ozogamicin: (108); lixisenatide: (108); omalizumab: (108); bacillus calmette-guerin: (101); pegfilgrastim: (94); pegaspargase: (89); denileukin diftitox: (84); influenza virus vaccine: (84); aflibercept: (80); atezolizumab: (80); interferon beta-1b: (79); brentuximab vedotin: (78); eculizumab: (75); immune globulin: (74); peginterferon alfa-2a: (74); ramucirumab: (72); certolizumab pegol: (70); pancrelipase: (70); abatacept: (68); mepolizumab: (66); follitropin alfa/beta: (60); insulin degludec: (60); pegvisomant: (60); avelumab: (56); dulaglutide: (56); botulinum toxin type b: (52); albiglutide: (51); tenecteplase: (49); imiglucerase: (48); rasburicase: (48); sipuleucel-t: (46); olaratumab: (9); raxibacumab: (9); antihemophilic factor (human): (8); asfotase alfa: (8); beractant: (8); immune globulin (human): (8); ocriplasmin: (8); salmonella typhi ty21a: (8); anti-thymocyte globulin (rabbit): (7); antihemophilic factor/von willebrand factor complex (human): (7); brodalumab: (7); cat hair: (7); factor ix complex: (7); galsulfase: (7); choriogonadotropin alfa: (6); dinutuximab: (6); human c1-esterase inhibitor: (6); latrodectus mactans: (6); sacrosidase: (6); varicella virus vaccine live: (6); velaglucerase alfa: (6); von willebrand factor (recombinant): (6); antithrombin iii (human): (5); somatropin [rdna origin]: (5); alglucosidase alfa: (4); antihemophilic factor, recombinant: (4); antihemophilic factor, recombinant): (4); calfactant: (4); desirudin recombinant: (4); ecallantide: (4); equine thymocyte immune globulin: (4); hepatitis a vaccine, inactivated: (4); idursulfase: (4); isatuximab-irfc: (4); methoxy polyethylene glycol-epoetin beta: (4);

TABLE 14.1 (Continued)
Patents Protecting Biopharmaceuticals

evolocumab: (19); vedolizumab: (19); antihemophilic factor (recombinant): (18); laronidase: (18); sarilumab: (18); anti-inhibitor coagulant complex: (16); antihemophilic factor human: (16); inotuzumab ozogamicin: (16); interferon alfa-n3: (16); secukinumab: (16); benralizumab: (15); hepatitis a vaccine: (15); insulin glulisine recombinant: (15); metreleptin: (15); abobotulinumtoxina: (14); ambrosia artemisiifolia: (14); histamine phosphate: (14); human papillomavirus quadrivalent (types 6, 11, 16, and 18) vaccine, recombinant: (14); incobotulinumtoxina: (14); dupilumab: (13); corticorelin ovine triflutate: (12); immune globulin intravenous (human): (11); capromab pendetide: (10); collagenase clostridium histolyticum: (10); dornase alfa: (10); ixekizumab: (10); pneumococcal vaccine polyvalent: (10); tuberculin purified protein derivative: (10); ziv-aflibercept: (10); antihemophilic factor recombinant: (9);
a and hepatitis B (recombinant)
vaccine: (2); idarucizumab: (2); immune globulin infusion (human): (2); insulin glargine recombinant: (2); insulin glargine); lixisenatide: (2); insulin recombinant human); insulin susp isophane recombinant human: (2); isatuximab: (2); meningococcal group b vaccine: (2); neisseria meningitidis group A capsular polysaccharide diphtheria toxoid conjugate antigen: (2); ovine digoxin immune fab: (2); pneumococcal 13-valent conjugate vaccine: (2); rotavirus vaccine,

peginterferon beta-1a: (4); poractant alfa: (4); rho (d) immune globulin: (4); smallpox (vaccinia) vaccine, live: (4); talimogene laherparepvec: (4); coagulation factor IX (recombinant): (3); fremanezumab-vfrm: (3); house dust mite, dermatophagoides pteronyssinus: (3); human plasma proteins: (3); imciromab pentetate: (3); mecasermin rinfabate recombinant: (3); plasma protein fraction (human): (3); ravulizumab-cwvz: (3); sebelipase alfa: (3); taliglucerase alfa: (3); technetium tc-99m albumin colloid kit: (3); asparaginase erwinia chrysanthemi: (2); bezlotoxumab: (2); clostridium tetani toxoid antigen (formaldehyde inactivated),: (2); diphtheria and tetanus toxoids and acellular pertussis adsorbed and inactivated poliovirus vaccine: (2); Adsorption of diphtheria, tetanus, and acellular pertussis toxoids, as well as hepatitis B (recombinant) and inactivated poliovirus vaccines:(2); Adsorption of diphtheria and tetanus toxoids, as well as the acellular pertussis vaccine: (2); guselkumab: (2); hepatitis
live, oral: (2); coagulation factor IX recombinant human: (1); coagulation factor VIIa (recombinant): (1); elosulfase alfa: (1); human fibrinogen, human thrombin: (1); human papillomavirus 9-valent vaccine, recombinant: (1); influenza vaccine, adjuvanted: (1); insulin aspart); insulin degludec: (1); insulin degludec); liraglutide: (1); obiltoxaximab: (1); pegademase bovine: (1); polatuzumab vedotin-piiq: (1); poliovirus type 1 antigen: (1)

14.1.1 GUIDE

Guide to the BPCIA's Biosimilars Patent Dance

First-Wave Litigation
42 U.S.C. § 262(l)(2)-(7)

FDA Accepts aBLA

Within 20 Days

Applicant provides a copy of aBLA and manufacturing information to the Reference Product Sponsor (RPS)
(l)(2)(A)

Within 60 Days

§ 262(l)(3)(A) and § 262(l)(7)

RPS provides Applicant with a list of potentially infringed patents
(l)(3)(A)(i)

RPS identifies any patents on list that RPS is willing to license to Applicant
(l)(3)(A)(ii)

RPS must supplement its list with relevant newly issued or licensed patents within 30 days of issuance or licensing. Any newly issued or licensed patents listed on the RPS supplement will be subject to the second wave of patent litigation
(l)(7)

Within 60 Days

§ 262(l)(3)(B)

Applicant may provide RPS with list of patents Applicant believes could reasonably be asserted by RPS
(l)(3)(B)(i)

Applicant responds to each patent on RPS's (l)(3)(A) list with:
i) Detailed statement of invalidity, unenforceability or noninfringement
OR
ii) Statement that Applicant will not commercially market product before patent expiration
(l)(3)(B)(ii)(I)-(II)

Applicant responds to RPS's licensing offers, if any
(l)(3)(B)(iii)

Within 60 Days

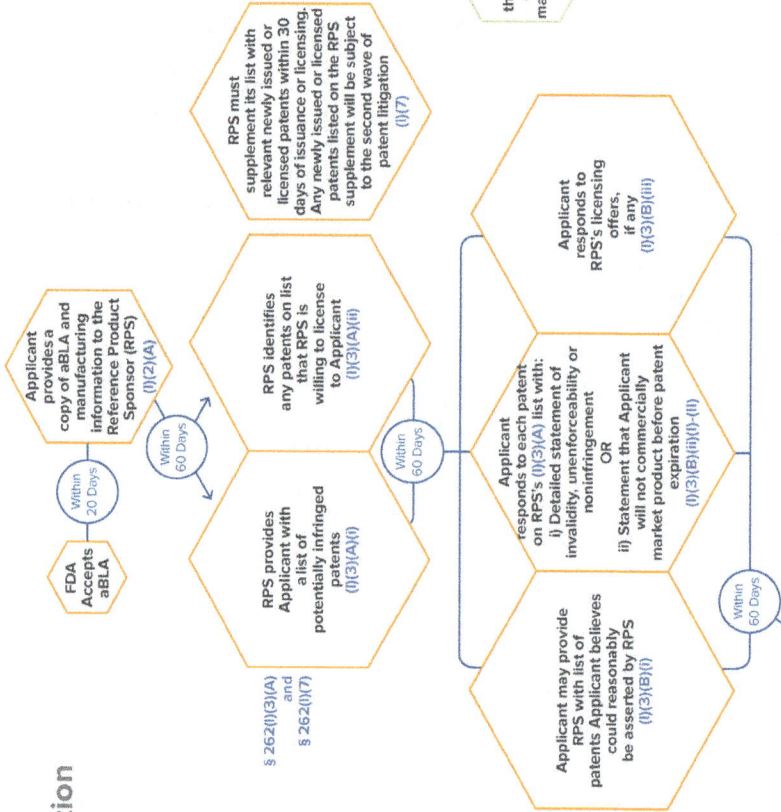

Second-Wave Litigation
42 U.S.C. § 262(l)(8)

The Court of Appeals for the Federal Circuit has held that regardless of whether an Applicant provides the RPS with a copy of its aBLA and manufacturing information pursuant to § 262(l)(2)(A), it must provide the notice of commercial marketing pursuant to § 262(l)(8)(A), *Amgen Inc. v. Apotex Inc.*, 827 F.3d 1052, 1061 (Fed. Cir. 2016), *cert. denied*, 137 S. Ct. 591 (2016). As to when the Applicant can provide notice of commercial marketing, the Supreme Court has ruled that the aBLA Applicant need not wait until FDA approval to provide such notice. Rather, the aBLA Applicant "may provide notice either before or after receiving FDA approval." *Sandoz Inc. v. Amgen Inc.*, 137 S. Ct. 1664, 1668 (2017).

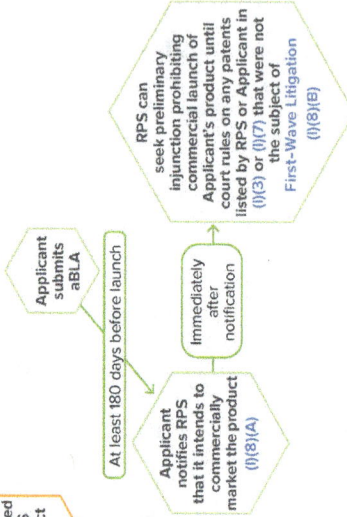

Applicant submits aBLA

Applicant notifies RPS that it intends to commercially market the product
(l)(8)(A)

At least 180 days before launch

Immediately after notification

RPS can seek preliminary injunction prohibiting commercial launch of Applicant's product until court rules on any patents listed by RPS or Applicant in (l)(3) or (l)(7) that were not the subject of First-Wave Litigation
(l)(8)(B)

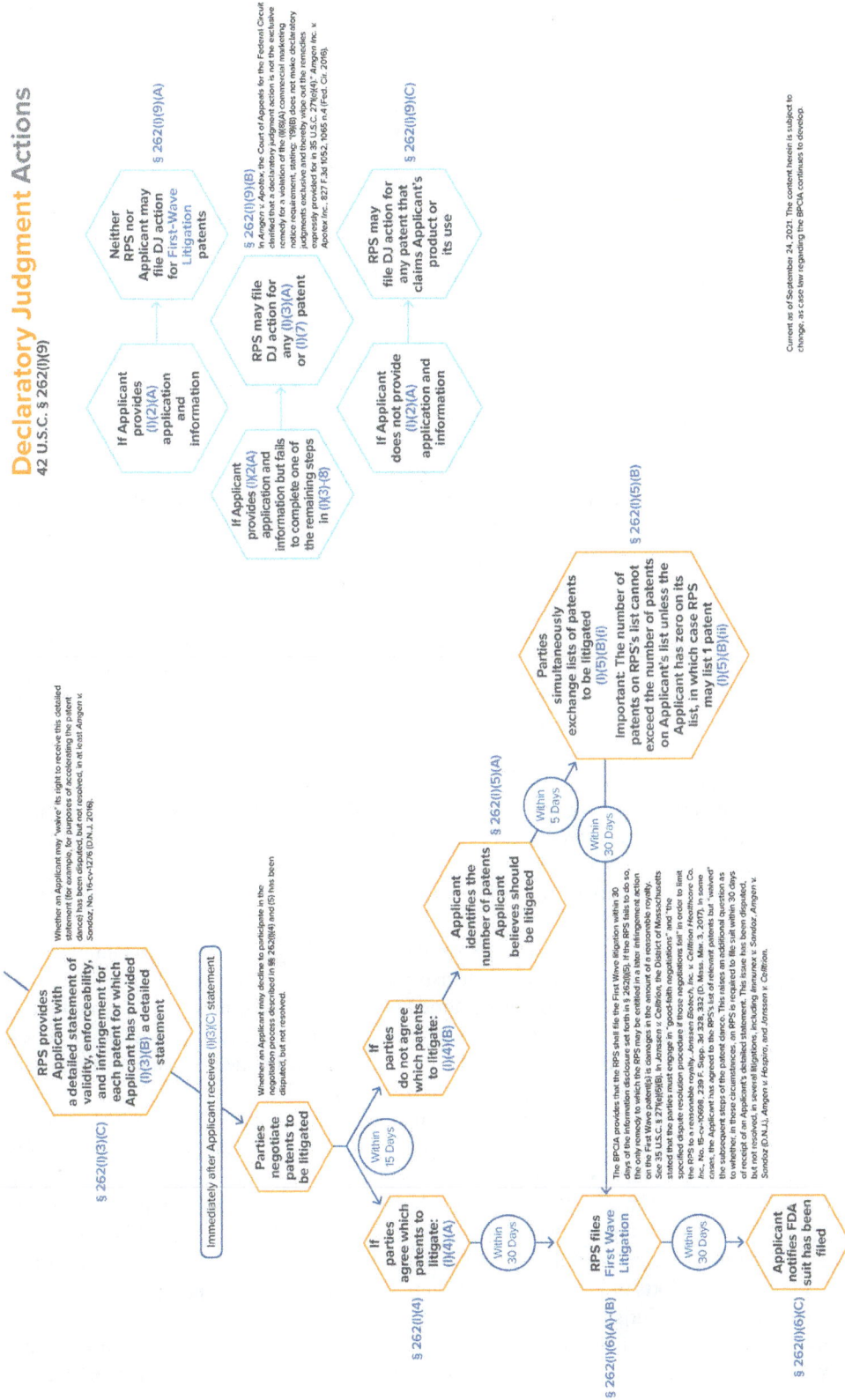

FIGURE 14.2 Overview of the "Patent Dance" under the Biologics Price Competition and Innovation Act

Source: Courtesy Big Molecule Watch. https://www.bigmoleculewatch.com/wp-content/uploads/sites/2/2022/12/Patent-Dance-Guide-December-2022.pdf

14.2   THE PATENT DANCE

The emergence of biosimilars has advanced healthcare by offering more accessible treatments. However, developing and commercializing biosimilars present challenges, notably patent disputes between manufacturers and reference product sponsors. The "patent dance," established under the Biologics Price Competition and Innovation Act (BPCIA) in the United States, aims to resolve these challenges. This essay comprehensively explores the patent dance, discussing its history, current status, resolved and pending cases, and its impact and future prospects.

The patent dance began with the BPCIA in 2010, aiming to balance competition while protecting reference product sponsors' intellectual property rights of reference product sponsors. The BPCIA introduced a regulatory framework for biosimilars and outlined the patent dance process as a means of resolving patent disputes. Over time, legal challenges and court rulings, particularly the land-mark Amgen v. Sandoz case in 2017, have shaped the interpretation and implementation of the patent dance.

This process continues to evolve, guided by regulatory directives and ongoing legal developments. The US Food and Drug Administration (FDA) has issued guidance documents clarifying aspects of the patent dance, such as information exchange and timing, streamlining the process to efficiently resolve patent disputes.

Additionally, the patent dance has led to an increasing number of resolved cases. Both biosimilar manufacturers and reference product sponsors have utilized this process to negotiate settlements, exchange patent information, and occasionally proceed to litigation. These resolutions showcase the effectiveness of the patent dance in resolving patent disputes and facilitating the entry of biosimilars into the market.

Resolved and Pending Cases: Several significant cases have found resolution through the patent dance process, highlighting its effectiveness. Examples include the legal disputes between Amgen and Sandoz over Zarxio and Genentech and Celltrion over Truxima. These cases have not only influenced the interpretation of the patent dance but have also established legal precedents, offering guidance for future disputes.

However, it is important to note that the number of resolved cases through the patent dance is relatively low compared to overall biosimilar applications. Many disputes are settled through negotiations outside this formal process. Several cases remain pending, awaiting resolution through continued negotiations or potential litigation. These pending cases underscore the ongoing importance and necessity of the patent dance in balancing competition and intellectual property rights.

The patent dance plays a crucial role in the biosimilar landscape by providing a structured frame-work to resolve patent disputes. From a comprehensive standpoint, it presents both advantages and challenges. It serves as a platform for communication between biosimilar manufacturers and refer-ence product sponsors, enabling the exchange of patent information and potentially reducing uncer-tainty surrounding disputes. Moreover, it offers an avenue for early resolution of patent infringement issues, thereby facilitating more efficient market entry for biosimilars.

However, challenges persist, notably the complexity and costs associated with the patent dance process. Critics argue that its intricacies can be time-consuming and burdensome, potentially delaying biosimilar market entry. As the biosimilar market expands and new disputes arise, striking a balance between safeguarding intellectual property rights and promoting competition for the benefit of patients and the healthcare system becomes increasingly critical.

In the future, refinements and modifications to the patent dance may address these challenges and streamline the process. Efforts toward international harmonization of patent dance procedures could promote consistency across jurisdictions.

Furthermore, as the field of biosimilar evolves, monitoring the evolving legal landscape and regulatory developments remains crucial. Ongoing court cases and potential legislative changes can significantly impact the effectiveness. It is important for stakeholders, including biosimilar manufacturers, reference product sponsors, regulatory authorities, and policymakers, to collaborate and actively engage in discussions to ensure that the patent dance process continues to strike an appropriate balance between competition and intellectual property protection.

From a broader perspective, the patent dance stands as a significant component of the regulatory framework for biosimilars. It not only fosters innovation and biosimilar product development but also safeguards intellectual property rights, encouraging continued investment in research and development. Ultimately, an effective patent dance process can foster a vibrant and competitive biosimilar market, enhancing patient access to affordable therapies.

The patent dance has become a pivotal process for settling patent disputes within the biosimilar sphere. Its history, characterized by legal hurdles and significant court decisions, has heavily influenced how it is understood and executed. While the procedure is still developing, regulatory advice and resolved cases showcase its efficacy in resolving patent conflicts and enabling the introduction of biosimilars into the market. Nevertheless, hurdles persist, necessitating ongoing endeavors to strike a delicate balance between fostering competition and upholding intellectual property rights. The future trajectory of the patent dance hinges on continual refinements, global coordination efforts, and the capacity to adapt to the shifting biosimilar landscape. Successfully navigating these challenges could see the patent dance bolster a thriving biosimilar market, delivering advantages to patients, healthcare providers, and the pharmaceutical industry.

Pending U.S. District Court BPCIA Litigations
Aflibercept+
Denosumab+
Natalizumab+
Tocilizumab
Resolved U.S. District Court BPCIA Litigations
Adalimumab+
Bevacizumab+
Epoetin alfa+
Etanercept+
Filgrastim+
Infliximab+
Pegfilgrastim+
Rituximab+
Trastuzumab+
Ustekinumab+

Source: Courtesy of Big Molecule Watch, https://www.bigmoleculewatch.com/ bpcia-patent-litigations/, Last updated: June 1 2023

The history of the patent dance for biosimilars traces back to the enactment of the Biologics Price Competition and Innovation Act (BPCIA) in the United States in 2010, as part of the Affordable Care Act (ACA). It aimed to establish an abbreviated pathway for biosimilar product approval and market entry.

The patent dance provisions in the BPCIA aimed to balance competition and protect the intellectual property rights of reference product sponsors. Although the legislation doesn't explicitly mention the term "patent dance," it outlines the process for resolving patent disputes between biosimilar manufacturers and reference product sponsors.

The key milestones in the history of the patent dance are as follows:

1. Enactment of the BPCIA (2010): Introduced a regulatory framework for biosimilars and included provisions for the patent dance, aiming for an efficient approval pathway while allowing reference product sponsors to assert patent rights.

2. Legal Challenges and Interpretation: Post-enactment, legal debates arose about interpreting BPCIA provisions, particularly the patent dance. Scrutiny focused on aspects like timing and requirements for exchanging patent information.

3. Amgen v. Sandoz Case (2015–2017): A significant event involving a dispute between Amgen and Sandoz regarding Zarxio, a biosimilar of Amgen's Neupogen. The case reached the U.S. Supreme Court, leading to a landmark ruling that clarified certain patent dance aspects.

In Amgen v. Sandoz, the Supreme Court addressed whether the biosimilar applicant was obligated to complete the entire patent dance process and if the reference product sponsor could file an infringement lawsuit before the biosimilar product was commercially marketed.

The Supreme Court ruled that biosimilar applicants aren't obligated to complete the entire patent dance process and can opt out of certain steps. Moreover, the Court held that the reference product sponsor could file an infringement lawsuit even before the biosimilar product was commercially marketed. This ruling offered crucial guidance and clarification on the patent dance process.

4. Subsequent Legal Developments: Following the Amgen v. Sandoz ruling, subsequent legal cases and disputes have arisen regarding the patent dance, contributing to the ongoing evolution of this regulatory process. These cases have played a significant role in shaping the interpretation and understanding of the patent dance provisions.

5. Continued Refinement and Regulatory Guidance: In the years after the Amgen v. Sandoz case, regulatory authorities and organizations have offered additional guidance to further refine the patent dance process. The US Food and Drug Administration (FDA) has issued draft and final guidance documents addressing various aspects of the patent dance, such as information exchange, timing, and dispute resolution.

These regulatory guidance documents aim to bring more clarity and predictability to the patent dance process, providing stakeholders with a clearer framework for resolving patent disputes. They cover issues such as the types of patents involved in the exchange, the timing of information exchange, and the consequences of non-compliance with the patent dance provisions.

6. International Perspectives and Harmonization Efforts: While the patent dance is primarily associated with the United States, other countries and regions have developed their own procedures for settling patent disputes related to biosimilars. International perspectives on patent dance-like processes differ, with some jurisdictions adopting similar steps, while others use different mechanisms.

Efforts to harmonize patent dance procedures have emerged to streamline processes across different jurisdictions. Organizations like the World Health Organization (WHO) and the International Federation of Pharmaceutical Manufacturers & Associations (IFPMA) have engaged in discussions and initiatives to encourage global consistency in resolving patent disputes for biosimilars.

7. Ongoing Evolution and Future Directions: The history of the patent dance continues to evolve with new legal challenges, court rulings, and refined regulatory guidance. The patent dance process remains relatively new, and stakeholders are still gaining experience and adapting to its complexities.

Looking ahead, ongoing discussions and debates about the patent dance include suggestions for potential improvements, such as increased clarity, more defined timelines, and reduced litigation burdens. These discussions are likely to influence the future of the patent dance, along with possible legislative and regulatory changes aimed at improving its effectiveness and efficiency.

TABLE 14.2
Total Patent Applications and Awarded Patents at the USPTO from 1790 to 2019

Type of Application	Total Filed	Percentage Approved
Utility	19,774,364	53%
Design	870,770	69%
Plant	35,161	89%
All	21,064,418	54%
Foreigners	4,051,671	35%

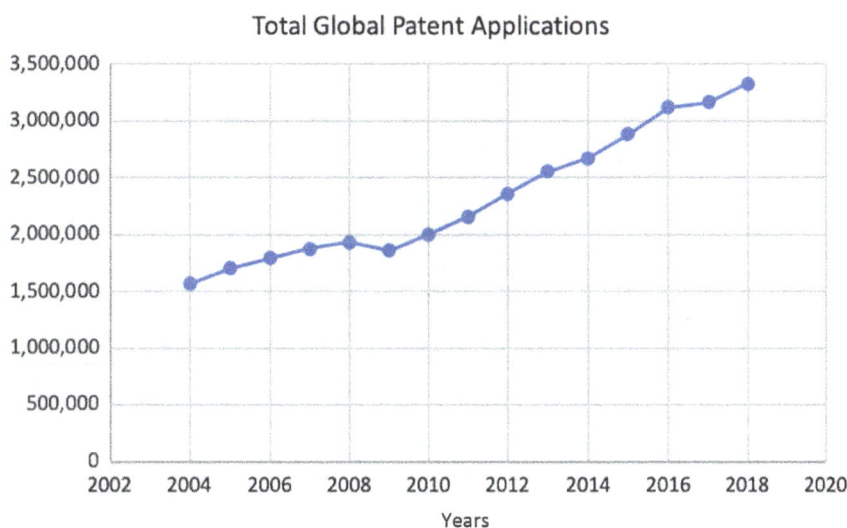

FIGURE 14.3 Yearly global patent filing 2004–2018

Additionally, the rising significance of biosimilars in healthcare and the increasing number of biosimilar approvals globally may prompt further international harmonization efforts and collaborations across jurisdictions to establish consistent approaches to resolving patent disputes.

Numerous patents on biological molecules pose challenges for scientists and technicians involved in developing and producing biopharmaceutical products, hindering the design of manufacturing procedures. A Freedom-to-Operate Document, as later described, sets the boundaries for technology used in creating a new process. Safeguarding patent rights entails formal actions such as non-disclosure agreements, validating inventions, and timely patent filings. Consequently, scientists and technicians require a basic understanding of intellectual property protection to collaborate effectively with legal teams.

14.3 PATENT LANDSCAPE

This chapter delves into patents, a pivotal aspect of intellectual property. Patents, commonly granted across various legal jurisdictions, primarily delineate invention boundaries concerning novelty, non-obviousness, and utility. Intellectual property encompasses additional components (Figure 14.1).

TABLE 14.3
Patent Search Resources

US:	http://www.uspto.gov
India:	http://www.ipindia.nic.in/
Europe:	http://www.european-patent-office.org
Japan:	http://www.jpo.go.jp/
Korea:	http://www.kipo.go.kr
Italy:	http://www.info-brevetti.org/
Canada:	http://strategis.ic.gc.ca/sc_mrksv/cipo/
Australia:	http://www.ipaustralia.gov.au/
African region:	http://www.aripo.wipo.net/
New Zealand:	http://www.iponz.govt.nz/
Singapore:	http://www.ipos.gov.sg/
UK:	http://www.ukpats.org.uk
WIPO:	http://www.wipo.int/patentscope/en/
PCT: Patent Cooperative Treaty	http://www.wto.org/english/tratop_e/trips_e/trips_e.htm http://www.pctlearningcenter.org/
Public Patent Foundation	http://www.pubpat.org/index.html
Intellectual Property Owners Association:	http://www.ipo.org/
Global: Espacenet	https://worldwide.espacenet.com/patent/
China	http://english.sipo.gov.cn
Trilateral: the US, Japan, the EU	https://www.trilateral.net/index
ASEAN	https://www.aseanip.org

As of May 2020, over ten million patents had been issued in the US. The initial US patent was granted in 1790 (three patents that year), and the first patent to a foreigner was not issued until 1836. The rate of patent rejections varies widely based on technology and, interestingly, on the inventor's US citizenship (Table 14.2).

"Everything that can be invented has been invented."

Charles H. Duell, United States Patent Office Director, telling
President McKinley to abolish the office in 1899

The global filing of patents is shown in Figure 14.2 from 2004 to 2018, as reported from 160 patent offices worldwide.

Table 14.3 lists links to patent search resources around the world. There are over 160 patent offices around the world.

14.4   PATENT LAW BASICS

Patents bestow the holder the right to prohibit others from producing, using, selling, or importing a patented invention in the United States (or the patentee's nation) for a specified period (usually twenty years from the patent application date). Unauthorized actions infringe upon the patent, leading to potential monetary penalties and legal repercussions. The purpose of patent exclusivity is to incentivize innovation by enabling the patent holder to recover research and development costs. Patentees benefit from exclusivity by shielding themselves from competition and setting higher prices for patented goods. This protection is particularly crucial for expensive-to-produce commodities like pharmaceuticals, which are easily replicable once on the market.

Pharmaceutical patents extend beyond the active ingredient, covering various facets of a medication or biologic. Among the claims of such "secondary patents" are

- Methods of employing the pharmaceutical (e.g., to treat a specific ailment); methods of manufacturing or technologies utilized to create the pharmacological
- Additional substances connected to the active ingredient, such as intermediates; or techniques or technologies for administering the pharmaceutical.

14.4.1 Pharmaceutical Patenting Practices

The practices outlined, perceived as legitimate exercises of patent rights by patent holders, are critiqued by opponents as exploitative strategies that misuse the patent system, contrary to Congress's intentions.

- Moreover, evergreening, also known as patent "layering" or "life-cycle management," is a process in which some drug firms allegedly attempt to extend their drug patent monopolies by acquiring new patents as old ones expire. It's noted that a single pharmaceutical product can be covered by numerous patents since different aspects of pharmaceutical goods are patentable. Critics of evergreening argue that secondary patents typically cover minor alterations or auxiliary components of a pharmaceutical product, effectively extending patent protection beyond the intended term set by Congress. However, defenders contend that additional patents must incorporate significant new discoveries or improvements to existing products, going through the same patentability and inspection procedures as any other patent.
- Furthermore, "product hopping" describes the process wherein a brand manufacturer leverages its dominant market position to encourage the shift from a drug with expiring patents to a newer version with later-expiring patents. This can involve introducing an extended-release form, a different dosage, altered administration methods, or slight chemical modifications to the medication. Marketing campaigns, discounts, and rebates are employed by the brand manufacturer to incentivize this transition, commonly in the form of a "hard switch" or a "soft switch." Critics of product hopping argue that the new product often provides minimal or no clinical benefit, primarily serving to delay generic competition. Conversely, defenders assert that manufacturers have legitimate reasons to develop and patent new products, often resulting in clinical advantages such as fewer side effects or improved patient compliance.
- Moreover, "patent thickets" refer to a brand manufacturer's strategy of acquiring multiple patents related to a single product, hindering competitors from entering the market or making it too costly and risky to do so. Manufacturers got an average of seventy-one patents on each drug, according to a recent survey of the top twelve drugs by gross US sales. Concerns about patent thickets are prevalent, especially in biologics versus small-molecule chemical medications, partly due to the complexities involved in developing drugs from living cells, offering various options for patenting novel techniques or the use of different mediums for cell growth or dosage changes. Critics argue that patent thickets are formed by patenting minor or secondary innovations, significantly delaying competition as generics or biosimilars must navigate or challenge each patent, incurring high costs and complexity. Proponents, however, argue that these patents represent advancements encouraged by patent laws, each validated during the patent examination process.
- "Pay-for-Delay" Settlements. When generic (or biosimilar) manufacturers submit shortened applications for products covered by certain unexpired patents, brand manufacturers may commence patent litigation under Hatch-Waxman and the BPCIA procedures. Some brand manufacturers have paid (or otherwise compensated) generic producers in exchange for the generic manufacturers agreeing to postpone market launch. The Supreme Court has ruled that this method, known as "reverse payment" or "pay-for-delay," may be a legal exercise of patent exclusivity in some cases but may violate antitrust laws in others. Pay-for-delay agreements, according to critics, are used by brand manufacturers to safeguard weak patents

from invalidation; yet, because pay-for-delay agreements end the litigation, patent validity and infringement problems remain unanswered. As a result, critics argue that pay-for-delay harms competition by allowing the brand manufacturer to (1) avoid the danger of having its patents invalidated, (2) postpone generic competition from entering the market, and (3) extend the company's exclusive marketing rights for the specified medicine. Defenders argue that settlements are a reasonable means to decrease the cost and risk of litigation, pointing out that most claims are settled in all areas of law. Furthermore, defenders claim that the case might end with the brand maker winning, thereby barring competition until the patent period expires. Defenders argue that settling the case ensures generic entry before the patent period expires.

- Lastly, despite being discussed separately, opponents argue that these strategies can be combined. For instance, brand manufacturers might use a pay-for-delay settlement along with product hopping to postpone generic entry. By transitioning the market to a new product protected by patent exclusivity, the brand manufacturer can effectively delay competition.

14.4.2 UNITED STATES PATENT ELEMENTS

A patent functions as a license that restricts others from using or practicing an invention. If an inventor's creation infringes on other inventions even in part, they cannot practice their own invention. For instance, when patenting a new application of an unexpected drug, others are barred from using that drug for the specific treatment the inventor has devised. However, if the drug molecules are safeguarded under a chemical patent, the inventor retains the right to use the drug for the treatment they've developed. Essentially, a patent inherently restricts the usage of an invention.

For an invention to be eligible for a patent, it must satisfy certain criteria: uniqueness, non-obviousness, and significant utility. The term "new and novel" signifies that the invention must not have been publicly disclosed anywhere globally more than a year before the patent application's filing date. Importantly, this one-year grace period isn't applicable in other countries. Uniqueness and non-obviousness necessitate a creative process in the innovation's development.

A utility invention, distinct from utility filing in the EU, can fall under various definitions:

- A kit for achieving a useful purpose
- A method or process of synthesis or processing
- A machine
- An article of manufacture
- A matter composition (such as a chemical compound), or
- Enhance any of the above categories.

The specification, a comprehensive description of the invention, also includes instructions for its creation and utilization. It should be articulated in a manner that enables an expert in the field to replicate and apply the innovation. For current regulations and methods on preparing a patent application, the US Patent Office's URL (https://mpep.uspto.gov/RDMS/MPEP/current) should be consulted, current as of June 2020, the publication date of this book.

Patents are granted to individuals in the United States, who may subsequently transfer them to others or file patents in other jurisdictions. An individual artistic contribution from each co-inventor is required for at least one argument of the patent, excluding co-authorship on a research paper.

A patent application is a structured document encompassing various elements, following a typical format across most patent offices globally but may differ in naming of headings and presentation order.

14.4.2.1 Title of Invention

The title of the invention should be concise, limited to 500 characters, and as precise as possible.

14.4.2.2 Cross-Reference to Related Applications
In a non-provisional utility patent application claiming benefit from prior-filed co-pending applications, a reference to each prior application must be provided in the specification after the title, as per laws 120, 121, or 365(c).

14.4.2.3 Statement Regarding Federally Sponsored Research or Development
If applicable, a declaration concerning rights to innovations developed under federally financed research grants or intramural programs should be included.

14.4.2.4 Background of the Invention
This segment encompasses a statement about the intended use of the invention, along with a summary of the relevant US patent classification definitions or the subject matter of the invention. This part was previously referred to as "FIELD OF INVENTION" or "TECHNICAL FIELD." This part should also offer a summary of the information.

14.4.2.5 Brief Summary of the Invention
This section should present the alleged invention's content, purpose, or general concept in its summarized form. The benefits of the invention and how it addresses previously known problems in the specification will be highlighted in the overview. The description is not the same as the abstract.

14.4.2.6 Background of the Invention
Elements to be included in the invention's background are as follows: (1) Invention's Field: Describing the art form to which the invention belongs, potentially summarizing relevant patent classification definitions from the United States. This should specifically pertain to the subject matter. (2) A description of the relevant art, as well as a data disc where applicable.

14.4.2.7 Brief Description of the Drawing
In cases with accompanying drawings, a numbered list of all figures (e.g., Picture 1A) is presented, accompanied by clear explanations delineating the content of each figure.

14.4.2.8 Detailed Description of the Invention
The description within the specification is distinct from the abstract. Here, a detailed, yet precise explanation of the innovation, its creation, and application is provided. This section should differentiate the invention from previous works and other inventions. Biomedical patent descriptions frequently integrate experiments involving materials and procedures.

14.4.2.9 Claim or Claims
These arguments serve as the defining features of the invention, forming the legal basis for its defense. The claims or arguments must specifically identify and assert the subject matter regarded as the invention. They establish the extent of the patent's protection.

The most crucial part of a claim include:

- Scope: Each argument should contain one sentence, which can be broad or narrow, but not simultaneously both. Narrow claims provide more specific details than wider ones, potentially enabling legal ownership of various parts of the invention through multiple claims with distinct scopes.
- Characteristics of Significant Importance: When formulating the claim, consider various factors:

- Patent examiners assess each claim's validity, approving or rejecting it based on its merits. Therefore, the language used in claims often repetitively emphasizes the novelty of the invention.
- The initial phrase in a claim defines the innovation's category and, in some instances, its purpose, like "a diagnostic test kit" or "a cancer-treating composition."
- Claim Evaluation: Each claim is individually assessed by the Patent Examiner. Crafting claims covering various aspects of the invention maximizes coverage. Creating an initial claim and referencing it in narrower scope claims ensures the inclusion of specific inventive features in some or all claims.

14.4.2.10   Abstract of the Disclosure
The abstract summarizes the disclosure found in the introduction, statements, and drawings; the summary must indicate the technological area to which the invention relates, providing a clear understanding of the technical issue, the gist of the invention's solution to a technical problem, and the primary application or use of the invention.

14.4.2.11   Drawings
If sketches are necessary to understand the subject matter for a patent, they must be included in the patent application. Every feature of the invention, as stated in the claims, must be depicted in the sketches. An application may be considered incomplete if drawings are missing. In each patent drawing, every aspect of the invention listed in the claims must be shown.

14.4.2.12   Oath or Declaration
An oath or declaration must include the following information: (1) the legal name of the inventor or joint inventor executing the oath or declaration; (2) the application to which it is directed; and (3) certification that the person administering the oath or announcing the true inventors is one of the declared or joint inventors. The declaration, a brief document, is required for each inventor to claim ownership of the invention.

14.4.2.13   Sequence Listing (When Necessary)
Amino acid and nucleotide sequences, considered conceptual, must be used if part of the invention. This section must disclose a nucleotide and amino acid sequence, complying with patent rules 1.821, 1.822, 1.823, 1.824, and 1.825 (37 CFR 1.821 Nucleotide and amino acid sequence disclosures in patent applications and WIPO Standard ST.25 (1998)).

14.4.3   TYPES OF PATENTS

Utility patents cover novel methods, formulations, or gadgets, while a design patent protects a new decorative design for a manufactured item. Plant patents provide protection for any asexually reproduced distinct and novel type of plant.

Patents for utility and plant inventions typically last 20 years from the date of issuance. The appropriate maintenance payments must be made on time. Design patents are granted for 14 years from the date of issuance, without ongoing maintenance expenses.

A patent is personal property, allowing the owner to sell, assign, or transfer it at any time. Differences may be arbitrated by competent authorities or jurisdiction in cases of infringement. Sanctions and compensation for the rightful owner may be decided upon identifying a violation.

In the 1990s, the World Trade Organization established a minimal set of rights for all patent owners, including a 20-year patent duration from the application filing date.

14.4.4 UNPATENTABLE INVENTIONS

Natural products that remain unaltered cannot be awarded patents. Natural chemicals, genes, proteins, or unmodified animal or plant species cannot be patented. However, a modified version of a natural object could be copyrighted if the alteration is beneficial. Natural ingredients used in useful devices, chemicals, or diagnostic tests may be patented.

In summary, rather than attempting to patent a gene or protein as a composition of matter, patent claims should focus on the non-obvious functional use or altered form of the gene or protein.

Nature's laws, physical facts, abstract notions, and various artistic works are exempt from patent protection. Such elements are not copyright-protected but can be replicated. Patents will not be granted for technologies considered non-useful, technically impossible (e.g., perpetual motion machines), or objectionable to public morality by the USPTO.

Section 101 of the Patent Act (the "congressional categories") allows the patenting of any process, machine, manufacture, or composition of matter. However, certain inventions, such as abstract ideas, natural facts, and natural laws, do not fall into these categories and are considered judicial exceptions.

Since 2012, the Supreme Court has issued three significant rulings prohibiting the patenting of certain types of inventions. These rulings outlawed patents on medical diagnosis and research (Mayo v. Prometheus), artificial DNA characterized by a natural nucleic acid sequence (Association with Molecular Pathology v. Myriad Genetics or Myriad Genetics), and computer hardware/software used in financial transactions or other "abstract concepts" (Alice ruling). While some anti-patent factions, notably Silicon Valley and the generic drug industry, have welcomed these decisions (collectively known as the "Alice" decisions), organizations reliant on creativity, such as research universities, solo inventors, and biotechnology firms, have criticized them. The Alice trifecta overturns long-standing legal precedent, diverges from international patenting standards, and breaches TRIPS Section 5 Article 27 Part 3. Although Congress has introduced legislation to address the Alice trifecta, no tangible progress has been made at the time of this writing.

Molecular profiling and customized therapy offer new insights into illness management, providing novel tools and treatments. Although genomic and proteomic research isn't new, the patentable knowledge derived from these molecular insights constantly challenges existing health and patent rules.

The economic well-being of every country hinges on advancements in software, medical methods, and business methods. It is widely acknowledged that sustained investment in these fields necessitates fair compensation for innovators. However, the grant of patents for such ideas requires meticulous consideration, and many governments are still deliberating on how to handle such requests.

14.4.5 SOFTWARE PATENTS

The basic theory in the United States is that a software invention is patentable if it meets two criteria:

- It's one-of-a-kind, which means it's something different.
- It's connected to a computer, in the sense that the type of hardware platform on which the program runs is defined, ensuring that a patent isn't awarded for the interpretation of an abstract process but rather for something that necessitates a particular type of physical hardware. (As we'll see, this is a little more open-ended than the machine specifications in other countries.)
- However, there are three forms of applications that aren't patentable:
  - An algorithm is not patentable.

- It is impossible to copyright a scientific law.
- Patenting an abstract concept is impossible.

In the European Union, software cannot be patented as a standalone entity. Patents are granted only to "computer-implemented inventions," which are defined as software programs performing innovative and beneficial functions within a patented hardware system.

Countries such as Japan, India, and South Korea typically align with the EU's stance, allowing software patents solely as part of a physical invention. China previously held a similar position on software patents. However, newly introduced patent review rules indicate a shift in China's perspective, showing a growing inclination towards patenting software as an independent entity. The State Intellectual Property Office (SIPO) of China has guidelines permitting the patenting of both storage mediums and computer program executions. Some researchers suggest that these two components—storage devices and software—may be individually patentable.

14.4.6 MEDICAL METHOD PATENTS

In the United States, a medical procedure qualifies for a patent if it meets three criteria:

- Specificity: It is detailed enough to reveal its flaws.
- A way of treating a specific condition with a specific medication is referred to as a practical application.
- It has a primary transformative effect, meaning it fundamentally changes the goal's nature.

The European Patent Office (EPO) approves medical technique patent applications if they are novel, creative, and don't involve surgery, therapy, or diagnostics. Denying patents for medical, pharmaceutical, and diagnostic processes aims to relieve clinicians of the fear of inadvertently infringing on a patent while treating a patient.

Japan, akin to the EPO, approves medical patents unless they obstruct the practices of physicians. China has allowed pharmaceutical patents since 1992. Surprisingly, Chinese examiners don't seek a patent claim adhering to approved medical technique standards. Instead, they maintain a database of non-patentable medical operations. South Korea does not accept patents for medical procedures. India also disqualifies such patents, prohibiting methods for human or animal treatments that render them disease-free.

14.4.7 BUSINESS METHODS PATENTS

In the United States, business process patents have been granted since 1988, but the Alice judgment casts uncertainty on their future validity. For a business method to be patented, it must generate a "useful, measurable, and observable outcome" with real-world value—not merely a theoretical or investigational procedure.

Running a specific hardware system or device combination in an obvious, current, and inventive manner falls within patentable bounds.

Japan allows the patenting of business processes applied using hardware, while China does not. South Korea protects novel technologies enhancing the technological aspects of automated systems. However, India doesn't permit the patenting of business processes.

14.4.7.1 Utility Model in the European Union
- A utility model, similar to a patent, safeguards tinventions. Although many nations offer this protection, the United States, the United Kingdom, and Canada don't provide utility models. Utility models are akin to patents but are typically more affordable to obtain and

maintain. They usually have shorter durations (6 to 15 years), quicker grant times, and fewer patentability requirements. They are applicable only to specific technologies in certain countries, often referred to as second-class patents.

- Unlike copyright or trademark treaties, no international treaty mandates utility model protection. Yet, the Paris Convention covers them under the Protection of Industrial Property. This mandates adhering countries to rules like national treatment and priority. Utility models can also be accessed through the Patent Cooperation Treaty (PCT) for foreign patent applications in countries with utility model systems.
- Utility models grant a statutory exclusive right for a limited time in exchange for providing sufficient information for an ordinary person in the related field to replicate the invention. Utility model laws grant privileges similar to those granted by patent laws, but they are more suited to "incremental inventions." A utility model is a "right to prohibit anyone from commercially using a protected invention without the permission of the right holder(s) for a limited period."
- Various terms such as "petty patent," "innovation patent," or "minor patent" describe utility models. The "Gebrauchsmuster" from Germany and Austria has inspired similar models in countries such as Japan.
- Many countries with utility model rules require novelty in technology. However, some offices do not conduct substantive reviews and grant utility models based only on meeting formal requirements. This process is often termed "utility model registration." Certain subject matters like methods (processes), chemical substances, plants, and animals may be exempted from utility model protection in some countries.
- In the EU, innovation can also be protected under utility models
  - IP right with a territorial registration.
  - Only in a few countries is it available.
  - In Europe, there is no central filing.
  - Up to 10 years of defense.
- Only some countries have a search report after a few months, it was registered and released.
- In most cases, there is no in-depth investigation (novelty, inventiveness, industrial applicability).
- Only invalidation or violation cases are checked.
- The following are some of the methods for safeguarding the utility model:
  - Contractual obligations.
  - Job arrangements with restrictive covenants.
  - Non-disclosure agreements (NDAs).
- Convenient "Need to know" knowledge is only available to a limited number of people.
- Encryption is the process of encrypting data.

14.4.8 Provisional Application

In the United States, a provisional application for patent may be filed, providing extensive details about the invention, though not to the same extent as a standard (or non-provisional) application. Within one year, a regular patent application based on the provisional application must be filed.

A provisional application establishes an earlier registration date for an innovation than the final date of patent issue for a regular application. Unlike a regular utility patent, a provisional patent expires within a year and does not commence a 20-year patent term.

Provisional applications are primarily filed to establish priority dates when urgently needed. Reasons for filing a provisional application include overall reduced expenses and a shorter waiting period for patent issuance (prosecution only begins upon the utility application). Under US patent law, a provisional application can be upgraded to a utility patent application.

A disclosure document serves as proof of concept for a new idea or product. It should not replace a provisional or standard utility patent application. Filing a standard patent application within two years of receiving the disclosure document at the USPTO allows the applicant to establish a registered proof of the date of conception for a fee of USD 10. However, unlike a Provisional submission, the date of the Disclosure Document cannot be used as an effective filing date. Due to the earlier filing date it offers, most intellectual property offices prefer the Provisional application over the Disclosure Document.

14.5   COMPARISON OF PATENT LAWS

14.5.1   JURISDICTION

A patent in the United States doesn't grant the holder an absolute right to utilize the creation. Under 35 USC 271(a), the patent owner has the right to prevent others from making, using, selling, or importing the patented invention.

Patents are limited to specific territories and must be applied for in the country where protection is desired. A U.S. patent solely safeguards an inventor's rights within the United States, necessitating separate patent applications in other countries or regional patent offices for international protection. Virtually every country has its own patent laws, requiring individuals seeking patents in multiple countries to adhere to each country's regulations.

Patent rules in many nations differ from those in the United States in a variety of ways. In most foreign countries, publicizing an innovation before the filing date can invalidate the right to a patent. Maintenance expenses are typically mandatory, and many countries demand the technology's production within their borders after a specified period. Failure to produce may invalidate the patent in certain countries. Additionally, providing obligatory licenses to any patent applicant is possible in many countries.

14.5.2   THE PATENT COOPERATIVE TREATY

To secure coverage in a particular jurisdiction, it is imperative to hold a patent awarded by that country. Consequently, many new patent applications are submitted under an international agreement that allows countries to pool patent applications. PCT Learning Center (http://www.pctlearningcenter.org/) is a non-profit organization that educates people about PCT. The Patent Cooperation Treaty, or PCT, is an international treaty that controls the filing of patent applications in 117 nations. Although the PCT scheme does not grant foreign patents, its primary aims are to streamline the process of filing in multiple countries, defer costs associated with seeking international patent protection, and afford inventors more time to assess the commercial viability of their inventions.

Submitting a PCT application doesn't mean filing separate applications in each covered country. The invention must be independently filed in each jurisdiction, adhering to their regulations. Though PCT application standards mirror those for US patent applications, each country has unique requirements. Filing fees for PCT applications are substantial, and additional fees are due for each foreign nation filing. Moreover, patent claims accepted in different countries may vary.

Signed in June 1970 and effective from January 24, 1978, the Patent Cooperation Treaty has been ratified by over 160 countries, including the United States (as of May 2, 2020). The treaty streamlines filing procedures and offers a common application format, making it easier for member countries to file patents for the same invention. Upon timely foreign application filing, the applicant receives an international filing date in each covered country, an invention search, and an extended deadline for national patent applications. Many patent attorneys specialize in obtaining patents abroad. Seeking treaty immunity within one year of filing in the US allows up to 30 months to file in other signatory nations.

For inventions originating in the United States, prior permission from the Director of the USPTO is necessary before applying for patents in other nations. A license grant is mandatory unless a filing receipt with a license grant has been provided earlier. This requirement applies when an overseas application is submitted before a U.S. application or before the six-month period following the U.S. application filing expires. Upon filing a patent application, a license request is made, and its approval or denial is indicated on the filing receipt sent to each applicant. Unless the innovation has been classified as secret, a license is unnecessary after 6 months from the filing date in the United States. However, if an order of secrecy has been granted for the invention, the USPTO Director's consent is required for filing outside the United States while the secrecy order is in effect.

14.5.3 FIRST-TO-INVENT RULE

In the US, the patent is granted to the first inventor who conceives and implements the innovation, be it a functional prototype or a well-defined concept. Conversely, other countries adhere to the first-to-file rule, awarding the patent and all rights to the first person to submit a patent application for an invention.

Clause 101 of US Code 35 states, "Whoever invents or discovers any new and useful technique, system, manufacturing, or composition of matter, or any new and useful improvement thereof, may acquire a patent therefor..."

On January 1, 1996, Clause 104 of US Code 35 was amended to permit World Trade Organization member countries to utilize the "first to invent" approach in determining innovation precedence in the United States.

One way to establish the date of invention is through the inventor's logbook. Ideally, the inventor's logbook should be a distinct book or a collection of highlighted pages or entries in a continuous laboratory notebook. It should contain detailed records of ideas, test findings, and other aspects of the invention process. Look for pre-printed numbered pages, non-fading backgrounds, spaces for signing and dating by the inventor and a witness. Avoid using loose-leaf notebooks, 3-ring binders, taped-together legal pads, or notepads. Opt for a notebook with bound or sewn-together pages. The binding ensures that, in the event of a valid patent dispute, it can be proven that the notebook record was not added or backdated later.

14.5.4 FIRST-TO-FILE RULE

In cases where two individuals apply for a patent on the same invention, the patent is awarded to the person who filed their application first (assuming the invention is patentable). This holds true even if the second person created the invention first. The filing date is the decisive factor. In 2013, the United States adopted the first-to-file system. Under this system, the first applicant has a prima facie claim to the patent. However, if two parties claim the same invention under the first-to-invent scheme, the USPTO will conduct an interference proceeding to evaluate evidence regarding creation, reduction to practice, and diligence. This process of interference is time-consuming and costly.

If the technology was publicly available before the patent application was filed, the application may be rejected. "Publicly accessible" refers to selling the idea, giving a talk about it, displaying it to an investor without a non-disclosure agreement (NDA), publishing it in a journal, etc. It doesn't matter whether the disclosure was made by the inventor, a neutral third party, or another individual.

In the United States, there exists a one-year grace period (35 US Code section 102). This means that the inventor can publish their innovation without fear of losing the patent. However, this rule only applies within the United States. If an inventor does so, they forfeit all future European patent rights (as well as rights in many other countries worldwide). This grace period is effectively limited under the Leahy-Smith America Invents Act to publications made by the inventor or those who directly obtained the inventor's knowledge. A third-party publication might jeopardize the novelty of the innovation (though this is debatable and may require legal resolution).

Article 30 of the Japan Patent Act provides a six-month grace period for disclosures made by experiments, publications, presentations at study conferences, exhibitions (trade fairs or the World's Fair), or if the invention becomes publicly known against the applicant's will. These types of disclosures are not considered prior art. This exemption is significantly broader than that provided by European patent law (Article 55 EPC) but narrower than that offered by US patent law.

In Japan, the person who first applies for a patent for an invention is entitled to obtain the patent, not necessarily the individual who first invented the same thing. Existing inventions do not receive exclusionary protection under Japanese patent law, as they do in other countries. Article 29(1) of the Patent Act stipulates that an inventor may not obtain a patent for inventions that were publicly used ("publicly used") (Item ii), or inventions that were described in a distributed publication or made available via electronic communication in Japan or abroad.

14.5.5 BEST MODE REQUIREMENT

According to US patent law (35 US Code section 112), the inventor must disclose the best mode for carrying out the patent application. This prevents the inventor from obtaining a patent while concealing an essential or valuable feature. Failure to include the best mode before the Leahy-Smith America Invents Act could result in the invalidation of the patent. Even though this Act is no longer in force, it still must be formally included.

Contrary to US law, European patent law (Article 83 EPC) doesn't contain such a clause. It requires that the proposal includes at least one method of carrying out the invention, although this method doesn't necessarily have to be the best one.

14.5.6 PATENT PUBLICATION

Public disclosure, making copies available to the public, is mandatory for most plant and utility patent applications. Patent applications are also published by the World Intellectual Property Organization (WIPO) and the United States Patent and Trademark Office (USPTO). When filing a U.S. plant or utility application, the applicant can request non-publication if the invention has not been or will not be part of a foreign application necessitating publication 18 months after filing or under the PCT.

Both the USPTO and WIPO/PCT publish patent applications 18 months after the applicant's earliest successful filing date or priority date. Once a patent application is published, the US Patent and Trademark Office (USPTO) and the World Intellectual Property Organization (WIPO) no longer keep it confidential. Any member of the public can request access to the entire file history of the application.

Until 2001, patents in the United States were only issued upon obtaining them. Unless withdrawn or accompanied by a non-publication order stating that the application is solely for the United States, US patent applications are now published 18 months after submission.

This is similar to the European approach, where all patent applications are published 18 months after filing unless they are withdrawn. If the novelty search has been completed by that time, the search report is published along with the application.

Filing a patent application doesn't determine the patentability of the invention; it simply indicates that the application has been open for 18 months. People familiar with the US system, which only publishes granted patents, may mistake anything published by the EPO as a granted patent.

The distinction between a patent application and a granted patent can be seen in two ways. A publication with a "A" in the top-right corner denotes an application, while a "B" indicates a granted patent. Additionally, European patents that have been granted do not have an abstract on the front cover.

As a result of publication, an applicant can claim provisional rights. These rights enable a patentee to sue a third party who infringes on a claim in a published application for lawful royalties. Consequently, anyone who infringes on one or more claims of the invention before the patent is granted can face penalties.

14.5.7 RIGHTS CONFERRED

A US patent is a legally enforceable property right in the United States. It grants the patent holder the authority to prevent others from making, using, or selling the patented invention within the United States. This holds true due to the federal statute outlined in the US patent law (35 US Code).

In contrast, the European Patent Convention (EPC) stands as a treaty signed by 27 European countries, including Austria, Belgium, Bulgaria, Switzerland, Cyprus, the Czech Republic, Germany, Denmark, Estonia, Spain, Finland, France, Greece, Hungary, Ireland, Italy, Liechtenstein, Luxembourg, Monaco, the Netherlands, Portugal, Romania, Slovenia, Slovakia, Sweden, Turkey, and the United Kingdom. The EPC patents are issued by the European Patent Office (EPO), headquartered in Munich.

For the chosen nations within the EPC, a European patent issued under the EPC bestows the same rights as a national patent. Essentially, a European patent represents a compilation of national patents. After obtaining a European patent, it can only be invalidated in each selected country. Anyone can file an opposition with the EPO for the first nine months after the patent is awarded to have the patent canceled in all of these countries at the same time.

14.5.8 OPPOSITION AFTER GRANT

Anyone can file an opposition with the EPO within nine months of the issuance of a European patent, arguing why the patent should not have been granted (as expected, with arguments and evidence). After that, the patent holder and the opponent will debate each other. Finally, the EPO will decide based on all parties' evidence and arguments.

Typically, the parties involved present their cases during Oral Proceedings held at the EPO in Munich following the submission of their arguments in written form. Although the EPO generally reaches a final decision during these hearings, the proceedings may continue in written form. Both parties have the right to appeal the ruling, which entails further exchanges of letters and the possibility of additional Oral Proceedings.

In the United States, while there exists a re-examination procedure, it lacks the efficacy of the opposition process. In a re-examination, any individual may challenge the validity of a granted patent by presenting reasoning and facts to the USPTO. However, in this process, the patent holder engages in discussions with the USPTO examiner to assess the validity of the arguments, while the challenger remains uninvolved.

The Leahy-Smith America Invents Act introduced an "inter partes" review where the challenger participates in the hearing. The continuation of this investigation remains uncertain.

14.5.9 INVENTIVE STEP

Two primary requirements under European patent law demand that an invention be both patentable and novel, as well as inventive (Article 52 EPC). This aligns with similar criteria in the US, where innovation must be novel and non-obvious (35 US Code sections 102 and 103). The Patent Cooperation Treaty specifies that innovation must be both original and inventive, streamlining the filing process across participating nations. Notably, being non-obvious is sufficient to necessitate a creative step.

Contrarily, the EPO adopts a more stringent approach. A European patent application is deemed inventive if it addresses a technical challenge in a non-obvious manner. It's crucial to highlight two additional requirements: the invention must present a solution to a technical problem (lack of a problem solved implies no inventive step), and the problem must be technical (solving purely economic issues lacks an inventive step).

The process of determining a technical issue involves establishing the novelty of the invention. Once established, the closest prior art document, sharing the most features with the invention or most closely resembling it in some manner, is selected. Then, the differences are assessed to identify the problem that the invention resolves.

For instance, if the technological challenge is to enhance a driver's visibility in low-light settings, and the innovation pertains to a bike equipped with a reflector while the closest prior art is a bike without lights, the issue is rectified by attaching a reflector to the bike. This enables other road users to see the driver in the dark due to the reflected light.

The subsequent query revolves around whether the solution to a technological problem would be obvious. Adding a headlight to enhance visibility, akin to vehicles or signal towers, is a common choice. A professional can conventionally install a headlight on the bike. Consequently, the answer to the obviousness question would be negative, necessitating a creative phase in the innovation process.

It's essential to note that in patent law, the terms "qualified individual" and "obvious" hold distinct meanings compared to everyday usage.

Additionally, the determination of a technical issue doesn't occur retrospectively. Initially, when confronted with an invention, the initial perception might be that it's obvious because the solution appears naturally apparent. However, this perception doesn't reflect the effort required to actualize the invention. Consider a scenario where everyone settles for a mediocre solution (e.g., a bike with a headlight powered by human effort through a dynamo). Recognizing that a particular method would be desirable in such a situation can be considered innovative.

For a patent to be granted in Japan, it must first hold industrial relevance. Article 29(1) of the Patent Act in Japan specifies that innovations involving genes, chemical substances, or species must identify a concrete, appropriate usage. The term "industry" encompasses manufacturing, agricultural, fishing, forestry, mining, commercial, and service industries but excludes medical enterprises. Consequently, patents for medical care discoveries aren't accepted as they lack industrial significance. This prohibition is grounded in the ethical principle that patent rights shouldn't restrict the diagnosis and treatments available to medical practitioners caring for patients. While there's no explicit constitutional provision barring patent rights for medical care acts, patent rights can be obtained for medical practice fields such as drugs, medical equipment, and their manufacturing, with pharmaceutical patents subject to certain limitations under Article 69(3) of the Patent Act.

14.5.10 Two-Part Claim

European patents and applications frequently utilize two-part claims, initiating with a list of traits followed by the phrases "characterized in that" or "with an augmentation containing," and additional attributes. These latter characteristics define the innovation (often termed characterizing features). The prior art encompasses the first two qualities.

In the scenario of submitting an application for a single-part allegation, the Examiner may suggest delimiting the argument from the closest prior art (text most similar or sharing the most features with the invention).

Conversely, one-part claims are almost always present in US patent applications and patents. If a US patent contains a two-part argument, it is likely held by a European corporation. In the US, utilizing two-part claims places anything before the characterizing portion within prior art (also known as "Jepson claims" after the first patent attorney to use them). If a novel feature is erroneously included in the pre-characterizing part, it is deemed prior art, potentially jeopardizing patentability.

Consider a scenario where an applicant includes a feature in the pre-characterizing section not found in the closest prior art in Europe. In such cases, relocating the feature to the characterizing section suffices. This situation commonly arises when the applicant initially begins with a document designated as the closest prior art. However, during review, it's determined that another text represents the closest prior art, necessitating an amendment. Nonetheless, this typically doesn't impact patentability significantly.

14.6 PATENT ASSIGNMENT

Transferring or selling a patent is akin to selling a house; the patent no longer belongs to the original owner. Licensing a patent, however, is akin to renting a home; if the licensee breaches the terms, eviction follows.

In patent law, a written agreement known as an "assignment" facilitates the transfer or sale of a patent, passing the full interest in the patent to the assignee. Consequently, the assignee becomes the patent owner, enjoying identical rights as the original patentee. Partial interest in a patent, such as half, fourth, or fifth interest, can also be assigned, often related to specific aspects of the invention or certain application areas.

The US Patent Office maintains records of assignments, grants, and similar instruments, providing public notice. If a patent or interest in a patent remains unassigned, granted, or conveyed within three months after documentation at the US Patent Office, subsequent buyers cannot claim ownership.

Patent licensing and joint ownership offer alternatives. Joint inventors or assignees of a portion interest in a patent can hold patents jointly. Each joint owner, regardless of their ownership share, has rights to create, use, offer for sale, sell, and import the invention independently of other joint owners. They can sell their stake or grant patent licenses without needing approval from other joint owners.

When a licensee signs a patent licensing agreement, the Licensor agrees not to sue the licensee for patent infringement. This agreement can take any written form containing mutually agreed terms, including royalties.

14.7 PATENT INFRINGEMENT

According to patent law, transferring or selling a patent involves a written agreement called an "assignment," which transfers the full interest in the patent. Once the patent is given to the assignee, they become the patent owner and possess the same rights as the original patentee. Patent law permits the assignment of a partial interest in a patent, such as half, a quarter, or a fifth. Assignments can relate to specific aspects of an invention or certain application areas.

The US Patent Office records assignments, awards, and similar documents, serving as formal notification. If a patent or interest in a patent (or a patent application) isn't transferred, granted, or conveyed within three months after the transaction at the US Patent Office, subsequent buyers cannot claim ownership.

Patent licensing and joint ownership are viable options. When a patent is shared among joint inventors or a portion of a patent is assigned, it can be owned by multiple individuals. As long as they don't infringe on others' patent rights, each joint owner has the right to use, sell, import, or offer the invention for sale, regardless of their share. They can also sell their stake or grant patent, regardless of how little their portion of ownership, may create, use, offer for sale, sell, and import the invention for profit. Without regard for the other joint owners, they may sell the stake or any portion of it, or grant patent licensing to others.

A patent licensing agreement involves the Licensor pledging not to sue the licensee for patent infringement. It doesn't have a set format and is a written agreement incorporating terms agreed upon by the parties, such as royalties.

14.8 BIOLOGICAL PATENTS

Gene patenting raises ethical concerns in bioethics. Three main arguments against genetic patenting exist: ethical objections to treating life as a commodity, the argument that living elements cannot be patented as they are naturally occurring, and concerns that patenting genetic material could compromise the integrity of human and other species by allowing external ownership of their genes. International agreements such as the Agreement on Trade-Related Aspects of Intellectual Property Rights (TRIPS) mandate intellectual property protection for most biological inventions, making outright bans on gene patents unlikely for many governments.

The usage of gene patents ethical use of gene patents post-issuance is a significant concern. Patent owners' restrictions might make utilizing proprietary products and processes extremely expensive or even impossible. Furthermore, considering the vast markets for these goods, the innovators construct a wall around their composition patent in order to profit well beyond the initial exclusivity period, innovators often build barriers around their patented composition, contradicting the fundamental purpose of patents to benefit humanity until expiration.

In Australia, patents on naturally occurring DNA sequences are valid.

In the United States, natural biological compounds (along with related methods or uses) sufficiently "isolated" from their natural state can be patented. Previous patents on adrenaline, insulin, vitamin B12, and various genes exemplify this. However, the United States Supreme Court reached an opposing conclusion in a landmark ruling in June 2013, stating that naturally occurring DNA sequences are not eligible for patents, unlike the stance taken by the European Patent Organization, which allows protection for such sequences if they are "isolated from [their] natural environment or generated using a technological approach." However, the United States Supreme Court concluded in a landmark ruling in June 2013 that naturally occurring DNA sequences are not patentable.

European patents cannot be granted for treatments that require the termination of human embryos, according to the European Patent Office.

In the case of Diamond v Chakrabarty (447 US 330; 1980), the Supreme Court ruled that discoveries involving live organisms altered by humans were eligible for patents. The Court's interpretation of section 101 expanded the scope, providing the embryonic biotechnology industry with the impetus to begin and drive an intense period of growth.

Biotechnology patent claims, like all invention claims, delineate a patentee's enforceable rights. Failing to offer the widest claim breadth could pose a significant obstacle for a patentee defending their rights. Considering the critical role of claims in understanding and utilizing patent rights effectively, it's worth exploring how claims function in the biotechnology field to protect breakthroughs. Imagine a scenario where a patent claim, though broad, is poorly worded and rejected due to formal defects; this leaves the patentee with a defense scope barely larger than the actual developed protein species. Competitors can then make minor adjustments to circumvent the literal meaning of the claims. According to the Federal Circuit, the purpose of claims is to determine the enforceable breadth of patent rights. For patents to continue fostering innovation, they must continue fulfilling this role.

The counterparts' theory, on the other hand, provides a reasonable foundation for discouraging the alleged infringement by preventing minor alterations to evade the claim. In exceptional cases, it seems reasonable for a patentee with excessively narrowed protein patent claims to bypass the limitations imposed by the literal scope of the claims, safeguarding against "the unscrupulous copyist" who makes insignificant changes and substitutions in the patent that add nothing substantial (Graver Tank, 339 U.S. at 607).

Before 1995, the expiration dates of various biotech invention components could be years apart. Most patents now expire 20 years after filing in the US, unless extended due to office or regulatory delays or pediatric exclusivity extensions.

14.8.1 Monoclonal Antibody Technology

Biotechnology medications are derived from the immune system's processes that produce white blood cells, known as lymphocytes. In the thymus gland, these cells originate as stem cells in the bone marrow, then differentiate into B-lymphocytes (B-cells) or T-lymphocytes (T cells). B-cells' primary role is to create antibodies in response to encountering foreign materials through interactions with B-cell surface receptors. Following activation, the activated B cell rapidly divides, generating an identical clone of plasma cells that release antibodies with the same antigen specificity as the original B cell. Antibodies, also referred to as immunoglobulins or Ig molecules, are intricate proteins with antigen-binding sites on their branches, resembling the structure of the letter Y. These antibodies attach to antigen molecules, forming a cross-linked, insoluble complex that prevents the spread of the antigen. Antigens are proteins located on the surface of invading cells, like bacteria. When antibodies bind to the cell's surface, it exposes them to macrophages and other immune system components (opsonization).

Antibodies isolated from human blood, specifically immunoglobulin-G (IgG or gamma-globulin), have long been used to treat viral infections. The efficacy of these antibodies varies based on the recentness of the donor's infection. They can also serve in disease diagnosis and distinguishing between biological species. Hybridoma lines were initially included in patent disclosures because early inventions were unable to characterize the amino acid sequence in antibody molecules. However, as more sophisticated methods became available, antibody sequencing replaced or supplemented cell line deposits. Characterizing antibody amino acid sequencing enabled the production of antibodies using recombinant DNA methods. A concern with clinical use of monoclonal antibodies was the potential interaction of mouse proteins, after repeated injection, with the patient's immune system, reducing their potency or potentially inducing a severe allergic reaction. To address this, antibodies produced by recombinant (rDNA) methods used chimeric MAbs with murine variable regions (Y arms), while the constant portions (the Y's base) remained human. Another technological advance replaced all hypervariable regions with specificity, resulting in a humanized antibody.

Further technological advancements allowed segments of antibody genes to be produced on a carrier's surface, like a bacteriophage. This approach enabled the selection of hypervariable sections of specific specificity, combining them into genes that can be expressed to produce entirely human monoclonal antibodies. However, by the time the first of these medications entered the market, the technology for chimeric and humanized antibodies had become obsolete. Phage display also aids in discovering compounds, large or small, that bind to a given structure, such as a receptor or its ligand. Antibodies with unique properties often serve as catalysts, facilitating processes by maintaining two reagent molecules in the correct conformation.

Claims to the nucleic acid encoding the antibody protein, vector constructs, cell lines harboring vectors expressing the protein, methods of harvesting the antibody, purifying the protein from cell line components, formulation for administration, and the device for antibody administration can all protect a monoclonal antibody product.

14.8.2 Antisense Technology

If the genetic code of a disease-causing gene is identified, it could be entirely avoided. Genes consist of double-helical DNA. When a gene is activated, the genetic code in that DNA portion is transcribed as messenger RNA (mRNA). mRNA, often called a "message" sequence, can be translated into amino acids to create a protein. In a DNA double helix, the "antisense" strand is the complementary strand (T pairs with A, C pairs with G, and G pairs with C). Using the antisense coding sequence of the disease gene, short antisense DNAs can be developed as medicines. These molecules attach to disease gene messenger RNAs, preventing the production of disease-causing proteins.

Normally, a 20-base fragment only influences one gene's expression and does not affect other genes. However, antisense medications face obstacles such as in vivo instability of single-stranded DNA and the necessity for effective delivery vehicles. To address stability issues, chemical modifications to the DNA chain, like replacing phosphate groups with less readily hydrolyzed groups, can be employed and potentially copyrighted.

14.8.3 Transgenic Plants

Plant cells, unlike animal cells, possess a sturdy cell wall, making it challenging to introduce genetic information. Additionally, the cellular environment restricts the movement of vectors within the cell. Therefore, unique methods are employed, such as directly delivering DNA molecules onto micronized glass bead surfaces. Once transformed, plants can be conventionally bred. Enhancing yields, improving nutritional quality, and reducing production costs are objectives of transgenic plants.

14.8.4 Exclusivities for Biological Products

The three primary sources of market exclusivity for biological products are regulatory exclusivities, patents, and trade secrets or proprietary knowledge. Patents and regulatory exclusivities safeguard a product's market for a specified duration. According to the BPCIA, innovative biologic drugs filing a complete BLA receive 12 years of regulatory exclusivity. Typically, a "twenty-year period" begins upon patent award and ends twenty years after the application was filed in the United States. (The "twenty-year term" does not apply to patents that were in force on June 8, 1995, or that were issued from an application filed before that date.) The greater of the "twenty-year term" or seventeen years from the grant date determines the length of a patent in this category. (See 35 U.S.C. 154(c) for further information.) Pediatric exclusivities, patent term extensions, and patent term amendments can extend baseline exclusivity periods further.

Regulatory exclusivities offer market protection for innovative products, even without patent protection. In the absence of patents, generic drugs can enter the market after the regulatory exclusivity period. Thus, a biopharmaceutical company's economic strategy necessitates a strong patent portfolio acquisition and maintenance.

Patents can be granted at any stage of drug development. For instance, patents claiming the drug product itself might be issued before or concurrently with NDA or BLA submission. Other patents, such as those for commercial formulation, tailored delivery systems, or comprehensive treatment regimens, would likely be granted post-completion of human clinical trials. Additionally, life cycle management strategies might result in "submarine patents," inadvertently extending patent exclusivity.

A submarine patent was filed pre-1995 but issued later due to a delay, such as an interference proceeding. Remaining hidden in the patent office before the application publishing deadline, it unexpectedly surfaces years later. Consequently, the patent remains hidden at the patent office because it was filed before the deadline to publish the application, and it unexpectedly appears submarine. As a result, a patent is given years after technology has advanced, and the patent is valid for 17 years from the issue date, as per the prior statute's laws.

Moreover, as product development inherently involves innovation, subsequent advancements— such as improved purification processes or application methods—may offer additional patent exclusivity. Consequently, regulatory market and patent exclusivity may run concurrently or independently.

Trade secret laws differ across states but share a common requirement: the information must offer economic benefit to the owner. The owner has taken and continues to take appropriate measures to safeguard this information from public disclosure.

Biopharmaceutical companies often exclude certain information—deemed exclusive trade secrets—from patent disclosures that demand public revelation.

Confidentiality under trade secret laws is not limited by statute and can furnish organizations with a competitive edge. For instance, a biologic manufacturer could monitor critical process controls used in manufacturing or downstream bioprocess steps for creating a reference product. Keeping such proprietary knowledge hidden grants the producer a competitive advantage. Manufacturing process controls, tailored for each product/process, significantly influence the quality and purity of biological medicinal products.

14.8.5 Broad Coverage

Numerous patents may cover various aspects of a single biological product, including nucleic acid and amino acid sequences, expression vectors, production methods, formulations, administration devices, methods of use, and indications. It's not uncommon to witness 50 to over 100 patent filings for one biological product due to the breadth of patentable subject matter. Table 14.4 summarizes the potential patent arguments applicable to an antibody product.

TABLE 14.4
Possible Patent Claims for Antibody Products

Antibody Product	Possible Patent Claims
Amino acid sequence	Complete heavy and light chains
	Heavy and light chain variable regions
	CDR regions
	Modifications made to the framework, CDR, or Fc regions
Analytical methods	Assays developed to monitor the quality or purity of the product
Culture conditions	Media components
	Culture method/feed media
	Optimized culture conditions
Device	Device for administration and use thereof
Diagnostic methods and kits	Methods and kits used to identify select patents that are more or less likely to respond to treatment
Expression system	Host cells engineered to express the product
Expression vector	Every individual element and combination of the vector elements express the sequence in a suitable host cell, including promoter, enhancer, other regulatory sequences, and selection marker
Formulation	Pharmaceutical compositions comprising the drug product
Methods of use	Broad mechanism-based methods of use
	Disease-specific methods of use
	Indication-specific treatment regimens corresponding to the product label
Nucleic acid sequence	Nucleic acid sequences encoding any or all of the above-listed amino acid sequences
Platform technology	Platform technologies and assays used to discover or optimize the structural and functional features of the product or processes used to manufacture or purify the product
Purification	Chromatography methods claiming the use of resins alone or in series
	Optimized conditions
	Compositions having a defined level of purity or homogeneity

14.9   PURPLE BOOK

On September 9, 2014, the FDA introduced the first version of the biologic equivalent of the Orange Book, known as the "Purple Book" is formally known as "Lists of Approved Biological Products with Reference Product Exclusivity and Biopharmaceutical Interchangeability Evaluations," and it contains a list of biological products, including biopharmaceuticals and interchangeable biological products licensed by the FDA under the Public Health Service Act (PHS Act). Unlike the Orange Book, it does not contain patents unique to the biological innovator product. The lists include only the date a biological product was approved under section 351(a) of the PHS Act and if the FDA reviewed the biological product for reference product exclusivity under section 351(k)(7) of the PHS Act. The FDA has determined whether a biological product approved under section 351(k) of the PHS Act is biopharmaceutical or interchangeable with a reference biological product, according to the Purple Book (an already-licensed FDA biological product). The reference product that exhibited biopharmaceutical or interchangeability will be classified under the biopharmaceutical and interchangeable biological products authorized under section 351(k) of the PHS Act. Separate listings for biological goods controlled by the Center for Drug Evaluation and Research (CDER) and the Center for Biologics Evaluation and Research (CBER) will be updated on a regular basis (CBER).

14.10   PATENT TERM EXTENSION

Patents related to human "drug products," including biological products, might qualify for a regulatory delay extension in the United States. A patent claiming a prescription product, usage technique, or production method can be extended if it meets six criteria outlined in 35 U.S.C. 156. However, only one patent term extension is allowed per "drug product."

Another aspect of the extension is that the patent can be reinstated for up to five years, considering a constitutional limit on total patent duration. The product's total patent life with the extension cannot exceed 14 years from the approval date. If the product's patent life post-approval is already 14 years or more, no extension is granted. The extension must be requested within 60 days of the product's initial commercial marketing or use permission; it's not automatic.

14.10.1   PATENT TERM ADJUSTMENT

14.10.1.1   Factors Affecting a Patent Term

GENERIC VARIATIONS: Although 20 years is the accepted modern standard for patent terms, not all countries hold to it yet, and other factors cause variation in terms. These include:

- Foreign legal sanctions and their effect, for example, a TRIPS Council decision, required Canada to extend the duration of some patents issued under 17-year term legislation to 20 years.
- Delays in obtaining a patent before it is granted (which can shorten or lengthen a term).
- Nonpayment of annuity payments, whether on purpose or by mistake, results in a premature lapse.
- Changes in the law can affect the duration of all pending or active proceedings.
- Only a subset of pattents is affected by targeted legal changes (special provisions in the law for pharmaceutical patents).

14.10.1.2   Pharmaceutical Patent Variations

The pharmaceutical industry commonly receives limited patent term extensions, with some countries allowing extensions for medical devices and agrochemicals. These extensions compensate patent owners for sales time lost due to mandatory registration requirements (testing safety and efficacy). These provisions prevent patent owners from infringing their patent property between the award of the patent and the approval of the marketing authorization, a penalty that no other industry faces. Different countries have implemented different mechanisms, but they all follow the same strategy to recover part of the lost exclusivity period.

There are essentially two mechanisms to receive a term extension: expanding the original patent's scope (as done in the US and Japan) or introducing a new legal instrument that takes effect after patent expiration, as in the European Union's Supplementary Protection Certificate (SPC).

The United States (Hatch-Waxman Act), Japan (19814), and the European Union have enacted comprehensive term extension provisionsfollowed by Japan in 19814. Two laws from the European Union date from 1992 and 1996. Unfortunately for knowledge specialists, putting those provisions in place was not easy. However, implementing these provisions was complex, especially due to existing national legislation in France and Italy preceding the EU regulations, potentially affecting certain goods covered by those laws rather than the EU regime.

Several nations, including Australia, Bulgaria, Cyprus, Czech Republic, Estonia, Hungary, Iceland, Israel, Latvia, Mexico, Moldova, Norway, South Africa, South Korea, Switzerland, and Taiwan, have enacted or are contemplating patent term extension legislation. Most countries have adopted a variable-term extension, allowing a maximum extension of 2–7 years.

14.10.1.3   Annuity Fees and Term Computation

In most developed countries, patent security relies on post-grant payments (annuity fees). In the United States, these are due at 3.5, 11.5, and 14.5 years after the grant, while in Europe, they are payable on the third anniversary of filing, even if the patent is still pending. A public registry usually records payment notices. Annuity payments in many countries increase with patent age, following a sliding scale.

National patent laws significantly determine a patent's duration. For instance, in the United Kingdom, a patent remains valid for 20 years from the application date. Thus, a UK patent issued on April 1 would generally expire on March 31, 20 years later. Conversely, in Germany, a patent is valid for 20 years from the date of the application's filing for the invention. Though seemingly minor, this distinction in calculation can be crucial in certain scenarios.

14.10.1.4   Information on Aspects of Patent Term

When dealing with legal status information, it's crucial never to rely solely on one source. Actual information and inclusion timelines can vary between sources. Some references may be less updated due to differing coverage and updating policies. Furthermore, certain sources might only provide partial details, necessitating careful selection by users.

National registers, if available in searchable formats, hold authoritative information. However, be cautious about format discrepancies; machine-readable documents within the patent office may not fully align with public web copies. The INPADOC file, now accessible via the esp@cenet® website (http://ep.espacenet.com), remains the most comprehensive single source for multinational data. Additionally, note that certain online implementations of these data sources might not directly link relevant records (such as US reissue or reexamination cases) or other legal instruments (such as SPCs) to their parent records.

14.10.1.5   USPTO Web Sources

The basic public legal status source of the US Patent and Trademark Office is the PAIR service (http://pair.uspto.gov). This contains some annuity payment data (although it may be incomplete) and some information on Hatch-Waxman extensions under 35 USC § 156. A specific part of the website (www.uspto.gov/web/offices/pac/dapp/opla/term/156.html) discusses these actions. Hatch-Waxman extensions are issued as a Certificate of Correction to the "master" patent. They are available in facsimile form (as TIFF files) in the main patent search area of the website.

14.10.1.6   Other Web Registers

Many patent offices increasingly provide legal status data on the internet. The web version of the European Patent Office (EPO) Register is free and accessible under the epoline® umbrella (www. epoline.org/register.html). However, this site lacks data on any SPC applications citing a European Patent as the "basic patent" because the granting or refusal of an SPC is solely within the purview of individual national governments in Europe. There's no obligation to feed data back to the EPO for inclusion in its register.

Other patent offices with websites that contain legal status information include those in the United Kingdom (www.patent.gov.uk), Germany (www.dpma.de/index.htm), The Netherlands (www.bie. nl), and Australia (www.ipaustralia.gov.au). Typically, such sites are free, but they may require you to register for a user ID before using them. A limited amount of English-language legal status information is from the free Japan Patent Office website (www.jpo.go.jp). Still, more comprehensive information is only on the fee-based Patolis-e-service.

14.10.1.7   Commercial Online Files

In addition to the web-based sources described above, many electronic files are available on commercial host systems. Most of them have a mixture of general legal status and some actions specific to the pharmaceutical industry.

14.10.2   Non-Patent Office Sources

It is vital to note that drug exclusivity is not totally regulated by patents. Other government agencies have the authority to grant or deny marketing exclusivity. The US Food and Drug Administration's Center for Drug Evaluation and Research, for example, maintains approval listings on its website (www.fda.gov/cder/orange/adp.htm). The record of medicine patent expiration can be found in the electronic edition of the so-called Orange Book (www.fda.gov/cder/ob/default.htm). Based on the same dataset, there are new versions or derivatives. Minesoft (London, UK, www.minesoft.com) has created an alternative to the Orange Book, and FOI Services Inc. (Gaithersburg, MD, www.foiservi ces.com) publishes Drugs under Patent.

A second mechanism exists in the United States for extending the term of a patent. This second extension, known as Patent Term Adjustment (PTA), was established by the American Inventors Protection Act of 1999 (AIA). The AIA empowers the United States Patent and Trademark Office (USPTO) to meet specific deadlines during the patent examination phase. Failure by the USPTO to meet one or more of the AIA's time constraints (such as issuing the first Office Action within 14 months of the filing date, responding within four months of an appeal or board decision, and issuing patents within four months of the issue date) is a common reason for obtaining a patent term extension. The AIA also stipulates that the initial patent application procedure should be completed within three years of the actual filing, unless ongoing applications and appeals by the filing party cause delays. If these deadlines are not met, patent applicants may receive compensation for USPTO administrative delays in the form of a day-for-day extension of the patent term resulting from the prolonged examination process. Patent holders can acquire term extensions ranging from a day to several years. Any time spent responding to USPTO conduct during the patent application will be subtracted from the PTA granted.

14.11   FREEDOM-TO-OPERATE OPINIONS

All patents and patent applications relevant to the manufacture, use, or sale of a product, such as a biopharmaceutical product, undergo comprehensive examination in Freedom to Operate (FTO) decisions. The assessment scrutinizes each patent/application to determine infringement, invalidity, or potential expiration before the product's release. The FTO serves various purposes in biopharmaceutical applications. Its primary function is to provide a well-considered opinion that prevents courts from imposing treble damages in the event of a biologic product infringing on a patent. Additionally, it creates a competitive environment for designing around potentially infringed patents and provides a list of patents that the Reference Product Sponsor (RPS) might claim during the patent exchange process, as mandated by legislation.

The gene sequence responsible for expressing the substance is part of the composition of matter, making these patents challenging to avoid. Fortunately, most of these patents are nearing expiration. Although their expiration dates vary widely, there is concrete data available for evaluation. It's typical for a span of 2–4 years to pass between major markets, and therefore, the date of the composition of matter will determine the manufacturing location for the initial launch.

14.11.1   SUBMARINE PATENTS

Submarine patents may emerge just as the first composition of matter patent is close to expiring, owing to a complex system of cross-licensing and overlapping patent applications filed before 1995. Examples such as interferon-alpha and etanercept illustrate this, both enjoying decades of exclusivity despite contradicting the spirit of patent law. They exploited a flaw in the US patenting system, which has now been rectified. The patent period is currently 20 years from the date of the first filing, instead of the 17 years exploited by the submarine patents. Outside the United States, this risk doesn't exist, and these patents are impossible to circumvent.

14.11.2   SYSTEM EXPRESSION PATENTS

Patents cover fundamental speech technology, like the Cabilly patents; these are broader patents. In this scenario, a biosimilar developer might acquire a license unless Genentech manufactures the product. This particular patent was due to expire in 20114, and getting around these patents is unfeasible.

14.11.3   PROCESS PATENTS OF ORIGINATOR

While much focus centers on composition of matter patents, process patents prove to be the most challenging. This challenge surfaces as major market cap products like adalimumab and etanercept approach their expiration dates. Despite potential contests and invalidations of these patents, their highly detailed specifications for protected areas are remarkable. For instance, concerning etanercept, one must demonstrate that the amino acid composition during upstream processing doesn't match the stated distribution. However, most upstream processes don't track amino acid composition. The scope of these patents includes media selection, upstream conditions, buffer pH and structure, downstream purification columns, their order of use, and even claims of higher purity.

With a significant number of bioprocessing patents held by both the originator and third parties, defining a suitable manufacturing method has proven to be exceedingly difficult and technically challenging. Patents that specify amino acid composition during upstream processing demonstrate the challenges; ironically, this is not a standard examination. Even the media's composition remains unknown to the producer. However, upon publication of such patents, it becomes the developer's responsibility to research this aspect.

14.11.4 THIRD-PARTY PROCESS PATENTS

While bypassing originator process patents is difficult, third-party patents referencing a specific product or product class are also potential hurdles. In certain instances, a biosimilar developer must devise an alternative manufacturing route to circumvent the originator patent and then conduct a thorough review of third-party patents.

14.11.5 FORMULATION COMPOSITION

Early biological product pioneers underestimated the significance of these patents, but now we observe formulation patents aimed at raising the bar for demonstrating similarity. Despite the intention of keeping biosimilar developers out of the market, this approach hasn't succeeded if agencies require equivalent quality. Agencies, recognizing this, might allow alternative formulations.

14.11.6 LIFECYCLE FORMULATION PROJECTIONS

As a composition of matter patent nears expiration, a recent trend involves altering the formulation, such as shifting from a lyophilized formulation to a solution or adopting a high-concentration sub-cutaneous formulation instead of an intravenous solution. This change aims to make the product more user-friendly, posing a challenging marketing task. However, once the new formulation is launched, obtaining reference samples for biosimilar product testing becomes challenging, assuming any intellectual property issues are resolved.

14.11.7 ALTERNATE OFFERING

Even though the original product might have had limited presentations initially, these can evolve over time, mostly to enhance usability, like the use of prefilled syringes or injectors instead of vials. Such changes impact marketing and delivery, complicating reimbursements.

14.11.8 INDICATIONS AND DOSAGE

Initially disregarded by early biological drug pioneers, patents specifying particular product uses, like indications, have become standard. Several patents will cover almost any large molecule approaching expiration, including specific doses, conditions of use, and dosing schedules. For instance, AbbVie holds a patent prescribing precisely 40 mg of adalimumab every other week. These patents aimed to prevent biosimilar products resembling those already on the market, assuming regulatory authorities wouldn't permit different dosing or indications. However, realizing the risk, regulatory agencies are open to alternative suggestions. Nevertheless, these can pose significant challenges. Recently emerged patents have surprised major biosimilar developers who may have heavily invested in clinical trials only to find out they can't market the drugs after the trials. A biosimilar developer doesn't need to investigate existing intellectual property but rather anticipate potential future developments.

14.11.9 DELIVERY DEVICES

Since these devices are unique to the product, even if they are distributed by software manufacturing firms to many customers, the originator may hold multiple patents on the delivery device. The chosen device significantly impacts the biosimilar's marketability.

14.11.10 DEVELOPING FREEDOM TO OPERATE

Determining the freedom-to-operate for a biopharmaceutical firm requires a multifaceted strategy to identify all relevant patents and patent applications. Starting with a list of search terms is crucial. At a minimum, this list should include parties involved in discovery and substance manufacture, as well as alternate names for the biologic used in the development process.

Given the convoluted history of biologic products involving multiple parties, it's feasible that several parties hold patents covering a single product. A university or a cutting-edge biotech company may discover a molecular target or lead molecule, subsequently choosing whether to license, sell, or partner with a pharmaceutical company for product development. As the medication research continues, any or all involved parties could possess patents on the final product.

To identify patents claiming the amino acid sequence used to express the biologic product, one can scan sequence databases after identifying the specific amino acid sequence. The Basic Local Alignment Search Tool (BLAST) available at http://blast.ncbi.nlm.nih.gov/Blast.cgi is a public sequence database suitable for such searches. Additionally, commercial databases like GenomeQuest are available as alternative search providers.

A comprehensive search of a patent database is necessary once the search criteria are determined. Although several publicly accessible databases like the USPTO and the EPO exist, they lack support for open-ended operators, making information retrieval more challenging compared to paid databases with more powerful search capabilities. In addition to product-specific patents/applications, it is crucial to check for generic methods for producing the biologic, such as media and conditions for cultivating the cell line and expressing and purifying monoclonal antibodies and proteins. For example, Genentech obtained a general process patent (enter 6331415 at http://patft.uspto.gov/netahtml/PTO/srchnum.htm) known as Cabilly II for monoclonal antibody expression. This patent, obtained after a lengthy prosecution involving interference actions and re-examination, was issued in 2001 with a priority claim dating back to 1983. Despite this priority, the patent expired on December 18, 2018, after 17 years in effect. Its claim 1 specifically involves a technique for producing an antibody molecule in a single host cell comprising at least the heavy and light chains' variable domains.

After entering the search criteria into the chosen database, hundreds, if not thousands, of patents will need to be sifted through. Relevant patents concerning the biopharmaceutical applicant's cell line, media, production technique, bioreactor technology, purification process, formulation, and tests should be selected from the search results. Analyzing these patents claim by claim is crucial to assess their relevance to the applicant's market freedom, forming the foundation for the Freedom-to-Operate (FTO) final opinion.

Determining the expiration dates and total number of patents to be examined is essential. This involves considering the filing date of claims, any patent term adjustments by the USPTO, impact of terminal disclaimers, patent term extensions due to regulatory approval delays, and the timely payment of maintenance fees. Identifying the expiration dates is critical as patents expiring before the planned product launch may become irrelevant to the study.

The FTO opinion must evaluate each argument to ascertain whether current processes, products, or therapeutic indications breach the patent. The latest set of claims needs examination to gauge the likelihood of infringement based on the claims' interpretation at the time and the probability of patent issuance for patent applications. It is assumed that the patent application is likely to be violated. Consequently, this application should be included in a watch list to monitor prosecution during the development of a biopharmaceutical product.

If patents are not due to expire before launch and are likely to be found infringing, the biopharmaceutical applicant must strategize upon receiving the FTO opinion. If designing around patent claims is unfeasible due to cost, time, or product alteration issues, challenging the patent or requesting a license from the patent owners becomes an option. If the decision is to contest the patent, an invalidity opinion must be drafted. This opinion can be utilized to craft a post-grant appeal against a patent or used as a negotiating tool during the patent exchange process under the provisions of the BPCIA legislation.

After the USPTO has granted a patent, three avenues for contesting it are available: ex parte re-examination, inter partes review, and post-grant review. Each option has its own set of advantages and disadvantages. Ex parte re-examination is the most cost-effective method as it does not require the challenger to be named. However, once the initial appeal is filed, the challenger cannot participate further, and the re-examination is conducted solely by the patent reviewing corps, taking approximately two years to complete.

Early in the product lifecycle, a strategy for managing the product's lifecycle is developed. As the product advances through multiple production and regulatory approvals, a comprehensive and intensive intellectual property strategy becomes imperative. Proposals for specific treatments and doses arise following the success of numerous clinical trials. Patents continually emerge, especially when composition or gene sequence patents are nearing expiration. The authors anticipate that limitations on drug manufacture, formulation, and use will dissuade biopharmaceutical companies from entering the market. They also speculate that product design modifications might lead the FDA to no longer classify them as biopharmaceuticals.

14.12 CONCLUSION

In the formulation of biopharmaceutical products, intellectual property plays a significant role. Despite being a legal concern for most, the complexities in biological drug technology make it a concern for all scientists involved in biopharmaceuticals. Given the potential patentability of the process and high financial stakes, litigation is common among biopharmaceutical companies. This chapter aims to educate team members in development, manufacturing, and marketing on avoiding litigation, a prime contributor to the high cost of development and market entry delays.

Bibliography

Aa S, Gottschalk U (2013). Single-use disposable technologies for biopharmaceutical manufacturing. *Trends Biotechnol.* 31(3), 147–154. DOI: 10.1016/j.tibtech.2012.10.004

Akbarzadeh A, et al. (2019). Recent advances in biopharmaceutical production in plants. *Biotechnol Lett.* 41(9–10), 1077–1095. DOI: 10.1007/s10529-019-02717-6

Al-Fageeh MB, et al. (2018). Challenges and strategies for the production of therapeutic proteins in plant cells. *Plant Biotechnol J.* 16(5), 1006–1024. DOI: 10.1111/pbi.12894

Arnold L, Lee K, Rucker-Pezzini J, Lee JH (2019). Implementation of fully integrated continuous antibody processing: effects on productivity and COGm. *Biotechnol J.* 14(2), e1800061. DOI: 10.1002/biot.201800061

Baeshen MN, Al-Hejin AM, Bora RS, et al. (2015). Production of biological medicines in *E. coli*: current scenario and future perspectives. *J Microbiol Biotechnol.* 25(7), 953–962. DOI: 10.4014/jmb.1412.12079

Baghban R, Farajnia S, Rajabibazl M, et al. (2019). Yeast expression systems: overview and recent advances. *Mol Biotechnol.* 61(5), 365–384. DOI: 10.1007/s12033-019-00164-8

Bakeev KA (2010). Process Analytical Technology: Spectroscopic Tools and Implementation Strategies for the Chemical and Pharmaceutical Industries: Second Edition. John Wiley & Sons Inc.

Balasundaram B, et al. (2019). Recent advances in the expression of recombinant proteins in Pichia pastoris. *Bioengineered* 10(1), 441–455. DOI: 10.1080/21655979.2019.1645827

Baur D, Angelo JM, Chollangi S, et al. (2018). Model assisted comparison of protein A resins and multi-column chromatography for capture processes. *J Biotechnol.* 285, 64–73. DOI: 10.1016/j.jbiotec.2018.08.014

Belongia B, Blanck R, Tingley S (2003). Single-use disposable filling for sterile pharmaceuticals. *Pharm Eng.* 23, 26–134.

Beni V, Nilsson D, Arven P, et al. (2015). Printed electrochemical instruments for biosensors. *ECS J Solid State Sci Technol.* 4, 3001–3005. DOI: 10.1149/2.0011510jss

Berlec A, Strukelj B (2013). Current state and recent advances in biological medicine production in Escherichia coli, yeasts and mammalian cells. *J Ind Microbiol Biotechnol.* 40(3–4), 257–274. DOI: 10.1007/s10295-013-1235-0

Berrie DM, Waters RC, Montoya C, et al. (2020). Development of a high-yield live-virus vaccine production platform using a novel fixed-bed bioreactor. *Vaccine.* 38(20), 3639–3645. DOI: 10.1016/j.vaccine.2020.03.041

Biopharmaceutic Market. www.alliedmarketresearch.com/biological medicine-market#:~:text=Biological medicines%20Market%20Overview%3A,13.8%25%20from%202018%20to%202025

Bisschops M, Frick L, Fulton S, Ransohoff T (2009). Single-use, continuous countercurrent, multicolumn chromatography. *BioProcess Int.* 7, S18–S23.

Boedeker B, Goldstein A, Mahajan E (2018). Fully single-use manufacturing concepts for clinical and commercial manufacturing and ballroom concepts. *Adv Biochem Eng Biotechnol.* 165, 179–210. DOI: 10.1007/10_2017_19

Bohonak D, Mehta U, Weiss ER, Voyta G (2021). Adapting virus filtration to enable intensified and continuous mAb processing. *Biotechnol Prog.* 37(2), e3088. DOI: 10.1002/btpr.3088

Bracewell DG, Brown RA, Hoare M (2004). Addressing a whole bioprocess in real-time using an optical biosensor-formation, recovery and purification of antibody fragments from a recombinant E-coli host. *Bioprocess Biosyst Eng.* 26, 271–282.

Branco C, et al. (2018). Microalgae for recombinant protein production: current trends and prospects. *Pharm Bioprocess.* 6(6), 385–394. DOI: 10.1208/s12249-018-1122-6

Brestrich N, Briskot T, Osberghaus A, Hubbuch J (2014). A tool for selective inline quantification of co-eluting proteins in chromatography using spectral analysis and partial least squares regression. *Biotechnol Bioeng.* 111, 1365–1373.

Brestrich N, Sanden A, Kraft A, et al. (2015). Advances in inline quantification of co-eluting proteins in chromatography: process-data-based model calibration and application towards real-life separation issues. *Biotechnol Bioeng.* 112, 1406–1416.

Briskot T, et al. (2021). Cell-free protein synthesis for the development of biopharmaceuticals. *Curr Opin Biotechnol.* 68, 12–19. DOI: 10.1016/j.copbio.2020.08.006

Brower M, Hou Y, Pollard D (2015). Monoclonal antibody continuous processing enabled by single-use. In: Subramanian G, ed. Continuous Processing in Pharmaceutical Manufacturing. Wiley VCH. pp.255–296.

Brown J, et al. Scale-Up of Microbial Fermentation Using Recombinant E. coli in HyPerforma 30 L and 300 L Single-Use Fermentors. Thermo Fisher Scientific: San Jose, CA, 2014; www.thermofisher.com/content/dam/LifeTech/Documents/PDFs/CO29180-SUF-Launch-AppNotes-Scale-Up%20of%20Microbial-Global-FLR_V2.pdf. Application Note CO29180.

Capito F, Skudas R, Kolmar H, Stanislawski B (2013). Host cell protein quantification by fourier transform mid infrared spectroscopy (FT-MIR). *Biotechnol Bioeng.* 110, 252–259.

Carrondo MJT, Alves PM, Carinhas N, et al. (2012). How can measurement, monitoring, modeling and control advance cell culture in industrial biotechnology? *Biotechnol J.* 7, 1522–1529.

Chaudhuri RK, et al. (2021). Recent advances in mammalian cell culture technology for recombinant protein production. *Biotechnol Genet Eng Rev.* 37(2), 191–210. DOI: 10.1080/02648725.2021.1966385

Chemmalil L, Prabhakar T, Kuang J, et al. (2020). Online/at-line measurement, analysis and control of product titer and critical product quality attributes (CQAs) during process development. *Biotechnol Bioeng.* DOI: 10.1002/bit.27531

Chen C, et al. (2016). Engineering next-generation antibody therapeutics using artificial intelligence. *Front Immunol.* 7, 295. DOI: 10.3389/fimmu.2016.00295

Chen PH, Cheng YT, Ni BS, Huang JH (2020). Continuous cell separation using microfluidic-based cell retention device with alternative boosted flow. *Appl Biochem Biotechnol.* 191(1), 151–163. DOI: 10.1007/s12010-020-03288-9

Chisti Y (2018). Bioconjugates and biologics: from discovery to manufacturing. *Biochem Eng J.* 138, 204–212. DOI: 10.1016/j.bej.2018.07.010

Chu L, et al. (2021). Continuous manufacturing of biologics: current status, opportunities, and challenges. *Engineering* 7(12), 1492–1500. DOI: 10.1016/j.eng.2021.09.017

Chuah SH, et al. (2020). Advanced technologies for improved recombinant protein production in bacteria. *Bioengineered* 11(1), 438–452. DOI: 10.1080/21655979.2020.1751549

Chusainow J, et al. (2009). Transient protein expression in suspension mammalian cells for accelerated early stage recombinant protein detection. *J Biotech.* 139(3), 203–211. DOI: 10.1016/j.jbiotec.2008.11.009

Contreras-Gómez A, Sánchez-Mirón A, García-Camacho F, et al. (2014). Protein production using the baculovirus-insect cell expression system. *Biotechnol Prog.* 30(1), 1–18. DOI: 10.1002/btpr.1842

Costa AR, et al. (2021). Cell-free systems for recombinant protein production: Strategies, challenges, and opportunities. *Biotechnol J.* 16(2), e2000127. DOI: 10.1002/biot.202000127

Datar RV, et al. (2019). Emerging trends in biomanufacturing: Implications for the future of medicine. *Pharm Res.* 36(1), 4. DOI: 10.1007/s11095-018-2542-2

De Jesus M, Wurm FM (2011). Manufacturing recombinant proteins in kg-ton quantities using animal cells in bioreactors. *Eur J Pharm Biopharm.* 78(2), 184–188. DOI: 10.1016/j.ejpb.2011.01.005. Epub 2011 Jan 20. PMID: 21256214.

De Luca C, Felletti S, Lievore G, et al. (2020). Modern trends in downstream processing of therapeutic proteins through continuous chromatography: the potential of multicolumn countercurrent solvent gradient purification. *Trends Anal Chem.* 132, 116051. DOI: 10.1016/j.trac.2020.116051

Dhara VG, Naik HM, Majewska NI, Betenbaugh MJ (2018). Recombinant antibody production in CHO and NS0 cells: differences and similarities. *BioDrugs.* 32(6), 571–584. DOI: 10.1007/s40259-018-0319-9

Dingermann T (2008). Recombinant therapeutic proteins: production platforms and challenges. *Biotechnol J.* 3(1), 90–97. DOI: 10.1002/biot.200700214. PMID: 18041103.

Donini M, Marusic C (2019). Current state-of-the-art in plant-based antibody production systems. *Biotechnol Lett.* 41(3), 335–346. DOI: 10.1007/s10529-019-02651-z. Epub 2019 Jan 25. PMID: 30684155.

Donini M, Marusic C (2019). Current state-of-the-art in plant-based antibody production systems. *Biotechnol Lett.* 41(3), 335–346. DOI: 10.1007/s10529-019-02651-z. Epub 2019 Jan 25. PMID: 30684155.

Dorival-García N, Bones J (2017). Monitoring leachables from single-use bioreactor bags for mammalian cell culture by dispersive liquid-liquid microextraction followed by ultra high performance liquid chromatography quadrupole time of flight mass spectrometry. *J Chromatogr A.* 1512, 51–60. DOI: 10.1016/j.chroma.2017.06.077

Dumont J, Euwart D, Mei B, et al. (2016). Human cell lines for biological medicine manufacturing: history, status, and future perspectives. *Crit Rev Biotechnol.* 36(6), 1110–1122. DOI: 10.3109/07388551.2015.1084266

Dyson MR (2016). Fundamentals of expression in mammalian cells. *Adv Exp Med Biol.* 896, 217–224. DOI: 10.1007/978-3-319-27216-0_14

Elich T, Goodrich E, Lutz H, Mehta U (2019). Investigating the combination of single-pass tangential flow filtration and anion exchange chromatography for intensified mAb polishing. *Biotechnol Prog.* 35(5), e2862. DOI: 10.1002/btpr.2862

Esbensen K, Kirsanov D, Legin A, et al. (2004). Fermentation monitoring using multisensor systems: Feasibility study of the electronic tongue. *Anal Bioanal Chem.* 378, 391–395.

Farid SS (2007). Process economics of industrial monoclonal antibody manufacture. *J Chromatogr B Analyt Technol Biomed Life Sci.* 848(1), 8–18. DOI: 10.1016/j.jchromb.2006.07.037. Epub 2006 Aug 8. PMID: 16899415.

Farid SS, et al. (2018). Economic considerations in the production of recombinant therapeutics in mammalian cells. *Proc IEEE.* 106(9), 1537–1562. DOI: 10.1109/JPROC.2018.2846686

Feidl F, Vogg S, Wolf M, et al. (2020). Process-wide control and automation of an integrated continuous manufacturing platform for antibodies. *Biotechnol Bioeng.* 117(5), 1367–1380. DOI: 10.1002/bit.27296

Fernández FJ, Vega MC (2016). Choose a suitable expression host: a survey of available protein production platforms. *Adv Exp Med Biol.* 896, 15–24. DOI: 10.1007/978-3-319-27216-0_2

Fischer S, Handrick R, Otte K (2015). The art of CHO cell engineering: a comprehensive retrospect and future perspectives. *Biotechnol Adv.* 33(8):1878–1896. DOI: 10.1016/j.biotechadv.2015.10.015. Epub 2015 Oct 31. PMID: 26523782.

Fisher AC, Kamga MH, Agarabi C, et al. (2019). The current scientific and regulatory landscape in advancing integrated continuous biological medicine manufacturing. *Trends Biotechnol.* 37(3), 253–267. DOI: 10.1016/j.tibtech.2018.08.008

Flickinger MC (2013). Upstream Industrial Biotechnology. Equipment, Process Design, Sensing, Control, and cGMP Operations. John Wiley & Sons Inc.

Fogle JE, et al. (2021). Emerging trends in viral vectors for gene therapy. *Curr Opin Biotechnol.* 68, 268–275. DOI: 10.1016/j.copbio.2020.11.014

Fu H, et al. (2021). Intensified processes in downstream bioprocessing: Current status and future perspectives. *Biotechnol J.* 16(3), e2000259. DOI: 10.1002/biot.202000259

Fuller M, Pora H (2008). Introducing disposable systems into biomanufacturing: a CMO case study. *BioProcess Int.* 6, 30–36.

Gagnon M, Nagre S, Wang W, et al. (2019). Novel, linked bioreactor system for continuous production of biologics. *Biotechnol Bioeng.* 116(8), 1946–1958. DOI: 10.1002/bit.26985

Gagnon M, Nagre S, Wang W, Hiller GW (2018). Shift to high-intensity, low-volume perfusion cell culture enabling a continuous, integrated bioprocess. *Biotechnol Prog.* 34(6), 1472–1481. DOI: 10.1002/btpr.2723

Gallihere PM, Hodge G, Guertin P, et al. (2011). Single use bioreactor platform for microbial fermentation. In: Regine E, Dieter E, eds. Single-Use Technology in Biopharmaceutical Manufacture. John Wiley & Sons Inc. pp. 241–250.

Garnick RL (1997). Specifications from a biotechnology industry perspective. *Dev Biol Stand.* 91:31–36. PMID: 9413680.

Ge X, et al. (2022). Recent advances in protein glycoengineering. *Curr Opin Chem Biol.* 69, 73–81. DOI: 10.1016/j.cbpa.2022.02.019

Ge X, Hanson M, Shen H, et al. (2006). validation of an optical sensor-based high-throughput bioreactor system for mammalian cell culture. *J Biotechnol.* 122(3):293–306. DOI: 10.1016/j.jbiotec.2005.12.009

Ghaderi D, et al. (2018). Emerging trends in cell and gene therapy manufacturing. *Ther Deliv.* 9(4), 303–315. DOI: 10.4155/tde-2018-0004

Goussen C, Goldstein L, Brèque C, et al. (2020). Viral clearance capacity by continuous Protein A chromatography step using sequential multicolumn chromatography. *J Chromatogr B Anal Technol Biomed Life Sci.* 1145, 122056. DOI: 10.1016/j.jchromb.2020.122056

Graumann K, Premstaller A (2006). Manufacturing of recombinant therapeutic proteins in microbial systems. *Biotechnol J.* 1(2), 164–186. DOI: 10.1002/biot.200500051. PMID: 16892246.

Grillberger L, Kreil TR, Nasr S, Reiter M (2009). Emerging trends in plasma-free manufacturing of recombinant protein therapeutics expressed in mammalian cells. *Biotechnol J.* 4(2), 186–201. DOI: 10.1002/biot.200800241. PMID: 19226552; PMCID: PMC2699044.

Grilo AL, Mantalaris A (2019). Apoptosis: a mammalian cell bioprocessing perspective. *Biotechnol Adv.* 37(3), 459–475. DOI: 10.1016/j.biotechadv.2019.02.012

Gupta RD, et al. (2019). Emerging trends in antibody drug conjugates: Recent advances in payloads, linkers, and conjugation chemistries. *Bioconjug Chem.* 30(2), 249–261. DOI: 10.1021/acs.bioconjchem.8b00635

Gupta SK, Shukla P (2017). Microbial platform technology for recombinant antibody fragment production: a review. *Crit Rev Microbiol.* 43(1), 31–42. DOI: 10.3109/1040841x.2016.1150959

Gupta SK, Shukla P (2017). Sophisticated cloning, fermentation, and purification technologies for an enhanced therapeutic protein production: a review. *Front Pharmacol.* 4(8), 419. DOI: 10.3389/fphar.2017.00419. PMID: 28725194; PMCID: PMC5495827.

Hacker DL, Balasubramanian S (2016). Recombinant protein production from stable mammalian cell lines and pools. *Curr Opin Struct Biol.* 38, 129–136. DOI: 10.1016/j.sbi.2016.06.005

Hacker DL, De Jesus M, Wurm FM (2009). 25 years of recombinant proteins from reactor-grown cells - where do we go from here? *Biotechnol Adv.* 27(6), 1023–1027. DOI: 10.1016/j.biotechadv.2009.05.008. Epub 2009 May 20. PMID: 19463938.

Hansen SK, Jamali B, Hubbuch J (2013). Selective high throughput protein quantification based on UV absorption spectra. *Biotechnol Bioeng.* 110, 448–460.

Health USD, Services H (2004). Pharmaceutical CGMPs: Guidance for Industry PAT – A Framework for Innovative Pharmaceutical Development, Manufacturing and Quality Assurance. Food and Drug Administration.

Heidemann R, Lünse S, Tran D, Zhang C (2010). Characterization of cell-banking parameters for the cryopreservation of mammalian cell lines in 100-mL cryobags. *Biotechnol. Prog.* 26(4), 1154–1163.

Helal NA, Elnoweam O, Eassa HA, et al. (2019). Integrated continuous manufacturing in pharmaceutical industry: current evolutionary steps toward revolutionary future. *Pharm Pat Anal.* 8(4):139–161. DOI: 10.4155/ppa-2019-0011

Hesse F, Wagner R (2000). Developments and improvements in the manufacturing of human therapeutics with mammalian cell cultures. *Trends Biotechnol.* 18(4), 173–180. DOI: 10.1016/s0167-7799(99)01420-1. PMID: 10740264.

Hilbold NJ, Le Saoût X, Valery E, et al. (2017). Evaluation of several protein a resins for application to multicolumn chromatography for the rapid purification of fed-batch bioreactors. *Biotechnol Prog.* 33(4), 941–953. DOI: 10.1002/btpr.2465

Hogwood CE, Bracewell DG, Smales CM (2014). Measurement and control of host cell proteins (HCPs) in CHO cell bioprocesses. *Curr Opin Biotechnol.* 30, 153–160.

Huether-Franken CM, et al. (2013). Scalability of Parallel E. coli Fermentations in BioBLU® f Single-Use Bioreactors. Eppendorf AG. www.eppendorf.com/product-media/doc/en/70274/DASGIP_Fermentors-Bioreactors_Application-Note_293_BioBLU-f_Scalability-Parallel-E-coli-Fermentations-BioBLU-f-Single-Bioreactors.pdf. Application Note 293-I.

Hughson MD, Cruz TA, Carvalho RJ, Castilho LR (2017). Development of a 3-step straight-through purification strategy combining membrane adsorbers and resins. *Biotechnol Prog.* 33(4), 931–940.

Ichihara T, Ito T, Gillespie C (2019). Polishing approach with fully connected flow-through purification for therapeutic monoclonal antibody. *Eng Life Sci.* 19(1), 31–36. DOI: 10.1002/elsc.201800123

Ivarie R (2006). Competitive bioreactor hens on the horizon. *Trends Biotechnol.* 24(3), 99–101. DOI: 10.1016/j.tibtech.2006.01.004. Epub 2006 Jan 30. PMID: 16445998.

Jacquemart R, Vandersluis M, Zhao M, et al. (2016). A single-use strategy to enable manufacturing of affordable biologics. *Comput Struct Biotechnol J.* 14:309–318. DOI: 10.1016/j.csbj.2016.06.007

Jafari P, et al. (2021). CRISPR technologies for improving recombinant protein production in mammalian cells. *Biotechnol Adv.* 52, 107813. DOI: 10.1016/j.biotechadv.2021.107813

Jagschies G, et al. (2019). Recombinant protein bioprocessing strategies. Handbook of Process Chromatography: Development, Manufacturing, Validation and Economics, 2nd Edition, CRC Press, 145–178. DOI: 10.1201/9780429198515

Janarthanan OM, et al. (2021). Emerging trends and technologies in cell-free protein synthesis. *Biotechnol Bioprocess Eng.* 26(6), 823–836. DOI: 10.1007/s12257-021-0405-0

Jazayeri SH, Amiri-Yekta A, Bahrami S, et al. (2018). Vector and cell line engineering technologies toward recombinant protein expression in mammalian cell lines. *Appl Biochem Biotechnol.* 185(4), 986–1003. DOI: 10.1007/s12010-017-2689-8

Jiang B, et al. (2021). Emerging trends in bioprocess monitoring and control for biopharmaceutical manufacturing. *Biotechnol J.* 16(10), e2100005. DOI: 10.1002/biot.202100005

Jiang R, Monroe T, McRogers R, Larson PJ (2002). Manufacturing challenges in the commercial production of recombinant coagulation factor VIII. *Haemophilia.* 8(Suppl 2), 1–5. DOI: 10.1046/j.1351-8216.2001.00115.x. PMID: 11966844.

Johnson SA, Chen S, Bolton G, et al. (2022). Virus filtration: a review of current and future practices in bioprocessing. *Biotechnol Bioeng.* 119(3), 743–761. DOI: 10.1002/bit.28017. Epub 2022 Jan 11. PMID: 34936091.

Jordi MA, Khera S, Roland K, et al. (2018). Qualitative assessment of extractables from single-use components and the impact of reference standard selection. *J Pharm Biomed Anal.* 150, 368–376. DOI: 10.1016/j.jpba.2017.12.029

Juturu V, et al. (2021). Emerging trends and challenges in upstream bioprocessing: a review. *J Ind Microbiol Biotechnol.* 48(3–4), 351–364. DOI: 10.1007/s10295-020-02450-9

Kadlec P, Gabrys B, Strandt S (2009). Data-driven soft sensors in the process industry. *Comput Chem Eng.* 33, 795–814.

Kamga MH, Cattaneo M, Yoon S (2018). Integrated continuous biomanufacturing platform with ATF perfusion and one column chromatography operation for optimum resin utilization and productivity. *Prep Biochem Biotechnol.* 48(5), 383–390. DOI: 10.1080/10826068.2018.1446151

Kateja N, Agarwal H, Hebbi V, Rathore AS (2017). Integrated continuous processing of proteins expressed as inclusion bodies: GCSF as a case study. *Biotechnol Prog.* 33(4), 998–1009. DOI: 10.1002/btpr.2413

Kelley B, Kiss R, Laird M (2018). A different perspective: how much innovation is really needed for monoclonal antibody production using mammalian cell technology? *Adv Biochem Eng Biotechnol.* 165, 443–462. DOI: 10.1007/10_2018_59. PMID: 29721583.

Kelley B, Kiss R, Laird M (2018). A different perspective: how much innovation is really needed for monoclonal antibody production using mammalian cell technology? *Adv Biochem Eng Biotechnol.* 165, 443–462. DOI: 10.1007/10_2018_59

Kelly PS, Dorival-García N, Paré S, et al. (2019). Improvements in single-use bioreactor film material composition leads to robust and reliable Chinese hamster ovary cell performance. *Biotechnol Prog.* 35(4), e2824. DOI: 10.1002/btpr.2824

Kim JY, et al. (2021). Emerging trends in glycoengineering of therapeutic antibodies. *Front Bioeng Biotechnol.* 9, 617962. DOI: 10.3389/fbioe.2021.617962

Klutz S, et al. (2016). Trends in biopharmaceutical drug development: targets, therapeutic classes, and indications. *BioDrugs.* 30(5), 409–418. DOI: 10.1007/s40259-016-0182-0

Koukourava A, et al. (2019). Recent advances in the development of plant factories and bioreactors for pharmaceutical proteins. *Front Plant Sci.* 10, 906. DOI: 10.3389/fpls.2019.00906

Krämer O, Klausing S, Noll T (2010). Methods in mammalian cell line engineering: from random mutagenesis to sequence-specific approaches. *Appl Microbiol Biotechnol.* 88(2), 425–436. DOI: 10.1007/s00253-010-2798-6

Kreyenschulte D, Paciok E, Regestein L, et al. (2015). Online monitoring of upstream processes via non-invasive low-field NMR. *Biotechnol Bioeng.* 112, 1810–1821.

Krishnan R, Chen H (2012). Overview of single-use technologies for biologics production. *Am Pharm Rev.* 15(3), 15–19.

Kshirsagar R, et al. (2020). Recent trends in downstream processing of recombinant proteins: a review. *Protein Expr Purif.* 174, 105673. DOI: 10.1016/j.pep.2020.105673

Kuczewski M, Schirmer E, Lain B, Zarbis-Papastoitsis G (2011). A single-use purification process for the production of a monoclonal antibody produced in a PER.C6 human cell line. *Biotechnol J.* 6(1):56–65. DOI: 10.1002/biot.201000292

Kuglstatter A, et al. (2021). Recent advances in the design of bi-specific antibodies and antibody-drug conjugates for cancer treatment. *Antibodies* 10(4), 49. DOI: 10.3390/antib10040049

Kumar A, et al. (2020). Recent trends in process analytical technology for monitoring and control of bioprocesses. *Biochem Eng J.* 160, 107674. DOI: 10.1016/j.bej.2020.107674

Kumar R, et al. (2021). Emerging trends in the development of microbial bioprocesses for the production of recombinant proteins. *Appl Microbiol Biotechnol.* 105(10), 3925–3942. DOI: 10.1007/s00253-021-11339-x

Kumar V, et al. (2019). Recombinant protein production in insect cells: Challenges and strategies. *Crit Rev Biotechnol.* 39(1), 26–39. DOI: 10.1080/07388551.2018.1521679

Kunert R, Reinhart D (2016). Advances in recombinant antibody manufacturing. *Appl Microbiol Biotechnol.* 100(8), 3451–3461. DOI: 10.1007/s00253-016-7388-9. Epub 2016 Mar 3. PMID: 26936774; PMCID: PMC4803805.

Kunert R, Reinhart D (2016). Advances in recombinant antibody manufacturing. *Appl Microbiol Biotechnol.* 100(8), 3451–3461. DOI: 10.1007/s00253-016-7388-9

Kwon YM, et al. (2021). Advances in high-throughput screening technologies for antibody engineering. *Front Bioeng Biotechnol.* 9, 607674. DOI: 10.3389/fbioe.2021.607674

Lacki KM (2014). High throughput process development in biomanufacturing. *Curr Opin Chem Eng.* 6, 25–32.

Łącki KM, Riske FJ (2020). Affinity chromatography: an enabling technology for large-scale bioprocessing. *Biotechnol J.* 15(1), e1800397. DOI: 10.1002/biot.201800397

Lagassé HA, Alexaki A, Simhadri VL, et al. (2017). Recent advances in (therapeutic protein) drug development. *F1000Res.* 6, 113. DOI: 10.12688/f1000research.9970.1. PMID: 28232867; PMCID: PMC5302153.

Lalonde ME, Durocher Y (2017). Therapeutic glycoprotein production in mammalian cells. *J Biotechnol.* 251, 128–140. DOI: 10.1016/j.jbiotec.2017.04.028

Lamers ML, et al. (2020). Emerging trends in cell and gene therapies: a European perspective. *Mol Ther Methods Clin Dev.* 18, 751–757. DOI: 10.1016/j.omtm.2020.03.009

Langer ES, et al. (2021). Emerging technologies for the production of complex biologics. Trends in Biotechnology, 39(12), 1324–1339. DOI: 10.1016/j.tibtech.2021.04.008

Laukel M, Rogge P, Dudziak G (2011). Single-use downstream processing for clinical manufacturing. Current capabilities and limitations. *BioProcess Int.* S2, 14–21.

Lee HS, et al. (2019). Next-generation antibody therapeutics: discovery, development, and beyond. *Int J Mol Sci.* 20(20), 5137. DOI: 10.3390/ijms20205137

Levine HL (2013). Going beyond flexible single use facilities for achieving efficient commercial manufacturing. *Bus Rev Webinar.*

Li F, Vijayasankaran N, Shen AY, Kiss R, Amanullah A (2010). Cell culture processes for monoclonal antibody production. *MAbs.* 2(5), 466–479. DOI: 10.4161/mabs.2.5.12720

Lin H, Leighty RW, Godfrey S, Wang SB (2017). Principles and approach to developing mammalian cell culture media for high cell density perfusion process leveraging established fed-batch media. *Biotechnol Prog.* 33(4), 891–901. DOI: 10.1002/btpr.2472

Lin YH, et al. (2019). Emerging trends in cell-free protein synthesis. *Biotechnol Adv.* 37(1), 110–122. DOI: 10.1016/j.biotechadv.2018.11.001

Lopes A, et al. (2020). Recent advances in the glycoengineering of recombinant therapeutic proteins in plants. *Plant Biotechnol J.* 18(1), 31–45. DOI: 10.1111/pbi.13200

Lopes A, et al. (2021). Emerging trends in the production of therapeutic proteins in mammalian cells. *Biotechnol Adv.* 49, 107760. DOI: 10.1016/j.biotechadv.2021.107760

Lu H, Villada JC, Lee PKH (2019). Modular metabolic engineering for biobased chemical production. *Trends Biotechnol.* 37(2), 152–166. DOI: 10.1016/j.tibtech.2018.07.003. Epub 2018 Jul 28. PMID: 30064888.

Lubiniecki AS, Petricciani JC (2001). Recent trends in cell substrate considerations for continuous cell lines. *Curr Opin Biotechnol.* 12(3), 317–319. DOI: 10.1016/s0958-1669(00)00219-6. PMID: 11404113.

Luitjens A, Lewis J, Pralong A (2012). Single-use biotechnologies and modular manufacturing environments invite paradigm shifts in bioprocess development and biopharmaceutical manufacturing. In: Subramanian G, ed. Biopharmaceutical Production Technology. Wiley VCH. pp. 817–857.

Lute S, Kozaili J, Johnson S, et al. (2020). Development of small-scale models to understand the impact of continuous downstream bioprocessing on integrated virus filtration. *Biotechnol Prog.* 36(3), e2962. DOI: 10.1002/btpr.2962

Luttmann R, Bracewell DG, Cornelissen G, et al. (2012). Soft sensors in bioprocessing: a status report and recommendations. *Biotechnol J.* 7, 1040–1048.

Mahajan E, Ray-Chaudhuri T, Vogel JD (2012). Standardization of single-use components extractable studies for industry. *Pharm Eng.* 32(3), 1–3.

Mahalik S, Sharma AK, Mukherjee KJ (2014). Genome engineering for improved recombinant protein expression in Escherichia coli. *Microb Cell Fact.* 13, 177. DOI: 10.1186/s12934-014-0177-1

Matasci M, et al. (2019). Recent advances in the development of biocatalytic processes for the production of chiral intermediates and APIs. *Org Process Res Dev.* 23(5), 889–903. DOI: 10.1021/acs.oprd.8b00353

McElwain L, Phair K, Kealey C, Brady D (2022). Current trends in biopharmaceuticals production in Escherichia coli. *Biotechnol Lett.* 44(8), 917–931. DOI: 10.1007/s10529-022-03276-5. Epub 2022 Jul 7. PMID: 35796852.

Menegatti S, et al. (2022). Emerging technologies for the manufacturing of gene therapies. *Curr Opin Biotechnol.* 72, 66–72. DOI: 10.1016/j.copbio.2021.12.011

Merhar M, Podgornik A, Barut M, et al. (2001). High performance reversed-phase liquid chromatography using novel CIM RP-SDVB monolithic supports. *J Liq Chrom Rel Technol.* 24, 2429–2443.

Michalik M, et al. (2022). Recent advances in the manufacturing of antibody-drug conjugates. *Antibodies* 11(1), 8. DOI: 10.3390/antib11010008

Minow B, Rogge P, Thompson K (2012). Implementing a fully disposable MAb manufacturing facility. *BioProcess Int.* 10, 48–57.

Mire-Sluis A (2011). Extractables and leachables. *Bioprocess Int.* Forums/extractables-and-leachables. 2016/04/11/2016;311844.

Mohamed A, Anoy MI, Tibbits G, et al. (2021). Emerging trends in process analytical technology for biopharmaceutical manufacturing. *Biotechnol Bioeng.* 118(9), 3509–3523. DOI: 10.1002/bit.27794

Molowa DT, Mazanet R (2003). The state of biopharmaceutical manufacturing. *Biotechnol Annu Rev.* 9, 285–302. DOI: 10.1016/s1387-2656(03)09008-2. PMID: 14650933.

Montesinos-Seguí JL, et al. (2019). Recent advances in the application of microfluidic systems in biopharmaceutical production. *Biotechnol Adv.* 37(2), 180–201. DOI: 10.1016/j.biotechadv.2018.12.001

Mora-Montes HM, et al. (2019). Advances in the recombinant protein production in yeasts. *Front Microbiol.* 10, 2683. DOI: 10.3389/fmicb.2019.02683

Moreira JL, et al. (2021). Upstream process intensification in recombinant protein production: advances and future perspectives. *Front Bioeng Biotechnol.* 9, 665833. DOI: 10.3389/fbioe.2021.665833

Moro S, et al. (2021). Recent advances and future perspectives on recombinant protein production in insect cells. *Cells* 10(5), 1174. DOI: 10.3390/cells10051174

Munro TP, Mahler SM, Huang EP, et al. (2011). Bridging the gap: facilities and technologies for development of early stage therapeutic mAb candidates. *MAbs.* 3(5), 440–452. DOI: 10.4161/mabs.3.5.16968

National Academies of Sciences Eg, and Medicine, Studies DoEaL, Technology BoCSa. Continuous Manufacturing for the Modernization of Pharmaceutical Production: Proceedings of a Workshop (2019).

New single-use sensors for online measurement of glucose and lactate: the answer to the PAT initiative. In: R E, D E, eds. Single-Use Technology in Biopharmaceutical Manufacture. John Wiley & Sons Inc (2011) 295–299.

Nicholson P, Storm E (2011). Single-use tangential flow filtration in bioprocessing – an approach to design and development. *BioProcess Int.* 9, 38–47.

Nørholm MH (2015). A mutant Pfu DNA polymerase designed for advanced uracil-excision DNA engineering. *BMC Biotechnol.* 15(1), 34. DOI: 10.1186/s12896-015-0148-y

Noui L, Hill J, Keay PJ, et al. (2002). Development of a high resolution UV spectrophotometer for at-line monitoring of bioprocesses. *Chem Eng Process.* 41, 107–114.

Odman P, Johansen CL, Olsson L, et al. (2009). Online estimation of biomass, glucose and ethanol in Saccharomyces cerevisiae cultivations using in-situ multi-wavelength fluorescence and software sensors. *J Biotechnol.* 144, 102–112.

Oh I, et al. (2021). Advances in the glycoengineering of therapeutic antibodies: implications for antibody functions and human health. *Biomolecules* 11(6), 826. DOI: 10.3390/biom11060826

Oh SK, Yoo SJ, Jeong DH, Lee JM (2013). Real-time estimation of glucose concentration in algae cultivation system using Raman spectroscopy. *Bioresour Technol.* 142, 131–137.

Omasa T, Onitsuka M, Kim WD (2010). Cell engineering and cultivation of Chinese hamster ovary (CHO) cells. *Curr Pharm Biotechnol.* 11(3), 233–240. DOI: 10.2174/138920110791111960

Oosterhuis NMG, Van Den Berg HJ (2011). How multipurpose is a single-use bioreactor? *BioPharm Int.* 24, 51–56.

Orellana CA, et al. (2020). Recent advances in the development of microbial hosts for recombinant protein production. *Microorganisms* 8(6), 830. DOI: 10.3390/microorganisms8060830

Ötes O, Flato H, Vazquez Ramirez D, et al. (2018). Scale-up of continuous multi-column chromatography for the protein a capture step: from bench to clinical manufacturing. *J Biotechnol*. 281, 168–174. DOI: 10.1016/j.jbiotec.2018.07.022

Ötes O, Flato H, Winderl J, Hubbuch J, Capito F (2017). Feasibility of using continuous chromatography in downstream processing: comparison of costs and product quality for a hybrid process vs. a conventional batch process. *J Biotechnol*. 259, 213–220. DOI: 10.1016/j.jbiotec.2017.07.001

Oyola-Reynoso S, et al. (2021). Advances in bioprinting technologies for tissue engineering applications. *Front Bioeng Biotechnol*. 9, 717788. DOI: 10.3389/fbioe.2021.717788

Pais DA, Carrondo MJ, Alves PM, Teixeira AP (2014). Towards real-time monitoring of therapeutic protein quality in mammalian cell processes. *Curr Opin Biotechnol*. 30, 161–167.

Papaneophytou CP, et al. (2021). Recent advances in the optimization of recombinant protein production in Escherichia coli. *Bioengineering* 8(3), 33. DOI: 10.3390/bioengineering8030033

Papathanasiou MM, Quiroga-Campano AL, Steinebach F, et al. (2017). Advanced model-based control strategies for the intensification of upstream and downstream processing in mAb production. *Biotechnol Prog*. 33(4), 966–988. DOI: 10.1002/btpr.2483

Parashar D, et al. (2021). Advanced process monitoring and control strategies for biomanufacturing. *Biotechnol Bioeng*. 118(12), 4833–4848. DOI: 10.1002/bit.27923

Patel M, et al. (2021). Emerging trends in glycoengineering of therapeutic proteins. *Front Bioeng Biotechnol*. 9, 693736. DOI: 10.3389/fbioe.2021.693736

Patil R, Walther J (2018). Continuous manufacturing of recombinant therapeutic proteins: upstream and downstream technologies. *Adv Biochem Eng Biotechnol*. 165, 277–322. DOI: 10.1007/10_2016_58. PMID: 28265699.

Pegel A, Reiser S, Steurenthaler M, Klein S (2011). Evaluating disposable depth filtration platforms for MAb harvest clarification. *BioProcess Int*. 9, 52–56.

Pidgeon T (2010). Disposable technologies for fill-finish of clinical trials materials. *Pharm Technol*. 34, s22–s25.

Pollard DJ, Richardson D, Brower M (2017). Progress toward automated single-use continuous monoclonal antibody manufacturing via the protein refinery operations lab: innovative technologies and methods. In: Subramanian G, ed. Continuous Biomanufacturing - Innovative Technologies and Methods. Wiley VCH. pp. 107–130.

Pollock J, Ho SV, Farid SS (2013). Fed-batch and perfusion culture processes: economic, environmental, and operational feasibility under uncertainty. *Biotechnol Bioeng*. 110(1), 206–219.

Porowińska D, Wujak M, Roszek K, Komoszyński M (2013). [Prokaryotic expression systems] Prokariotyczne systemy ekspresyjne. *Postepy Hig Med Dosw (Online)*. 67, 119–129. DOI: 10.5604/17322693.1038351

Porse A, et al. (2018). Genome-scale analysis of recombinant protein production in Escherichia coli. *Biotechnol J*. 13(8), e1700594. DOI: 10.1002/biot.201700594

Rajendran A, Paredes G, Mazzotti M (2009). Simulated moving bed chromatography for the separation of enantiomers. *J Chromatogr A*. 1216(4), 709–738. DOI: 10.1016/j.chroma.2008.10.075

Rajendran V, et al. (2018). Advances in downstream processing of monoclonal antibodies: From high-throughput screening to continuous manufacturing. *J Chem Technol Biotechnol*. 93(2), 306–319. DOI: 10.1002/jctb.5421

Rathore AS, et al. (2019). Advances in continuous bioprocessing for the manufacture of biopharmaceuticals. *Biotechnol J*. 14(9), e1800432. DOI: 10.1002/biot.201800432

Rathore AS, et al. (2020). Emerging technologies for continuous biomanufacturing. *Biotechnol J*. 15(6), e1900340. DOI: 10.1002/biot.201900340

Rathore AS, Kumar D, Kateja N (2018). Recent developments in chromatographic purification of biopharmaceuticals. *Biotechnol Lett*. 40(6), 895–905. DOI: 10.1007/s10529-018-2552-1. Epub 2018 Apr 27. PMID: 29700726.

Rathore AS, Kumar D, Kateja N (2018). Recent developments in chromatographic purification of biological medicines. *Biotechnol Lett*. 40(6), 895–905. DOI: 10.1007/s10529-018-2552-1

Ravisé A, Cameau E, De Abreu G, Pralong A (2009). Hybrid and disposable facilities for manufacturing of biopharmaceuticals: pros and cons. *Adv Biochem Eng Biotechnol*. 115, 185–219. DOI: 10.1007/10_2008_24. PMID: 19623478.

Rawlings B, Pora H (2009). Environmental impact of single-use and reusable bioprocess systems. *BioProcess Int*. 7(2), 18–25.

Riesen N, Eibl R (2011). Single-use bag systems for storage, transportation, freezing and thawing. In: Single-Use Technology in Biopharmaceutical Manufacture. John Wiley & Sons Inc. pp. 14–20.

Ritacco FV, Wu Y, Khetan A (2018). Cell culture media for recombinant protein expression in Chinese hamster ovary (CHO) cells: history, key components, and optimization strategies. *Biotechnol Prog.* 34(6), 1407–1426. DOI: 10.1002/btpr.2706

Roque AC, Lowe CR, Taipa MA (2004). Antibodies and genetically engineered related molecules: production and purification. *Biotechnol Prog.* 20(3), 639–654. DOI: 10.1021/bp030070k. PMID: 15176864.

Roque ACA, Pina AS, Azevedo AM, et al. (2020). Anything but conventional chromatography approaches in bioseparation. *Biotechnol J.* 15(8), e1900274. DOI: 10.1002/biot.201900274

Roy I, et al. (2018). Recent advancements in biopharmaceutical process development. *Trends Biotechnol.* 36(9), 936–948. DOI: 10.1016/j.tibtech.2018.05.004

Saeed AFul H, Awan SA (2016). Advances in monoclonal antibodies production and cancer therapy. *MOJ Immunology.* 15(4).

Sanchez-Garcia L, Martín L, Mangues R, et al. (2016). Recombinant pharmaceuticals from microbial cells: a 2015 update. *Microb Cell Factories.* 15(1), 1.

Schofield M (2018). Current state of the art in continuous bioprocessing. *Biotechnol Lett.* 40(9–10), 1303–1309. DOI: 10.1007/s10529-018-2593-5

Shukla AA, et al. (2017). Advances in large-scale production of monoclonal antibodies and related proteins. *Trends Biotechnol.* 35(12), 992–1004. DOI: 10.1016/j.tibtech.2017.06.011

Shukla AA, Hubbrard B, Tressel T, Guhan S, Low D (2007). Downstream processing of monoclonal antibodies. *J Chromatogr B.* 848, 28–39.

Siddiqui K, et al. (2020). Current trends and challenges in the downstream processing of recombinant proteins. *Curr Protein Pept Sci.* 21(12), 1199–1212. DOI: 10.2174/1389203721999200309143146

Sinclair A, Leveen L, Monge M, Lim J, Cox S (2008). The environmental impact of disposable technologies – can disposables reduce your facility's environmental footprint? *BioPharm Int.* 6, 4–15.

Sinclair AM, et al. (2021). Current trends in antibody manufacturing. *Antibodies* 10(3), 31. DOI: 10.3390/antib10030031

Singh N, et al. (2020). Emerging trends in upstream and downstream process development for antibody manufacturing. *Bioengineering* 7(3), 81. DOI: 10.3390/bioengineering7030081

Singh N, Herzer S (2018). Downstream processing technologies/capturing and final purification: opportunities for innovation, change, and improvement. A review of downstream processing developments in protein purification. *Adv Biochem Eng Biotechnol.* 165, 115–178. DOI: 10.1007/10_2017_12. PMID: 28795201.

Singh R, et al. (2020). Emerging trends in the development and optimization of vaccine manufacturing processes. Biotechnology Journal, 15(4), e1900448. DOI: 10.1002/biot.201900448

Sonnleitner B (2013). Automated measurement and monitoring of bioprocesses: key elements of the M(3)C strategy. *Adv Biochem Eng Biotechnol.* 132, 1–33.

Stanke M, Hitzmann B (2013). Automatic control of bioprocesses. In: Mandenius CF, Titchener-Hooker N, eds. Measurement, Monitoring, Modelling and Control of Bioprocesses. Springer. pp. 35–63.

Stepper L, Filser FA, Fischer S, Schaub J, Gorr I, Voges R (2020). Pre-stage perfusion and ultra-high seeding cell density in CHO fed-batch culture: a case study for process intensification guided by systems biotechnology. *Bioprocess Biosyst Eng.* 43(8), 1431–1443. DOI: 10.1007/s00449-020-02337-1

Stoger E, Sack M, Nicholson L, Fischer R, Christou P (2005). Recent progress in plantibody technology. *Curr Pharm Des.* 11(19), 2439–2457. DOI: 10.2174/1381612054367535. PMID: 16026298.

Stutz H (2023). Advances and applications of capillary electromigration methods in the analysis of therapeutic and diagnostic recombinant proteins - a review. *J Pharm Biomed Anal.* 222, 115089. DOI: 10.1016/j.jpba.2022.115089. Epub 2022 Oct 1. PMID: 36279846.

Sugimoto MAA, Toledo VPCP, Cunha MRR, et al. Quality of bevacizumab (Avastin®) repacked in single-use glass vials for intravitreal administration. Arq Bras Oftalmol. 2017 Mar-Apr 2017;80(2):108–113. doi:10.5935/0004-2749.20170026

Tao Y, Shih J, Sinacore M, et al. (2011). Development and implementation of a perfusion-based high cell density cell banking process, *Biotechnol. Prog.* 27(3), 824–829.

Tharmalingam T, et al. (2021). Advances in cell line development technologies for therapeutic protein production. *Biotechnol Adv.* 49, 107740. DOI: 10.1016/j.biotechadv.2021.107740

Thomas JA (1995). Recent developments and perspectives of biotechnology-derived products. *Toxicology.* 105(1), 7–22. doi: 10.1016/0300-483x(95)03122-v. PMID: 8638286.

Thorne BA, Waugh S, Wilkie T, Dunn J, LaBreck M (2012). Implementing a single-use TFF system in a cGMP biomanufacturing facility. *BioPharm.* 25, s20–s26.

Tiwari R, et al. (2021). Recent advances in the production of therapeutic antibodies in plants. *Biotechnol Lett.* 43(10), 1311–1328. DOI: 10.1007/s10529-021-03151-x

Tripathi NK, Shrivastava A (2019). Recent developments in bioprocessing of recombinant proteins: expression hosts and process development. *Front Bioeng Biotechnol.* 7, 420. DOI: 10.3389/fbioe.2019.00420

Tscheliessnig A, et al. (2021). Emerging trends in therapeutic antibody manufacturing. *Biotechnol J.* 16(8), e2100013. DOI: 10.1002/biot.202100013

Türkanoğlu Özçelik A, Yılmaz S, Inan M (2019). Pichia pastoris Promoters. *Methods Mol Biol.* 1923, 97–112. DOI: 10.1007/978-1-4939-9024-5_3

Ullrich KK, Hiss M, Rensing SA (2015). Means to optimize protein expression in transgenic plants. *Curr Opin Biotechnol.* 32, 61–67. DOI: 10.1016/j.copbio.2014.11.011

Vachette E, Fenge C, Cappia JM, et al. (2014). Robust and convenient single-use processing: superior strength and flexibility of flexsafe bag. *Bioprocess Int.* 12(5), 23–25.

Vázquez-Rey M, et al. (2015). Advances in the production of antibody fragments in E. coli: from the inclusion bodies to the bioreactor. *Antibodies* 4(1), 12–41. DOI: 10.3390/antib4010012

Vazquez-Rey M, et al. (2018). Characterization of IgG aggregates and evaluation of aggregate impact on product quality and immunogenicity. *Pharm Res.* 35(8), 141. DOI: 10.1007/s11095-018-2449-y

Voss C (2007). Production of plasmid DNA for pharmaceutical use. *Biotechnol Annu Rev.* 13, 201–222. DOI: 10.1016/S1387-2656(07)13008-8. PMID: 17875478.

Wagner R, et al. (2021). Emerging trends in viral vector manufacturing. *Biotechnol Adv.* 47, 107679. DOI: 10.1016/j.biotechadv.2021.107679

Walsh G (2014). Biopharmaceuticals: approval trends in 2013. *Biotechnol J.* 9(2), 221–222. DOI: 10.1002/biot.201300561

Walsh G (2018). Biopharmaceutical benchmarks 2018. *Nat Biotechnol.* 36(12), 1136–1145. DOI: 10.1038/nbt.4305

Walsh G, et al. (2021). Accelerating the development of novel technologies and improving their manufacturing readiness for biopharmaceutical manufacturing: a perspective. *Biotechnol J.* 16(4), e2000195. DOI: 10.1002/biot.202000195

Walter JK (1998). Strategies and considerations for advanced economy in downstream processing of biopharmaceutical proteins. In: Subramanian G, ed. Bioseparations, Processing, Quality and Characterisation, Economics, Safety and Hygiene. pp. 447–460.

Walther J, Hwang C, Konstantinov K, et al. (2015). The business impact of an integrated continuous biomanufacturing platform for recombinant protein production. *J Biotechnol.* 213, 3–12.

Wang Q, et al. (2021). Cell-free protein synthesis: Recent advances in bacterial and eukaryotic systems. *Bioengineering* 8(1), 10. DOI: 10.3390/bioengineering8010010

Warikoo V, Godawat R, Brower K, et al. (2012). Integrated continuous production of recombinant therapeutic proteins. *Biotechnol Bioeng.* 109(12), 3018–3029. DOI: 10.1002/bit.24584. Epub 2012 Aug 6. PMID: 22729761.

Wells E, Robinson AS (2017). Cellular engineering for therapeutic protein production: product quality, host modification, and process improvement. *Biotechnol J.* 12(1). DOI: 10.1002/biot.201600105

Westbrook A, et al. (2014). Application of a two-dimensional single-use rocking bioreactor to bacterial cultivation for recombinant protein production. *Biochem Eng J.* 88, 154–161. DOI: 10.1016/j.bej.2014.04.011

White T, Ott K (2015). Management, notification and documentation of single-use systems change orders: challenges and opportunities. *Bioprocess Int.* 13(9): 24–29.

Wolton D, Heaven L, McFeaters S, Kodilkar M (2015). Standardization of disposables design: the path forward for a potential game changer. *Bioprocess Int.* https://bioprocessintl.com/manufacturing/supply-chain/standardization-of-disposables-design-the-path-forward-for-a-potential-game-changer

Wong WJ, et al. (2021). Emerging trends in continuous bioprocessing for viral vector production. *Front Bioeng Biotechnol.* 9, 660689. DOI: 10.3389/fbioe.2021.660689

Wurm FM (2020). Recombinant protein production in mammalian cells. *Methods Mol Biol.* 2070, 15–30. DOI: 10.1007/978-1-4939-9857-2_2

Xiao-Jie L, Hui-Ying X, Zun-Ping K, Jin-Lian C, Li-Juan J (2015). CRISPR-Cas9: a new and promising player in gene therapy. *J Med Genet.* 52(5), 289–296. DOI: 10.1136/jmedgenet-2014-102968

Xu J, Xu X, Huang C, et al. (2020). Biomanufacturing evolution from conventional to intensified processes for productivity improvement: a case study. *MAbs.* 12(1), 1770669. DOI: 10.1080/19420862.2020.1770669

Xu S, Gavin J, Jiang R, Chen H (2017). Bioreactor productivity and media cost comparison for different intensified cell culture processes. *Biotechnol Prog.* 33(4), 867–878. DOI: 10.1002/btpr.2415

Xu Y, et al. (2018). Continuous manufacturing of biologics: Integration of upstream and downstream processes. *Curr Opin Biotechnol.* 53, 127–136. DOI: 10.1016/j.copbio.2018.03.012

Yadav DK, et al. (2020). "Recent advances in cell-free protein synthesis and their applications. *Biotechnol Lett.* 42(7), 1303–1317. DOI: 10.1007/s10529-020-02919-6

Yang M, et al. (2021). Recent advances in genome engineering applications for the production of recombinant therapeutic proteins in mammalian cells. *Biotechnol Bioeng.* 118(3), 778–791. DOI: 10.1002/bit.27504

Yang Y, et al. (2021). Current trends and challenges in viral vector manufacturing for gene therapy. *Biotechnol J.* 16(10), e2000362. DOI: 10.1002/biot.202000362

Yang Y, et al. (2021). Emerging trends in bioprocess intensification for recombinant protein production in mammalian cells. *Biotechnol Bioeng.* 118(3), 766–777. DOI: 10.1002/bit.27500

Yilmaz D, Mehdizadeh H, Navarro D, et al. (2020). Application of Raman spectroscopy in monoclonal antibody producing continuous systems for downstream process intensification. *Biotechnol Prog.* 36(3), e2947. DOI: 10.1002/btpr.2947

Yongky A, Xu J, Tian J, et al. (2019). Process intensification in fed-batch production bioreactors using non-perfusion seed cultures. *MAbs.* 11(8):1502–1514. doi:10.1080/19420862.2019.1652075

Yu X, et al. (2021). Advanced glycosylation modification and its biotechnological applications. *Front Bioeng Biotechnol.* 9, 620853. DOI: 10.3389/fbioe.2021.620853

Zhang H, et al. (2019). Advances in cell line development technologies for recombinant protein production. *Pharmaceuticals.* 12(3), 138. DOI: 10.3390/ph12030138

Zhang H, et al. (2021). Advances in CRISPR/Cas-based gene therapy in human genetic diseases. *Theranostics.* 11(5), 2219–2237. DOI: 10.7150/thno.53922

Zhang X, et al. (2019). Continuous downstream processing of biologics: a comparative study of current technologies. *Biotechnol J.* 14(9), e1800428. DOI: 10.1002/biot.201800428

Zhang X, et al. (2019). Emerging trends and advances in the microbial production of bioactive peptides. *Trends Biotechnol.* 37(12), 1302–1315. DOI: 10.1016/j.tibtech.2019.04.007

Zhang Y, et al. (2020). Advances and prospects of CRISPR-Cas systems in gene therapy. *Biotechnol Adv.* 40, 107502. DOI: 10.1016/j.biotechadv.2020.107502

Zhang YP, Sun J, Ma Y (2017). Biomanufacturing: history and perspective. *J Ind Microbiol Biotechnol.* 44(4–5), 773–784. DOI: 10.1007/s10295-016-1863-2. Epub 2016 Nov 11. PMID: 27837351.

Zhao M, Vandersluis M, Stout J, et al. (2019). Affinity chromatography for vaccines manufacturing: finally ready for prime time? *Vaccine* 37(36), 5491–5503.

Zhao R, Natarajan A, Srienc F (1999). A flow injection flow cytometry system for online monitoring of bioreactors. *Biotechnol Bioeng.* 62, 609–617.

Zhou Y, Lu Z, Wang X, et al. (2018). Genetic engineering modification and fermentation optimization for extracellular production of recombinant proteins using Escherichia coli. *Appl Microbiol Biotechnol.* 102(4), 1545–1556. DOI: 10.1007/s00253-017-8700-z

Zhu J, et al. (2018). Emerging next-generation sequencing-based discoveries for understanding human immunodeficiency virus diversity, drug resistance, and cure. *J Virol.* 92(12), e00630–18. DOI: 10.1128/JVI.00630-18

Zhu J, et al. (2018). Engineering next-generation antibody therapeutics using artificial intelligence. *Front Immunol.* 9, 3016. DOI: 10.3389/fimmu.2018.03016

Zhu J, Hatton D (2018). New mammalian expression systems. *Adv Biochem Eng Biotechnol.* 165, 9–50. DOI: 10.1007/10_2016_55

Zhu MM, et al. (2022). Harnessing machine learning and artificial intelligence for bioprocess optimization and control. *Trends Biotechnol.* 40(3), 213–226. DOI: 10.1016/j.tibtech.2021.11.007

Index

Note: Page locators in **bold** and *italics* represent tables and figures, respectively.

For Product Safety Concerns and Information please contact our EU
representative GPSR@taylorandfrancis.com
Taylor & Francis Verlag GmbH, Kaufingerstraße 24, 80331 München, Germany

www.ingramcontent.com/pod-product-compliance
Lightning Source LLC
Chambersburg PA
CBHW080655220326
41598CB00033B/5211